The Neuroses

DIAGNOSIS AND MANAGEMENT OF FUNCTIONAL DISORDERS AND MINOR PSYCHOSES

By WALTER C. ALVAREZ, M.D.

Emeritus Consultant in Internal Medicine, Mayo Clinic;
Emeritus Professor of Medicine,
University of Minnesota, Mayo Foundation

W. B. SAUNDERS COMPANY

PHILADELPHIA AND LONDON

Preface

WHEN A PHYSICIAN has had the privilege of a large experience and has picked up along the way hundreds of little secrets of diagnosis and treatment, he ought to publish them, and make them available to the younger men who are starting out in Medicine. He should not carry his knowledge to the grave; he should share it with others before illness or death comes along to put an end to his teaching days.

Seeing that for long I have had the good fortune to work in a place to which each year now come some 140,000 sick persons, many of them with those puzzling neuroses and functional troubles that have always fascinated me, I decided a while ago that I ought to be recording some of this experience, and that it was high time that I got at the job. So I started, and this book is the fruit of two and a half years of writing. A little of the material presented here has appeared in articles; a little has gone into books, and the rest of it is new.

As I started writing I felt a bit of an inferiority complex, wondering what I, an internist, was doing, writing on neuroses and minor psychoses; wasn't that a job for a neurologist or a psychiatrist? But gradually, as I gathered together my material and as I read some of the newer books on neurology and psychiatry, I came to see that the ideal book on neuroses for a non-psychiatrist would have to be written by a fellow-non-psychiatrist: a man who for long had dealt with the everyday problems of all physicians, and especially with the problems of diagnosis. He would know better than anyone else what these problems are, and he would be most likely to write about them in simple speech. He would know what it is to struggle daily with the problems of differentiating largely functional and largely organic disease, and worse yet, of identifying chronic organic disease after it has become heavily encrusted with neurosis. He, more than anyone else, would know what it is to struggle with the problem of selling nervous persons the idea that what they have is only a neurosis.

These problems are somewhat different from those of the psychiatrist. A psychiatrist, when he tries to write a book for non-psychiatrists, naturally tends to write a text on psychiatry or a book on the weird mental quirks of the many queer persons whom he sees. Their queer ideas are much queerer than those that we non-psychiatrists hear about, and few of us can get interested in them.

About the only interest in psychiatry we non-psychiatrists can develop is just enough to help us in understanding the mental peculiari-

iii

ties and the worries, strains, and life-problems of our patients. Every one of us must be, to this small extent, a psychiatrist. As William J. Mayo used to say, every specialist must know how to take care of most of his own "neuros"; much as he might like to, he cannot dump them all onto someone else.

Today most thoughtful physicians realize that they need more information on the neuroses, the minor psychoses and the functional troubles. In this field their training in college was woefully inadequate. Some wish to remedy the defect, but where can they get the desired information? Unfortunately, much of what has been written on the subject is almost inaccessible to them; it is scattered through journals and books which they rarely see. To help them, I have here summarized some of the best of that information. For the rest, I have drawn from that rich hoard of information which, through the years, I have picked up from patients and from my fellow-specialists at the Mayo Clinic.

Here in this book are hints for recognizing nervous, neurotic, or slightly psychotic persons, and for diagnosing the many functional syndromes from which they tend to suffer. Particularly helpful, I hope, will be the descriptions of the neuroses as they are met with by the several specialists, such as the surgeon, the gynecologist, the urologist and oto-laryngologist. There is even a section here on psychosomatic medicine for the anesthetist!

Under the heading of treatment are chapters on the handling of nervous persons, on the art of convincing them that their trouble is a neurosis, and on the art of teaching them what they can do to help themselves. Many writers say, "Use psychotherapy," but there they stop; they do not go on to tell what it is. Here is detailed information on what to say and what not to say to a troubled patient. Patients ask, "What can I do now to help myself?" Here is a chapter full of suggestions for them.

I regret that here and there I must criticize some of the practices of the profession which I love, but I cannot tell what I think are desirable improvements without first pointing out those practices of ours which have proved to be mistaken and unfortunate. Some of the things I say here I would not have dared say thirty-five years ago, but as Montaigne wrote, as a man grows older he should gain courage to express ever more of the truth as he sees it. Also, as he approaches three score and ten he should feel ever less concern over whether other men disagree with him, or like what he says. If in his consultant practice he sees what the common medical mistakes are, it is his duty to warn against them. All that need concern him is that he speak truly and kindly and humbly, and with a full realization of the fact that in his ignorant youth, he made most of the mistakes which he now asks his readers to avoid.

We physicians must always be dissatisfied with the gaps in our knowledge, and distressed over the mistakes that we cannot help making, especially in the fields not well known to us. Most of these mistakes are made simply because no one of us can ever know all that he needs to know; he just cannot know all the fine points of specialties other than his own.

There is duplication here and there in this book, but this is easier on the reader than frequent references to some other chapter or page. Most men, when they pick up a book like this, do not read it through. They are searching for information on a particular case, and hence they read only a part of some one chapter.

Many a young physician today wishes he could get a graduate course in the diagnosis and treatment of functional troubles: He wishes that in this field he could fit himself to be a better diagnostician and a better therapist. This book was written for him: It is dedicated to his needs. It contains the best of what I have been able to glean during forty-five years of busy practice.

700 N. Michigan Ave.,
Chicago, Illinois

WALTER C. ALVAREZ

Contents

Part I

Introduction: The Need for a Better Recognition of Neuroses and Minor Psychoses

CHAPTER 1

A Part of Medical Practice
Needs to Be Improved

MEDICAL PRACTICE TODAY is in many ways excellent, and everywhere in the land it is improving. Examinations of patients are being made ever more thoroughly, and surgery is becoming ever safer and more brilliant. Physicians are being better educated; those who would be specialists are undergoing special training and passing stiff examinations, and the general practitioner is becoming ever more skillful and proud of his wide specialty. In every community better clinics and laboratories and hospitals are being built, and, as a result, even in small mountain cities the local physician or surgeon can get for his patients the tests and roentgenograms he needs.

This is splendid, and we physicians can be proud of it. The only sad feature is that there is a part of our practice that is still unsatisfactory. It is improving but not yet as fast as it might. What I am referring to is the difficulty many of us are having in recognizing and treating the neuroses and minor psychoses. It would not be so bad if this difficulty were being encountered only by poorly trained and poorly equipped doctors, but this is not the case; the city consultant is having as much trouble as is the country doctor—perhaps more.

All of us are getting ever more skillful at finding *organic* disease, but this very fact has caused many of us to expect to find it too often —in almost every patient we see. Many of us think, as our patients do, that an examination, if thorough enough, should reveal a focus of infection or of organic disease. We fail to think of the brain as a possible source of pains, discomforts, and feelings of illness, and we fail to think of the possibility that the patient before us is ill because of a bad nervous heredity, overwork, great strain, unwise living or thinking, or some personal tragedy.

As I shall emphasize again and again, many of us practice medicine largely oblivious of these great possibilities; we fail to think of the enormous amount of illness-producing unhappiness which is round about us, and, as a result, we miss diagnoses, and occasionally we order an operation that cannot do any good. At this point the reader may say, "But, no; many of us are constantly telling patients that their examinations showed nothing; we often tell them that there is nothing the matter with them." True; we often do this, but in doing it we commonly commit still another serious fault and one that I will have occasion to discuss in several chapters.

On telling patients there is "nothing the matter" with them. Rarely is it enough to tell a patient that there is nothing the matter with him. We should go on to find out exactly why he consulted us, and why he is ill, uncomfortable, in pain, or perhaps unable to work. If we do not do this we do not do much for him, and we must not be surprised if he goes away dissatisfied. Some of the most meticulous internists I have known hated to bother any more with a patient after an examination had revealed no organic disease. If a woman persisted in coming back and asking questions and demanding help, the doctor became annoyed, and showed it. To illustrate: A pleasant intelligent woman of forty came to see me after an associate professor of medicine at a fine university had had a "run-in" with her. As he wrote me, he had lost all patience with her because "she was a tartar and a nuisance and an ingrate." He felt that because, during her examination, he had run onto a malignant polyp in her rectum and had had it fulgurated and destroyed, she should have been satisfied, but, instead, she had kept coming back to fuss.

Her version of the matter was that she had gone to him complaining of prostrating headaches, insomnia, distressing sensations of fatigue, and an inability to work. She had been so ill that she had had to give up a fine position as an executive secretary. When the professor found only the polyp and started to dismiss her, she said to him, "But you have not yet even touched on the problems which led me to consult you. I am truly grateful for what you have done, but my head is still splitting, I cannot sleep, and I cannot work. I have to support my aged father; my savings are fast disappearing, and I am getting panicky for fear I will go broke before I can get back to work. I am all the more scared now that you have been unable to find the cause of my trouble." Aside from saying that her troubles were functional and that he had done his job, the doctor did not have any suggestions to make. Next day the woman returned to beg him to refer her to someone who was interested in headaches; but he was busy and had no suggestions. When she returned the following day, to beg again for help, the doctor refused to see her.

I found a fine, sensible, able woman who had broken down nervously because of a severe migraine made disabling by much strain in her job, plus much unhappiness in a marriage that had ended in disaster. Obviously, the woman was in much need of counsel; she needed medicine to help her to sleep, she needed an understanding of her migrainous constitution; she needed help in identifying the exciting causes of the acute attacks, and she needed gynergen to block the headaches when they started. There was much that could be done for her, and she was very grateful for the help she got.

When a doctor looks up from a sheaf of negative reports and tells a woman that there is nothing the matter with her, *his work is not done; it should be just beginning.* If he does not go on to really tackle her problem, if he does not find out exactly what type of neurosis or functional trouble she has, and if he does not fit appropriate treatment to it, he must not be angry if she leaves disgruntled and feeling that she has received nothing for her money. Actually, she may not have received much. It is a fine and a creditable thing to have given her a good examination and to have refused to send her for much useless treatment or an operation, but this is not enough; the doctor must go further and must take the sort of history which will tell him which one of the many functional troubles described in Chapter 3 is present. Why must he do this? Because the treatment that might help indigestion due to an ordinary sore colon will not help that due to smoking three packages of cigarettes a day, or to eating too many eggs, or to fighting with an alcoholic husband.

The world of psychogenic disease which many physicians have not yet discovered. One afternoon, after I had seen three persons who, so far as I could make out, were ill purely because of great worry or unhappiness or personal tragedy, I got to thinking. These patients had all been examined several times by internists in their home cities: men who had apparently failed even to suspect what was really wrong. Now, why had they missed it? It wasn't because the problem was at all difficult; in every case it was easy enough to solve.

The first of these persons was a matron who complained of bloating. This bloating evidently was not due to gas, because when the abdomen went down she never passed flatus. Since I knew that this syndrome is hysterical in type and commonly due to sexual unhappiness (see Chapter 16), I asked the woman if she was happy. After crying a bit she told me that two years before, when the trouble started, her husband's old sweetheart from college days began writing and telephoning to him. Naturally, this was deeply resented by the wife, especially as the husband seemed rather to appreciate the compliment, and soon she was threatening divorce. When I found that neither she nor her husband really wanted to separate, that both were tired of bickering, and the old sweetheart had long since given up and disappeared, I got them to make up, and soon sent them off smiling and on their way to happiness again.

The next patient, a middle-aged salesman, gave a ten-year history of going from one internist to another, complaining of digestive discomforts and panicky spells. Most of the doctors he had seen had diagnosed an ulcer, although most of the roentgenologists and gastroscopists who had studied him had been unable to find one. I soon learned that he was a manic-depressive who had had several spells of depression. That was the trouble.

The third patient was a middle-aged woman who came with the diagnosis of a "slowly-emptying gallbladder." Her local surgeon was all set to operate but she had decided to have the work done by one of my colleagues. She wanted to go right into the hospital and get the job over with and hence was annoyed when I insisted on a preliminary check-up. Eventually, after ten days of refusing to admit that she had any psychic strain, she confessed that her distress began when she fell into the clutches of a blackmailer. She had bought the woman off for a while, but, naturally, she was still filled with anxiety as to the future.

These three are samples of the stories I keep getting week after week, not because I am any better a clinician than were the good men who had previously studied these patients but, perhaps, because I am more aware of the existence of such tragedies all around me, and more inclined to ask about them and to keep asking even after I have been rebuffed.

My experience has shown me that in this land of ours there must be thousands of physicians who, each day, while seeing many troubled patients, never even suspect the existence of the tragedies which produced the illness.

The need for asking, "What did you really come to talk about?" I know that every so often, with all my interest in people, I, too, fail to help someone with a neurosis because it never occurs to me that the syndrome complained of is due to some tragedy, or perhaps is just the patient's excuse for coming into the office to talk about some psychic or sexual difficulty. Thus, I remember a stout, unattractive, middle-aged widow living on a Dakota farm who came twice to the Clinic complaining of a vague abdominal pain. Because she was of cancer age, each time I examined her thoroughly, but I could find nothing. Later, she wrote to say that I had failed her. All her trouble was that, with her husband's death, she, a very passionate woman, had had to suffer tortures from sexual deprivation. She had hoped that some operation, perhaps the removal of the clitoris, would calm her down. Unfortunately, she was too shy and embarrassed to come right out and tell me what the trouble was. She had kept hoping that I would make it easier for her to confess by asking about sexual difficulties. Because of her age and unattractiveness it never occurred to me that she could have a sexual problem.

Cases like this have taught me the great need for asking many a patient, especially when his or her story is rambling and vague, "What did you really come here to find out? What frightened you, or what is on your mind?" Often, then, the important story is told.

The physician who is not interested in his patient as a human being. Patients often resent our lack of interest in them as human beings. Many a person has said to me: "That surgeon may have saved my life, but I dislike him and always shall because he had no interest in me aside from my gallbladder; every time during those three weeks when I tried to be friendly, he rebuffed me, or he coldly walked away without a word." In answer, many a surgeon will say, "How, during my hurried morning rounds, can anyone expect me to stop for a chat?" That is true, but I cannot get over the fact that some of the busiest surgeons I have known did manage often to stop for a moment to ask a kindly question or to say a comforting word. And, with this, some of them did grip their patients to them with bonds of affection and lifelong devotion. Evidently, it can be done.

Internists may say, "Why should a patient expect any friendly interest from me? Why should he expect it any more than if I had sold him my old car?" Perhaps the answer is that a patient has little right to expect friendly converse when a physician is treating organic disease, but he has some reason to hope for it when he is being treated for a neurosis. Why? Because, usually, without friendly interest in a patient it is very difficult for a physician to get an adequate history, and without some rapport it is hard to induce the person to mend his or her ways and to pick up hope again. Many a time I have helped a woman more easily because she wanted to please me and be a credit to me. Often I ask a patient to write me in six months and report, because I will be so interested to know how she is coming along. And I will be interested.

Probably there is nothing that can ever be done to change a physician who does not like people, but God grant that these paragraphs may serve to put even more humanity and kindliness and sympathy into the hearts of those young doctors who already do feel kindly toward their patients and are showing it, and who are just beginning to see what a wonderful help in the healing art this interest in people can be. Such sympathy helps many a man to achieve great success in the practice of medicine.

Medical men sometimes fail to recognize a neurosis or psychosis even in their own loved ones. Osler was so distressed one day when a physician brought in his little daughter to find out why she did not grow. There she stood, the textbook picture of a chubby little cretin, and the father had never even heard of the disease! As Osler said, if this could happen within a few miles of Johns Hopkins Medical School, how great must have been the need all over the country for more graduate education. The same thought comes to me every so often when a fine old physician brings in his wife, suffering from an unrecognized melancholia or the mental deterioration that has followed an unrecognized stroke. Only as I draw out the typical story does a great light break over the doctor, so that he suddenly sees what the trouble is. As he then says, at college no one taught him to recognize such things, or even to think of them.

I remember a fine old surgeon who came with his favorite niece from whom, when she started regurgitating, he promptly removed the appendix. When she got no better, he did not know what to do because no one had ever taught him to recognize the typical picture of nervous regurgitation with anorexia nervosa, and no one had taught him to associate this syndrome with the sort of spiritual struggle through which the poor girl had been passing. Happily she got well as soon as she was helped to solve her problem.

Even the person with organic disease may have a serious psychic problem. As Karl Menninger once pointed out, even when organic disease is found and the physician thinks his diagnosis is made and his job done, he may not even have suspected the presence of the really important problem. This is the patient's reaction to the diagnosis he or she has received. For instance, a spinster of Puritan upbringing came with a chancre on her lip. So far as the syphilologist could see, all she needed was some penicillin. But, as Menninger said, much worse and more serious than the syphilis was the poor woman's shock at learning what she had, and at thinking of how she got it, of her defilement, of her misplaced trust, and of her bitter awakening from a dream of love and marriage. Full of thoughts of suicide, she was for the moment far more in need of psychiatric care than of medicine. The sad fact is that it may not have occurred to the syphilologist that he should have sat down to talk to the woman for a while like a kindly big brother. He may just have hurried on to see the patient in the next room.

A while ago a physician described the case of a young woman who was hurt slightly in an automobile accident in which her sister was killed. The physician at the emergency hospital dressed her bruise and moved on. He thought his work was done. But it was not. If he had only sensed that the woman was overwhelmed with a feeling of guilt for the accident he would have stopped to talk to her and try to get her to see that she could not hold herself responsible simply because she had insisted on her sister's going on the ride. But he did not sense the need, or react to it, and so the young woman went to a window and dived out to her death.

Today the man or woman who is going insane commonly gets operated on. If one takes a group of psychotic patients as they reach an asylum, and goes back over their histories to see how they were treated during the years in which they were going insane, the records make one sad. I remember a thin young woman whom I saw one day. She had the pinched sullen face of a schizophrenic, and on her abdomen the scars of a half-dozen successive operations, performed in an attempt to cure a regurgitation of food which, almost certainly, was just a part of her psychosis.

Or, I remember a hysterical bloater with her abdomen well scarred and on her back two more white lines representing futile splanchnicotomies. Or, I think of a woman with a depressive psychosis who, besides the usual five or six abdominal operations, had had her thyroid gland and her coccyx removed. Or, I remember the woman who went into a melancholia when her aviator son was killed. Because she complained of gas and abdominal pain and a little "fever" she was treated extensively with injections of millions of units of penicillin! From a letter received from her physician, it was evident that it had never occurred to him that he was treating insanity.

The following case report by Lloyd Ziegler (1929) shows what sort of treatment a patient with a beginning psychosis was likely to get in the last twenty years, even at the hands of unusually able physicians and surgeons in a large clinic.

A laborer, thirty-nine years of age, was seen first in June, 1921. He was a serious, gloomy fellow who had always been much worried about his health. He complained mainly of gassy distress in the epigastrium. He would have spells of this lasting for several weeks. Although a duodenal deformity was reported by a roentgenologist, a medical consultant doubted that he had an ulcer, and diagnosed a neurosis. Later, an ulcer type of regimen was tried.

During the years that followed the man kept coming back. In October 1921, another Sippy regimen was tried which failed to help. In May 1922, the man was apprehensive, and complaining of epigastric burning which had no relation to eating. This doubtless was a paresthesia in the skin. He complained, also, of alternating constipation and diarrhea. Then pyloroplasty was performed and the appendix was removed. In August 1922, he returned with vague epigastric distress and hypersecretion of gastric juice. In January 1923, he complained of epigastric numbness and loss of weight. In April 1923, because of the regurgitation of sour food, he was taught to wash out his stomach. In August 1924, his physician became suspicious of his sanity and sent him for a neurological examination which was reported as negative because there were no positive Babinski or Romberg or Chvostek tests. In April 1925, he complained of gas, constipation, numbness of the abdominal wall, and more loss of weight. Because a roentgenologist thought that there might be an ulcer, in May 1925, gastroenterostomy was performed. The man was now unable to work, and his financial and domestic troubles became acute. He was still complaining of abdominal misery.

Then, a psychiatrist was added to the staff and he saw the patient. He immediately noted that the man's complaint was that his stomach was *"rotting out."* This statement was a give-away, because it was so typical of the interpretations schizophrenics put on their discomforts. He probably had previously said such things to the young assistants who had taken his history but, because they had had no training in psychiatry, the significance of the man's wording had escaped them. At last the basic cause of the man's long illness was recognized, and he was sent to a psychopathic hospital, the place toward which he had long been drifting. On going back over the story, the psychiatrist suspected that, from the start, his troubles had all been due to the psychosis.

In another case of this type that I ran onto, a frail little postal clerk had had nine abdominal operations, all designed to cure a duodenal ulcer that was never demonstrated. On going back over his history it became clear that, from the start, all his troubles were purely those of a neurosis combined with a high degree of constitutional inadequacy. He never had any symptoms of ulcer, and his first operation was performed for a slight duodenal spasm.

It would be helpful if every so often, in big institutions, a number of overly long records were to be pulled out of the files, analyzed by a psychiatrist, and their lessons hammered home to the staff at their monthly meetings.

Some men may say, "But Ziegler's patient had his troubles twenty years ago." Yes; but one could easily fill a book with recent reports of this type to show that the present-day recognition and handling of psychotic patients is not so much better that we can brag about it. They are still being operated on. As I write this chapter, I keep seeing one psychotic patient after the other who has been treated for a supposed abdominal disease.

Bennett and Semrad (1936), when they studied 100 cases of psychoneurosis, found that in seventy-two, mistaken diagnoses had been made of organic gastro-intestinal disease, and 179 surgical operations had been performed, probably half of them unnecessary. In 1946, Bennett reported another 121 cases of women with psychiatric syndromes. Some 111 had been treated for supposed gastro-intestinal disease, eighty-eight for supposed endocrine disorders, thirty-one for supposed disease of the genito-urinary organs, and thirty-nine for supposed heart disease. Six had had all their teeth removed; fifty-seven had been given long periods of bed-rest, thirty-one had been given many sedatives, and three were suffering from chronic bromide intoxication; fifty-eight had gone to irregular practitioners. Only seventeen had had some psychiatric treatment such as they all needed. Some 205 operations had been performed, eighty-four on the pelvic organs, forty on the appendix, eleven on the gallbladder, sixteen on the thyroid gland, five on adhesions, three on the kidney, twenty-one on the rectum, and twenty-four on the tonsils and nasal sinuses. One woman, suffering from melancholia, had had her clitoris unhooded to relieve frigidity!

In a review of 1,000 consecutive cases of the common irritable colon syndrome, it was discovered by Collins and Van Ordstrand that 204 of the patients had had 302 operations without relief of symptoms; 163 had had a "chronic appendix" removed.

Physicians need to know that abdominal pains can be due purely to trouble in the brain. All internists and surgeons need to know that a neurosis or psychosis can, *all by itself,* produce abdominal aches and pains and miseries. This is a most important point, but one about which not all of us feel sure. I can sympathize with those who do not feel sure because I know how hard it is sometimes to cling to the faith that is in me, especially when a woman goes on suffering for weeks or months. Even with all the experience I have had with patients who have had the abdomen explored futilely several times, occasionally I have wavered, and, against my better judgment, I have allowed the woman to have another exploratory laparotomy. Practically always later I have had to apologize to the surgeon for getting him into an embarrassing situation. The trouble is that when for months one has had a woman on one's hands complaining of an ache in her right loin and begging for relief, it is hard to keep saying, "This is a mild psychosis with a sort of thalamic syndrome," or, "This is the result of an unhappy home situation, and an exploration will not show anything." I know what a terrible pressure is put on the home physician to do something for such women, and I do not blame him when, in desperation, he consents to an abdominal exploration.

I remember a case like this in which, after thirteen years of "misery" in the right loin, the patient talked a surgeon into exploring his abdomen. When nothing was found, the young physician who had examined the man said, "I will bet something was there but they missed it." A while later the patient obligingly died of an accident, and a most careful necropsy was made. It, too, showed nothing to explain the pain. Years ago I saw a woman whose experience taught me the futility of even eviscerating one side of the abdomen in the hope of curing *certain types of* pain met with in certain types of patients. She showed that surgeons can remove the right half of the colon, the uterus with tubes and ovaries, and the gallbladder, and can cut all the sensory nerves leaving the abdomen, and the pain will go on unchanged. One must remember that abdominal pain can be due purely to a brain tumor, to a stroke, to epilepsy, or to migraine. I remember a physician who gets abdominal pain just from tension due to driving through heavy traffic. Another gets severe abdominal pain whenever he is frightened by illness in his family.

With neurotic patients the family doctor may be more correct than the consultant. Many a time I have seen the wise old family physician or general practitioner in the right about a neurosis when the eminent consultant was in the wrong. From wisdom gained through years of experience with families, the old doctor had recognized a neurotic type of girl and a neurotic clinical picture. Perhaps, also, he knew that in the girl's family there had been a great tendency to psychopathy and chronic illness, or he knew from local gossip that the patient had had an unhappy love affair. He may have known, also, that from childhood onward the girl was sickly and constantly ailing, just like her mother and grandmother before her. Naturally, then, he felt that the trouble should be functional in nature.

And yet he may have hated to come out definitely and say that it was a neurosis for fear that some young doctor newly come into the community might see the patient, might carry out much laboratory and roentgenologic work, and might make some fancy diagnosis of brucellosis, low blood sugar, or a slowly emptying gallbladder. Then the old doctor would be blamed and accused of ignorance. The patient and her family would be sore at him all the more so because they did not like his diagnosis. For a time they might be delighted with the new diagnosis of organic disease; they would feel that at last the new doctor with his new methods had found the hidden cause of all the trouble. Only after a few months would they be disillusioned.

As many an old country doctor has said to me, when I told him that I thought his patient's trouble was a pure neurosis, and not the fancy disease diagnosed in a big city, "I was fairly certain of that, but who am I to argue with my betters?" My hunch was that, in many ways, the consultants had not been his betters.

Patients commonly do not go to the right specialist. It is unfortunate that when a person gets a pain in what he thinks is his heart he is inclined to consult a heart specialist. If he thinks the pain is in his stomach he goes to a stomach specialist, and if he thinks it is in his kidney he goes to a kidney specialist. If each of these specialists were quickly to take a history good enough to reveal the fact that the patient has a mild psychosis, and were then to send him right off to a psychiatrist, all would be well; or at least it would be well until the supply of psychiatrists gave out. *But we non-psychiatrists usually accept the patient and his self-made diagnosis, and worse yet, we tend to hold onto him and to keep examining him and treating him and operating on him, perhaps for years.*

When a woman has pain in the region of her liver she spends her days with gastroenterologists; when it is in her loin she spends her time with urologists, and when it is in or around her pelvis she goes to gynecologists. The woman with a great mental conflict and resulting giant urticaria or a neurodermite will spend her days with dermatologists and allergists; and so it goes.

An occasional patient with a mild psychosis and all the distress in thorax or abdomen or face eventually gets into the hands of psychiatrists, so that the syndrome he or she has becomes known to them, but most of such patients never reach a man interested in mental problems and this is bad for them and for psychiatry. For instance, I doubt if psychiatrists often see the type of psychopath who hawks and clears his throat for an hour or more every morning for fear that if he swallows any of the mucus he will become poisoned and his brain will be damaged. He will spend his life in the offices of nose and throat specialists, never suspecting that he does not belong there, and never being told where he should go to get real help. Recently I saw one of these patients and suspected what was wrong but I had to talk to the family before I could know how badly depressed and psychotic the fellow was.

Some day we specialists must learn that all is not grist to our particular mill. We must learn to recognize (1) the person with a functional disturbance whom we can reassure and send away happy, and (2) the person with a psychosis so bad that our reassurance will never convince or satisfy him. Such a patient ought often to be gotten promptly into the hands of an able and kindly psychiatrist. Even this doctor may not be able to help much, or to cure, but at least he can get an idea as to how serious the man's condition is and can warn his family.

The best specialist is one who recognizes in his clientele the greatest percentage of patients who do not belong to him. Obviously, one of the best signs of a fine, wise, and idealistic specialist is a tendency to tell a high percentage of the patients who come to him —because they think they have the disease that he is best trained to treat—that they are mistaken, and that they do not belong in his office.

Another sign of a really fine, scientific, and well-trained specialist is an ability to recognize quickly the clinical picture of constitutional inadequacy, or of the "persistently unwell," or of the woman who aches and hurts all over, or who is always tired.

No one should confine himself too narrowly to a specialty. I am glad that early in my career I learned that no man can be purely a kidney specialist or a stomach specialist. He must first be a physician, knowing much about disease in all parts of the body; and then, whether he likes it or not, if he is to help many of his patients, he must spend much of his time being a physician to the troubled mind and the bruised spirit.

How poor a gastroenterologist a man would be if every time a half-crazy air-swallower and belcher came in he should start treating him with diets, antacids, and belladonna. How poor a physician he would be if he did not stop to ask and find that the man had no indigestion, and that his spells of air-gulping came only when he got panicky and perhaps filled with an awful fear that he was going insane like his mother before him!

The fact that most belchers are suffering from a neurosis and not a gastric lesion is not well taught in medical school, and it is not sufficiently emphasized in texts on gastroenterology. Some day, and this is important, the description of a number of syndromes will have to be moved from books on digestive diseases, where they do not belong, to books on neuroses where they do belong.

THE NEED FOR REMEMBERING THAT THE BRAIN HAS SOME DISEASES ALL ITS OWN

If one did not know that most of us older physicians had never received any college training in the recognition of neuroses or psychoses, it would be a puzzle why we so rarely think of the brain as the seat of discomfort or disease. We seldom think of it as an important organ of the body which can have some diseases all its own, or which can determine whether the person usually feels well and full of energy, or feels tired and ill and weak, or fearful of disaster and death.

Until a few years ago, even the pathologist, who should have known better, would sometimes look up from the necropsy table and say, "I don't know why this man died." And it did not seem to bother him that he had not examined the brain. If he had only opened the skull he might have been astonished to find there a hemorrhage, a tumor, an acute meningitis, or an acute encephalitis.

The state of the brain often determines the feelings of the patient. From a medical point of view, the brain is the most important organ in the body because its state determines the nature of a patient's response to his illness. On its good or poor functioning depends the man's feelings of good or poor health, the amount of concern he feels about his discomforts, and the degree to which he complains.

Surely, every thoughtful physician must have marveled at the great difference that exists between the mental reactions of individuals to their illnesses. Some, very ill and facing death, are stoical, unconcerned, or without complaint of pain or distress; and others, with no organic disease, are always complaining, and full of the fear of death. I remember an able, hard-driving business man who had never known illness until one day when he noticed a little blood on the toilet paper. A few days later a carcinoma of the colon was found and quickly removed. Two years later the man returned, jaundiced, and with his liver filled with cancer. The remarkable fact is that during the next six months he continued to feel well, to walk briskly, to work hard, and to enjoy three meals a day. He could hardly believe he was ill, and he felt well up to the day when his home surgeon explored his abdomen and threw him into his final coma. It was remarkable that a man so riddled by disease could be so free of any sensation of illness. He was not very sensitive and he certainly was not a worrier.

I remember, also, a stocky man with an active duodenal ulcer and a very painful jejunal ulcer. His wife had dragged him in because she was tired of watching him walk the floor at night. But he would not stay to have anything done because he felt no concern about his pain and did not care to do anything about it; as he said, "Lots of people have worse troubles than that!"

On the other hand, we physicians are constantly seeing patients with nothing discoverable to explain their utter misery and prostration. Greatly depressed, they feel so awful that they can hardly get out of bed in the morning. They say their suffering is more than they can bear, and they keep going from one physician to another. I remember even some football stars who belonged in this group: big husky fellows whom I took care of for years. Because of an inherited tendency to depression, they were always miserable and apprehensive. It was the sight of these men with their powerful but uncomfortable bodies that started me thinking that it must be the state of the brain that determines whether a man feels fine and full of energy, or miserable and tired and weak.

One reason we physicians seldom think of the brain as the seat of disease. One reason we physicians today so seldom think of disease in the brain is that during the four years we spent working in the wards of a big charity hospital, we kept seeing mainly physical wrecks—men and women in the final stages of the several degenerative diseases. Daily we saw patients suffering from decompensated disease of the heart, the kidneys, and the liver. We saw the end-results of chronic alcoholism, arteriosclerosis, encephalitis, prostatism, arthritis, emphysema, bronchiectasis, tuberculosis, rheumatic fever, the degenerative nervous diseases, syphilis, and carcinoma. After years of living alongside of this human wreckage, is it any wonder that when we went out into a downtown practice, we found ourselves in a new world, filled with sick men and women such as we had seldom seen or heard of before?

The idea that it is disgraceful to diagnose functional disease. Some medical graduates tell me that during their college years they were given the impression by a few of their teachers that it was a sign of incompetence or laziness to diagnose functional disease. A certain professor of surgery used to begin his course of lectures with the statement, "Gentlemen, I would have you know that in this department there is no such thing as a functional disease; if you will only keep examining long enough and carefully enough you will find organic disease." By this I presume he meant easily visible disease that could be removed. Naturally, a man who has been taught this sort of thing in college is likely to go on believing it when he gets out into practice.

The failure to teach much about neuroses in college. One of the bad features of medical education today is that each week in the college amphitheater the students are shown examples only of the rare diseases which they will not see after they are graduated. Seldom are they shown examples of the common diseases which they will see every week. I maintain that the professors should often show nervous women with multiple complaints and no positive findings. These are the patients whom the students will see when they get out into practice. I cannot remember ever in my college days seeing in the amphitheater a woman with migraine, or a mildly psychotic woman with a fibrositis or a constant abdominal pain of psychic origin, yet today I am constantly seeing such patients.

The results of early training. With our college training what it was, is it any wonder that when we physicians saw our first pampered and oversensitive wife of a well-to-do man, complaining perhaps of nausea and vomiting and a pain over one eye, our only thought was to search diligently through her body for an ulcer or a gallstone? Is it any wonder that we failed to ask and learn that the woman was migrainous by nature, and that her spells came whenever she got too tired, or distressed because her husband was too busy ever to give her a little of his time? Furthermore, is it any wonder that when, in a case such as I have just described, the laboratory technician reported the finding of a few amebas in the stools, or the roentgenologist reported a harmless ptosis or diverticulosis of the colon, we grasped at these diagnostic straws and were satisfied with them?

The failure even of consultants to recognize the man whose brain has been injured by arteriosclerosis or encephalitis. Sometimes when I have pointed out to a physician what seemed to me obvious signs of brain disease in his patient, I have been discouraged to see his reluctance to entertain the diagnosis. He could not think of the brain as the seat of disease. The distress complained of was in the abdomen and hence he was determined to find the lesion there.

Often what impresses me is that even if the patient had had the supposed coronary injury or cholecystitis or spasm in his colon these things *could not have produced his mental deterioration.* We physicians should remember that there is no abdominal disease, except perhaps carcinoma of the pancreas, that will quickly produce a picture of a nervous breakdown with premature aging.

Many a time, when I have called attention to a patient's mental deterioration, his relatives have said, "Oh, he has just been worrying so much over his indigestion that he hasn't had time or energy for his work; if you can only get his bowels to moving, or his gas to passing he will be all right." Actually, I have never cured one of these patients by working along these lines.

Today an insane person can undergo a thorough examination and be given a report of perfect health. As I shall point out again and again in this book, today a patient suffering from a psychosis, if he is quiet in the physician's office, can emerge from a thorough medical examination with a clean bill of health! I have seen many a manic-depressive or schizoid person come with a sheaf of reports from good clinicians, all of whom evidently had failed to notice his mental disease. Often it is only the family physician who writes that the man has been behaving queerly.

I remember the professor's wife who, with a typical melancholia, went through the local university hospital and came out with a diagnosis of amebiasis! No one had drawn out the story that she, who had always been a fine wife and mother and housekeeper, had suddenly lost all interest in her husband and family and home, and had taken to sitting in a room alone. No one had learned that her father was in an asylum, also suffering from melancholia.

I have seen many a physician who did not recognize manic-depressive insanity, even in his own wife. During her hypomanic spells, the doctor thought she was a fine hard-working woman who did too many kind things for her family and her community; but in her depressed spells he thought only that she was cantankerous, suspicious, unreasonable, jealous, and mighty hard to live with.

The inability of some physicians to recognize insanity even when it is pointed out to them. One of the discouraging features of the situation is that sometimes even when a physician is told that his patient is psychotic he cannot believe it. His idea of an insane man is of someone who is irrational or raving mad. Time and again, when I have told a new first assistant that the trouble of the woman whom we had just seen was a psychosis, I have sensed his unbelief; and later, after he had dismissed the patient, I noted that all he had put down on the line for the diagnosis was some such inadequate label as "chronic nervous exhaustion."

HOW BIG IS THE PROBLEM OF NERVOUS AND MENTAL DISEASE IN THE UNITED STATES?

Statistics are often boring, but perhaps, here, with a few figures, I can startle some of my readers into a greater interest in the problem facing us all. I will try to do this by showing what a tremendous number of mentally weak and ill and troubled persons are living among us here in America. This incidence is bad enough; what is worse is that from the fringes of this horde of mentally weak and disturbed people there spreads out another horde of chronic complainers. They are the people who fill our waiting rooms and take up most of our time. They are the "chronics" and the "often unwells." (See Chapter 13.)

The high incidence of mental defects in the population. I can remember how shocked I was, years ago, when I heard that in New York state a baby just born had one chance in twenty of eventually being committed to a public institution for the insane, the feeble-minded, or the epileptic. I promptly looked up the figures and found that several agencies had gathered them and all had agreed fairly closely.* Similar figures have since been computed for Sweden. Actually, in America, especially for boy babies, the chances of hospitalization for mental abnormality is somewhat greater than one in twenty; in New York and Massachusetts the figure was fifty-seven per 1,000, or one in 17.5. As Tietze showed, if one takes all commitments, including those of old persons with senile psychoses, the expectation would be 85.5 per 1,000 born, or one in twelve! Worse yet, with the now steady increase in numbers of persons older than sixty-five years, the expectation of senile types of mental deterioration must increase. But these figures are for the years from 1929 to 1931, and it looks now as if the incidence of mental disease is rising.

Estimated Number of Mentally Disturbed Persons in the Country

Dr. Parran once estimated that one in every thirteen persons in the United States is either mentally unbalanced or has a serious problem of adjustment. Cobb estimated that there are some 2,500,000 psychotic persons in the country, with another 4,000,000 more or less incapacitated by nervous and psychic troubles.

Idiots and dullards. According to Cobb, in this country there are some 100,000 idiots and imbeciles. Stevenson, of the National Committee for Mental Hygiene, once stated that from 1 to 3 per cent of the population is substandard in intelligence. From the experience of the draft boards and the Army, the problem would appear to be even more serious than this. Certainly there must be some 1,500,000 dullards in the country: persons who cannot be counted on to support themselves.

Perhaps included with the 1,500,000 dullards, are some 500,000 children who do not get on well in school. They either haven't enough intelligence to learn, or they are too undisciplined or psychopathic to fit into the routine of a classroom. Some 15 per cent of all school children are so badly handicapped mentally that they need special attention. Even in our colleges 15 per cent of the students have to apply to counselors for psychiatric help!

Epileptics, alcoholics, and criminals. It is estimated that in this country there are some 650,000 persons with epilepsy and that for each of these there are perhaps ten relatives with a dysrhythmic electroencephalogram, and perhaps a violent temper or some other nervous problem.

According to Kolb, there are 2,500,000 Americans so addicted to alcohol that their efficiency in life is poor, and some 200,000 of them

---

* W. Ogburn and E. Winston, 1929; Pollock and Malzberg, 1928 and 1929; The Metropolitan Life Insurance Company Statistical Bulletin, 1937; H. F. Dorn, 1938; Tietze, 1943; Mental Health Statistics, Federal Security Agency, Sept., 1949.

are decidedly psychopathic. Then, there are some 50,000 persons, mainly men, who are handicapped by habituation to morphine and other crippling drugs (J.A.M.A., Dec. 4, 1948).

There are the perhaps 2,000,000 criminals in and outside of our prisons, most of them somewhat psychopathic. J. Edgar Hoover is reported as saying that one in seventy-eight of our people is criminal and has to be watched. There are, also, hundreds of thousands of prostitutes, professional gamblers, hoboes, eccentrics, recluses, and other undesirables.

Stutterers. There are some 1,200,000 persons handicapped by stuttering and other speech defects. According to several surveys made in schools and colleges about 1 per cent of our young people have trouble talking. Stuttering is often the person's share of a psychopathic inheritance.

Nervous problems in general hospitals. Harold Wolff and some of his colleagues once studied 500 patients in general hospitals and found that at least 30 per cent of those with ordinary medical and surgical problems had personality disturbances that were serious enough to modify the course of the illness or to interfere with a return to work. Interestingly, the duration of convalescence in the group with the personality disturbances was much lengthened; they stayed in the hospital three times as long as they should have.

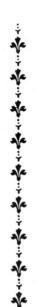

CHAPTER 2

Classifications and Definitions

I SHALL NOT SAY much about classifications and definitions, partly because this subject is of such little interest to non-psychiatrists, and partly because no two psychiatrists appear ever to agree on these subjects. This is unfortunate because as the Chinese say, "The beginning of wisdom is the calling of things by their right names." One finds most of the ablest teachers in the field expressing dissatisfaction with even their own classifications, and wondering if any system can ever be devised that will be satisfying. Douglas Campbell some years ago said, "In no branch of medicine is there such astonishing variation in terminology, and therefore apparently in theory, as in contemporary psychiatry!" He thought this condition was to be expected because of the lack of knowledge as to the nature of mental disease.

Three or four psychiatrists, seeing the same patient, commonly make different diagnoses, such as anxiety neurosis, obsessional neurosis, compulsion neurosis, or psychopathic personality. Similarly, one internist, on seeing a patient with a mild manic-depressive psychosis, may diagnose chronic nervous exhaustion; the next one may say constitutional inadequacy; another, biological inferiority; and another, an anxiety neurosis, a fatigue state, or brucellosis.

After reading definitions of the words "neurotic" and "psychoneurotic" given by many authorities, I am sure of only one thing and that is that they do not all agree. As Ross pointed out, the words "neurosis" and "psychoneurosis" have been used in so confusing a way that one cannot be sure of any difference between them. Because of this uncertainty, I avoid the use of the word "psychoneurosis."

In many cases the important point is not so much to give the disease a name as to be able to guess correctly that it is (1) more a neurosis than a psychosis, (2) more functional than organic, (3) not likely to end up in a psychosis, and (4) likely to be amenable to simple forms of treatment.

Probably all the non-psychiatric physician will want to know about a highly nervous man is exactly what the patient wants to know himself, and that is, is he ever going to go crazy? I remember an intelligent man who years ago used to come and say, "Chat with me for half an hour and tell me if I am still sane." Actually, he never went insane. I think most physicians of large experience, after chatting with a patient, can say in a few minutes that: (1) "Here is a sane, essentially normal person who for good reasons has become very tired and nervous, or (2) here is a person who has always been abnormally nervous, jittery, and worrisome, but eminently sane; (3) here is a flighty 'screwball' who worries insanely and might perhaps someday go over the edge into a psychosis; (4) here is a fine person who, in spite of repeated hereditary depressions, is at present sensible and fine and working like a good citizen; (5) here is a psychopathic character who goes from one scrape to another but who will never get so illogical as to get himself shut up in an asylum, and (6) here is a person who is so manic that he is likely soon to have to be committed." I think most physicians of experience can usually sense quickly a difference between the person who is just nervous or neurotic and the one who has an insane or an alcoholic ancestry; whose worries are pathologic, and who is either close to a psychosis, or headed for one some day. (See Chapters 13 and 14.)

Some physicians may think that the difference between a psychosis and a neurosis is that the psychosis is more disabling, but this is not true. There are many psychotics who are working well, making money, and never complaining about their health, while there are many neurotics so disabled that they seldom work or enjoy life.

No one has ever found a satisfactory definition of psychosis. As someone once said, for a Haitian Negro to believe in voodooism is normal and sane, but for a Harvard professor to believe in it is suggestive of insanity.

The books say that when a man has a hallucination and knows it is unreal, he is sane; but if he believes the thing is real, he is insane. But this definition sometimes fails us. People who are definitely psychotic will at times discuss their problems with good insight and apparent sanity. Or they may be psychotic or violent with someone whom they dislike and distrust, and sane with someone they like and trust and respect.

T. A. Ross and others have maintained that a neurosis never turns into a psychosis. I think what they meant was that from the first interview they could recognize the nervous person who has no tendencies to psychosis. They could recognize other persons whose symptoms suggested that some day they would go into a psychosis. Not in agreement with Ross was Purves Stewart, who felt that there are transitional types between neurosis and psychosis: He knew of no dividing-line.

According to Strecker and Palmer, the psychotic is profoundly shaken in his whole personality, and sometimes that personality is disintegrated. There is a deep cleft between his self and his environment, and for him reality is disturbed, distorted, and even abolished. In the case of the psychoneurotic there is only a partial alteration of personality, and environmental contacts remain largely undisturbed.

As I have said, the trouble with all these definitions is that so often one sees a person who is mildly manic or too depressed to work and yet able to chat in the office as sensibly as anyone. He knows what is wrong with him, and he goes out to the hospital to get the shock treatments that he has read about.

A good example of the psychotic type of symptom that a sane person can have is the paralyzing fear that some fine and able women have of a harmless cat. The woman may be unable to go into a house where there is even a kitten! Another woman is made acutely ill by the sight of a mouse or even the picture of a mouse! This certainly is not sane behavior, and yet the rest of the woman's personality may appear to be excellent. Other sensible and able persons are unable to enter a telephone booth or a Pullman berth, or to sit in a theater anywhere except in the back row, near the door. Others are unable to go on a journey alone. Innumerable persons whom no one ever thinks of committing to an asylum worry insanely about fears which they conjure up. Some interesting and attractive women are "fey" or "psychic" all their lives, and occasionally they will have curious experiences with "ghosts" or evident hallucinations.

Insanity seems often just an exaggeration of some quirk of "normal" character. An important point is that every type of psychosis is an exaggeration of some quirk of "normal" human behavior. Manic-depressives, schizophrenics, and paranoiacs, as found in an asylum, are all suffering from exaggerations of moods which bother many people. Many of us are at times too blue and pessimistic, or too "lit up," or too shy, or too prone to think that something some-

.e did was directed against us. In other words, much of "insanity" is a quantitative increase in eccentricity. Purves Stewart used to explain this with a story. He said that let a person be just shy, reserved, dreamy, artistic, and philosophical, and he will be accepted as a normal member of society. Next, let him get a bit worse so that he goes in for some freak religion or "ism," and then he will be frowned on for being too eccentric or antisocial or "Red." Finally, let him get still worse so that he says he has been in the presence of Christ, or that he has been chosen for a Messiahship, and soon he may become so argumentative and obstreperous and troublesome that he has to be locked up.

Similarly, many a paranoiac person who is only mildly suspicious of people, and inclined to assume that many things that were done innocently were done with intent to annoy and thwart him, is tolerated by society and looked on as normal enough. But let him become a bit worse and he may start instituting foolish lawsuits. Later, as he gets still worse, he may some day become so enraged at a supposed annoyer that he shoots and kills him. Then he must be put away because he is so dangerous to society.

Compulsions. Thousands of persons with queer compulsions are otherwise normal enough; they are just overly neat or punctilious or fussy. They may wash their hands too often, or they may always be going back to make sure that the gas is shut off, or they may constantly be distressed with a feeling that they should give themselves up to the post office inspectors and go to prison for having inadvertently left some writing in a second-class parcel. Some will fear that they may start shouting or swearing in church. They may wear gloves to protect themselves from contaminations with germs; or because of their fear of germs, they may stop shaking hands. But they rarely go over the edge and get so bad that they have to be committed. Hysterical symptoms of a mild degree are commonly observed in the cases of men and women who are otherwise normal enough. A big businessman came in one day, so worried over an operation he had to have that he had marked tubular (hysterical) vision.

On differentiating neurosis and psychosis. Cobb believed that when a patient who is thought to be just neurotic later becomes psychotic, the chances are that the original diagnosis was wrong. As he said, "Who has not made such mistakes in diagnosis? The fact is that at present there is no accurate means of early differentiation in mild cases."

The trouble with psychiatry today is that so little is known about etiology. Until etiology is known there can be no logical classification.

Doubtless we physicians will have to go on for awhile using the terms "neurosis" and "psychosis" because they are convenient. There is no harm in using these terms so long as we do not fool ourselves into believing that they have some real etiologic meaning.

When a patient has to be committed, someone may say he became psychotic on such and such a day. Actually, he doubtless was ill for years, and all that may have happened was that on a certain day, society became alarmed at his behavior and insisted on locking him up. The distinction is only a legal one.

To me it seems obvious that most nervous persons are sane, while a few are not always well balanced or well controlled. Some persons with anxieties are sane; others are not. Some hysterical persons can hardly be called sane; some persons with anorexia are sane and others are not. Some hypochondriacs can hardly be called sane—in regard to their health; some alcoholics are saner than others, and some persons with psychopathic personalities are saner than others.

AVOIDING CONFUSION AS TO "FUNCTIONAL" AND "ORGANIC"

Today we physicians keep talking about functional and organic diseases as if they were very different. Actually, it is doubtful if there is much difference. Even when a woman is just worrying she may have made herself physically ill, and even the woman with a psychosis may have demonstrable disease in the brain or its blood vessels, or she may have some as yet unknown toxin circulating in her blood.

Often when we say that a man's pain is functional all we mean is that nothing grossly wrong can be found in the region where his distress is felt. There may be a microscopic or a chemical or a nutritional change there, or the pain may be referred out from the brain or the cord or some nerve.

For instance, a tabetic may have no demonstrable lesion in his abdomen to explain his crises of pain but he has plenty of disease in his spinal cord. I have seen many persons whose abdominal pain was due to a stroke, a brain tumor, encephalitis, or epilepsy.

Pain due to chemicals in the blood. In some types of "functional" illness the distress may well be produced by some chemical circulating in the blood. For instance, we know that a man who, after being bitten by a black widow spider, is writhing with terrible abdominal pain, has nothing in his abdomen that can be demonstrated by an exploring surgeon. And yet, obviously, his trouble is organic, and due to the toxin injected by the spider. The pain can be relieved by injecting calcium and antivenin.

Nervous strain may eventually produce organic disease. In some cases what starts out as a nervous strain seems to end up as organic disease. For instance, let a woman with a family predisposition to thyroid disease live for several years under great strain with an abusive husband. For a time she may have only an extra outpouring of hormones which will put stress on her thyroid gland, and then her trouble may be said to be functional. But, after months or years of the excessive stimulation of the thyroid gland, it may hypertrophy and change its structure, and then we will say that the woman has an exophthalmic goiter. The abnormal thyroid cells are now filling her body with toxins, and in time these may cause the woman to become mentally queer. Later on, after more years of the poisoning, she may drop dead, and at necropsy much damage will be found in her heart muscle and her liver.

A hysterical contraction, if maintained long enough, can end up as a bony ankylosis. A woman was told by good physicians that she had a psychogenic vaginitis because, whenever she became tired-out and run-down, she got a distressing discharge. But she really had a trichomonas infestation which flared up whenever her bodily resistance fell. John Stokes has described similar cases in which mental strain caused excessive sweating, and this caused a skin fungus to grow rapidly and get out of hand.

As I point out elsewhere in this book, emotion can even kill a man, quickly or slowly (Dunbar, 1946). I have seen many people who, I think, died of fright, and I once saw a man who died of hatred. In Chapter 23 I tell of some of the persons I have known who died, apparently of fright, as they went on the operating table. Among some primitive peoples a man will sit down and die when told he is being "prayed to death" by a witch. Many persons appear to die of sorrow or disgrace, and one often hears of dogs who pined away and died after the loss of a much-loved master. Animals and men will sometimes die suddenly of fright.

Some allergic men, after receiving an injection of antitoxin, may get a serum sickness with fever and a rash. In rare cases, the victim will die, and then, here and there throughout his body, the pathologist will find places where the wall of a small artery had sloughed out, with resultant serious injury to the surrounding tissues. Again, we have what appears to have been a transition from a functional to an organic disease. Raynaud's syndrome, at first brought on definitely by emotion, may eventually become so severe as to cause ulceration of the fingers.

Probably all one can say today is that "functional" means that one cannot demonstrate any gross or microscopic or chemical cause for the discomfort or disability. In many cases the difference between "functional" and "organic" may be only a quantitative one. Thus, for years, a man may suffer from a supposed "functional epigastric pain" until the disease in his pancreas becomes severe enough to produce diarrhea or changes in the blood levels of amylase, lipase, or sugar. Then, at last, the physician has enough evidence so that he can recognize organic disease.

When I think of the billions of cells in the body in which something could go wrong, or the millions of delicate chemical processes which might vary from normal and result in the production of some poisonous chemical, or in the elaboration of too little or too much of some common constituent of a body fluid, I marvel that any of us men and women are ever well. I marvel that we physicians can demonstrate changes as often as we do.

When it comes to trying to distinguish between functional and organic disease of the brain, as Cobb says, there is not a chance of doing it. There can be no thinking without a brain, and good or bad thinking depends on a good or bad brain. Even the symptoms of nervousness, irritability, or lethargy that come from a period of overwork or nervous strain probably arise from some defect in the metabolism of some part of the brain. As Dunbar has said, in dealing with a disease, we can only ask how much is on a physical basis and how much on a psychic basis.

WHAT IS PSYCHOSOMATIC MEDICINE?

What is psychosomatic medicine? Is it a new specialty? Is it something that everyone will eventually have to learn and practice to some extent, or is it a branch of medicine that can be left to the psychiatrists?

Psychosomatic medicine is not new. Psychosomatic medicine is nothing new. Probably 100,000 years ago it was being practised by the witch doctors of the Old Stone Age in their efforts to convince their patients that the demons of disease had been driven out of them, and hence recovery was at hand. Psychosomatic medicine was well known to an ancient Egyptian who, some 4,000 years ago, wrote a whimsical poem to the effect that his doctors were on the wrong track and did not know what was troubling him. Their diagnoses were wrong and their medicines were of no avail because, as so often happens today, they had not taken an adequate history. They did not know that his illness was due to the fact that his girl had left him and gone away. He knew that all of his symptoms were due to this, and that only the girl's return or a letter from her could cure him!

Psychosomatic medicine was known, also, to the ancient Greek physicians, but evidently not well practised by all of them, as shown by Plato's complaint that they had been making the mistake of trying to divorce the mind from the body. Away back there, before the time of Christ, Plato had seen that mind and body are inseparable and can never be divorced. Hippocrates emphasized the importance of the temperament. He used the rest cure, and in the temple sanatoria the priests used suggestion, supposedly coming from the god. Doubtless, much of the early Greek physician's reputation was based on cures obtained through psychotherapy.

The Greeks had evidently seen men who could become jaundiced when sufficiently enraged because they called violent-tempered persons "choleric" or full of bile. The old prophets who wrote the Bible must have noticed the marked effect of anxiety on the bowel because in it they placed the seat of the emotions and the soul. The same idea is found among many primitive peoples.

The effect of the mind on the body was known to the physician, Erasistratus, who practised around 290 B.C. We are told that he correctly diagnosed the illness of a certain young prince who wouldn't eat; he was pining away, and no one knew what was wrong. The physician noted that the youth's pulse rate shot up the minute one of his father's young and beautiful wives came into the room. Immediately realizing the significance of this, the doctor told the king that he could easily cure the lad if he loved him enough; all he had to do was to turn over to him the much-desired stepmother. This the king did, and all was well.

Through the ages there have always been two types of medical practice. One reads in many articles and books that at some unspecified time in the past there was an unfortunate divorce between the medicines of the psyche and of the soma. Actually, I doubt if they ever were properly married. Much study of the medicine of savages and primitive peoples has convinced me that ever since the Old Stone Age, in every land, there have always been two types of medicine practised by two very different types of practitioners. One group believed that all disease was due to demoniac possession or the evil machinations of hostile gods or demons or witches. To their way of thinking, if a man died otherwise than through accident or wounds, he must have been bewitched, or he must have been struck down by some god whose tabu he had broken. This is the medicine of Homer's *Iliad,* of the Bible, and of the pastors of churches in the United States during the influenza epidemic of 1918. At that time some ministers claimed that the way to stop the epidemic was for people to go into the churches and appease their angry God with prayer and penance. We encounter the same idea when a man says he had a stroke (from an angry God), and we are using this old medical theory when we say, "I wonder what possessed me," or "What got into me to do that?"

Obviously, when people, believing in such theories of disease, fall ill, they go to a shaman, priest, faith-healer, or witch: someone who can find out which god or demon was offended and why, or what witch is at work, and who is paying her to do harm to the sick man. Then the shaman or priest tells the invalid how to square himself with the god or demon. In Africa the priest may "smell out" the offending witch and his or her client, and then he may either have the witch killed or he may perform counter-incantations. He performs ceremonies designed to drive the demon of illness out of the sick man.

This type of "physician" needs no knowledge of the body or of disease. His success depends purely on his prestige and on his ability to put on a big show with plenty of ritual and hocus-pocus to make the patient feel he is going to get well: In other words, he practices a form of psychotherapy. The other type of practitioner, found among all primitive peoples, is the herb doctor, either a man or a woman, who takes care of simple diseases, such as coughs, indigestions, and diarrheas.

Today, in every community, one finds the descendants of the two main types of practitioners: on the one hand, faith healers, layers-on of hands, and quacks of many types; and on the other hand, all scientific physicians and surgeons and specialists.

The combination of hocus-pocus and good medicine. To me a curious and interesting fact is that all through the ages the two types of medicine have been combined and employed together. Thus, in the Ebers Papyrus, written some 3,400 years ago, the prescriptions all call for a mixture of some useful drug, such as opium or castor oil, and the dung of some animal! This dung was probably put in to make the devil of disease so disgusted that he would quickly get out of the patient's body. In addition, the medicine was to be taken while an incantation was being read.

Years ago, some archaeologists, digging in Mesopotamia, found several letters that had passed between an ancient king and a distinguished physician who had been called from a distance to consult with the local doctors. He left some medicine, but later the king wrote to say that he was no better. The consultant then sent more medicine but suggested that a soothsayer or magician be called in consultation to see what he could add to the treatment!

The beginnings of interest in organic disease. I suspect that the modern tendency to think only of disease of the soma began some two hundred years ago when, at necropsy tables, physicians began to see the ravages that many diseases work throughout the body. Later, they saw the microscopic changes in the tissues which are the result or cause of disease, and still later they learned of the chemical changes that account for certain disorders, such as diabetes and gout. Later came the knowledge of bacteria, viruses, glands of internal secretion, hormones, and substances that mediate the actions of the autonomic nerves. Along the way there came the marvels of surgery and what Osler called the discovery of the pathology of the living: that is, the discovery of the frequency with which abdominal pain is due to organic disease, such as acute appendicitis, cholecystitis, or peptic ulcer.

After watching the coming of all these marvels is it surprising that most physicians got the idea that all diseases would eventually be found to be due to some demonstrable cause, and usually a localized or focal one? Perhaps some day chemical and microscopic causes will be found to explain most diseases, but certainly gross macroscopic causes will never be found for many of them.

The idea of focal infection or focal disease. To some extent it was unfortunate when E. C. Rosenow and Frank Billings reported that the removal of foci of infection would sometimes relieve arthritis. For a time physicians became so enthusiastic over this conception of disease that every patient who went into a doctor's office was ordered to part with his tonsils and most of his teeth. Worse yet, out of this type of practice came the idea, still held by most intelligent laymen and many physicians, that whenever a person falls ill, all he has to do to get well is to have a thorough examination made: one which presumably will reveal somewhere a focus of infection or disease.

In the chapters that follow I shall present many facts to show that no practitioner of medicine can do without some knowledge of the effects of the mind on the body.

WHAT IS SOMATOPSYCHIC MEDICINE?

Many writers have failed to note that together with psychosomatic medicine the physician should be studying somatopsychic medicine or the influences of diseases of the soma, or body, on the psyche, or spirit. For instance, when in a case of chronic ulcerative colitis, psychic strain causes a flare-up in the diarrhea, that is a psychosomatic manifestation; but when a patient's diarrhea frightens him so badly as to make him worse, that is a somatopsychic manifestation.

We physicians need to remember that every serious disease of the body can have a disturbing effect on the brain. Every alarming, deforming, mutilating, humiliating, or painful illness is likely to have a disturbing effect on the victim's thinking, and if the distress lasts long enough, it is likely to deform his character and impair his mental health. Often one look at the patient's face and one can see what suffering has done to him. We physicians should more often think of this as we treat our patients.

Naturally, some persons are more likely than others to become depressed over an illness, a deformity, or a mutilation. Some fear illness and death much more than others do, and to some the intactness of the body is particularly important. Some, also, are shy and sensitive, and particularly distressed by the stares of people.

The psychic effects of a disease may be more important than the disease itself. Every week in his office the wise and kindly physician will be trying to minimize the somatopsychic effects of disease. Often these psychic effects are more important and disturbing than are the physical effects of the disease that has just been found in the thorax or abdomen. Thus, in thousands of cases the man who has survived an attack of coronary thrombosis with but little injury to his heart would be all right if he were not so badly disabled by fear. It is fear that is making him ill.

In many a case the physician should tell the patient all the encouraging things that he knows about him. After an operation for cancer it may be that the doctor can say that the pathologist reported that the grade of the malignancy was low and that there was no involvement of lymph nodes. These two facts so greatly increase the man's chances of a cure. Perhaps the test of liver function showed no sign of injury due to metastasis, and that is worth a million dollars. Perhaps the blood sedimentation rate was low, and that goes far to rule out any scattering of the growth. All these findings and their hopeful significance should quickly be explained to the patient. When the tumor has scattered he can be told that roentgenotherapy may well retard the growth of the malignant cells.

A person who is particularly in need of a good chat with a kindly physician is one who has a cancer of the lung or of the jaw and cannot make up his mind whether he wants to go to all the trouble of a tremendous operation when the chances are he will be left somewhat crippled and perhaps not cured. Some men are gamblers and others are not, and this may determine whether or not they accept the operation.

In trying to encourage persons with operable cancer the physician will often have to combat adverse suggestions that the patient has received from other patients, nurses, and "friends." Usually these Job's comforters are pessimists who delight in telling of the persons they knew who failed to recover. Too many of us physicians are not convinced that it is worth while to operate for cancer of certain parts of the body and we need to study the available statistics which are encouraging. Other patients who need encouragement are those suffering from hypertension, nephritis, diabetes, tuberculosis, arthritis, or a venereal disease.

The person who is to be mutilated. The person who is to be mutilated by some operation may need wise and friendly counsel.

Thus, the physician or surgeon should give encouragement to the woman who must have a breast removed. The fear of death may be disturbing her less than the fear of losing the beauty of her body. If unmarried, she will fear the effect of this on her chances of marrying, and if married, she may worry about the effect of the mutilation on her husband's love.

Similarly, a young-looking, sensitive, and attractive woman, and especially a childless one, who is to have a hysterectomy may be much disturbed psychically. A man who is to undergo prostatectomy may be worrying most about the possible destructive effect of the operation on his sexual life and on his ability to hold a wife, perhaps ten years younger. Again, he may be too ashamed to ask the question which is constantly on his mind. A man who has to have a testicle removed for tuberculosis is likely, also, to be worried, and full of questions which should be answered before he gets up courage to ask. During a war, soldiers whose external genitalia are often badly wounded by the explosion of a land mine should receive kindly psychiatric attention. A man who has become impotent due to some nervous disease is usually in need of psychiatric help.

It is curious how badly some persons react to a little mutilation. I remember once being puzzled over the great amount of mental distress suffered by a friend of mine who had to have three fingers amputated. He was so greatly ashamed of the deformity that always thereafter he hid his hand in a pocket. His constant mental distress seemed to pull him down a great deal.

The psychic disturbance produced by an ugly defect or deformity. No wise physician should ever fail to think how mentally disturbing to a person some ugly defect can be. Oftentimes today something can be done about it by a good cosmetic surgeon. I remember once putting back into industry a nice-looking woman who, for years, had had a paralyzing neurosis that took her from one psychiatric institution to another. Apparently the most important thing I did was to insist that she get rid of an unusually heavy moustache. Later, when she was well, she told me that her serious mental troubles dated from a moment when a two-year-old little girl, whom she had started to talk to, had run from her, screaming. Instead of assuming that the child was just afraid of strangers, she concluded that she must look so awful as to frighten little children into fits.

Those who would like to get a glimpse of the painful mental processes of a sensitive and brilliant girl who became a hunchback should read *The Little Locksmith,* and particularly *The Journals of the Little Locksmith.* Elsewhere in this volume I shall mention other books which describe the impact on a sensitive person's mind of a paralyzing poliomyelitis, deafness, blindness, spastic paralysis, tuberculosis, an early amputation, or confinement to a wheel chair or bed.

One of the commonest causes of humiliation is great overweight. Another source of unhappiness is excessive shortness, especially in men. The dwarf, and especially the homely big-headed achondroplastic dwarf, has an even harder road to go. Unhappy usually is the woman who is too tall or too big all over. The man who has feminine traits, such as a high-pitched feminine voice, suffers much. I remember an able physician, with a feminine voice, who, many times a day became enraged when someone hearing him answer on the phone, said, "Beg pardon, Ma'am; is the doctor in?"

Much is being done today to help the disfigured. Fortunately, today many bodily defects can be corrected early in life. It is good that no longer are we seeing children with a gaping harelip. But still there are too many persons going about with cross-eyes that could be straightened, flaring ears that could be drawn back, projecting rabbit teeth, a badly receding jaw, or an ugly nose that could be fixed. Physicians should urge the parents of children with such defects to have the deformity corrected early in life before humiliation, bitterness, resentment, and perhaps an inability to find a satisfactory mate have injured the victim's personality.

It should be remembered that the orthopedists, the cosmetic surgeons, and the makers of rubber noses, ears, and hands are becoming ever more skillful, and the deformed who so need their help should quickly be gotten into their expert hands.

Especially in these days of scanty bathing suits, any bodily deformity such as either flat or enormous breasts in a woman, or large ones in a man, bow-legs, or big legs and ankles is likely to be very disturbing. A big port-wine mark, or a scar from a burn, especially on the face, is a constant source of sorrow. The waddle of congenital dislocation of the hips, a bad limp as from a polio leg, or clubfeet, or a bad stammer, or a set of tics, a bad body odor, a bad breath, or a bad skin disease can all be distressing. Even a bald head or heavy glasses or a hearing-aid can greatly disturb some men. It would be bad enough to have these defects, even if everyone were courteous enough not to stare or jeer or tease.

The demoralizing effect of pain. There is another phase of somatopsychic medicine and this is the demoralizing effect of long-continued pain on a person's mind and spirit. Particularly demoralizing appears to be pain arising in the pancreas. Some men with carcinoma of the pancreas or with a duodenal ulcer eating into the head of the pancreas will behave in so psychopathic a way that they may even be put into an institution for psychotic persons. I have seen this happen a number of times.

The demoralizing effect of nausea. Perhaps the most demoralizing body sensation is that of nausea. It can be more demoralizing even than pain. Fortunately, now, it may be helped by dramamine (50 mg.). Very disturbing to the brain, also, can be the effects of severe diarrhea.

Some bodily diseases are more disturbing to the brain than are others. The old clinicians used to comment on the fact that in many cases severe tuberculosis does not seem to have much of a depressing or alarming effect on the brain. A person with his lungs full of cavities may remain optimistic and without the disturbing fears that come usually with a much less dangerous disease of the heart.

It would seem that particularly demoralizing should be any large hemorrhage, as in cases of ulcer. One would think it should frighten a man to see his life-blood flowing away, but many persons who have had several hemorrhages do not seem to be particularly fearful of them.

The importance of the bad effects of anxiety. Years ago, Fox, the pathologist at the Philadelphia Zoo, wrote on the injurious effects that the fear of impending death can have on the individual. Fox suspected that such fears have much to do with the disability and prostration seen in the last stages of fatal diseases. He suspected this because animals, from their inability to understand what is happening to them, do not get frightened; often they keep running about until the day of their death. One day a monkey will be climbing about his cage, apparently as well as ever, and next morning he may be found dead with every tissue of his body riddled with tuberculosis. The pathologist will then wonder how he ever kept going.

Similarly, many times at necropsies on the insane who died suddenly and were found to be riddled with cancer or tuberculosis, I have marveled at this same lack of a history of previous illness. Apparently, the man had been either so elated or so disorganized in his mind that he could neither notice discomforts nor worry about them. Just like the unconcerned and insensitive monkey, he kept going right up to the last minute when, perhaps, an internal hemorrhage or the rupture of some organ brought an end to his life.

Certainly these observations strengthen the impression that often comes to a physician, that if only his patient were not so alarmed over his disease he would hardly be ill. Sometimes one observes this in a person who is not upset by approaching death. Thus, I remember several able and dynamic and fearless men who, though jaundiced and with the liver full of metastatic cancer, felt well and worked cheerfully up to a day or two before their deaths.

The effect of disease of the brain on the mind and thought of the patient. Naturally, one would expect destruction of parts of the brain, or a serious impairment of its blood supply to affect the victim's mental processes and his character. And anyone who has studied many persons with brain tumors or vascular thromboses or hemorrhages knows how true this is. (See Chapter 12, also *Little Strokes* in Oxford Medicine and in Geriatrics.)

An interesting book on the curious changes in a man's thoughts which can take place as a tumor grows in his brain was written by Frigyes Karinthy, one of the leading newspapermen of Hungary (*A Journey Round My Skull*).

Part II

Diagnosis

CHAPTER 3

Hints for Recognizing in a Moment the Neurotic Patient, or the One Whose Troubles Are Likely to Be Functional

THE LETTER ASKING FOR AN APPOINTMENT. Often a secretary will recognize a nervous or psychotic patient just from the way in which he or she writes or telephones for the first appointment. The letter may be too long, or rambling or lacking in good sense, or full of insignificant complaints, or it may tell of many diagnoses made and futile operations performed. When the patient is somewhat psychotic, the letter is likely to be twenty pages long, written in pencil on both sides of cheap ruled paper. In an occasional case, it may even be written on butcher's paper!

The fact that the patient is a woman will, of course, suggest a neurosis, because women are perhaps ten times as subject to neuroses as men are. Some women, like spinsters, divorcees, and broken-down music teachers, are even more likely to have a neurosis. Some people, like the Jews, the Latins, the Irish, and the American Southerner, seem particularly subject to nervous complaints.

What the receptionist notes. Commonly, the doctor's receptionist recognizes a bad neurosis when the patient, often a woman, keeps coming to the desk every few minutes to ask why she cannot go right in. Soon she may get unreasonable and even abusive. She cannot sit still. She may keep going out to the toilet, or she may be in the hall much of the time smoking one cigarette after another. Sometimes in desperation the harried receptionist will beg the physician to take the woman right in before she drives everyone in the anteroom crazy.

What the physician can learn from the first glance. The observant physician will learn much from his first glance as the patient is ushered into the office. He will note in a moment the person's social status, and estimate his or her intelligence. He will notice if the patient is pleasant, wide-awake, bright, friendly, interesting, or perhaps a person of distinction, or even a "character." Or the newcomer may be obviously dull, uninteresting, uneducated, colorless, stupid, senile, or, worse yet, a bit unpleasant or "difficult." A man may be a thin typical little dyspeptic who looks as if he examined with suspicion every bit of food on his plate. Or he may be dissipated-looking, perhaps a gay dog with the women, perhaps with a little waxed moustache, or he may be an alcoholic with his red skin, his bloodshot moist eyes, his twitching facial muscles and his bad teeth. A woman may evidently be a fuss-budget, or a typical stout middle-class matron, or a typical old maid, or a keen, quick-witted, attractive, well-dressed little woman with migraine. In a minute the doctor will note the "screwball," the person who is nervous enough to jump out of his skin, or the person who is dying of anemia or cancer.

The doctor will quickly notice if the person steps quickly and firmly like a young healthy person, or slowly, insecurely and with short shuffling steps like an old sickly person. He will note if there is a limp or a gait characteristic of any well-known nervous disease. He will note if the person looks about quickly with bright, observant, attractive eyes, or if the eyes are dull and slow and unobservant.

A pen-picture of the patient. I am often disturbed when a new assistant writes, "Well-nourished woman about stated age" and lets it go at that. I wonder if he failed to observe the many interesting things about the person, or if, noting them, he did not appreciate their great significance. I think if he had known their tremendous importance he would have made note of them.

I like to see in the record some pen-picture of the patient as a human being; it can be so valuable. To illustrate: One day, on picking up one of my old records of a patient, I found I had written: "A pleasant, attractive woman of refinement and education, well preserved, comes in walking uncertainly and holding onto her husband. Evidently her sense of balance is poor. Her chin and mouth are trembling, and she raises the right eyebrow as she talks. She does not raise the left eyebrow. She is tense and anxious, and keeps smacking dry lips in an agony of worry as to what I will find. She gives the impression of a woman whose brain has been hit pretty hard, perhaps by encephalitis or a little stroke."

This woman came with a report from a neurologist who said that her central nervous system was normal. By that he must have meant that her skin sensations, muscle strengths and reflexes were within normal limits. He did not make note of what I did, or if he noted those things they did not influence his diagnosis. A little questioning revealed the fact that this woman of forty-five had had two sudden "dizzy spells" with nausea, in the second of which she lost all joy in life and lost her ability to write. She almost certainly had had two little apoplexies.

Picking up another record I found that I had written, "A strongly built, handsome woman of thirty-eight years comes in a wheel chair, evidently in much pain. She sits tilted over to her right. Her husband had to lift her onto the examining table. Every movement of her right thigh caused her to groan and wince with pain." As one might have expected, she had a badly displaced disc. In another record I had said, "A merry, middle-aged farmer walks in slowly, stepping gingerly as if walking on eggs. He is trying not to jar himself. He holds his spine rigid, and in order to save it from bending or jarring, when he sits down he takes hold of the sides of the chair and lowers himself slowly and carefully into it." He had a little tumor pressing on his spinal cord. Interestingly, in this case a well-trained hospital resident had failed to make note of these peculiarities, and had taken without question the roentgenologic diagnosis of duodenal ulcer previously accepted by the man's home gastroenterologists!

It is a sad commentary on medical education today that so often striking peculiarities of behavior of this sort are not noticed by young physicians. Often even when the oddity of behavior is pointed out, and its great significance is explained, the young man prefers to accept a roentgenologic diagnosis of some kind. He puts far more trust in what some laboratory person has found than in what he can see for himself.

Other things to be observed. A glance will often give the observant doctor a good idea as to whether the person is sane and well balanced, or if he has the pinched, narrow ascetic face and piercing eyes of a certain type of crank or psychopath. In the case of a sane, intelligent person the clothes should be clean, pressed, and suited to the person's station in life. Occasionally, one can make a correct diagnosis of a mild psychosis on one sign alone, the fact that a well-to-do woman, perhaps a college graduate, is wearing an old dress which her cook would not want to be seen in. It is important to notice grease spots on the coat or vest. Good grooming is as important a sign of nervous health in a man as in an animal or a bird. Any good farmer, cattle-man, shepherd or poultry-raiser can tell in a minute when an animal is ill, and we doctors ought to size people up in the same way. Rarely, the doctor will note that a man is wearing long hair, a flowing black bow tie, a waxed moustache, or spats and a cane, all showing that he is a bit of a character, and not likely to pay his bill!

An exaggerated state of nervous tension can be recognized in a moment when one sees trembling hands, perhaps a twitching face, restlessness, or a corrugated washboard forehead, with the eyebrows pulled far up. As the person talks the platysma muscles in the neck may be contracted, and, rarely, an associated retraction of the upper lip may bare the teeth. Later, the physician may note great rigidity of the abdominal muscles, or greatly exaggerated deep reflexes, or perhaps perspiration running down from the armpits in big drops.

Occasionally a patient will come in using crutches or sitting in a wheel chair, and in a few minutes the physician can see that these aids are not necessary. This, of course, tells much about the individual, and the nature of his or her illness. In rare cases, as the patient comes in, a hysterical type of walk or contracture can easily be recognized. The patient's gait or mode of walking should always be noted. Occasionally, it will point clearly to the diagnosis.

Masculinity and femininity. A normal man should be masculine in his appearance, demeanor, movements and dress, and a normal woman should be feminine in her appearance and dress, Commonly, one sees a stocky woman, heavy about her middle, clad in a mannish tailored suit, with a man's hat, a man's tie, woolen stockings, and low oxfords. She will have a man's haircut, she may walk with a sailor's rolling walk, and her voice may be a bit husky. The corresponding type of man will be carefully dressed, and perhaps he will have some feminine mannerisms, a beautiful complexion, and a distinctive walk.

Occasionally, one will see the peculiar, waxy-pale, old-looking, weazened and wrinkled face of the eunuchoid person, male or female. As Hippocrates pointed out ages ago, an elderly man of this type will still have all his hair, and none of it will be gray. His head will be small, his legs long, his pelvis wide, and his face almost devoid of hair. These things should be noted because such persons are handicapped; although they marry and have children, Nature has to some extent played them a dirty trick, and they are likely to be somewhat odd or neurotic.

The appearance of good health or ill health. As I have said, the physician should note if the patient looks healthy or ill or very ill, thin, anemic or in pain. The physician who would save himself from making humiliating mistakes about people who claim to be in pain should early learn to recognize the patient who is suffering great distress. He should notice the postures he or she gets into trying to get relief.

Perhaps the patient looks depressed and slowed-up, or his clothes may be hanging loosely about him, showing a recent marked loss in weight. Or he may be abnormally stout. Because of nervousness, he may want to keep smoking steadily in the office, or he may be unable to sit down and stay quiet. He may stand through the interview. Occasionally, the physician will note the poker face, the stooping posture and the tremor, or the "pill-rolling" movements of the encephalitic, or the characteristic position of the forearm close to the body of the man who has had a little stroke. Characteristically, also, the patient may keep looking down toward the floor. Or often he will be speaking out of one side of his mouth. This important fact often goes unnoticed and, as a result, the story of the all-important stroke is not obtained. Occasionally the doctor can instantly diagnose a stroke when he notices trophic changes in one hand. This hand will be a bit stiff or clumsy, and the skin may have a red, shiny, tightly stretched appearance. Rarely, in winter, one will see the white fingers of Raynaud's disease, usually a sign of highly overactive sympathetic nerves.

Often the physician should diagnose probable migraine the minute he sees a trimly built, full-breasted, pleasant, wide-awake, bright-eyed, quick-thinking and quick-moving little woman, perhaps with a heavy head of hair. Usually his hunch will be correct. He will then know why she is hypersensitive, headachey, easily nauseated, sometimes dizzy, often ill, and easily and suddenly fatigued.

Ugly and embarrassing physical defects. The doctor should note whether the person is nice-looking, well-built, and sexually attractive, or poorly proportioned, awkward, or a clumsy slob. Sometimes the hand of the Potter slipped and the body was botched. Poor materials went into it, and it may look as if it were made up of odd parts. The abdomen, buttocks, thighs, or breasts may be too large for the rest of the body. Poor physique is seen often in schizoid persons, in persons with a poor nervous heredity, and in persons with a low intelligence. Sad to see is the type of botched person who, old and gray, is still working as a messenger boy, a "peanut butcher," a newsboy, or a busboy in a restaurant. As the Bible says, these sad persons were doomed by Nature to be "hewers of wood and drawers of water."

Ugly defects should always be noted: defects such as great homeliness, flaring ears, an ugly nose, protruding teeth, a mouse jaw, a bad squint, a port-wine mark, an acne rosacea, a bad facial scar from a burn, a hunchback, clubfeet, bow-legs, smallness and great shortness in a man, or bigness and great tallness or huge breasts or big legs and ankles in a woman. There may be a short polio arm or leg, or an amputation, or a stiff leg, or the waddle of dislocated hips. Great overweight, especially in women, with the resultant constant teasing, causes much mental distress. Because it is so easily curable, its retention shows a lack of adult mentality, or of self-control, or sexual pride on the part of the person involved. All of these defects which cause life-long embarrassment and shame are likely to have some warping effect on the mind and the soul.

Some day we physicians may understand better the physiologic significance to the individual of a severe acne that leaves the face pitted and unattractive. Because it is primarily a disease of puberty and can be produced in older women by the giving of male hormone, it must have some relation to the internal secretions. It must be significant, also, that it usually clears up by the age of twenty-two. It causes much mental torture in boys and girls.

The sexual and general attractiveness, social poise, and self-assurance of a youth or girl means much, in two ways. If a person during the mating years is attractive, interested in the opposite sex, and easily accepted by that sex, it suggests sanity and a good nervous heredity. On the other hand, if the person is not attractive, not interested in or acceptable to the opposite sex, it suggests psychic abnormality, and it means that the victim must throughout life put up with much loneliness and unhappiness, many rebuffs, and perhaps eventually an unsatisfactory marriage with a similarly handicapped mate: another person left behind on the matrimonial counter.

The fact that a person past thirty-five is unmarried should cause the physician to wonder why, and perhaps to ask why. Often this question will open the way to an important part of the patient's history.

What is noted on shaking hands. Much can be learned from the way in which a patient greets the physician and shakes hands. The normal person does this in a simple, easy, friendly way without effort or embarrassment. He or she looks the doctor in the eye, with interest and perhaps with a searching glance to see what sort of person he is. The shy man may not look the doctor in the eye or may do so only for a moment. He may be either diffident or else painfully nice, making a great effort to seem friendly. Or he may have a peculiar shy handshake, or he may give the bone-crushing grip of a man who is trying to cover up the fact that he has an inferiority complex. One can sometimes recognize in a minute the earnest pupil of Dale Carnegie!

The doctor should note instantly the overly warm hand of the person with hyperthyroidism and a high basal metabolic rate, or the flabby, soft, "boneless" hand of some asthenics or persons with a peculiar nervous system; or the commonly met with cold wet hand of the person with much anxiety and an overly active set of sympathetic nerves. Often the presence of this clammy hand practically makes the diagnosis of neurocirculatory asthenia with a number of added neuroses.

Easily recognizable is the overly shy, quiet, reserved and apparently uninterested, schizoid young man or woman who, when the doctor comes into the room, hardly looks up at him, and does not rise to greet him. Perhaps the person goes on looking out of the window, and lets a relative give the history. Perhaps the patient is a girl with anorexia nervosa or some form of hysteria. From her disinterested behavior, one can see that she came only at the behest of her mother, and not because she was concerned about her illness or wanted to do anything about it.

Other things noticed during the first interview. During the first interview the physician will be keeping his eyes open and noting many things, most of which will have much meaning for him. For instance, he may note that the patient has a number of tics of face or neck or shoulders, all signs of a nervous nature. Or with some words there may be a relic of an almost cured stutter, and this shows the man has a nervous heredity.

Occasionally, a nervous person will keep sniffing, or clearing his throat or cracking knuckles, or using a benzedrine inhaler, or rubbing the skin of the end of his thumb with another finger. An arteriosclerotic oldish man may keep making curious little whistling or swishing sounds with his lips. His facial muscles may be twitching because of vascular changes in his nervous system. There may be a little egg on his chin, or a little drooling at one corner of his mouth, all signs of some injury to the brain.

Rarely one will meet a hypomanic patient who will keep talking at a great rate. One will suspect mild mania, also, if the man is supernormally friendly, affable, and "pally." Another curious type of patient, perhaps with a brain tumor, will keep wise-cracking, or he may keep his hat on, or he may urinate in the hall. Often one can recognize a probably migrainous woman the minute she starts shading her eyes because of light coming from a window.

Occasionally, especially in the northwestern tier of states, one will note prominent or shining eyes with a full neck and perhaps the dark reddish skin of the person with exophthalmic goiter. Such a person is likely to fidget about and to wink the eyes frequently. Sometimes one has to ask and find out if a slight exophthalamos runs in the family or was always present. Occasionally one will see the scar of a thyroidectomy and this will go far to explain the woman's nervousness. It may also explain a lack of interest in sex and a failure to have held the husband. One can often recognize the person with marked hypothyroidism and the pudgy anemic-looking face, the slow answers, perhaps a hoarse voice and some overweight. One can recognize in a moment the man with pituitary disease with his distinctive raucous voice, his massive homely features, and his large hands and feet.

Often, at a glance, one can recognize the patient with heart disease, with his shortness of breath, or his bluish lips. He will get short of breath trying to undress. One can suspect the man with ascites because of his only partially buttoned pants; or the asthmatic with his wheezy, labored breathing, his barrel-chest, his contracted neck muscles, his clubbed fingers, and his nasal voice with a wide nose full of polyps. One can recognize, also, the scarred neck of a person who once had tuberculous glands. Occasionally a deep-set eye on one side will point to a Horner's syndrome and a lesion in the cervical sympathetic nerves on that side. Rarely one can be led quickly to a diagnosis of primary anemia by noticing premature gray hair. A diagnosis of fibrositis or arthritis can be made as the patient gets up stiffly from his chair.

As one talks to the patient, one may note constant air-swallowing and belching, or the regurgitation of food into a handkerchief: all signs of a neurosis. A woman's chin muscles may quiver, showing that she is under great emotional strain and trying hard not to cry, or from time to time she may actually cry. Then she will deny that she is nervous! Her fingers may be badly stained from smoking, her breath will be heavy with tobacco; she will have a cigarette cough, and her nails may be bitten to the quick. Her teeth may be full of big cavities and in terrible shape. In women this usually means lack of good sense or of good discipline, or a great fear of pain. In men it often means alcoholism.

As many a nervous red-headed woman talks to the physician, especially about painful emotions, red blotches will form on the side of the neck and will spread downward.

As one comes near an overanxious patient one may note a fecal type of bad breath due to great anxiety, or one may note the bad breath of bad teeth, pyorrhea, tabagism, alcoholism, eating much garlic or pork, diabetes, carcinoma of the esophagus, ozena, or some one of the unknown metabolic disturbances that give rise to halitosis.

Occasionally a patient will be wearing heavy dark glasses in the office where obviously they are not needed. Many a time this will immediately make the diagnosis of a neurosis or even a hysterical syndrome. In older persons who have had a little stroke one may be able to recognize the thick or uncertain speech. One can also recognize the whisper of a person suffering from a hysterical aphonia.

Peculiar behavior of a patient. In a few minutes the physician may recognize types of behavior which point clearly to a peculiar kind of personality. For instance, a neurotic woman may refuse to have her examination started by an assistant; she wants immediate attention from one of the senior men. Another patient may begin by demanding all known tests, and another may seem to be desirous of submitting to uncomfortable examinations such as gastroscopy, bronchoscopy, cystoscopy, or duodenal drainage. From this the doctor will suspect he is dealing with a type of psychotic person.

The physician will quickly recognize the type of patient who does not listen, but keeps breaking in all the time to do the talking. This is a most important observation because it reveals a type of person whom no one is likely ever to help. How is psychotherapy ever to affect a woman if she never pays attention or listens to anyone? She is so absorbed in herself and her problems that she cannot think of anyone else. Other patients are evidently of such low intelligence, or so rattled, confused, anxious, or senile that they cannot take in what is told them, even when it is repeated several times.

A type of undisciplined scatterbrain was the wealthy woman who came a thousand miles to get my opinion about a disease which she said was going to kill her unless someone saved her. She came with her meek husband, her physician, and her nurse. Because she arrived on a Saturday morning I had to tell her that I could not get much of her examination started until Monday. With this, she said to her entourage, "I can't wait; I am homesick; we are going home right now." And home she went. Her diagnosis was obviously, "Stupid, spoiled, and undisciplined, grade IV." Another spoiled young woman of this type came with a diagnosis of chronic ulcerative colitis. In the hospital she could not be bothered to save samples of feces or urine. Instead of taking the prescribed diet she ran out several times a day to get candy bars and ice cream. She would not stay in bed, and she kept smoking one cigarette after the other. As I expected from this, she did not have an ulcerative colitis; her diarrhea was due to a stormy love affair with a gay dog who, apparently, from her account, was as hard to pin down as she was.

What can be learned from watching the relatives with the patient. Often, when relatives come with a patient, one can learn much from observing what they are like and how they behave with the invalid. Perhaps some are odd or poorly adjusted. Perhaps a bossy wife wants to give her husband's history, and angrily he tries to shut her up. Or one can see that the wife is afraid of her husband, or one is shocked to see how discourteous he is to her. Or, one may get a hunch that the terms of endearment used are shams that conceal a lack of love or even a deep resentment. Or, if a mother comes with her sick daughter, one can see signs of friction between them: efforts at enslavement on the part of the mother, and resentment on the part of the daughter. One can see, perhaps, the contempt of the girl for a silly mother or for a father who lacks education and refinement. Many a time I have learned most of what I needed to know about a patient by watching how he and his wife and mother-in-law got along and spoke to each other.

Observations made as the Chief checks over the history taken by an assistant. When, after the preliminary study by an assistant, the Chief comes in, there will be several things he will quickly note. For instance, what is the patient's age in years, and does he or she look older or younger than that? What is the person's occupation, and does he or she look the part? I was once led quickly to a diagnosis simply because an old-looking man past fifty was listed as a boiler-maker's *apprentice.* I immediately wanted to know why he had never been promoted. From his answers I learned that when he lost his health he was a successful farmer with a big place. While caring for a number of horses sick with encephalitis, he apparently took their disease and had a fever with somnolence. This left him so disabled mentally that he could no longer run the farm; he sold it and moved to the city. There his son, who ran the roundhouse for the local railroad, gave him a little job working around the boilers. The internists who had seen him before I did had been so satisfied with a roentgenologic diagnosis of duodenal ulcer, based on the finding of an old scar of one, that they had failed to get the all-essential story and thereby to make the correct diagnosis.

Hints that can be obtained quickly from the way in which the history is given. Most that the physician needs to know about a patient can often be learned in a minute from the way he or she starts to give the history. A man with organic disease, such as peptic ulcer, is likely to begin by saying he has pain in a certain spot, while a neurotic woman will be unable to say what is her principal complaint. One may never be able to get a satisfactory history out of her.

The physician can discount much of what a person says about the severity of his pain and his illness if he spends most of his time in the office telling about inconsequential things, such as little blisters on his fingers, spots before his eyes, or freckles on his face! Obviously, a man who fusses over such trifles is likely to be exaggerating what few real symptoms he has.

The heart of every physician of experience sinks when an old school teacher or professor's wife pulls out a long list of her symptoms or even a notebook full of them. The doctor knows then what he is in for. The woman wants to be sure that now that she has reached a consultant *all* of her troubles will be discussed and cured. She does not want to forget a single one of the questions she intended to ask; she does not want to get back home and have her husband ask, "While you were at it, why didn't you find what makes that 'click' in your neck?"

The physician will suspect a neurosis when the disability is great, the results of the examinations are negative, and the patient is well nourished. He will suspect a psychotic temperament when there have been more than six or eight operations. He can be almost certain of a neurosis when there are many aches and pains and sorenesses from the head to the feet, especially on one side of the body. He will think first of a neurosis when there are a number of odd symptoms, such as a mental haziness, a confusion when going out on the street, some loss of the feeling of contact with the world, or an inability to read or to go to a movie. All these things cannot possibly come from a uterine myoma or a movable kidney; they must come from the brain.

The patient who does not answer the questions asked. Particularly instructive, often, is a patient's habit of not answering the questions that are being asked. The answer is often irrelevant. For instance, a fluttery-looking woman said that her sufferings were so great that unless something were soon done for her, she would have to do away with herself. The physician said, "Well, what seems to be the main trouble?" Her answer was, "I have so many troubles that I don't know where to begin."

"Well, let's begin somewhere."

"All right," said the patient, after thinking a while. "You wouldn't call these little brown, liverish spots on my hands normal, would you?"

"No," said the doctor. "But I wouldn't worry about them. Let's now get down to business. What is your outstanding symptom?"

"I have had it a long time."

"Yes; but what is it?"

"I had my gallbladder out."

"No, we'll go into that later; what I want to get straight is, what is bothering you most right now?"

"My doctor said he was looking for bleeding."

"No," said the doctor, now deciding that, as a bit of research, he'd like to see how long this sort of thing could be kept up. "No, I asked what your worst symptom is."

"They put me on a milk and toast diet."

"No, let's get back to the question, 'What would you say bothers you most?' "

"Ulcers, I guess."

"No, that is someone's diagnosis: I want to know what your worst symptom is."

"I still have the same symptoms!"

"Now, perhaps we are getting somewhere; what are those symptoms?"

"In the last few years I have been eating everything."

"No, again we are straying from the subject: What is your main trouble?"

"Do you think I should be so constipated?"

"We will take that up later: What is your main symptom?"

"My sister says that no one should ever be as constipated as I am."

"No, that is not what I want. I want to know what is bothering you most."

" I went to the store to see a customer. She said, 'Take some herb tea and you'll be better.'"

"No, just for fun, let's stick to the question until we find out what is bothering you most."

"My doctor said the ulcer was active on its outer edge."

"No, that does not help me; what is your main trouble?"

"My doctor gave me a bottle of green medicine. Would you like to see it?"

"No, that wouldn't tell me anything; can't you tell me what is bothering you most?"

"I should say I was just sick."

T. A. Ross said that persons who answer in this way have such a disorganized brain they must be psychotic, and I suspect he was right. They certainly are scatterbrained. Nielsen and Thompson thought this behavior suggests a mild schizophrenia. Some persons also have a curious way of talking without ever finishing their sentences. Again, this shows a poorly organized activity of the brain.

A certain type of "smart aleck" patient when asked, "What is the trouble?" answers, "That is for you to find out." Other curious self-centered persons will not let the doctor say much. They do not listen, but break in with what they want to say. Such persons can hardly be helped.

The common symptoms of a neurosis. Suspicious of a neurosis or minor psychosis are the following well-known complaints. First is chronic ill health, perhaps with much fatigue, loss of energy, and lack of joy in life. A woman will have to force herself to work, especially in the morning. By evening she feels better. Usually she is tense and jittery, perhaps so much so that at times "she could jump out of her skin." Her nerves are constantly playing tricks on her as is described in Chapter 13. She sleeps poorly. She may be unable to stand crowds or to drive a car in traffic. She may have such claustrophobia that she cannot go into a telephone booth or a Pullman berth. She may be full of a number of silly compulsions, and she may worry without reason.

The woman with a sore colon and much fear of autointoxication may be taking several enemas a day. She may have an exaggerated fear of illness and death and disaster. She may be so suggestible that she thinks she has all the diseases she hears about. She may rush to a doctor whenever slightly ill, and she may want to be filled with sulfonamides and penicillin.

Some anxiety or uncertainty may cause her to urinate every twenty minutes during the day, but not at night. When panicky she may suffer from diarrhea. She may vomit or faint easily with emotion; she may perspire freely when tense, or even when writing a letter. She will probably at times get air-hunger, or a feeling that she is smothering or cannot take in a big enough breath. Occasionally she may feel a globus in her neck, and often she is likely to have palpitation, headache, and backache. There may be weak spells or feelings of giddiness or swimming in the head. The woman almost certainly will be constipated, and she is likely to suffer from mucous colics. She may also complain much of painful menstruation, or a lack of sexual feeling, or perhaps epigastric burning, heartburn, regurgitation of food, nausea, air-swallowing and belching, abdominal quivering and throbbing, and a feeling of "butterflies" or a "tying of the bowel in a knot."

Diagnostic often is the fact that a person lost all symptoms the day he or she left home to go to see a consultant. Furthermore, it is significant that while visiting the consultant the patient ate indigestible foods in an effort to bring on one of his or her attacks, and nothing happened. This suggests that at home it was strain and annoyance that produced all the trouble. The doctor will be the surer of this when a blow-up occurs the day the person buys a ticket to go home or receives an annoying message from spouse or boss.

The dyspeptic never can eat much at a time; his capacity is so small. The food-crank can quickly be recognized. He is often a "screwball" who is a vegetarian, an eater of nuts, or a drinker of a quart of carrot juice a day. He leaves out foods by groups; that is, he eats no acids or no pastries or no desserts or no fried foods or no warmed-over foods. He loves vitamins and drugs, and tries out new patent medicines.

The abuse of drugs. It is helpful to know that a person uses much tobacco, alcohol, and much sleeping medicine because this shows he has a restless, undisciplined, and perhaps uncomfortable type of nervous system.

The significance of hypersensitiveness. It is helpful to know that a person is abnormally sensitive to smells, sounds, light, and other stimuli. Some women can even sense an approaching storm by the aches it produces in the head or the joints or the abdomen. Many of these persons are highly sensitive to foods and drugs, dust, and pollens. They vomit if they suspect that some food eaten was spoiled or if, while eating, some unpleasantness arises. Some say they are made ill by infinitesimal doses of certain drugs. It is highly diagnostic that barbiturates and morphine affect them wrongly and distressingly. Some persons are so sensitive to nervous influences that they faint at the sight of blood or even of a hypodermic syringe. Others nearly get sick on going down in an elevator.

A woman may be so sensitive that brushing her back teeth will cause her to retch, or the eating of something a bit too sweet will bring vomiting; the taking of a drink of cold water or pop may cause sudden bloating or a feeling of impending diarrhea, or the taking of an enema or even a douche will cause nausea.

Some persons show what sort of human beings they are by telling queer stories like that of the woman who said she belched day and night for nine days after her mother died. Another woman said she cried for three weeks when her brother lost his money. A man was ill for three days after an unpleasant argument; another took to his bed when his only son flunked out of college, and another ran a temperature of 102° F. whenever he lost his temper.

Observations made during the physical examination. A psychopathic woman will sometimes be abnormally prudish about undressing and getting examined. Another type may be somewhat exhibitionistic. Schizoid persons sometimes have a greasy, unpleasant type of skin with an unpleasant odor. Often it helps in the diagnosis of a functional trouble to notice on the neck or arm or leg a scaly and itchy neurodermite.

A rattle-brained person, when asked to look at the physician so that the pupillary reflexes can be checked, will keep looking about the room: everywhere but at the doctor! It is important to note if a patient cannot get up on the step of the examining table without the help of the hands. Such quadriceps weakness is common in cases of hyperthyroidism, and it is seen occasionally in cases of mild hysteria.

It is important to note an asthenic bodily build, with a long narrow thorax, a narrow costal angle, a flat, apelike pelvis, and perhaps long thin arms and legs and long hands and feet. The woman with "toothpick" legs and ankles is inclined to neuroses. One should look particularly for the person with neurocirculatory asthenia who, especially on cold days, has cyanotic and mottled legs and feet, and perhaps large leg veins. Poor materials went into that cardiovascular-renal system. Such a person's pulse may race, and there may be a tremor, some dyspnea, and a little hypertension.

The asthenic, somewhat psychopathic woman often has small tender breasts, with large "shotty," glandular units, and perhaps a small infantile uterus with a long conical cervix. She is likely to have hair around the nipples and up the abdomen, like a man. Rarely, she will have one breast considerably larger than the other. I doubt if I have ever seen this except in girls with a poor nervous inheritance. Rarely, such a girl will have a ticklish abdomen which, again, points to a poor sexual development and a poor nervous inheritance. In girls of this type an attempt by the physician to examine the pelvis may cause much mental distress with a marked defensive reaction in which the thighs are forced together. A rectal examination usually does not excite any such distress.

These nervous girls sometimes have a vaginal discharge, perhaps with a bad odor. Usually it is made up only of mucus which appears to be excreted to excess. In these girls other glands, such as those which secrete perspiration and the fat of the skin, often work excessively.

It is well, especially in these days when unmarried women are so free sexually, to note if the hymen is virginal. The more schizophrenic and untouchable the girl, the more likely she is to be a virgin! Sometimes the fact that a fine type of "unmarried" woman has a marital introitus will lead the physician to inquire and learn of an unhappy and nerve-wrecking "affair" or a broken marriage.

In the cases of some nervous women the examiner can suspect a "mucous colitis" instantly on seeing on the abdomen brown scars of hot water bottle burns. One suspects a neurosis, also, when one sees several operative scars. I am always interested to note that a woman who has had children has either marked striae gravidarum or else a remarkable absence of them. Their absence suggests that the woman "has good rubber in her" and my hunch is that she will retain her youth and will live longer than will the girl whose abdominal wall gets badly marked by the first pregnancy. Occasionally one sees ugly striae on the hips and breasts of a girl of eighteen who was fat and then reduced weight. That looks as if she had "poor materials" in her.

I make particular note of the intensity of the knee jerks because, as I once showed in a statistical study, greatly exaggerated deep reflexes are commonly associated with curious nervous syndromes.

As I examine a man or woman I am on the watch for signs of hyper-sensitiveness which will point to the presence of a neurosis. Occasionally a woman will have tissues so sensitive that she will cry out over a little pinch or will even object to the pressure of the sphygmomanometer cuff. I notice, also, how much or how little a woman complains of pain as I examine her pelvis and her rectum. A correspondingly hypersensitive man will flinch and object when I try to pass a finger up through his scrotum and into the external ring. Teeth full of caries usually suggest that the person is very fearful of the dentist.

Signs of an overly reactive nervous system. A nervous, apprehensive person, perhaps with a neurocirculatory asthenia, may have on the first day a fast pulse, some tremor, a slight hypertension, and a temperature of 99.6° F. A few days later, when he has become used to the physician, these slight abnormalities will be gone.

I make note of large lymph nodes because I think they are found oftenest in a frail hypersensitive type of person who is subject to repeated and long-lasting colds and other infections. I note if a man lacks hair on his chest and nipples and if he has a feminine type of pubic hair, but for lack of a large series of cases studied statistically, I do not know how much these things mean. They do not consistently indicate a lack of masculinity or sexual power. Rarely one will see a woman with her pubic hair shaved off. If asked why she did it, she may say she likes it that way or she feels cleaner. Some physicians state that this sign, together with a hyperemic introitus, indicates homosexualism.

Rarely one will see on a person's forearms the many pits of old abscesses that tell of morphinism. Rarely, also, one will note a kyphosis that has come recently, due to the menopause or a tumor of the parathyroid glands. Or one will note the dark pigmentation of parts of the skin due to Addison's disease, or the massiveness of bones and the hoarse voice of a person with a pituitary adenoma, or the hairiness and coarseness of a girl with a Cushing's syndrome, or, in a young man, the soft fat bodily contours and small external genitalia of a Fröhlich's syndrome.

On the need for learning to recognize the person who is in pain. A useful faculty for the physician to acquire is that of recognizing the patient who has real pain. Many an old doctor will reach into his bag for his hypodermic syringe and a large dose of morphine the minute he walks into a room and finds a patient lying over a bed or a chair, or walking around on his hands and knees or hunched over with his knees near his chin and his hands clasped around them. One look at his drawn face and the sweat on his brow and the doctor does not ask questions: He gives morphine, and takes the history later when the patient is able to talk. Some physicians have not yet learned this wisdom, and hence occasionally a man with a posterior perforated ulcer gets locked up in a psychopathic ward.

I do not mean to say that one can always be sure that a certain person is in real pain, but as a physician grows older his skill in this regard should grow. Some day he should be able to recognize migraine the minute he sees a woman in an attack, or he should suspect that a man has a pancreatic cancer, or a stone going down the ureter, or a gastric crisis of tabes. The doctor will feel fairly certain of these things because of the way the person acts and from the positions he or she gets into, trying to find relief.

Hints obtained from other examiners. Much can often be learned about a patient from the notes made by special examiners. The proctologist often remarks that the patient had a fit over his examination and could hardly "take it," and the girl in the gastric laboratory reports that a great fuss was made over swallowing the stomach-tube. A barium enema may also have caused the patient to act up and complain bitterly. These notes show that the individual is either hypersensitive or else lacking in stoicism and self-control. Many a person who is almost unable to stand the mask of the apparatus for measurement of the basal metabolic rate is evidently subject to claustrophobia. The woman who complains that she could hardly stand the smell of the rubber mask is usually migrainous.

Observations made at the final interview. Much becomes obvious about a patient when he get angry because nothing was found wrong with him. Perhaps he tries to argue with the physician and to catch him in some inconsistency of statement. A normal person is pleased and reassured with a good report, but here is a man who, when told he is all right, acts as if he had been cheated. Of course, in some cases in which the person's suffering and disability are great, one can understand and sympathize with his disappointment and perhaps alarm, when it looks as if he will have to go home without a definite diagnosis and, worse yet, without any prospect of a cure.

Typical is the reaction of the woman who, when told that a few weeks of rest in bed would probably cure her, says, "Why, I'd go crazy if I had to stay in bed." This tells how jittery and restless she is. Curious is the behavior of some persons who do not bother to stay and finish their tests, or who do not stay to get their report. Other odd persons will stay around a clinic for weeks, only occasionally taking a test.

Many wise old physicians could doubtless add to this collection of significant things to be observed, but I think I have gathered here enough material to show that the eyes and ears of the physician can often make the correct diagnosis. What I would urge is that physicians more often trust to the information they obtain in this way. Today they are too inclined to distrust the diagnosis made by their eyes and ears, and to accept only what some laboratory girl writes on a piece of paper. The girl's report may be good, but the hunch of a wise physician can be even better.

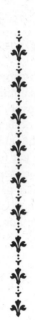

CHAPTER 4

Hints for the Taking of a History

IN SPITE OF ALL the great advances that have been made in recent years in laboratory and roentgenologic and special methods of diagnosis, a good history, well taken and well interpreted, is still the most important factor in the making of most diagnoses. Certainly it is the all-important factor in the making of diagnoses of neuroses, psychoses, and functional troubles. Often an able diagnostician knows he is dealing with a neurosis just because the patient tells his story in a certain typical way.

Often a physician could get the story of the nervous suffering that produced the illness if he would only give the patient a little time in which to tell it. Then he would hear of the overwork or unhappiness or strain which caused all the trouble, and with this it would be obvious that the removal of the appendix or the gallbladder couldn't possibly work a cure. Unfortunately, most good physicians are very busy, and the amount of time allotted to a patient must represent a compromise between what the doctor can give and what he would like to give.

It is sad that in many cases, without a good history, the physician cannot make the diagnosis, and without a wide knowledge of medicine he cannot take an adequate history.

The diagnosis of a neurosis must not be made by exclusion. Many physicians today have the idea that they can make the diagnosis of a neurosis or functional trouble by exclusion, but in this they are often wrong: The trouble with this method is that they are too likely to become satisfied with some unimportant finding which shows up during the examination. Chapter 7 is filled with hints for recognizing these findings which have nothing to do with the production of the patient's symptoms. Elsewhere in this book I show, also, that a psychotic person, if he only remains quiet and well behaved, can go through an extended examination in the office of a top-flight internist and come out with a clean bill of health. Unfortunately, there is no laboratory test which will show the presence of a neurosis or a psychosis.

On recognizing known neuroses and telling one from the other. It is highly important that the physician know well the several neuroses and functional troubles so that he can begin to recognize one as soon as he gets a bit of the story; then he can go ahead to get the rest of it; he can ask questions which will either confirm or disprove his hunch. Repeatedly in this book I shall plead for such training of the young physician that, for the rest of his days, he will be able to make the diagnosis of neuroses and functional troubles positively and surely, just from hearing the typical story, or from hearing the story and noting the appearance and behavior of the patient as he or she goes through the tests. He may go on to put the patient through the usual series of tests, but, then, if he finds gallstones or even a beginning cancer, he will know that the finding has nothing to do with the symptoms. The gallstones and the cancer can be removed and the patient will be left just as ill as before.

Let us say that a woman has been having "dizzy spells." The doctor immediately should want to know what she means by dizziness. He should know that there are a number of symptoms such as wooziness, giddiness, top-heaviness, "swimming," "floating away," or loss of a sense of good balance which are different from vertigo with its feeling that the patient or the room is spinning around. These vague symptoms are not so likely to be associated with disease in the inner ear or with organic disease in the brain. The doctor will be thinking of the several conditions which might cause a loss of the sense of balance, and he will keep asking questions which will give him an idea whether the patient is just nervous or hysterical or migrainous or has suffered an edematous injury in the internal ear or an arterial thrombosis in the brain, or is getting a brain tumor, or has a low blood sugar, or has an overly irritable carotid sinus, or has been smoking too much, or is slipping into the menopause.

Perhaps a woman has come in, evidently restless and nervous, and complaining that she is urinating every fifteen minutes. The physician will immediately ask and determine the fact that she does this only during the day. Her urine is clear, like water; there is no urethral burning with urination, and there is no fever or any sign of toxicity. A few more questions will bring out the fact that the woman started running to the toilet when she was faced with a difficult decision, and then the diagnosis is practically made. The trouble is all due to nervousness and anxiety and indecision. If the urine is found to be without a pus cell or a bacterium, one hardly needs to go any further with the examination.

The great need for cross-questioning the patient and making sure what he means by each complaint. When taking a history hurriedly, as one so often has to do, and especially when the patient is slow and vague in his answers, the physician is very likely to jump to conclusions and to write down something that the person did not actually say. The temptation to do this is so great that after forty-six years of fighting it, I still find that I have constantly to be on my guard against it. For instance, a man will say that he brings up blood, and if I do not look out I may put down that he is "coughing up" blood. Actually, more questioning may show that he is regurgitating it from his esophagus, or hawking it down from his nose, or getting it from diseased gums. A woman may say she is short of breath and I may start to write that she has dyspnea. Actually, her wind may be splendid, and all she has is a feeling, when very nervous, that the room is close and that the air does not contain enough oxygen. All she has, then, is a psychic air-hunger.

As Liveing said so well in 1873, "One way in which error in such matters is propagated is . . . by our faulty methods of interrogation. We are too apt to accept in the hurry of routine the inferences of patients for statements of fact; we often wring from them conformity to our views by pressing them with leading questions or anticipating what they have to say."

One of the most important points in taking a reliable history is to write nothing until one has cross-questioned the patient and pinned him down, making sure just what he meant by a certain statement. If the physician fails to cross-question well, he will surely make many distressing mistakes in diagnosis. For instance, many a time a thin young woman comes in and says she is vomiting. The assistant may put this down and be satisfied with it. But the Chief will ask, "What do you mean by vomiting? Do you mean that you wait until 11 o'clock in the evening and then, after a spell of nausea, bring up all your dinner, or do you mean that, without nausea, you start bringing up mouthfuls of food either at the table or later, a few minutes after you finish your meal? Do you mean that the food comes up easily, without effort or retching?" If this last is the case, the patient is not vomiting, she is *regurgitating,* and this distinction makes the diagnosis. If the girl has no obstruction in the esophagus or at the cardia, she has a disease which is practically always functional.

Another patient may say she has "gas," and the assistant may put this down and be satisfied with it. But he shouldn't be, because the woman may only be swallowing air or perhaps just pushing her abdomen forward hysterically (see Chapter 18). She hasn't any gas. Another patient may give the impression that she has abdominal pain, but the assistant must not put this down. All she may be talking about is "butterflies," or a burning in her skin, or a hallucination of feeling "something in there."

To satisfy an able diagnostician who knows the significance of every little symptom, every history must be taken with care. Commonly, once he has secured a really adequate history he can make a diagnosis without any help from the laboratory worker and the roentgenologist. He may even go against their evidence and be correct.

One of the best stories to illustrate the tremendous need for cross-questioning patients was that of my experience with a stout woman of forty whose history had been taken on three different occasions by three different assistants. It appeared at first glance to be typical of stones in the common duct. Four years before I saw her, after suffering from what the record said were colics, the woman had been operated on and a gallbladder full of stones had been removed. Following this, according to the record, she went on having the same old "colics," sometimes with a chill, some fever, and a little jaundice.

Because this story was so typical of a stone in the common duct, I was about to send her into the hospital for an exploratory operation when I realized that I was breaking my rule and was not cross-questioning her. When I did, to my astonishment, I found that she had never had a bit of pain, even before the operation. She had never had a colic. What she had had were two-day spells of vomiting with unilateral headache: In other words, she had had typical attacks of migraine. More questioning then showed that the gallstones had never given any symptoms, and so, naturally, their removal had made no change in her condition. On asking about the chills she said she once had had a nervous one after a quarrel with her husband. The so-called fever was a temperature of 99.6° F. when she was nervous, and the story of jaundice did not stand up under cross-questioning. It was only a vague sallowness. Next, it was helpful to learn that morphine had not stopped her attacks, but injections of gynergen had. Evidently, the three assistants who had written her history had all jumped to the conclusion that any attack suffered by a woman who had gallstones could be put down quickly as a "colic."

When asked why she had told about the chills, fever, and jaundice, she said the Fellow had been so insistent on getting this story that finally she had given it to get rid of him! This habit we physicians have of insisting that a patient confess to some symptom is unfortunate, and many of us must fight against it. A teacher of mine who stood 6 feet 1 inch and weighed 200 pounds used to look menacingly at a woman and say, "You have jaundice at times; don't deny it." It never occurred to him that it was only a person of strong character who dared stand up to him and maintain that she never was even sallow. A much better technic would have been *to ask her* and her husband if, after one of her spells, anyone had ever noticed that the whites of her eyes were a bit yellow. One might then go further, and if they said, "Yes," try to talk them out of it! I hate to see on records that common statement, "Patient denies she has syphilis." It makes me suspect that the history was taken badly.

I remember a case in which I missed the diagnosis because I was too quickly satisfied with a story which suggested that a prominent society matron was having gallstone colics. When her gallbladder failed to function with the dye, I thought the diagnosis had been made and stopped questioning her. I was almost ready to have her operated on when, fortunately, I asked Dr. Snell to go over the story. He brought out the all-important fact that the woman was drinking in sprees and that the "colics" came with the drinking. A year later, after she had stopped drinking and her liver function had improved, the gallbladder filled well with the dye, and she had no more "colics!"

I could go on telling story after story of this type to show how often we physicians must guard against being satisfied with a short history and some laboratory report apparently confirming the presence of the disease we expected to find. If we had only asked a few more questions we would have made another diagnosis.

Patients who do not tell their story twice the same way. It is a curious fact that many patients, and especially neurotic and somewhat psychotic ones, do not mention the essential and most important symptoms, or do not tell their story twice the same way. This changing of the story suggests the diagnosis of a scatterbrained person. In dealing with such a man or woman, it is well that the history be taken on two or three occasions, preferably by two or three different men. The first day a woman may complain of a pain in her stomach; four days later she may say her trouble is really a backache, and a few days later she may say that what she came about and wants cured is a great sense of fatigue or a pressure in her head.

One day a woman came to consult me with a roentgenologic diagnosis of peptic ulcer and a hemoglobin reading of 50 per cent. She gave no history of bleeding from the stomach or bowel. Because such a low hemoglobin reading is practically never met with in the case of a nonbleeding ulcer, I asked her if she had ever menstruated excessively, and she said, "No." The next man who questioned her, probably more pertinaciously, got her to admit that at times she menstruated for two days rather heavily. The gynecologist who was next called got the story that sometimes she menstruated steadily for two weeks and flooded badly part of that time! Her myomatous uterus appeared then to be the cause of her anemia, and probably of all her troubles. One can only wonder why she did not give the history straight the first time.

A detailed history is necessary, not only for diagnosis, but also, later, for treatment. I often have to point out to an assistant that although he has done well to diagnose a neurosis he has not yet taken a good enough history so that he or I can tell what type of neurosis it is. And without this information we cannot give the patient any intelligent or satisfactory treatment. We must know which one of the many abdominal neuroses described in Chapter 18 is present. But even after we have established the fact that the woman's trouble is a severe migraine and nothing else, we may not be able to help her until we have taken another long history. We may have to question for a half-hour on each of several days before we can find out why she is having her attacks so frequently. We will have to find out what sort of strain she is going through, and what can be done to ease it.

For instance, a woman of forty-five years complained that an old migraine had recently come back to strike her down twice a week. She said she had a happy home and a kind and devoted husband whom she loved deeply. She told me she hadn't a care in the world. It was only after three interviews that I drew from her the admission that because of unwise credit allowances, her husband had been losing large sums of money in his business, and this was worrying her and "burning her up." Her great resentment against the people who were taking advantage of his trusting and easy-going nature was causing her headaches. Obviously, in such a case it would have been useless to fit new glasses or to eliminate foods or treat constipation. My prescription was that she become credit manager for the firm, and to this the husband agreed!

The danger of accepting unquestioningly the diagnosis with which the patient comes. One of the worst features of our modern hurried and mechanical practice of medicine is the willingness of many physicians to accept unquestioningly the patient's statement that he has "stomach trouble" or "heart trouble" or "kidney trouble." As I pointed out in Chapter 1, this sort of thing leads commonly to the specialist's accepting the patient's case and going ahead to examine and treat him. With a little thought or some taking of a history he might see that the man belonged in the office of another type of specialist.

The great advantage of quickly making a diagnosis from the history. As I said before, it is highly desirable that the diagnosis of a neurosis be made from the history when the patient comes in. Why? Because then the physician will be less likely to be led astray by little things which may happen to show up during the examination; things such as a deformity in the duodenal cap, produced many years before, or a peculiar-looking appendix, or some diverticula on the colon. If the physician already knows from the history that the patient's essential trouble is migraine or an epileptic equivalent he is not likely to be led astray by the reports of these little peculiarities in the abdomen. Other great advantages of a quick diagnosis are that the patient with a neurosis is not then frightened by much examining and hospitalization, and reassuring psychotherapy can be started more promptly, at a time when it will do the most good. In many cases much money can be saved by not ordering many needless tests.

What is the patient's principal or most troublesome complaint? As I have remarked before, *much can be learned from the way in which the patient starts telling the story.* A man with organic disease generally knows what is bothering him most, and usually he tells about it in a few words. The woman with a functional trouble is more likely to be vague and rambling and verbose.

On the value of getting a history down in proper order. Adolph Meyer used to teach the importance of getting the long story of a "chronic" patient's illnesses in proper order, year by year. Sometimes it is almost impossible to make a good diagnosis until this is done. In the worst cases the physician will have to make notes on scraps of paper, and then put them in order before he can write the whole story.

Why women lie to the physician. Often a woman lies or conceals facts when the physician asks her if she is happy with her husband. She will say, "He is a fine, able, kind man who gives me and the children a good home, and a place of respect in the community." She will not go on to say that she married him without love, or that he is twenty years older, or a cripple, or that for long she has been desperately unhappy and contemplating divorce. Asked later why she did not mention these important facts which could have thrown so much light on her illness, she says she did not know they were significant, or she felt that so long as she ate his bread she had no right to complain about him, or that since she went into a poor marriage with her eyes open she ought now to put up with it.

The need for satisfying a woman that her secrets will be kept inviolate. Often a woman will not talk of sorrows or sins unless she feels sure that her confidence will be respected. Many a physician, especially in a small city, cannot get the essential story because the patient does not trust the office nurse. The local physician will be handicapped, also, if the woman meets him socially. She may not want to tell her sexual secrets to a man with whom she dances at the country club.

Often a physician is wise if he does not even mention to his wife that a particular friend of hers is coming to his office for consultations. Then, if the patient should remark about this to the wife she will be surprised, and this will relieve the woman's mind of any fears she may have had that her problem was being discussed in the physician's home.

It is a good thing when asking about secret matters to push the history blank away and to do no writing. Hundreds of patients have begged me not to write down secret things and not to file certain letters with the history. One can easily sympathize with their feelings in the matter.

How long has the trouble been present? It is well to find how long a pain has been present because often its long duration alone will rule out the presence of a cancer, a metastasis, an intestinal obstruction, a brain tumor, or multiple sclerosis. The patient himself may be able to see that if he had had a cancer, by now he should be operated on or dead. If the trouble has been recurring at intervals since childhood this suggests a functional cause or some very chronic disease, such as migraine or fibrositis. It often rules out a psychic cause because one is not likely to have the same worry from childhood to middle age.

If intermittent attacks of abdominal pain were due to mild intestinal obstruction, as suggested by the home physician, the chances are that, long before, in some spell, the patient would have gone on to complete obstruction, and would have had to be operated on. The fact that he never came to grief, and that all attacks soon quieted down, leaving no residue, suggests that they were due to some stormy emotion, or that they were equivalents of migraine or epilepsy. When a man has an obstructing disease in his sigmoid colon, the fact that he had two similar spells some years before speaks strongly in favor of diverticulitis and much against carcinoma.

The importance of knowing what was happening to the patient when the disease started. It is very helpful often to know that the first attack of pseudo-angina or pseudo-intestinal obstruction came at a time when the situation was perfect for an attack of hysteria or fright. For instance, a woman remembered that her first attack of air-hunger and palpitation woke her out of sleep about 2 o'clock one morning. The evening before had been spent in wrangling with a recently widowed sister-in-law in an effort to talk her out of trying to break her former (divorced) husband's will. On reaching home at midnight the woman found that, without permission, her seventeen-year-old daughter had gone out with a young man, and when she returned there was another unpleasant argument. One could easily see, then, why later, when the woman woke with a start, she went into hysterics.

An excitable South American man of fifty came in a wheel chair, much frightened, with the story of what sounded like that of a cardiac neurosis. The man and his brother had remained unmarried so as to consecrate their lives to the care of their widowed mother. One evening the brother dropped dead and shortly after, when the mother got the news, she followed suit. Then my patient went to pieces and concluded that he, too, was dying. When his local physician arrived and agreed with him, he was in a bad way. Fortunately, with much reassurance, he got out of his wheel chair and went back to work.

The significance of a story of shortening intervals between attacks. Persons who have suffered for years from a functional type of pain often tell a characteristic story. This is that years before, the first attack came out of a clear sky. The next came perhaps a year later, and the next, some six months later. After that the interval between attacks kept getting shorter and shorter until perhaps the attacks fused and the pain became constant. In my experience, this story usually points to the type of pain for which the surgeon will never find a cause.

A good history may be enough to rule out a diagnosis made elsewhere. Often, if the history is only taken well enough, a diagnosis made elsewhere can promptly be ruled out. For instance, a patient came with a letter from a well-known internist saying that her spells were due to hyperinsulinism. But in a minute I learned that her syndrome had no relation to hunger; it never appeared in the morning before breakfast when the titer of blood sugar is lowest, and it was not relieved by the taking of sugar or the eating of a meal. The piece of pancreas removed at operation showed no adenoma. Obviously, her spells were not due to hyperinsulinism. A little more questioning and it became clear that the spells were migrainous headaches due to fatigue and excitement. Many of the diagnoses that patients bring with them can be quickly demolished in this way.

The importance of a chance remark. Time and again, after a long history has been taken and retaken, many examinations have been made, and I have remained puzzled, a chance remark of the patient has suddenly given me the diagnosis. This is why, when I cannot make a definite diagnosis, or I am not satisfied with the one given me by the laboratories or some specialist, I like to sit and chat a while with the patient. A cat may come out of the bag. For instance, I tell else-

where of a woman seen in what looked like an ordinary c
who one day remarked that her sister had had the same di
had been cured by a thyroidectomy. A little study then sh
the patient also had a mild thyrotoxicosis, and with thyroidect
got well. Oftentimes I have been puzzled about a case until the woman
happened to mention a scintillating scotoma, or sudden fatigues, and
then in a few minutes I had the story of a lifetime of suffering from
migraine.

A businessman came with letters from internists who had been
treating him for a supposed heart disease which I could not find. Then
he happened to remark that for some time he had been unable to sign
a document or a check if anyone was watching. He would become self-
conscious and jittery, and would go to pieces nervously. Obviously,
he had a big nervous and psychic problem, and soon he confessed that
he felt himself on the edge of a bad nervous break, and his "heart
trouble" had been used only as an excuse to get into my office. Once
there, he had not had the courage to go on and tell me of his insane
mother, and his fear that he, too, was about to lose his mind.

For days I had been puzzled over a question of a common duct
stone, until the patient spoke of some "fainting spells," and soon I
had the story of a severe epilepsy equivalent. Another woman's case
had me puzzled for days until she let fall the information that she did
not dare go on the street because there she became disoriented and
panicky. Soon I had the story of a mild psychosis! Another woman,
who at first complained of a stomach-ache, finally admitted that her
real trouble was that "life had gotten too much for her": It "had just
gotten her down." Another said that her main distress was a feeling
of constant anxiety, as if there were a lot of things she should be
doing but she could not remember what they were. In another case of
a nervous woman, I was unable to decide about the nature of a loin
ache until she remarked that her worst trouble was that she had a "sick
feeling all over." I was then all the more inclined to leave her normal-
looking kidney alone, and to treat her as a tired and nervous person.
With rest and reassurance she became much better. Still another
woman's case seemed just a simple one of gallstones until she told me
that on many occasions she had refused operation because her family
had paid the surgeon to cut an artery and let her bleed to death on
the table! Evidently she was a paranoiac.

Could it be that? Many a time, after I have drawn from a patient the
story of some psychic trauma, a light has dawned and he or she has
said, "Could it be that?" Often all one has to do is to satisfy an intelligent patient that the symptoms were due to "that," and he or she
goes home to straighten out and get well.

Patients often draw on their imagination. The physician must remember that some neurotic persons have such a wonderful imagination, with such difficulty in telling truth from fancy, or such a desire to impress their doctor favorably or to tell him what they think he wants to hear, that occasionally the story he gets is either much embroidered with fancy or it is made out of whole cloth. A. D. Hart once wrote of a woman who at first denied she had any psychic problems, but later got into the spirit of things and told a weird tale of worry over the ill health of a sister. From the family Hart learned that the sister lived 3,000 miles away; that she was well, and that, the patient had not seen her for fifteen years! One of my patients, a well-educated scientist with insane ancestry, spun me a different yarn every time he came into the office. Why he went to this trouble I do not know.

I remember an unusual patient of mine, a clever writer, with a vivid personality, who was undergoing psycho-analysis. One afternoon she dropped in at my office in San Francisco, chuckling to herself, and after a while said that she had just come from a session with her psychiatrist. There, her imagination and her desire to pull the man's leg had so carried her away that she had made up a Freudian tale of sexual fantasy that "had raised his hair," and had delighted him so much that he had said he would soon publish it!

The need for the physician's noting signs of emotion. Many a time I have obtained a story of great unhappiness only because, as I talked to the woman, I saw signs of strong emotion. Perhaps her chin muscles quivered or she cried a bit or fought back the tears. Perhaps, when pressed, she said, "Yes, I am unhappy, but that is my private problem, and I do not wish to discuss it." Later she broke down and told me what had caused her neurosis.

Helpful questions a physician should often ask. One of the best questions one can ask of many persons whose story is vague is, "What actually did you come here to talk about?" Sometimes I say, "Surely you didn't travel a thousand miles to tell me about this little ache," and then, perhaps, the real story comes out. Often it is about some fear or anxiety which is wrecking nerves, yet the patient was about ready to go home without saying a word about it. Perhaps a woman, on discovering that her husband has been unfaithful, gets the idea he may have picked up syphilis and given it to her, but she is ashamed to ask for a Wassermann test. Or her husband is talking of leaving her because she is frigid, and she would like to know if anything can be done to cure that.

Occasionally, if the physician is wide awake he may suspect from something a woman says that she wants to discuss some secret worry. She sort of leads a low card, hoping that the doctor will follow suit.

Many a woman uses an unimportant symptom as a sort of calling card to get into the physician's office. She may not have known how else to get in. Sometimes a mother will bring her child, when it is really she who wants advice about some secret matter, Often, when I suspect a woman wants to talk of some sexual difficulty, I tell of some such troubles seen in practice, so as to get her to talking. It helps her to see that I can discuss such matters in a dispassionate way. Once she is sure of this, she will quickly tell her story without fear of being embarrassed or blamed or scolded.

Many a time I get the patient to talking by asking just one short question, *"Are you happy?"* This may bring out the essential history. Often I ask a married woman, "How do you and your husband get along?" If she says, "Oh, I suppose well enough," I make her tell me what is wrong, and often "it is plenty!" If only surgeons were to ask many of their patients if they are unhappy there would be thousands fewer futile operations performed each year.

Other good questions are, "Did something frighten you?" "Did someone suggest that you had a tumor or cancer; did some relative or friend die suddenly or have a coronary attack or discover a cancer?" "Have you discovered a lump somewhere?" or, "Have you spat up or passed a little blood?" Another good question is, "What do you think is causing your illness?" Sometimes this will bring out the essential fact that the physician should know. Or, one can learn much by asking the spouse, "What do *you* think is the trouble?" Many a time a husband or wife has given me the diagnosis I could not make for myself. I remember a big husky farmer whose attacks of nausea had me stumped. When I asked the wife what his trouble was she said angrily, "He knows perfectly well what the trouble is; he gets sick when he goes on a binge of chewing tobacco." The man admitted his wife was right, but he said he had hoped I would find some other cause so he could go on chewing!

Another important question in many cases is, "What were you doing when this started?", or "What terrible thing happened to you about the time this began?" Often I have obtained the essential story quickly just by looking the person in the eye and asking, "What broke your heart just before you fell ill?" Perhaps a loved one had dropped dead, or a beau had married another girl, or a partner had been caught cheating so as to draw more money each month.

On handling reticent persons. A most useful technic for dealing with reticent persons is to tell a story like the one one suspects the patient would like to tell. After this a woman may say, "Well, my husband did even worse than that," and then she will pour out her tale of sorrow and strain. Sometimes, when discussing intimate matters, it may be helpful to sit beside the patient and not on the other side of a desk. Many a nervous woman will talk more freely if she is allowed to smoke during the interview.

Oftentimes, when the physician runs up against a wall of reticence, or when he sees that his probing is causing pain, and especially if he feels he has obtained enough information to tell him what sort of problem the patient is facing, and what can be done about it, he might as well stop. A good surgeon knows when not to probe further for a bullet, and a good physician should know also when to stop probing with questions. Perhaps, later, if it seems necessary, the patient can be turned over to a good psychiatrist who can decide whether or not to go deeper into the analysis.

Oftentimes I realize that if only I had more time in which to probe and listen I could get much more information in regard to the patient's temperament and his or her strains, tragedies, or unhappinesses. If I thought this information were essential to the diagnosis or cure of the person, I might try to find time in which to get it, but often I doubt if it is essential. If it is essential to a real cure I may have to get the patient into the hands of a psychiatrist at home *for months of interviews*. When there are grave defects of personality in a patient one cannot hope to work any miracle with two or three talks.

The need for looking further sometimes even after a good diagnosis appears to have been made. Occasionally, when a physician thinks he has made a good diagnosis he hasn't yet reached the core of the matter. For instance, one day I thought I was pretty good because I had recognized the signs of alcoholism in a man who had denied any drinking. I went ahead and showed him that he had injured his liver and that he had better stop his potations. Later, I learned from his sister-in-law that I had missed the essential point which was that he had been driven to drink by his psychopathic devil of a wife.

In another instructive case the home doctor was proud because he had diagnosed a fibrillating heart. I was pleased with myself because I went further and recognized the exophthalmic goiter that had produced the fibrillation. Later, when after thyroidectomy the woman did not get well fast enough, I discovered that I had missed the first cause. Apparently the husband's infidelity had so upset the woman for years that she had become hyperthyroid!

Sometimes, toward the end of what will probably be the final interview, one of the best questions one can ask of the patient is, "Is there still something that you would like to talk about or that I haven't yet asked you about?" Perhaps, then, the real complaint will come out. Often the most important thing to do is to find what the patient fears and, then, why he fears it so much. For instance, he may be terribly afraid of cancer of the stomach because several of his relatives died of it. Or he may fear coronary heart disease because his father and two brothers dropped dead in their early fifties.

Special subjects. The subject of pain is so important that I have devoted a special chapter (Chapter 5) to the diagnosis of the several types of distress. There, I give hints for taking a history that will bring out the diagnostic points.

While learning to take better histories the young physician might study, also, the sections on diseases of the heart, digestive tract, urinary tract, pelvic organs, and other parts of the body to get help in asking those questions that will enable him to make skillful differential diagnoses.

On recognizing the person whose trouble suggests more a psychosis than a neurosis. The symptoms that make me think more of a mild psychosis than a neurosis are a senseless type of extreme worry, feelings that suggest hallucinations (Chapter 15), marked hypochondriasis, marked hysteria, alcoholism, a tendency to drug addiction, and behavior of the type seen in the cases of persons with a psychopathic personality: I refer to such things as great selfishness and unkindness to loved ones, feelings of a lack of reality or of loss of contact with people, or an inability to feel interest in or love for them, fear of killing a child, somnambulism, with a tendency to attack persons or to wreck the room, certain types of inability to concentrate or work, an unexplained nervous breakdown, schizoid symptoms of shut-inness, or paranoid symptoms of suspicion, severe claustrophobia, an inability to travel alone, poor "insight," feelings of great apprehension, much fear of going insane, or a tendency to suicide.

THE ART OF GETTING THE HISTORY OF A DEFECTIVE NERVOUS INHERITANCE

Often the most important fact that can be learned about a highly nervous person is that he or she has a poor nervous inheritance. As a routine, the assistant asks about this, and is usually told that there is no insanity in the family. Perhaps the Chief will ask again later but if he does it too bluntly, he, too, will be told that the nervous inheritance is good. Usually, if he is to get the true story, he must question with tact, skill, kindliness, and pertinacity. Most people are so reluctant to face the implications of insanity in the family that the physician must approach the topic in such a way as to produce the minimum of alarm and resentment.

I may begin by asking if members of the family were able and useful and respected and well-to-do. Then I ask if anyone was very nervous. This does not frighten, and the patient may admit that one or more

members of the family were very nervous. Often it soon becomes clear
that the curse of poor nerves came down on only one side of the family.
Then I will ask particularly about nervous illnesses in that branch of
the family. I will ask about "nervous breakdowns," and if I hear of
any, I will ask quietly what the symptoms were. I may then learn of
spells of depression when the relative would hardly talk to anyone.
Perhaps there was a visit to a sanatorium, or the relative was "not quite
right." Later I may draw out the fact that there were several nervous
breakdowns, or that the person had a few shock treatments. Helpful
is the admission that the invalid committed suicide.

In many cases I learn only that some of the relatives were irascible,
eccentric, unemployable, unsocial, too queer to marry, or perhaps unwilling to get out of bed for months at a time. Other relatives dropped
out of sight for months or years. A woman one day sent her husband
to the corner for a loaf of bread. He returned with the loaf of bread and
the change—two years later! Sometimes the patient will finally admit
that the opinion of the community was that a certain relative was "a bit
off." A schizoid woman assured me repeatedly that her nervous heredity was good until I asked specifically about her father. Then she
wept, saying that he who had been a successful lawyer, one day when
he was forty sat down, "sort of quit living," rarely spoke, and never
went to work again. His poor wife had to take boarders so as to support
the family.

Sometimes one can hear of a psychotic relative only if one asks if
anyone in the family was driven into a breakdown by the cruelty of
someone. The patient will then admit that an aunt or a sister went
insane, but he will want it clearly understood that she was *driven into it*.
Perhaps a sister became depressed for a year because her beau left her.
From other relatives one then learns that the beau left because he began
to see that she and some of her family were a bit "queer."

Occasionally one learns that the patient's father deserted the family,
or one will learn of some eccentric or ne'er-do-well relative. Others may
have been "not all there," or hard to get along with, or fond of getting
into lawsuits. Commonly, one can find that some relative was an
alcoholic and perhaps a bad dipsomaniac. As I point out in Chapter
15, the experience of hundreds of persons has taught me that to have
a drunken ancestor can be just as significant of an odd nervous heredity
as it is to have a psychotic or feeble-minded or epileptic ancestor.

The doctor must be tactful, again, if he is to get the story of relatives
with a convulsive disorder. He must never mention the word "epilepsy"
but must ask about persons who fainted easily or had violent tempers,
or were hard to get along with, or who had curious short dreamy or

forgetful spells, or who walked in their sleep, or who in childhood had convulsions when feverish.

The physician should suspect something wrong when several members of a family failed ever to get married. I remember an odd-looking woman who told me that no one of her seven sibs had ever married. Some appeared to be schizoid, others homosexual, and others just uninterested in sex, or too "difficult" to live with. The physician should ask, also, about stutterers, or persons who wet the bed late, or children who, after several attempts, could not get through grade school.

On explaining to a man why he should know about his family history. Sometimes, when dealing with an intelligent patient, the physician can get the information he wants only by explaining why he needs it. The patient can be told that some day he or his children may be helped to understand some curious disease they have by knowing that there are certain trends toward nervous disease in the family. Such information may help not only in making a diagnosis but in making the prognosis. Thus, if there is no insanity in the family, a nervous breakdown is not likely to be so serious or lasting as it might be if several of the forebears had been melancholiacs. The patient may have to be assured, also, that the fact that he has a "screwy" grandfather does not mean that he or his children have to go insane. They may be untouched by the heredity, granting that the disease of the grandfather was inheritable.

Furthermore, if there is insanity in the family, the patient's children should know it so that some day they can avoid marrying into families with a similar tendency. Perhaps, by explaining the matter in this way, the physician can enlist the interest not only of the patient but of some of his older relatives. Perhaps the old mother will then tell a remarkable story of a family curse. She may take from the family closet skeletons that the patient had never heard of.

The patient often does not know enough about his family. Oftentimes, the story can be obtained only from the spouse, parents, friends, or the old family physician. I remember once being asked to see a girl who was not developing mentally. Noting that the mother was odd, I asked about her family. She said that hers was the grandest family imaginable. Her father was an eminent lawyer, her older sister was a distinguished educator, and her many brothers were all big handsome, able men. Later, she admitted that one of the brothers was a dipsomaniac. Then I sent for the older sister and learned that, as I had suspected, the mother of the defective child had been acting at times in a psychotic way. I learned, also that on a ranch in the Ozarks their father's brother, an old bum, lived with a caretaker who supplied him with his two quarts of whiskey a day. He was the signpost pointing to a bad streak of heredity in an otherwise fine family.

The statement on the history sheet, "No family history of insanity" means little. To show how little the statement on the history sheet usually means when it says, "No family history of epilepsy or insanity" I here append some samples of family histories obtained after a good assistant had been assured that nothing was wrong. This failure to get the story is not necessarily a reflection on the assistant's zeal or skill. His Chief, with years of experience behind him, may also fail to get it. He is more likely to get it if only because he will go after it for a special reason. The assistant was just filling a space on the history sheet. The older man, after having noted signs of psychopathy or equivalents of psychopathy wanted so particularly to know about the patient's antecedents that he could not be turned away easily with a denial. Even he may have obtained the story only after several interviews, or a year or so later when the patient had become more trustful and friendly.

Following are a few histories that were obtained after the intern had written, "No insanity or epilepsy in the family."

A rather odd woman, who at first was hostile to the idea that she had a poor nervous heredity, later told me that her father was a drunkard with a terrible temper, "the meanest man I ever knew." He once shot and killed a man because of unjustified jealousy, and was let off by a jury because "everyone in town knew he was crazy." This man's father was also a violent person, and his brother, the patient's great-uncle, was often arrested for beating his wife. As one would have expected, my patient's mother led a terrible life. She attempted suicide during her last pregnancy, and was depressed again during the menopause. She also had a poor nervous heredity as shown by the facts that her father was a hard drinker, one of her sisters was a morphine addict, a brother was a drunken vagrant, and a sister drank a quart of whiskey a day. This sister once attempted suicide and was finally murdered by her husband! The patient had three sisters, one of whom is a microcephalic idiot. The woman said that this was only part of the family story of alcoholism and degeneracy; she could have told me more if she had put her mind to it! She later wrote me a twenty-page letter from which any psychiatrist would, I am sure, have diagnosed some form of psychosis. It was not the writing of a sane person. A sad feature of this case was that many surgeons, not recognizing the woman's psychopathic makeup, had performed several futile abdominal operations.

Another woman, a migrainous regurgitator, who told my assistant that she had a perfectly good family, later admitted that her father's people were nearly all notorious souses. Her great-grandfather drank himself to death; her father drank terribly all his life and ended his days in an insane asylum. Three of his brothers were souses, as were two of his half-brothers and several of his nieces and nephews!

An odd solitary "character," a man with severe headaches, at the first interview would admit only that his father was a queer miser. On returning a few years later the patient was more friendly. He then told me that his father died insane as had his mother's sister and her son. One of his brothers was "a bit off," another brother "cracked up nervously" and another was "off his head part of the time." The patient finally admitted that he realized that he himself had a manic-depressive personality. His daughter was like him in being at times abnormally worrisome and moody. This patient eventually built himself a house on a lonely little island and became a hermit.

Another man, when first seen, would say but little about his family history. I told him I felt that with his troubles he should have a poor nervous heredity, but he would not talk. A few years later he made a special trip in order to tell me that since I had seen him a sister and a nephew had gone violently insane, and the patient's mother had gone into a depression and had shot herself. The father was unstable and a heavy drinker.

As Goddard said, "Oftentimes a second, a third, a fifth, or a sixth visit has been necessary in order to develop an acquaintance and relationship with these (degenerate) families which induced them gradually to relate things which they otherwise had not recalled or did not care to tell. Many an important item has been gathered (only) after several visits to these homes."

Some persons hide a bad nervous heredity to their own detriment. Somewhat amusing was the case of a queer-looking woman with a convulsive disorder who, years ago, came with a letter from a neurologist saying that he favored surgical exploration of the brain partly because there was no history of any convulsive disorder in the family. This was before the days of electroencephalography. Because I thought the woman looked like a mentally degenerated epileptic, I started asking about the family history and I kept doing this in spite of her repeated and indignant denials. Finally the husband said, "Don't you think you should tell him at least about your screwy Uncle Bill, who has those funny dumb spells, when he lies down wherever he is and won't talk to anyone?" She countered angrily with the remark that his Aunt Lizzie was nothing to brag about, and soon a violent family row was on. In the course of the exchange of personalities and insults I heard of five of her relatives who were suffering from what sounded like equivalents of epilepsy!

On learning about the early home life. It is often helpful to ask if, during the patient's childhood, the atmosphere of the home was pleasant or unpleasant. The answer can tell much about the parents. Was the home a comfortable one? Was there always enough money and food? Did the parents get along well together or were they always fighting, and did they eventually separate? Were the parents calm, cheerful, kindly, affectionate, tolerant, and indulgent people or were they morose, domineering, strict, overly religious, or too inclined to punish? Did they neglect the children? Did they have friends in often or did they keep people out of the home? The schizophrenic is not inclined to invite people to his house.

SYMPTOMS THAT SUGGEST A PSYCHOSIS

The general practitioner or the internist is not likely ever to take the searching type of history that a psychiatrist would take. In many cases it would be well if he did know how to take it, and it would be helpful if he would take at least some of it: enough so that he could recognize right off that he was dealing with an unstable or definitely psychotic person. It is unfortunate that only a very few physicians in the land can quickly appraise a patient's sanity or insanity.

The non-psychiatrist usually trusts to his ability to size up the patient in the office. He can probably recognize quickly the nervous, fussy, demanding, time-wasting, and overly apprehensive person, such as is described in Chapter 14, but usually he fails to recognize the early signs and symptoms of a psychosis, partly because he does not know them, or think of them, and partly because, in the office, the psychotic patient is on his good behavior. Thus, I remember a man who, in my office, was friendly, pleasant, intelligent, and well behaved. The only signs that gave him away were his restlessness, the rapid flow of his ideas, and his wise-cracking. He was evidently on the edge of mania, and I soon learned from his father that he had had several wild escapades. On the way out through the waiting room, the fellow suddenly became excited and created a scene; then he offered to beat up the doorman, and later, after a few drinks, he had a grand fight with three policemen. That evening, at the city jail I found him, again pleasant and friendly, and with such a good insight into his problem that he readily promised me that next day he would enter a sanatorium for a period of treatment. This he did, and in six months he was well enough to be discharged.

The physician who wants a good history must spend time, and he must be willing to listen. He must show no sign of hurry. Perhaps the worst offense of the would-be psychiatrist is to do all the talking. The next serious offense is to start right in telling the patient what he is thinking, and why.

Efforts to recognize quickly the psychopathic or the dull person.
During World War II, much effort was made to screen quickly the
psychopaths among the drafted men. Often the psychiatrist had only
a few minutes in which to make his decision, and, naturally then, he
had to depend on rough tests. For instance, in estimating intelligence
he had to depend partly on how far the man had gone in school, and
partly on what type of occupation he followed. A man's I.Q. has much
to do with determining his level in the world of labor. Thus, a
plasterer has a higher I.Q. than has his hod-carrier, a tool-maker has a
higher I.Q. than an ordinary factory mechanic; and a certified public
accountant has a higher I.Q. than an ordinary bookkeeper.

Several questionnaires that can be marked easily by "Yes" and "No"
have been devised for the "screening" of large groups of men.

The Canadian test. In the Canadian Army they used a brief ques-
tionnaire including such questions as (1) Do you think you're in good
health? (2) If you're not well, what is wrong with you? (3) Do you
often take medicine? (4) Have you stomach trouble? (5) Have you
dizzy spells? (6) Have you fainted more than twice in your life? (7)
Have you had any fits or convulsions? (8) Have you ever stuttered?
(9) Was your mother very nervous or high-strung? (10) Are any of
your brothers and sisters very nervous? (11) Do you think you are
very nervous? (12) Were you thought to be a delicate child? (13)
Have you ever wet the bed at night since you were ten years old? (14)
Have you had more than six jobs in the last two years, not counting
those which were finished? (15) Do you get up often at night to pass
water? (16) Did you ever quit a job because it seemed bad for your
health? (17) Do you get drunk oftener than once a month? (18) Do
you ever go on drinking sprees which last longer than a whole day and
night? (19) Have you ever been arrested and sentenced? (20) Would
you rather be by yourself most of the time? (21) Do you get along
well with other people? (22) Do they treat you fairly, as a rule? (23)
Do you worry about people talking about you behind your back? (24)
Have you any relatives who were ever in a mental institution or insane
asylum? (25) Were you ever a patient in a mental institution? (26)
Have you ever felt so blue that you did not go to your work as usual?
(27) Did you ever have a nervous breakdown? (28) Do you ever have
spells of sadness in which you cry?

Questions about childhood. The physician will want to find out
something about the childhood of some patients. Was there late bed-
wetting? This commonly is a sign of nervous heredity; or was there
late walking or talking (not always a bad sign); were there temper
tantrums, fever convulsions, bad nightmares, sleep-walking, or a violent
temper? All are signs of a tendency to epilepsy. Was the person as

a child nervous, high-strung, cruel, or overly destructive? Was he solitary or did he have friends? Solitariness suggests schizophrenia. Did he steal? Did he get into many fights? How did he do in school? How far did he go? Why did he stop? As a youth, did he accept discipline or was he incorrigible? Did he ever get arrested? Did he drink? Was he irresponsible, or was he reliable? Did he early get girl-crazy or did he scorn girls? If the patient is a woman, did she, as a girl, come home from school vomiting? This is a sign of migraine. Was she ever in love? To be able to love deeply is a fine sign of sanity.

The work record. One wants to know if a man likes his work or if he is unhappy about it. How does he get along with his superiors? Is he ambitious? Does he feel the work is too hard or the hours too long? Does he have to work evenings? That may be bad because so often it is the extra work at night that breaks a man down. Is he steady in his work, or is he often changing jobs?

The marriage record. If the patient is married one will want to know if he is happy and well adjusted to life with one woman. Is he full of strains and resentments? Is his sexual life satisfactory? If not, why? Has the patient become interested in someone else, and, if so, are there strong feelings of guilt over this?

If the patient is over twenty-five or thirty and is not married, why not? A failure to marry may suggest ill health, homosexualism, or a schizoid temperament. Some men and women fail to marry because of heavy financial responsibilities in their youth, or a mother-fixation; others fail because of a bad temper. Many an unmarried man will say that he was always too concerned about his health to take on the extra responsibility of a wife. A few fail to marry because of syphilis contracted early in life. They are never sure they are cured enough to marry and have children. In Chapter 15 on the relatives of the psychotic it will be noted that an abnormally high percentage were unmarried.

It is hard for an untrained physician to get a story of homosexualism, and the non-psychiatrist had better not probe into this. Often he can be fairly sure of the patient's nature just from a glance (Chapter 14).

Social adjustments and trends toward a psychosis. One will want to know about social adjustments. Does the man like to have guests in his home? The schizoid person does not bring friends home, and he may not even let his children do it. Do other people treat him right, or do they talk about him behind his back? Do they do things just to annoy him or do they try to harm him? Has he enemies? These questions reveal paranoid trends.

Questions to reveal the manic-depressive. Has the person wide swings of mood or has he blue spells lasting days or weeks or months? Did he ever have a nervous breakdown? If so, what were the symptoms, and what brought them on? How long did the spell last? Did it come suddenly and go suddenly? Was there any thought of suicide? Does a woman cry often and for no good reason? These questions may expose a manic-depressive temperament.

The early symptoms of a psychosis. One of the best things a non-psychiatric physician could do would be to pick up a book on psychiatry occasionally and look through the list of the early symptoms of the several psychoses. Especially if he is an internist with his main interest in gastroenterology, he will be surprised to see that some of *the early symptoms of a manic-depressive psychosis are the ones he is treating every day in his office.* For instance, Weiss and English said (1949), "The depressed patient feels terrible, and has countless aches, pains, and other distresses in his body. Almost always there are gastro-intestinal symptoms, such as constipation and loss of appetite, and to these may be added headache, backache, fatigue, abdominal distress, belching, and joint pains." Actually, these are the complaints of many of the patients who consult the gastroenterologist and the internist. Perhaps after reading this, a great light will break over a physician, and he will say to himself, "That Mrs. S. who keeps coming back all the time must be depressed; perhaps that is why she was so slow in getting up after her operations; I would not wonder if she has been psychotic for years, and I have never suspected it!"

Similarly, after reading what the psychiatrists write about schizoid persons, the doctor may say, "Why, I have a number of those quiet, uncooperative women in my practice; but I thought they had just anorexia nervosa or bad ovaries."

The symptoms of psychoneurotic patients. According to Fox and Schnaper in a study of psychiatric casualties (1944), the commoner complaints of a group of psychoneurotic patients were: nervousness, fatigue, nausea, vomiting, abdominal pain or discomfort, diarrhea, constipation, indigestion, pains and stiffness in the extremities, backache, twitches and tics, neck pains, headaches, palpitation, shortness of breath, chest pain, "heart pain" or a pressure, peculiar skin sensations, eye complaints, ear complaints such as buzzing and ringing, frequency of urination, loss of sexual power, pain in the penis, weakness, dizziness, frequent fainting, weight loss, excessive perspiration, poor sleep, shakiness, restlessness, excessive worry, poor appetite, poor ability to concentrate, irritability, loss of initiative, feeling dazed, crying spells, feeling disgusted, fear of insanity, hopelessness, a premonition of death, and bad nightmares. (See also Chapters 14 and 15.)

Suicide. It is well to ask neurotic patients if they ever think of suicide. Physicians fear to do this, but depressed persons do not seem to mind discussing the subject. Many say they think of it but will not do it; others say they fear doing it, and others say it would be a logical way out of their trouble, if they only had the courage.

The person in greatest danger of suicide is usually the depressed patient to whom life is an unbearable burden. He or she may be utterly miserable or weighed down with feelings of guilt and unworthiness. The following note left by a person who took his life well reveals the mental processes of these persons and shows how much they suffer.

"I'm terribly sorry to do this to you and Harry, but it's better that it happens now when you both are young and beautiful, rather than spend your youth, beauty and devotion on someone like me.

"Believe me, Honey, I'm not doing this because of anything you have done or haven't done. I love you both terribly. That's why I'm doing it.

"I've livcd with this thought for years. . . . The thoughts keep coming to me. What's the use? Why don't you commit suicide, why don't you end it all—no more worries, no working, no playing, no nothing. Just a blessed blank.

"That's what I've wanted and wanted. Now I'm going to have it.

"This way, Honey, with my life, I'm stopping the wrecking of three lives. One neurotic life for two normal, happy, beautiful ones is a cheap price to pay."

Hallucinations or delusions. Sometimes, if the physician is sympathetic, a patient will tell him of times when he saw things or heard things which seemed preternatural and uncanny, and frightened him. Or the patient will tell how his neighbor on the next farm directs radar at him and forces him to think unpleasant thoughts.

Sexual sins. It is said that if a patient appears too eager to tell of his sexual sins he may be psychotic. Persons of both sexes who are not well adjusted or are feebly inhibited, or are manic-depressive in temperament will sometimes get into difficulties because of their sexual drives and their poor choice of partners. I remember a mildly manic-depressive physician who, during each of his manic phases, ran off with some other man's wife; each time during his depressed spell, the woman left him! Neurotic women without good self-control often get mixed up with alcoholic or psychopathic men who are unsatisfactory either as husbands or lovers. Neurotic men, even when very successful in business, may get into one marital mess after another. They may have good judgment in choosing men to work with them, but they have no sense when it comes to choosing a woman. I remember one of America's ablest and wealthiest men who, for his first wife, chose a difficult, miserable, schizoid woman, and for his second, chose "a devil," with a psychopathic makeup.

Feelings of unreality. Important often is a feeling of unreality, perhaps with feelings of detachment from the world, a lack of interest in it, and a lack of love for anyone. This symptom always suggests the coming of serious trouble. Most persons of this type lose interest in the movies because they say they no longer feel any emotional response to the acting on the screen. They do not care what those people up there are doing.

Failure to concentrate or an inability to read. One of the most important symptoms complained of by many tired or mildly psychotic patients is an inability to concentrate and think. They will say, "My brain does not work as well as it used to." Or they will say, "I can't read." If they try to read their brain soon tires and they cannot take in or retain what they are reading.

These symptoms always indicate to me a brain which is either very tired from overwork or illness, or becoming disorganized by a mild psychosis. Conversely, when a nervous or tired patient can read comfortably I do not worry much about him. His brain is in good shape. Obviously, the physician will want to find out if the condition followed overwork or if it comes with fatigue, and goes quickly after a bit of rest.

On differentiating an anxiety or fatigue state and a melancholia. Often the physician needs quickly to differentiate an anxiety or a fatigue state and a true depression. The diagnosis ought to be made quickly and correctly because the patient with an anxiety state should be encouraged to keep at work; the person with a fatigue state should be given some rest, and the person with a spontaneous depression should perhaps be given a few electric shock treatments. Certainly no time or effort should be wasted on exhorting him to cheer up.

Ross felt that the following points are helpful in the diagnosis. The depressed person often slips into a spell rather suddenly with no reason that he or the family can see. Some of these patients say, "The curtain came down." Occasionally, however, a man with a familial tendency to depression will get a spell following some disappointment or tragedy, but then it is out of proportion to the amount of unhappiness, or it lasts a year or more. A woman may go into a depression after the break-up of a love affair or the birth of a child or the coming of the menopause. Oftentimes it helps much in the diagnosis to learn that the patient had two or three previous attacks of unexplained depression, with intervals of good health in between. I have often been led straight to the diagnosis by learning from the parents that when a woman was in college she had a nervous breakdown so bad that someone had to go and get her and bring her home. Another point that often helps me is that there are or are not manic-depressives in the patient's family.

The neurotic person usually has poor health most of the time; he likes to coddle himself, he likes to take medicine, and in the doctor's office he likes to tell a long tale of woe. He is likely to be wide-awake and talkative. He likes to go to doctors. The psychotic is often brought in by his relatives, and he may just sit and let his family tell most of the story. The neurotic is often quick in his reactions, while the depressed person may be slow. The neurotic also complains much about bodily aches and pains while the depressed person may say his suffering is mental, indescribable, and more than he can bear. Ross said that the neurotic person is more likely to behave emotionally, or to cry, while the depressed person often sits stolidly. The neurotic person may, at times, laugh and joke; the depressed person may smile, but he is likely to stick to his gloom. An interesting feature of the badly depressed person's trouble is that he has "hit bottom," and hence cannot feel further distress. Thus, I once had to tell a badly depressed man that I had found a cancer in his colon and would have to send him in for operation. As I expected, this did not bother him at all; without comment or concern he went and had the work done. He was like the "lifer" on a road-building gang who, one Sunday, was caught fishing without a license, with an over-the-limit catch. He wasn't worried when threatened with a week in jail!

In the office the depressed person can often discuss his problem in so intelligent and friendly a way that an assistant will never suspect that anything is mentally wrong.

Sudden changes in character. As Griesinger said, one should always note with concern sudden changes in a person's character. "The temperate man gives himself to drunkenness; the frivolous pores over the Bible; the bashful becomes impudent; the moral, obscene." It is hard to recognize these changes when they come on gradually during the course of years. One is likely, then, to miss the point that an old harmless eccentricity has turned into a serious psychosis. Often it is only a spouse or other relative of the patient who can say, "With this act he passed the bounds of sanity. In his right mind he never would have used obscene language or walked into church with his hat on— not him." That is the important point—"not him."

INVALUABLE INFORMATION OBTAINABLE FROM FAMILY AND FRIENDS

A blind spot in medical thinking. During the years in which I was gathering material for this book I read scores of articles written by psychiatrists on the technics of finding out why a patient is nervous or psychotic. I found reams on psycho-analysis, on the interpretations of dreams, and on the efforts that should be made to unearth the story of early sexual or mental traumas and unhappinesses and resentments. What surprised me was that rarely did I find a word to show that often in a few minutes a doctor can gather more information, more reliable information, and actually all he needs to know, by talking to the patient's relatives and business associates. He may not have been able to get a bit of this from the patient.

Information obtainable from relatives and friends. Many a time, a few minutes' conversation with a relative, business partner, or neighbor has given me more important facts about a patient's psychopathic makeup, sudden change in character, abnormal behavior, sins, life tragedies, little strokes, or bad nervous inheritance than I had obtained in hours of questioning of the invalid himself.

For instance, hours of questioning of a lovely young woman with a severe digestive neurosis, unrelieved by four operations, got me nowhere. Five minutes with her chum, and I learned that the trouble all started when she was cruelly cheated out of her savings and then jilted in a most humiliating way by a man who, she later learned, made his living out of this sort of thing.

Ross used to say that the physician who expects to get the story of sins and follies, sexual escapades, or alcoholism should try to get it *at the first interview,* because after that the patient may have come to like him too much to be willing to demean himself or herself in his eyes.

I have known women, who, in spite of all my efforts to overcome their reserve, would not tell me the story of the tragic engagement, the illegitimate pregnancy, or the marriage to a scoundrel which, in a few days or months, had changed a happy girl into a chronic invalid. Sometimes I got the story from a relative, and then, of course, I had to respect the confidence. Sometimes, later, with the information in my possession, I was able to draw out the story from the patient.

The patient may not know what is happening to him. There are many cases of beginning psychosis or brain disease in which the patient appears to have no idea that he is changing in health and character and behavior. He may blame all of his difficulties on others. For instance, a brilliant internist who had always been eccentric, gradually became more so; formerly good natured, he became irascible and unreasonable and picked on his assistants until several left him. He blamed them for the estrangement, and accused them of having willfully changed in their demeanor toward him. About a year later he began to do such queer things that he had to be committed.

A minister of the Gospel was brought for examination by his senior deacon. The minister said he was perfectly well, but seeing that the members of the board of deacons were his employers, he had to humor them. When I asked the deacon what the trouble was he said the minister had taken to coming late to church without showing any sign of concern or contrition, and that he had made ritualistic mistakes in a baptismal ceremony! The first physician consulted did not think

tle things deserved notice, but he was wrong, and the deacon was
No normal minister would have done what this man had done,
ana a little examination showed that a tumor had started to grow in
his brain.

On getting important help from a fellow patient. Curiously,
many a time I have learned most of what I needed to know about a
nervous or mildly psychotic person from another patient who, for a
few days, had been sitting alongside him or her in the waiting room.
Sometimes I have been given the secret and essential story, or I have
learned that the patient was terribly fretty and fussy and hot-tempered,
or that he was drinking or gambling, or worrying terribly about a wayward son.

The neurotic person may blame others for his misfortunes.
It is hard to get a correct story out of some persons because they blame
others for their misfortunes. According to them, if only someone had
treated them with more consideration or understanding, things would
have gone all right. Such a person is likely to forget the other side of
the story, granting that he was ever able to see it. A person with a
psychopathic personality may tell a long story of a lack of consideration and love for him shown by members of his family, forgetting that
his many escapades, together with the family's attempts at rehabilitating him and keeping him out of jail, have cost them many thousands
of dollars. In such a case I would much rather listen to the family's
story than to the patient's.

Getting help in deciding which of two stories is correct. Sometimes I have had to go to the patient's business associates or friends
to find out which of two divergent stories given me, let us say, by husband and wife, was correct. To illustrate: An attorney with an odd personality came several times, complaining of abdominal pain, fatigue,
and insomnia. He told a story of great unhappiness and strain at home
with a wife who, he said, did little to conceal her many infidelities. He
said she neglected him, the children, and the home; she nagged, and
she was a terrible problem to him. The only observation that told me
there was something mentally wrong with the man was that he never
remained in Rochester to get his final summing-up and opinion; he
would always go home before he was dismissed.

When I got the wife off by herself I was favorably impressed by her,
and she seemed like a fine woman. She told an astounding tale of a
harrowing life with a cruel and dangerous paranoiac. He beat the children and threatened her with death if she ever told on him or tried
to leave him. She had talked to several lawyers about getting a divorce
or having him committed, but the man was so vindictive and dangerous
that no attorney or judge in his city cared to tangle with him. As I

expected, further investigation showed that the wife's description of the situation was the correct one.

A nice-looking woman, with multiple complaints, for a few days had me sympathizing with her as she told me of her husband's alcoholism and how it had wrecked her nerves and her life. Fortunately, soon afterward, I began to sense that she had a nasty and psychopathic side to her; she said bitter and mean things about fine physicians who, from their letters to me, had obviously tried hard to help her. Then, one day, she turned savagely on me when, as friendly as I could, I suggested that she attempt a little self-discipline. Later, her mother and sister told me of her psychopathic personality with all its cruel selfishness. They told me that the husband was a fine, kindly man who, after marriage, had let the woman run rapidly through his good-sized fortune. She lived most of the time at expensive private sanatoria, and got herself operated on again and again. In return for his impoverishment, he got nothing but abuse. Finally, he took to drink, but, as his mother-in-law said, "Poor fellow, if he can get any comfort and forgetfulness from his whiskey, I am all for it!" Obviously, no one could ever have obtained this story from the psychopathic patient. Later, I got a nasty letter of abuse from her, because I had not found any sign of organic disease. Still later, I heard that a physician had been so taken in by her story that he had induced her to sue the husband for divorce under the plea of extreme cruelty! Finally I heard that she had had to be committed.

On learning what the main characteristics of the patient are. Often one can learn best from the family if the patient is energetic, aggressive, self-confident, sociable, and affectionate; or withdrawn, passive, submissive, easily offended, shy, shut-in, a day-dreamer, a person hard to approach or to talk to about important matters; or eager for sympathy, or always demanding love or reassurance; or expressing feelings of inferiority, sinfulness, or inadequacy. One can learn if the man is frank or evasive, suspicious, overly envious or jealous, rigid, stubborn and obstinate, or easily amenable to reason.

One can learn if, when he offends, he ever apologizes or admits that he was in the wrong; if he is impulsive, violent, or poorly inhibited; if he has quick bursts of temper or if he is good-natured; if he is quarrelsome or easy-going; or if he is always anxious and worrisome, fearful and timid, and, if so, what he worries most about.

One can learn if he is a perfectionist, overly neat, orderly, and meticulous; if he carries responsibility well or is irresponsible; if he slides out of jobs and side-steps decisions; if he is phlegmatic and placid; if he long holds resentments or if he forgives quickly; if he is generous or niggardly, close, or selfish. One can learn if he respects authority and willingly complies with regulations or if he is rebellious at any "infringement of his rights" and is overly critical of others; if he is stoical or often complaining about little discomforts and panicky about little illnesses. One can find out if he mixes easily with people or is aloof or unusually resentful of criticism or attempts on the part of his superiors to teach him new ways. One can discover if he is tactful and politic in his dealings, if he gets along well with those who work with him, and if he has many friends.

If the patient is a woman it will be helpful to learn of marked premenstrual tension with signs of nervous instability, loss of emotional control, or depression. If the menopause has come it will be helpful to know what nervous or psychotic symptoms, if any, have appeared. Often, as I have already pointed out, only the relatives will tell the doctor how well or how poorly a patient is aging. Sudden changes are most important to know about. Perhaps the person has failed much, and rather suddenly become old. Perhaps a man has lost his old interests in his work, his friends, and his children.

WHAT CAN BE LEARNED FROM GOING INTO THE PATIENT'S HOME

Often in the office, when a patient hasn't been able to tell me what is tiring her out, making her nervous, or bringing frequent migraines, I will say that if only for a few hours or a day or two, I could visit her in her home or work beside her in her office, I could tell her what her hurtful sins and follies are. Actually, in several cases, I did later visit the woman in her home, and there in a few minutes I did learn all that I needed to know to explain her troubles. There, perhaps, was a husband who, although a good provider with many good points, was not at all suited to her. Perhaps he was too old and serious, or too silent, or dour, or moody, while she was gay and full of fun. Perhaps he came from the wrong side of the tracks and used poor English, while she was college bred; perhaps he was crude and unable to share in her refinement and intellectual life.

Often a brainy woman who in college was either so sickly or so intelligent or studious or "highbrow" as to be unattractive to men of her own age, in her thirties marries a man whose main asset is his ability to give her a good home. He is no answer to a maiden's prayer but, then, she never "dated" much and so cannot be choosy. Perhaps he swaps his wealth for her social position. Later, she can hardly stand him, and then if children have come and she cannot bring herself to demand a divorce, neuroses are likely to appear.

In rare cases, on going into the woman's home, I found that the husband was handicapped in some way, as by deafness, clubfeet, a frail twisted body or a large fat one, and this distressed and embarrassed the wife. In one case it turned out that in his youth the man had been a prize-fighter. Although he was a likable "good scout," his wife had become very resentful of his smashed nose and his cauliflower ears. In other cases I could see at a glance that the husband was an alcoholic, or a gay dog whom the wife could not trust to leave at home with her maid. In other cases he was so boisterous and fond of "kidding" that he embarrassed her and made her nervous. Or he was such a hard-driving sales manager type of man that he was too much of a dynamo for her: He made her tense the minute he came into the house. Perhaps he was too fond of having always a houseful of guests. Or he was so critical of what she said or did that she was afraid of him, and I caught her frequently shooting a look of inquiry to see if by any chance she had offended.

In some cases it was obvious that in spite of the fact that husband and wife used terms of endearment there was no love between them, but rather smoldering hostility. Or the wife was watching the man with great jealousy whenever he spoke to a woman guest or touched her arm. Or there was a good deal of bantering which was so pointed and bitter as to make the people in the room uncomfortable. Perhaps the two were telling unpleasant stories about each other and appealing for sympathy to those present.

In some homes I found an unwise mother-in-law, demanding that her son show her more attention than he paid to his wife, or I found a senile father who, with his constant demands for quiet, was interfering with the lives of the children and everyone in the house. In other homes I found a problem-child whom the wife was constantly protecting from the censure of the disgusted father.

In several instances, as soon as my patient served a meal, it was obvious that she was much too worried over having everything go just right, and much too upset over every little thing that went wrong with the service. Evidently, she was a fuss-budget and a perfectionist who kept wearing herself out trying to make the world run exactly as she would have it run. Or, perhaps she was a poor housekeeper, and it was the husband who was the fault-finding perfectionist.

Langdon-Browne once wrote of a physician who was puzzled about the cause of a distressing neurosis presented by a young woman. She could not tell him of any strain, but one day he called on her and found her apartment filled with pictures of a handsome, mannish looking woman. When told what was the matter with her the girl first flared in anger, but later calmed down and admitted that the physician was perfectly right. As so often happens in such cases, this homosexual girl with a tremendous "crush" was being torn to pieces by jealousy and the fear that her love affair would any day break up.

If a physician could only go into a nervous man's office or store and watch him at work for a day he might see all sorts of neurosis-producing and fatigue-producing factors at work. He might see stupid conflicts with others, needless bawlings-out of employees, needless tantrums of temper, needless refusals to delegate authority, needless making of work, silly fretting or fussing or delaying in the making of decisions, or foolish reopening of questions already settled. The doctor might note overconscientiousness, or signs of a great dislike of the work being done, or dislike or fear of the boss.

I have watched even physicians and surgeons who were more than doubling the strain of the day's work by snapping at patients and secretaries and nurses and assistants. In the operating room they went into such tantrums that they soon had everyone about them upset and angry. It was perfectly obvious why they were having trouble with their nerves.

The old family physician has such an advantage over the city consultant because he knows the family and perhaps even three generations of them. He knows the family skeletons; he knows what goes on in homes and offices; he knows about unfortunate engagements, annulled marriages, heart-breaking children, unwise business enterprises, gambling and drinking and sexual escapades, and all sorts of worries and strains and dissatisfactions.

CHAPTER 5

Hints for Determining
the Causes of Pain

HAS THE PATIENT REAL PAIN? Often the first thing the physician must do is to make sure that what the patient is talking about is pain. An assistant may have put down that the man has *pain* but a few questions will show that what bothers him is a burning, or a vague "misery," or a feeling of distress. In the cases of women it is often a quivering, or throbbing, or "a feeling of something in there," or a mild constant ache. These milder distresses usually point to a functional trouble while real pain points often to organic disease. Sometimes a patient will say, "If I only knew what it was and that it would not turn into anything, I'd forget it."

How severe is the pain or ache? It is important often to find out how severe a distress or pain is, and hence how needful it is to do something strenuous to relieve it. Sometimes the question of exploring the abdomen turns on how desperate the patient is to get relief so that he can sleep and rest again.

Much can be learned about a patient and his pain by noting how he tells his story. From this alone an experienced physician may gain the impression that the man has real pain and that he has been suffering a great deal, or he may sense that the fellow is primarily a neurotic complainer. Often I want to know how sensitive to pain the man is, and so I ask him how he stands the dentist's drill. I will lift up a fold of skin and pinch it to see if he flinches or cries out. I will notice particularly how he behaves when he has a sigmoidoscope or a stomach tube passed. That will tell me how stoical and well controlled he is or how likely to make a great fuss over a little discomfort.

One can get an idea of the severity of a pain by learning if the person can work with it or sleep with it. A mild ache is forgotten during the day when the person is busy, and it gets bad as soon as he goes to bed and turns out the light. It helps to find out what relieves a pain. Will an aspirin tablet do it? If so, the pain is not bad. Will a drink of whiskey relieve? If so, again, the pain is not bad, and is probably due to nervous tension.

According to Susselman, Feldman, and Barrera (1946) and Ripley and Wolff (1947), sodium amytal, given intravenously in a dose of 0.10 gm., will often relieve pain and other symptoms, *if they are due purely to tension*. The significant point is that the dose is too small to give relief through any analgesic effect.

With a supposed severe abdominal pain I want to know if it has caused the person to lose much weight. Several times in the last forty years I have been deceived by persons who complained bitterly of abdominal pain. The fact that they had remained stout should have warned me not to let them be operated on. Actually, on opening the abdomen, the surgeon found nothing.

The severity of a pain can be estimated, also, from the amount of fear the patient has of it. For instance, a stout woman who has been having gallstone colics may so fear them that she will go without the rich foods that she craves, or a woman with tic douloureux will refuse to eat because chewing brings the spasms of unbearable pain.

It is very helpful to find out if morphine ever had to be used, and how it worked. If morphine had to be used for an abdominal pain it means that this was due probably either to gallstones, a ureteral stone, or a posteriorly perforating ulcer. The man with a cancer of the pancreas may need morphine after a while. Persons with acute appendicitis, acute pancreatitis, intestinal obstruction, or a rupturing aneurism need morphine but they usually present an acute problem that must soon be solved; they are not so likely to have a chronic pain.

Pain due to an embolus in an artery comes suddenly and is almost unbearable. The pain of angina pectoris may be unbearable. Facial pain due to an ulcerated pulp in a tooth may come in unbearable spasms especially when warm food or drink enters the mouth. The syndrome can resemble that of tic douloureux. Pain due to intestinal obstruction can be very severe, but it tends to come in waves like labor pains, and each spasm may end with a gurgle. The pain of pleurisy or a beginning pneumonia, or an acute lumbago, or an acute pleurodynia, or a slipped intervertebral disc may be very severe, and may make it impossible for the patient to lie down.

An estimate of the severity of the pain can be made sometimes by asking the patient if it is so bad that he will cheerfully accept an operation. If he says, "Yes, I don't care what you do so long as you give me some relief," he probably has a serious lesion like a cancer of the pancreas.

Another way in which to learn about the severity of a pain is to talk to the close relatives. I remember cases in which a daughter said, "Yes, mother has been complaining of pain and crying 'Wolf' all her life, but this time I think she is suffering acutely. This is different." Still another way in which to get the needed information is to put the patient in a hospital and ask the nurses to estimate the degree of pain. They will often give the correct answer. They can soon recognize the shammer, the whiner, the seeker after sympathy, or the woman who quiets down beautifully after an injection of pure water.

The nurses will recognize, also, the man with great pain who gets into peculiar positions in an effort to get relief. The sweat may roll off him and he may moan. With the severest pain he will be almost unable to talk. Persons with a bad stomach-ache usually walk bent over a bit like a patient just out of the hospital after an abdominal operation. The person with severe migrainous pain is utterly miserable, like a person who is seasick; the old woman with tic douloureux may have her head done up in a shawl to keep away drafts.

Pain that comes during sleep or out of a clear sky when the patient is happily occupied is likely to be organic in nature. The physician must be especially slow to diagnose a functional type of pain if the person is not neurotic in appearance or behavior, or if he has no unusual strain, or if he is past middle age and has recently begun to suffer. Neurosis is not so likely to come in later life as is organic disease. Any abdominal pain which suddenly strikes down a person past the age of forty must be viewed with alarm; it should not be ascribed to a newly developed "mucous colitis" or food allergy. Those are diseases of youth. As I wrote this, I saw a physician of sixty years who for a few months had been much distressed by an abdominal pain. He had always been well before. He so hoped it was due to "mucous colitis," but I said it couldn't be. Exploration of the abdomen showed the pancreatic carcinoma that we had both feared.

In puzzling cases it is often helpful to estimate the blood sedimentation rate; if that is high, and if there is no sign of arthritis, one had better search the body carefully from head to foot. The leucocyte count may also go up after an attack of pain, but a little rise can be due purely to the distress. The serum bilirubin may go up a little after a gallstone colic or in the presence of a carcinoma of the pancreas. Once I saw this slight bilirubinemia as the first sign of a pancreatic cancer. The blood sedimentation rate usually goes up after a coronary thrombosis, and this can help in the diagnosis. In all doubtful cases in which carcinomatosis is suspected one should check the liver function. Some dye retention often means that the liver is full of metastasis.

Is there soreness after a spell of pain? Pain due to some local inflammation should be associated with or followed by soreness and tenderness of the tissues. For instance, a man with an acute inflammation of an antrum should have soreness and tenderness of the cheek. A man who has just had an acute attack of cholecystitis should have soreness in the right upper quadrant of the abdomen, and the man with an acute duodenal ulcer usually has some soreness in his epigastrium. Such soreness is likely to be made worse by jolting, as in a tractor. Many a farmer, when his ulcer is active, is unable to ride over a plowed field. A woman with inflamed fallopian tubes may hate to step jarringly off a sidewalk.

Is the pain superficial or deep? Often it helps greatly to ask and find out if the patient knows that his pain is out in his abdominal wall; it helps, also, to know if he feels it deeply in. As I point out in Chapter 18, many so-called abdominal pains are superficial and due to fibrositis out in the abdominal wall. Under such circumstances, an operation is not needed. All one may have to do to make the diagnosis is to grasp a fold of skin and fat, lift it up and pinch it. Normal persons do not object to this, but others, with hyperesthetic tissues, may cry out with pain.

How long has the pain been present? Naturally, it is very helpful to find out that the person has had the same pain for twenty years or more. This immediately rules out diseases such as cancer or intestinal obstruction. Especially when a long-lasting distress is an ache which has been present day and night for years, one can be pretty certain that it is of central origin; it comes from up in the brain. See also the discussion of the mild thalamic syndrome in Chapter 12.

Has the pain always been the same? Often it helps to find out if the pain or ache has always been about the same. Occasionally, as in cases of duodenal ulcer, it will be found that the syndrome was typical and hence more easily recognizable in the first attacks which came years before. Later, complications came to obscure the picture. The ulcer may have perforated a bit and involved nerves which caused the pain to shift in its localization. Perhaps, also, in the early spells the pain was easily relieved by the taking of food, while in later years, after perforation took place or the pylorus contracted, food and alkalies no longer gave good relief.

How did the pain first come? Often one can learn much about a pain by finding out what the patient was doing the day it came. Perhaps he was under great strain, as when a loved one died, or he jumped from a height and hurt his spine, or he lifted something heavy and felt something tear in his spine or in his inguinal region. Oftentimes the person says that the pain came on so gradually that he cannot remember how or when it started, but in other cases he can date it from a certain hour of a certain day. That always helps. Perhaps it started with an attack of retching and diarrhea after eating food that made other people ill. In other words, he got infected with some dysentery organism. Perhaps he had a bad cold, or he received a blow in the stomach. It is very helpful to find that the first pain came under conditions which would favor an attack of hysteria. Perhaps it started with a severe sick headache, or an epilepsy-like attack, or an auto accident.

Especially when the first attack looked like one of appendicitis or gallstones, it is well to ask the patient what the physician said when he was called. Did he want to operate? If a surgeon saw the patient and said there was no sign of appendicitis or gallstones that is an important point. Did the doctor give morphine and did this stop the pain? Was the urine examined and was a leucocyte count made, and if so, what was the report? Was there fever? If an exploratory operation was performed, what did it show?

The exact location of the pain and the way it moves. One of the most important things a physician can do in the presence of pain is not to accept the patient's statement that it is in his *"stomach."* By this he may mean abdomen. The doctor should make the man strip and then show with his hand where the pain comes and how it radiates. I remember a man who lost his life because he told an internist's assistant that he had a pain in his "stomach." Actually, he meant his pelvis. The assistant sent him for a roentgenologic study of the stomach and when the report came back, "duodenal ulcer," the man was sent for futile Sippy treatments. The cancer in his rectum was not found until it was too late.

Once I was asked to give a clinic on peptic ulcer, and the assistant professor in charge of the meeting brought in for me an old Serbian laborer who walked with a cane. I asked him to pull up his shirt, drop his trousers and show the doctors with his hand just where the pain was in his "stomach." He ran his hands down the courses of his first lumbar nerves to the suprapubic region, indicating typical root pain! Turning to his films I found a tremendous deformity of his first two lumbar vertebrae due to arthritis. It was a wonder that the nerves emerging from the region were not entirely destroyed. At the time, the man had no symptoms of ulcer, and a little questioning showed that the deformity of the duodenum had been produced twenty years before!

One reason for noting exactly where the pain comes is that pain originating in the stomach, gallbladder, or pancreas is not likely to be felt below the navel, and pain originating in the colon or pelvic organs is not likely to be felt above the navel. Many a woman has long been treated futilely for ulcer when the location of her pain in the lower half of the abdomen should have told her physician that the trouble was probably in a sore colon or in the pelvic organs.

Pain arising in the small bowel is usually felt around the navel. Pain arising in the jejunum, as after the formation of a jejunal ulcer, is commonly felt to the left and a little below the navel. Because of a peculiar distribution of sensory nerves in some individuals, pains arising in the gallbladder will occasionally be felt in the left upper quadrant of the abdomen. Occasionally, also, pain due to an obstructing carcinoma in the descending colon will be felt in the cecum because of the back-pressure of gas into this weak-walled part of the gut. In the case of a gastric ulcer a sudden shifting of pain may be due to the penetration of the lesion into the peritoneal coat where it involves another set of nerves with a different area of reference in the skin.

Pains that arise in lesions around the cardia are generally felt in the epigastrium or in the middle back or in the thorax. Naturally, pains which arise in the pelvic organs, the bladder, the prostate gland, or the posterior urethra are likely to be felt in the pelvis or just above the pubis. Pains originating in the kidney or ureter are likely to begin in the flank and to run down toward the bladder, the penis, or the testicle. Pain arising in the pancreas is likely to be felt in the upper half of the abdomen, in the middle back, or in the lower part of the thorax. Depending on whether the tumor is in the head or the tail of the pancreas the pain may be more on the right or on the left. In rare cases it will be felt a little below the navel.

In acute appendicitis, as is well known, the pain should first be in the small bowel area just below the navel. Later, as the inflammation involves the peritoneal coat of the cecum, it affects spinal nerves, and this causes the pain to shift to the right lower quadrant of the abdomen. Occasionally, when the colon is filled with gas, it rises in the abdomen and pushes up against the parietal peritoneum so as to cause pain in the epigastrium. Such pain may be relieved in a moment if the patient will only hang over the side of the bed or will get into the knee-shoulder position.

It is very helpful often to see if a pain follows the distribution of some nerve or nerves or some segment. If it does not, it is not likely to be helped by the injection with procaine of any nerve or nerves.

Sometimes because of the bizarre and nonanatomic nature of the distribution of a pain one can tell that it must be of hysterical origin.

Pain in the groin which comes on standing may be due to a knuckle of bowel boring into the inner inguinal ring. Pain due to a diaphragmatic hernia may resemble that of angina pectoris or gallstones. It is likely to be worse when the person lies down soon after eating.

Does the pain shift about? It helps greatly to learn if the pain is always in the same place, because it then is more likely to be originating in an organic lesion in a certain spot. If it shifts around, and especially if it shifts out of the abdomen into the thorax or down the outer side of the thigh, it is much more likely to be produced in the spine or in the brain.

A shift in the location of a pain may tell much. For instance, after a gastroenterostomy for duodenal ulcer a shift of the pain to a point to the left of the navel and a bit below it nearly always means the coming of a new ulcer, now in the jejunum. The point of reference on the abdominal wall is lower for the jejunum than for the duodenum. Other shifts in pain may be due to a penetration of an ulcer into the pancreas, or to involvement of the peritoneum, as by an ulcer or a carcinoma. Pain coming at the tip of the shoulder means involvement of the diaphragm. Rigidity of the abdominal wall, in the case of a carcinoma of the stomach, is a bad sign, as it means involvement of the peritoneum. With a posterior penetrating ulcer the pain can be very severe, but the patient will show a soft abdomen because the peritoneum is not involved.

Is the pain constant or does it come in spells? Most pains of local organic origin tend to come in spells. Every physician knows that a pain due to gallstones is likely to come at intervals of months or years. The pain of peptic ulcer may be present for a month or two and then go away for six months or a year or two. Pain that is due to fibrositis in the thoracic or abdominal wall is likely to come and go.

The significance of the length of the attacks and the interval between them. Something can be learned by finding out how long the attacks last and how long the interval is between them. The rhythm of gallstone attacks is different from that of ulcer attacks or of gastric crises or migraines.

When gallstone colic comes it lasts usually only a few hours: An attack of ulcer pain may last for days or weeks, and a migrainous woman may vomit during much of a day, or even for two days. The pain of angina pectoris usually lasts only a few minutes until the person rests, while the pain of fibrositis in the chest wall may last for days. Pain in the liver, due to hepatitis, may last for months.

Characteristic in some states is the tendency of ulcer pain to come twice a year, in the spring and the fall. One can see why this sequence should be met with in the case of farmers who have the strain of sowing and reaping, but it is hard to explain it in the case of white-collar workers who have no extra strain in April and September.

How the pain comes on a typical day. Oftentimes it helps to ask a patient to describe a typical day, telling just when the pain comes and goes. Often an abdominal pain appears to be due mainly to a certain rhythm in the activity of the digestive tract; it may come just the same and at the same time even when no food is eaten.

Radiation of a pain. As everyone knows, some pains spread in certain directions. For instance, the pain of gallstone colic goes to the right scapula, kidney pain goes down to the penis or testicle or groin, and the pain of angina pectoris goes into the left arm or up into the mandible on one or both sides. The pain of a slipped disc often goes down one sciatic nerve.

The characteristics of a pain. Unfortunately, we physicians do not know as much as we would like to know about the significance of characteristics of a pain. A throbbing pain in the head is due to the opening up of an artery which enables blood to go pounding through. A scalding pain, felt in a small area of the skin of the neck or trunk is likely to be due to irritation of a spinal nerve. Intermittent labor-like pains suggest an intestinal obstruction, with strong peristaltic contractions. Colicky pains suggest uneven peristalsis in some muscular tube.

Persons speak of boring, cutting, stinging, distending, compressing, squeezing, viselike, rending, tearing, pressing, binding, or gnawing pains, but it is hard to say what these characteristics mean. Great constancy of an ache suggests a psychic origin.

Many a person feels that a distress in his abdomen is due to gas trapped in a segment of bowel, and he may well be right. Persons suffering from the pain of duodenal ulcer often say it feels as if it were due to gas. Perhaps it is. Taking food can cause gas to move onward. The pain of gallstone colic often interferes somewhat with breathing. Associated with heartburn there may be a rending feeling in the chest. Occasionally a person with pain says it feels as if it were due to a balloon being distended in his thorax or abdomen.

The pain of angina pectoris may be felt as a great pressure, or a rending or bursting feeling, or a feeling of a constricting band. A pain in the head may feel like a nail, or a tight band of iron.

Some pains are knifelike or needle-like, "neuralgic" jabs in thorax or abdomen. They appear to be due to irritation of a nerve by arthritis of the spine. They somewhat resemble the lightning pains of tabes. Some of the so-called pains in the chest are really sorenesses or aches in the thoracic wall.

A sudden change in the character of a pain. As already suggested, when a man has had, let us say, an ulcer distress off and on for years, and suddenly it changes for the worse, one must suspect the coming of a complication such as a perforation, or an involvement of the peritoneum, or penetration into the pancreas, or pyloric obstruction, or a change to a carcinoma.

A sudden let-up in a pain that is thought to be due perhaps to intestinal obstruction may be due to perforation of the bowel or to its slipping out of a hernia or to the untwisting of a volvulus. In cases of supposed acute appendicitis the let-up of pain can be due to rupture of the appendix.

Has the patient two pains? Often it is essential to diagnosis that the physician know that the patient has two or three types of pain. For instance, I remember a stout woman who had one pain due to angina pectoris, another due to a diaphragmatic hernia, and a third due to gallstones. Only with much questioning could my colleagues and I unscramble her story into its several constituents. Similarly, a person with a pain due to arthritis of the spine and some fibrositis in the abdominal wall can have other pains due to indigestion, food allergy, or a duodenal ulcer. Women who suffer from migraine commonly have two or three different types of headache, and rarely, also, a pain in the face or head.

The significance of symptoms that accompany the pain. It is sometimes helpful to find out if any symptoms accompany a pain. For instance, with a gallstone colic there may be nausea, a catch in the breath, perhaps vomiting, abdominal soreness and, some days later, a little jaundice. In between the acute attacks, there is usually flatulence. The woman will often rush home from a luncheon party to tear off her girdle and get relief from bloating.

When one suspects that a colicky pain is being produced by an irritative lesion somewhere in the digestive tract, one will expect (1) waves to run orad, producing nausea and perhaps vomiting or regurgitation or belching, and (2) waves to run caudad to produce diarrhea or a sensation that diarrhea is imminent.

With renal colic there may be frequency of urination and distress in the bladder and penis. With the pain of pleurisy there may be distress on taking a breath, or, with diaphragmatic involvement, a feeling of distressing sighing, hiccup or cough, fever, and what may be taken for lumbago. There may be considerable shortness of breath of a peculiar type; there may be a sore spot in the thoracic wall, and difficulty in lying down. With intestinal obstruction there should be some nausea, perhaps vomiting, perhaps bloating, borborygmus, perhaps visible peristalsis, constipation, or a little bloody diarrhea. There will usually be a loss of appetite, and if food is taken, it may immediately cause pain at the point of obstruction, because of the surge of peristalsis down against the obstructed segment.

Acute appedicitis is likely to be associated with nausea, vomiting of much intestinal fluid, a little fever, a fast pulse, and a drawing-up of the right thigh. There may be great prostration. Diagnostic is the fact that the patient cannot sleep. Often there will be a feeling that the bowels should move.

With angina pectoris there may be a fear of death with a great feeling of weakness. With gastric crises there may be severe nausea with retching and a pain which is not well relieved by morphine. There may be hyperesthesia of the thoracic wall on one side. There may also be pelvic crises and lightning pains in the legs. With the pain of pleurisy there is likely to be some cough, and often a chill or fever. I have seen attacks of pleurisy on the right with pain in the right upper quadrant of the abdomen resembling that of acute cholecystitis.

With lumbago or a slipped disc there may be some sciatica. In a case of zoster, after the patient has suffered a few days with a root-type of pain there may come the little blisters. The presence of urticaria or purpura, along with abdominal pain, will make one think of an allergic or vascular disturbance in the abdomen.

What seems to bring the pain on? Often the diagnosis can be made most easily by learning what brings the pain. For instance, angina pectoris is usually produced by anger or by walking too fast into a cold wind, and especially after eating a good-sized breakfast. The pain of pleurisy or of lumbago may follow an acute cold or cough with a little fever. The pain of cholecystitis may be brought on by eating some indigestible food, or by indulging in a tantrum of temper. A mucous colic is likely to be produced by some psychic strain, or by eating some allergen, by getting constipated, or by getting a cold. A flare-up of ulcer pain is likely to be due to some worry, or to lifting. An attack of migraine is likely to follow fatigue, psychic strain, or the eating of some food like chocolate.

A pain in the lower part of the thorax which is caused by lying down too soon after eating or trying to tie the shoes after a full meal may be due to a diaphragmatic hernia. A hunger type of abdominal pain may follow constipation which has been neglected. Pelvic pain which is due to disease of an ovary, tube, or uterus or to endometriosis is likely to flare up during each menstrual period. Pain due to a displaced disc is likely to come suddenly when the patient slips a bit and recovers himself, or when he lifts a trunk or heavy suitcase. Such a pain is likely to be felt acutely if the patient coughs or sneezes. This symptom is noted, also, with cord tumors. Pain due to an arthritic neck can be brought on in acute form by driving a car on a rough or winding road.

What lessens or stops the pain? One can often learn much about a pain by finding out from the patient what he has found that helps or stops the distress. For instance, if a woman says she can relieve her abdominal distress with an enema it is probable that it is arising in a sensitive colon; if it is relieved by taking food it is more likely to be due to a peptic ulcer. As everyone knows, ulcer pain is commonly relieved by taking food or alkalies. Occasionally, it is the better for vomiting or getting the stomach washed out. The pain of carcinoma of the stomach, of acute gastritis, or perhaps cholecystitis may be relieved for a while by fasting or by eating very little or by washing out the stomach.

The pain of angina pectoris can be stopped quickly by resting or by taking nitroglycerin. Pain that is arising in arthritis of the spine or fibrositis in the abdominal wall is usually relieved by the patient's getting up and walking around, or by getting into a tub of hot water. The pain is worse if the person remains quiet for some time. The pain of migraine is best helped by a hypodermic injection of gynergen or DHE 45. Pain due to gallstone colic or ureteral colic can usually be stopped by morphine. The distress of a sore colon may be helped by taking an enema or a little codeine or by applying heat to the abdominal wall.

Some persons say they can help an abdominal pain by applying pressure, but just what this means in a diagnostic way I do not know. Some get relief by assuming the knee-chest position, or by flexing the thighs on the abdomen. This decreases the tension in the abdominal cavity. Some persons get instant relief from nausea and abdominal pain when they bring up a big belch, or vomit a little. This must mean that there was some irritated or distended spot in the bowel or stomach which was sending off waves orad, and when one of these waves succeeded in running out, or distention was relieved, the ectopic focus quieted down. Pain due to a diaphragmatic hernia or to severe heartburn or a pancreatitis may be helped by sitting up. Pains due to having eaten an allergen and having filled up with gas are relieved as soon as the gas begins to move and to be passed. Such pains may be relieved a bit by the taking of food or whiskey, or crème de menthe, or the sipping of water or milk. It often helps to take a walk. All this causes waves to move down the bowel again.

Is the pain originating in the digestive tract? When a patient has a pain in the abdomen, one of the most important things the physician must do is to ask a few questions designed to determine if the pain is arising in the digestive tract. It probably does not arise in the tract if it is not influenced in any way by the taking of food, the emptying of the bowel, the taking of alkalies, belching, vomiting, passing flatus, or taking a laxative or an enema. Perhaps, if asked, the patient will say he has a stomach that can digest anything. He may say, also, that he is sure eating has nothing to do with his pain. If only more surgeons were to ask these questions there would be thousands fewer futile operations performed each year.

It helps greatly in making a diagnosis to find that the patient's pain, perhaps associated with bloating or a feeling of impending diarrhea, can be produced in a few minutes by drinking a glass of cold water. This shows that the trouble is not due to any particular food, and hence it cannot be relieved by any diet. The digestive tract is too irritable, and the peristaltic waves, as they run down the bowel, produce distress. In older persons such great irritability of the stomach with a tendency to spasmodic contraction can follow a small unrecognized stroke.

Especially in the cases of men, a pain which comes soon after eating is almost never due to an uncomplicated ulcer. One cannot be so sure of this in the cases of women because in them the syndrome of ulcer is often bizarre and unrecognizable. Epigastric burning and heartburn are probably never due to peptic ulcer, even when an ulcer is present.

It is well to ask if an epigastric pain ever comes before breakfast, because, in my experience, the pain of duodenal ulcer rarely comes before the first meal in the morning.

The diagnostic value of a Sippy treatment. More physicians ought to know the great diagnostic value of a few days of a Sippy type of treatment. If a patient gets no relief from staying in bed for forty-eight hours on frequent feedings and alkalinization, the chances are great that his trouble is not due to an ulcer. If it is due to an ulcer it must be a complicated one which is not likely to be helped by any form of medical treatment.

The significance of a pain which does not respond to morphine. Sometimes when I have been puzzled as to the nature of a pain I have given the patient a hypodermic injection of half a grain of morphine. Obviously, if the pain were due to such a thing as a gallstone or a ureteral stone the morphine would give great relief. The fact that in the case of a nervous woman with a constant ache the morphine gave no relief strongly suggests that the origin of the trouble was up in the brain.

Another thing that helps sometimes in diagnosis is to anesthetize with a solution of procaine the whole area in which a pain is felt. If, with the area numb, the pain is unchanged, the impression will be left that the trouble is up in the nervous system somewhere, well above the area in which the distress is felt.

Pains due to fear or anxiety or rebellion. The physician should remember always that there is such a thing as pain due to fear or acute anxiety or chronic worry. Persons will sometimes say, "Fear ties me in knots inside," or "Fear hits me in the pit of my stomach." Some say that when much frightened it feels as if someone were twisting the stomach at the cardia. I remember a woman who got a pain in the epigastrium the minute a big disappointment came to her. It disappeared later when she came to see how she got it. A nervous woman, when anxious, can get little "pinching" pains all through her abdomen.

Many women seem to interpret fatigue as pain. Elsewhere in this book I tell of two girls who got a sudden pain in the face when a psychic shock hit them. I have seen cases of severe abdominal or thoracic pain due to anger. I have seen many cases of peculiar thoracic or abdominal pain due to thrombosis of a small vessel in the brain, and I have seen abdominal pains due to a brain tumor.

Pains due to a neurotropic virus. The fact that for days before a crop of herpes comes out on the thorax the patient may suffer great pain makes me feel that some other pains felt in thorax and abdomen or elsewhere are due to a neurotropic virus which has involved the sensory ganglion on a nerve—without producing the usual blisters.

Pains due to chemical changes in the tissues. It seems probable that some obscure pains for which so far no organic cause can be found are due to chemical changes in the tissues. One thinks of the terrible pain of gout which is due to crystals of uric acid in the big toe joint. Some persons who have a sore and painful liver are suffering from hepatitis.

I have seen some cases in which, when a T-tube was in the common duct, a severe attack of pain came at a time when the bile changed from the normal thin golden yellow fluid to a thick, stringy, blackish substance. Apparently there was some change in metabolism in the liver associated with pain. This appeared to be due to food allergy.

I have seen typical colics, closely resembling those due to gallstones, in the cases of persons whose stoneless gallbladder had been removed and who were highly allergic to some food, such as coffee or egg. The colics stopped with the removal of a certain food from the diet.

Pains due to disease of the arteries. That changes in the small arteries can produce excruciating pain is known to anyone who has ever had to thaw out frost-bitten fingers. Severe pain can also be felt in some cases of chilblains.

As already noted, embolism in an artery can cause terrific pain. A patient of mine who, throughout her lifetime, suffered from crises of severe pelvic pain, was found at operation to have a dermoid cyst full of scars of old hemorrhages. After the removal of this cyst she had no more pain.

It is known today that pain in small areas can be due to arteritis nodosa. It is possible that with time some cases of arteritis in the abdomen will be recognized. It is known by physicians who have submitted to the puncture of arteries with a hypodermic needle that the pain produced in this way can be severe and sickening. It is well known now that some headaches are due to the distention of arteries in the brain. All this means that some of the pains which now go unexplained may be due to disease of small arteries. Often painful aneurysms are missed and not recognized until a necropsy is performed.

Pain due to exaggerated intestinal reflexes. Some of the abdominal pains which follow a little stroke appear to be due to a great exaggeration of reflexes in the abdomen which cause the bowel or stomach to cramp suddenly after the taking of food or water. Persons with such hypersensitiveness sometimes get a dumping syndrome after eating. Others have great distress or some pain right after defecation.

Equivalents of migraine or epilepsy and gastric crises. The consultant must always be on the watch for unusual cases in which the abdominal pain or distress or vomiting comes in acute episodes with, perhaps, a normal digestion in between. The doctor must always suspect a migrainous or epileptic equivalent when the patient has suffered from many severe spells, perhaps for years, without coming to any bad end. Sometimes the symptoms of nausea and vomiting are more prominent than those of pain. Perhaps there has been no pain. It helps in these cases to know that the patient's relatives are migrainous or that the patient had migraine in his or her younger years. In youth there may have been spells of "bilious vomiting." Perhaps as the person grew older the headaches largely disappeared, and the abdominal component remained or got worse.

In the case of epileptic equivalents one may learn of a relative with a convulsive disorder. Often the patient has a bad temper, or he had fever convulsions in childhood, and his electroencephalogram shows a typical dysrhythmia. In some cases, the pain is very severe; there may be much retching, and the clinical picture may be that of a gastric crisis. Against the diagnosis of an inflammatory lesion is the fact that during an attack the abdominal wall remains soft.

It must be remembered that gastric crises of tabes often come before the usual symptoms and findings of tabes are present. Sometimes the diagnosis can be confirmed only with the help of a spinal puncture. In one of my cases the diagnosis depended on one irregular pupil, an area of markedly hyperesthetic skin over the region of the liver and a "cord bladder." The man's knee jerks were normal and his Wassermann test was negative.

The important point in these cases is to see the person in an attack and then to sense the fact that the storm is much worse than that usually seen with a gallstone attack. Often it is different in that there is more nausea and retching and the storm does not quiet down entirely even with a big dose of morphine.

Pains due to abnormal peristalsis in the common duct or the ureter. There is considerable evidence to indicate that at times severe pain is due to a failure of waves to go normally over muscular tubes such as the common duct or the ureter. I remember a woman, previously well, who began to have typical left ureteral colics. Urologists could find nothing wrong with the ureter. Because her colics came with the menstrual period, she was operated on. An inflamed and obstructed fallopian tube was found lying near the ureter, and when it was removed, the colics ceased. This would indicate that there is such a thing as dyskinesia of the ureter. A similar dyskinesia of the common duct has been observed, and it is probable that there are dyskinesias of the esophagus and the vas deferens.

Pain that returns after an operation. When pain returns after a gastroenterostomy or a subtotal gastrectomy the physician will want to know its exact location. If it returns in the old place the trouble is probably due to a reactivation of the old ulcer, but if the pain is in a new place a little below and to the left of the navel, it is almost certainly due to a new jejunal ulcer.

Pain that returns after a cholecystectomy may be due to the presence of stones in the common duct or to spasm in the duct or perhaps duodenum. The physician must find out if the patient had stones and colics before operation. If no stones were found at the operation, the chances are slim that there now are stones in the common duct. If, however, the gallbladder was full of little stones it may well be that some were left in the ducts. It helps much to find out if the pain that returns is the same as that felt before the operation, and if it is felt in the same place. Such facts would suggest that the mechanism is the same. It helps to know if the common duct was drained, and if so, if the drainage kept up for more than six weeks. Long-continued drainage suggests the presence of a stone obstructing the papilla of Vater. After a supposed colic, if the amount of bilirubin in the blood rises, this fact adds to the suspicion that there is trouble in the common duct.

Pains due to disease in and around the spine. As pointed out in Chapter 18 many supposedly abdominal pains are really arising in an arthritis about the spine or in a fibrositis of the abdominal wall.

The diagnostic features of such pain are (1) that the patient often gives a story of having had backache, lumbago, sciatica, cricks, wryneck, or arthritis in many joints; (2) the pain gets worse when the patient rests or lies down or sits, and gets better if he gets up and walks around; (3) it gets better with heat and physiotherapy; (4) sometimes it gets the patient out of bed at six in the morning, and makes him walk the floor until he is "warmed up"; (5) sometimes it is worse as a storm approaches.

Sometimes it is helpful in diagnosing this type of pain to pick up a fold of the abdominal wall and pinch it. If it is too sensitive, and there is no deep tenderness, this will show that it is the wall that is the sore place.

It is possible that pains supposed to be due to chronic appendicitis are due sometimes to a myositis or fibrositis in the iliopsoas muscle.

"Nerve root pain." The so-called root type of pain can easily be recognized because it follows down the course of one or two spinal nerves. Sometimes, in such cases, a zone of hyperesthesia can be demonstrated by running the fingernail down over the skin of the back. Such pain may be due to disease of the spinal cord or of a spinal nerve. It may be due to involvement of a posterior root with the virus of herpes zoster.

Pains due to a slipped disc. A patient with a slipped disc commonly limps in with his body listed over to one side. He may be using a cane, or rarely he will be in a wheel chair. He often gives a history of a *sudden* attack of pain, perhaps when his foot slipped, or when he was lifting something. With this there may have come severe sciatica on one side, or a weakness of one leg or an inability to walk without help. Usually it hurts greatly to cough or sneeze. Sometimes one can get a history of several similar sudden attacks of the pain and disability. Strongly suggestive are the attacks that come suddenly and so weaken a limb as for a while to make walking difficult or impossible. Arthritis is not so likely to produce this picture.

Usually the differential diagnosis has to be made between a slipped disc and some arthritis. The difficulty is that the patient can have both a slipped disc and a long history of arthritis around the spine and in other joints. He or she may tell of attacks of wryneck, lumbago, cricks, and of jabs of pain in the thoracic region. Helpful are the special roentgenograms made with air or some opaque substance in the spinal canal. Helpful also are signs of nerve injury such as a loss of the ankle jerk on the affected side or signs of inflammation in the spinal fluid.

Pain due to the posterior perforation of a duodenal ulcer. There is a severe type of pain due to the posterior perforation of a duodenal ulcer or the penetration of an ulcer into the head of the pancreas. The story usually is that, some years before, the man suffered from hunger pain; later, perhaps, he suffered a sudden attack of severe pain, perhaps with retching for a day or two. This came with the perforation. Later the man could not get much sleep or rest because of severe pain which was not well relieved by the taking of food or alkalies. Often a person so affected goes down to skin and bones because of the pain and loss of sleep. Sometimes the ulcer cannot be seen with the roentgen rays, and then the diagnosis has to be made from the history. The diagnosis must often be made even when a good surgeon has looked at the duodenum and pronounced it normal. His mistake was not to explore behind it.

Pain due to disease of the pancreas. The medical profession is now coming to realize more and more that pancreatitis and carcinoma of the pancreas are fairly common diseases. Especially because persons suffering from the pain of carcinoma of the pancreas are often somewhat demoralized by it, the diagnosis commonly made is that of a neurosis.

Acute pancreatitis is likely to produce a severe abdominal attack with pain lasting several days and producing prostration and an "acute abdomen." The attack is likely to last much longer than a gallstone colic, and the patient should be much sicker. It is well, often, to get a scout film of the pancreatic region so as to rule out stones in the ducts. In an acute spell, a physician will want to get an estimate of the serum amylase and lipase to see if their titers shoot up. Occasionally the blood sugar and serum bilirubin will also be up a bit.

Abdominal pain due to angina pectoris. Occasionally pain due to a coronary thrombosis will shoot into the abdomen and then a mistake in diagnosis can easily be made. A little stroke can also produce abdominal pain.

Epigastric pain due to constipation. Some persons, when constipated, get a painful gaseous distention of the duodenum or upper part of the jejunum. On taking food they may get relief because the gas will then move onward, or they may get relief by taking a laxative or an enema. The syndrome resembles that of ulcer.

Pain due to regional enteritis or ulcerative colitis. There are rare cases in which abdominal pain associated with diarrhea should make one think of a beginning regional enteritis or ulcerative colitis. Sometimes the disease can be diagnosed by the roentgenologist or the proctologist. Helpful is the finding of a high blood sedimentation rate. In ruling out subacute appendicitis, one should note Crohn's statement that diarrhea is seldom present with this disease. An appendectomy, performed mistakenly for terminal ileitis, is likely to be unfortunate in that it may produce a fecal fistula.

Abdominal pain due to attacks of intestinal obstruction. Rarely, and especially in persons who have had abdominal operations, there will be attacks of threatening or mild intestinal obstruction which clear up perhaps with the help of suction through a long intestinal tube. The patient may suffer from flatulence and rhythmic labor-like pains, perhaps associated with the rising up of a loop of bowel. This then goes down with a gurgle. In older persons such symptoms usually indicate obstruction of the bowel due to carcinoma. Any old man or woman who begins to have marked borborygmus should be studied with the greatest of care, and in case of doubt, should have the abdomen explored. With intestinal obstruction there is often nausea and vomiting, and the taking of food may quickly cause pain due to the surging down of the intestinal contents against the sore obstructed place. Often a scout film of the abdomen will show a segment of bowel filled with gas.

Sometimes the patient is a woman who, after a hysterectomy, suffers from intermittent attacks which suggest intestinal obstruction. At operation one will find a knuckle of bowel almost closed because it is bound down so closely to the stump of the uterus. Rarely, intermittent attacks of intestinal obstruction are due to the twisting of a loop of gut around a point where it was fastened by a long "rat-tail" adhesion. There can also be volvulus of a long, loose sigmoid loop of colon.

Pain due to diverticulitis of the colon. In rare cases one will see a patient who has had one or more attacks of pain in the left lower quadrant of the abdomen, associated perhaps with fever and chills, and a doughy mass in the region of the sigmoid flexure. In such cases one should not give barium by mouth because it may cause obstruction. On passing a sigmoidoscope one finds that the tube will not go far because the bowel is bound down. Sometimes the urinary bladder is irritated, due to the adhesion to it or perforation into it of an inflamed diverticulum. The diagnosis can be made when air and feces come out with the urine.

The fact that a person has had two or three similar spells of pain and fever in previous years will go far to rule out carcinoma. A picture of the diseased region can be obtained by injecting a little barium into the rectum. This picture usually shows a narrowed segment about 7 cm. long where the descending colon turns into the sigmoid flexure. This segment is usually the one most thickly covered with diverticula.

There is a type of pain due only to spasm in the sigmoid region: spasm due apparently to the presence of a dozen or more diverticula on the short segment of bowel just described. Persons with such spasm show no signs of inflammation such as chills, fever, a high leucocyte count, a high blood sedimentation rate, and no mass.

Abdominal pains due to colds or infections. Some persons suffer from abdominal cramps for a few days before they come down with a cold or an attack of influenza. This pain may be of the hunger type, relieved by the taking of food, or it may be typical of a mucous colic, with a frequent desire to pass a little gas and mucus. The distress appears to be due to an irritation of the bowel by the toxins of the disease. This or a similar syndrome is often called "intestinal flu."

Pain due to cardiospasm or esophagospasm. Rarely one sees a patient with pain in the epigastrium which proves later to have been a forerunner of cardiospasm. It helps in the diagnosis if, at times, this pain runs up under the sternum and into the angles of the jaw or into the outer ear. It may also go down the arms and into the middle of the back. Helpful may be the observation that the pain is produced at times by the drinking of some iced beverage. Occasionally there may be a little spasm at the cardia with some difficulty in swallowing, which the patient fails to mention until he is asked about it. Rarely, pains are due to cramps in the esophagus, associated with painful emotion. In rare cases pain originating in the esophagus will be referred down into the abdomen, so severe that a surgeon will feel that he must explore.

Pain in the groin due to an incipient hernia. There are a few persons who complain of pain in the groin which comes when they stand much, especially in the evening when they are tired. The pain lets up in a minute as soon as they sit down or lie down. It is almost certainly due to a large internal ring into which a knuckle of bowel keeps boring. The surgeon should note that the pain is felt low in the groin, and he should then leave the appendix alone.

Suprapubic pain due to posterior urethritis. Rarely one will see a young man who, after gonorrhea, has pain above the urinary bladder. The urologist will find a posterior urethritis, and on treating this, he will give the man relief.

Pain and soreness in the xiphoid appendix of the sternum. A few persons complain of pain and soreness in the tip of the sternum. Usually someone diagnoses a peptic ulcer. Actually, all the patient has is a perichondritis, or inflammation of an arthritic type around the cartilage. The trouble usually disappears within a few days or weeks. Most of the patients have a long history of fibrositis or arthritis, and this helps in the diagnosis.

Distress arising in the abdominal aorta. Some stout women, with a flabby abdominal wall, complain of a throbbing or beating in the center of the abdomen, or of a soreness there which, on palpation, can be seen to be located in the abdominal aorta. Sometimes the aorta is tender to the touch. In these cases it is hard to say if the artery is inflamed. Certainly persons with an atheromatous and badly ulcerated aorta rarely complain of any distress.

Pain due to a gonorrheal patch on the peritoneum. In rare cases a young woman with a localized abdominal pain will be found to have an area of peritonitis due to a gonorrheal infection which probably went in by way of the fallopian tube.

A severe brief cramp in the perineum. Men sometimes complain of severe pain in the perineum which comes at rare intervals and lasts a few minutes. I think it is due to a cramp in the muscle of the prostate gland.

Abdominal pain due to desensitization by an allergist. Occasionally a person who is being desensitized to some pollen will suffer from abdominal pain. It will stop as soon as the injections stop. I do not know what the mechanism is.

Pains for which no operating should be done. There are quite a few persons who complain bitterly and repeatedly of a pain somewhere in the body: a pain for which they have undergone innumerable treatments and perhaps a few operations. For instance, a highly nervous man got an ache in the side of his neck. A physician electrocoagulated the tonsils and the man was worse. Another physician removed the tonsils and he was still worse. A surgeon explored the neck surgically and he was much worse. The ache then became centered in the scar. By this time the man was almost unable to sleep or to work.

In this type of case the longer a surgeon keeps operating in the region where the pain or ache is, the worse the patient is likely to get. Usually the only way one can help is to begin by prescribing enough of some barbiturate to give the man some rest and sleep. Then one must try to secure for him a good vacation. In this way one can raise his threshold for pain. Only then will he feel less distress. Some of these patients, after several futile operations, get into such a state that one fears that they will go on into a psychosis. Fortunately, they seldom do this; they just live on for years without getting much better or much worse.

Pains in the head. The reader should turn to Chapter 17 for a discussion of headaches and pains in the head.

Pains in the chest. In Chapter 19 the reader will find a discussion of angina and the various pseudo-anginas and their mode of production.

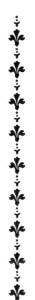

CHAPTER 6

The Ordering or
Not Ordering of Tests

A THOROUGH EXAMINATION IS ESSENTIAL BUT IT SHOULD NOT TAKE THE PLACE OF A GOOD HISTORY. Even forty-five years ago, when I went to work in a big city hospital, my fellow-interns and I often tried to get our diagnoses made quickly in the laboratory. But soon I saw that this practice was leading often to the making of poor diagnoses. I saw, also, that if long indulged in, the practice would lead to the making of a poor diagnostician, and so I started trying to avoid it. All through the years, however, the temptation to turn first to the laboratory has been present, and even yet I have to fight against it, especially on those days when I am tired and faced with more new patients than I can comfortably handle. Then I hope that the laboratory girl or the roentgenologist will make the diagnosis for me, and I am tempted to send the patient for tests so as to be spared the strain of struggling to get a clear history or one from which I can make the diagnosis.

Today I find my interns subject to the same temptation that afflicted me years ago. Worse yet, I see signs that suggest that even eminent consultants are sometimes overcome by it. In their offices, the patients all go through an extensive examination, but many are not given time in which to tell their story, and few are allowed time for an adequate discussion of the problems of treatment.

107

All patients should not be handled the same way. All of us physicians should keep remembering that the type of complete examination that has to be made when a man comes in with an obscure fever or loss of weight is not needed by a man who comes with an advanced Parkinson's syndrome or a typical Friedreich's ataxia, a typical familial epilepsy, or even a typical migraine. In such cases there is often no diagnostic problem at all, and then I do not believe we physicians are honorable if we act as if there were one. In many cases I hate to see my assistants ordering a repetition of all the tests that were made, perhaps only a few weeks before, by some able man. When a patient comes with a big envelope full of roentgenograms and long reports from a good internist at a fine clinic, all that is needed often is a review of the data, and then concurrence in the diagnosis, with perhaps some discussion of it to help the patient to understand it better.

I hate to see complete roentgenologic studies being made again and again of the digestive tract of a person who has perhaps a typical migraine and has just had a careful surgical exploration of the abdomen which showed nothing wrong.

In many cases the chances of learning anything from more tests and roentgenologic studies are very small, while the chances of making the diagnosis from an hour or so of history-taking and history-interpreting are large.

The needless running-up of large bills. What distresses me often is that we consulting internists will unthinkingly run up a large bill on a poor little salesgirl just because she wants her old mother, with a brain largely destroyed by a stroke, to have "the best examination money can buy." Sometimes I have had to do some of this type of examining because the girl insisted on it or begged for it, but at least, before I ordered the tests, I told her that I did not want them and that they would not teach me anything that would help me to help her mother. I felt I had to do this in order to keep my self-respect and my sense of common decency and honesty.

Sometimes, of course, we physicians have to order a score of tests out of simple kindness. For instance, a poor government clerk brought me his wife all the way from Puerto Rico. The minute I saw her, a poker-faced and trembling wreck, the result of a severe attack of encephalitis, I took the man aside and, as kindly as I could, told him what the situation was: why I did not care to examine her, and why I could not help her much. He said, "Go ahead and give her a lot of tests, because, otherwise, she will be terribly disappointed. I would not have the heart to take her back now without getting for her the thorough examination she has been longing for." He was right; I could see that: so we examined the woman; we extracted an abscessed tooth, and we sent her off happy with a bottle of artane tablets! But the husband and I knew why I had done what I had done: only out of kindness, and not for money or because I did not have sense enough to depart from a routine type of practice.

A lack of cerebration. I hate to see my desk girls and assistants getting the rigid idea that no patient can ever see me until he or she has gone through the whole diagnostic mill. And they can so easily slip into this habit. Many a time I can see that my head desk girl is troubled or personally aggrieved when I insist on seeing right off an old patient who has dropped in just to report progress or to ask me for a card to go to the oculist or the dermatologist. When I do not then put the patient through the whole mill the girl feels that the place is running down and its standards are slipping!

I once ran foul of a woman of this rigid type. I had asked a hypothyroid patient of mine, taking thyroid extract, to see a doctor friend in her city, and get a measurement of her basal metabolic rate. I gave her a note to my friend, asking if he would let his laboratory technician make the one test and mail the report to me. Later, the patient wrote in great distress to say that, on going to my friend's office, she had been unable to see him or to get the test. She had encountered a "hard-boiled" receptionist who had insisted that she go through all the tests again. This officious person said she was proud to work for the most thorough and scientific man in the city, and no one was ever seen by him until a score or two of tests had been made; that if Dr. Alvarez wanted to do slipshod medicine that was his affair, but no one could get that type of careless work done in that office!

I was upset to think that the practice of medicine was becoming so stupid and stereotyped as that, and then a woman, an old friend, came in and told me that she had had a similar experience in my own office! In order to get past my desk girl to tell me about her mother, about whose health I was concerned, she had had to register and be examined by one of my assistants! When I protested to the desk girl that she should not have done such a foolish thing, she maintained that she had been trying to protect me and save my time.

The best proofs I have had of how completely decerebrate the "thorough" practice of internal medicine can become were given my by a couple of my friends who work in large clinics. One of them told me how one day he was outraged when, on returning from a trip, he found sitting in his office a thin, pale, dying old man with, in his epigastrium, the fixed mass of an inoperable cancer of the stomach. The assistant, even after noting this mass and the roentgenologic report of extensive cancer sent by the home physician, had gone ahead and ordered a complete study of the man from his frontal sinuses to his prostate gland and his athlete's foot! When asked why he had done this thoughtless thing and had tired the poor old fellow to no purpose, the young doctor said he had been trained to examine all people that way, and he just thought it was the thing to do. Incidentally, since the senior physician refused to charge for all the needless tests, the institution had to bear the expense. Unfortunately, in some college hospitals, interns get the idea that tests do not cost anything. They just order them, with only a vague idea as to what they are to show or what they are good for.

Another example of decerebrate practice was that given me by a medical friend who one afternoon found his assistant handing out orders for a multitude of tests to a stenographer whose only complaint was insomnia. This seemed silly because what could the usual blood chemistry tests possibly reveal to explain insomnia? Besides, it took the doctor only a few minutes to learn that the girl's difficulty in sleeping had come four months before when she learned that her fiancé had started going out with another woman. He also learned that in two large clinics she had already been thoroughly examined for the insomnia. All the doctor did was to tell her to go right home and have it out with the fiancé. A few months later she wrote to say that she was happily married and sleeping perfectly! As a nice old doctor once said to me, "In this world a man has to be careful not to get so well educated that he acts like a darned fool."

Efforts should be made to teach interns not to waste money on tests. In every medical school a few "senior statesmen" should constantly point out to their younger colleagues and their interns and residents that in case after case many of the tests that were ordered were not indicated. Why, for instance, was an electrocardiogram ordered for a husky young lady who had sprained her ankle playing championship tennis? Did the intern expect to learn anything from this or was he just following some vague conditioned reflex? I find that most of the new assistants I get each quarter order red and white blood counts on every big husky patient who has come in with a hernia or a fibrositis. When I ask the young doctor what he expected to learn by this, he usually says, "I suppose nothing." And nothing is what he usually learns by ordering tests aimlessly.

A sad feature of such practice is that often the young doctor could have made the diagnosis with the help of a question or two. Doubtless, if the senior statesmen were to start preaching against useless tests, for a time the only reaction of the younger men would be to assume that the protester was an old fogey who hadn't kept abreast of medical advance, but gradually I think he would be able to earn the deep respect of the interns. He would keep showing them day after day that many of the diagnoses he made *from histories* were more accurate than the ones they made *from tests*.

The patients insist on tests. One day I saw a woman whose history showed that she had a typical migraine due to an irritable spot in her brain and an inherited tendency. The exciting cause was the effort of living with a mean husband. She had just been thoroughly examined in two large medical centers in the East. On her way back to California, she stopped off to see me. Finding that she could stay only a few days, I asked her if she would not like to let me decide how I was to use what time I had available to give her. I said I did not care to examine her again because, even if I should find something that had been missed by the other men, it would probably have no significance as regards the migraine. She agreed that my idea was a reasonable one, and so we spent some time each day discussing the nagging problems of her life and what might be done to somewhat solve some of them. A week later she returned shamefacedly to say that, when she got off the train at home, and her husband found I had not examined her, he was outraged, and had sent her right back with orders that I give her the biggest and most costly examination of her career. Evidently it had not occurred to him that if I had such knowledge of migraine that his home physician particularly desired my opinion, he might well have left me free to handle the problem in my own way. Actually, the new overhauling showed nothing more than the others had.

Some patients even resent it when a consultant shows that he knows what the diagnosis is before the results of the tests have come back.

Should we not refuse to give many tests to some patients? It is bad enough to order useless tests when the patient can afford to pay for what he demands and expects: It is worse when the patient cannot afford the expense. I remember the shiftless son of a poor share-cropper whose only outstanding achievement in life had been the begetting of eight children. He complained that he had always felt tired and sick and without energy, just like his parents and grandparents before him. He had been sent through several of the best clinics in the South, and, as he said, "no one had ever found what was wrong with him." Friends had taken up a collection and sent him to Rochester with the hope that at last the cause of his discomforts would be found and perhaps cut out by a surgeon.

One glance at him and his history, and the diagnosis of constitutional inadequacy was obvious. I wanted to send him right home but since this would have been against the tradition of the place in which I work, and would have angered him and the persons who sent him, he was given the thorough examination which he expected. When it showed nothing, he was outraged, and later when through some oversight he got a bill, he was angry clear through, and wrote a letter flaying me for stupidity and incompetence. As he said, "I don't owe you nuthin' because you didn't find out what is the matter with me." I agreed with him that I was stupid, but not for the reasons he gave. I was stupid because I had wasted my time in appearing to attempt what I knew I could not do, and I was stupid to do it for a man so ignorant that he could never understand that I had done what I had done only to avoid distressing him.

What I often wonder in these cases is, seeing that the man will probably go home angry and disgusted anyway, why should we doctors not let him go before we have wasted a lot of time and money and thought on him? That would be more logical than what we now do.

It bothers me that this problem which is so difficult to solve and so important to the future of medical practice is never discussed at our meetings or in our journals. Another thing that bothers me much is, that if the huge sums of money that are now being wasted on examining and re-examining and operating on people like this son of a share-cropper were only used for paying better salaries to professors, for educating gifted young men, and for maintaining fine research laboratories, some good could be done.

If we ever get socialized medicine in this country, and some wise provision is not made for the economical handling of the constitutional inadequates, the mildly psychotic, and the constant complainers, their demands will multiply by many times what the service would otherwise cost.

A complete examination will not reveal a neurosis. A bad feature of our having come so to worship tests, and tests alone, is that they do not reveal neuroses and psychoses. There is no test that will tell us that the woman sitting there on the other side of the desk is going insane, or dying of a broken heart, or is ill because she lies awake every night listening to the breathing of an asthmatic or epileptic child, or wondering where her dipsomanic husband is, or if he has gone on another bender, or smashed up the family car.

CHAPTER 7

*Disregarding Findings That Have
Nothing to Do with the Case*

I N THESE DAYS, when more and more of us physicians are looking to
the laboratory worker, the roentgenologist, and the specialist for
our diagnoses, one of the most useful courses that could be given in
every medical school would be one on the art of disregarding those
findings which either do not produce symptoms or, in the case of the
particular patient before one, have nothing to do with the illness.

**The present-day need for recognizing the unimportance of cer-
tain findings.** That such instruction is badly needed today would, I
feel sure, soon become obvious to anyone who, for a while, was to sit
back of some busy consultant, and note the number of cases in which
the diagnosis made by the home internist had to be rejected because
it was without significance and inadequate to explain the symptoms.
Oftentimes the objection to the diagnosis is not so much that it seems
wrong as that it cannot explain the patient's many discomforts or even
his principal one. It cannot explain perhaps his inability to work, or his
nervous breakdown, his inability to read, or to make decisions, or his
other mental or psychic difficulties.

A woman can have as definite a finding as a gallstone, and yet it
may have to be disregarded because she has no symptoms of cholecystitis, and all her complaints are those of worry, insomnia, fatigue,
fibrositis, headache, low backache, or an irritable bladder. Similarly,

a man may have a heart murmur but it may be due to a congenital lesion that obviously has never caused trouble. If his symptoms are all those of worry or a little stroke or a depression the murmur must be disregarded.

In many a case, for want of something better, the patient's physician grasps at what might be called "diagnostic straws": little harmless peculiarities or normal variations from the average. Often he makes much of a basal metabolic rate around minus 12 per cent, a hemoglobin reading of 75 per cent, a blood sugar value of 75 mg. per 100 cc., a systolic blood pressure of 98 mm., a low-lying kidney or stomach or colon, large tonsils, a small uterine myoma, or a long vermiform appendix, none of which findings are important or outside the range of normal.

Ranges of normal should be well known. Every so often I am distressed to learn that some internist or even some teacher of medicine was so naive as to treat a tense, nervous little woman for hypothyroidism because her basal metabolic rate was reported as minus 15 per cent. If that were logical then I should be taking treatment for gigantism because I am some 5 inches taller than the average native-born American. It would seem as if every physician should know that for every bodily measurement there must be a certain range of variation in which the figures are normal. These ranges should be well established, well publicized, and well known to all of us, but actually they are not well known, and few men have ever taken the trouble to work them out and publish them. For lack of such standards, many wrong diagnoses are made, and we physicians often give long treatments for what is normal.

I know that occasionally I get concerned about some laboratory measurement that seems to me to be too high or too low, and I may even propose to treat it. But when I discuss the matter with one of my laboratory colleagues, he says, "Of late we have so often been finding that degree of variation which you mention that we have decided it is within the range of normal; I would forget it."

A somewhat high leucocyte count. It should be remembered that fatigue and excitement can cause the leucocyte count to go up to even 15,000. Often if a second count is taken after the patient has rested, it will be found to have dropped to 5,000 or 6,000. Rarely I see a patient with a white count as high as 18,000 and no sign of serious disease. Expert hematologists tell me that such counts must sometimes be ignored, especially when the differential count and smears are normal, the blood sedimentation rate is low and the patient's symptoms are those of a neurosis.

Albumin in the urine. At a large clinic where many patients travel long distances to get an examination, many of the nervous men and women will be found on the first day to have a little albumin in the urine. Later, after they have rested, the urine will be normal. I suspect that this temporary albuminuria is of little significance. It certainly does not mean the presence of serious renal injury.

The need for repeating and checking questionable laboratory reports. Obviously, a measurement should always be repeated when the result does not fit with the symptoms or the other findings, and sometimes it should be repeated and checked even when it *does* support beautifully what at first glance appeared to be the logical diagnosis.

To illustrate: When one day a man came with a pulse rate of 130 beats a minute and several nervous complaints, I did not object when my assistant ordered an estimate of the basal metabolic rate, but I told him I much doubted if he was dealing with a case of hyperthyroidism. Why? Because the man was evidently a "screwball"; his hand was cool, his eyes were not prominent, his skin was not red, his neck was not full, he had no tremor, his eyes were not blinking, he did not have the fidgets, he was not perspiring, and he said he slept well; he had no excessive appetite, he had no diarrhea, and he had not lost weight.

Next day, when the report came back +35, my assistant thought he had me, but I asked the man if, when they put the mask on his face, he had gotten an acute attack of the "let-me-outs." He said he surely had, and the attendant reported that the test was not satisfactory. The next three reports were +5, —5, and —12 per cent. In the meantime I noted that as the man got to know me his pulse dropped to 85 beats a minute, and when his wife took it as he woke in the morning it was 60 beats a minute. Everything then showed that the pulse of 130 beats on the first day had been due purely to apprehension. The man's real trouble was that he was a borderline psychotic.

In the last twenty years we physicians have come to accept laboratory reports so unhesitatingly that it seldom occurs to many of us to question them and to say "This one must be repeated because it does not fit with the history or the results of the other examinations." For instance, one Saturday noon a stocky, ruddy-faced man, who had gone through a clinical check-up just to keep his wife company, was leaving for home with all his reports excellent except the hemoglobin reading which was 48 per cent. His red cell count was 5,000,000 and his differential count was normal. An assistant, accustomed to accept unquestioningly the reports of a usually very reliable laboratory staff, put down "secondary anemia" and prescribed some iron. But when I saw the man I said, "No, there must be something wrong; let us check the hemoglobin," and I called the chief of laboratories and asked him to look into the matter personally. In a few minutes he telephoned to say that the reading was 98 per cent. He could not guess what had gone wrong with the first test. Perhaps a girl had looked away for a minute and had lost some blood out of her pipette, or she had written a 4 when she meant a 9. I have run into a number of remarkable cases in which a patient received a most frightening diagnosis because a laboratory report was copied wrongly into the record. The sad feature is that an internist failed to note that the report as copied did not fit with the results of other tests.

One of my favorite stories to show the type of trap that Mother Nature sometimes sets for us physicians when we are not careful is that of the patient who went to a prominent teacher of medicine with the complaint of dysentery. The professor immediately sent him to the laboratory for a study of the stools, and when the report came back "amebiasis" the diagnosis appeared to have been made. But two courses of amebecides failed to influence the so-called dysentery, and then the professor sent the man to me. On shaking hands with him my assistant immediately noted a very warm hand and a scary look in the eyes, and made the diagnosis of hyperthyroidism. The patient was perspiring excessively, and he had a little tremor. I asked him what he meant by dysentery and he said he was having some twelve bowel movements a day. When I asked what they were like, whether they were watery or bloody, he said, "No," they were just little hard round balls! Evidently the man did not have "diarrhea"; he was just so nervous that he went to the toilet frequently. His basal metabolic rate proved to be $+65$ per cent, and a few days later, when a little highly toxic adenoma of the thyroid gland was removed, he was well.

It is distressing when, several times a year, I see a sprightly, vivacious, wide-awake, quick-thinking and quick-moving, thin little woman with a letter from her physician saying that her trouble is that she has a basal metabolic rate of -35 per cent. For a time he treated her for myxedema but then he was puzzled because she only got worse and more jittery. One must wonder how an able internist could have failed to see instantly that this hard-working woman could not possibly have had a basal metabolic rate so low. He should never have accepted the report from the laboratory. He should have sent her right back for more estimates, preferably by another and an abler technician. The fact that the woman could not stand thyroid substance should also have told the physician that she was not hypothyroid. But apparently no one had ever taught him to think about such things. When I sent the woman for several tests, the reports all showed normal figures. Every year I see several persons with such obviously wrong diagnoses of myxedema, and the sad fact is that good physicians accepted them without question.

After puzzling for years over the reason for these often-seen rates of —35 per cent, I got the answer one day from a young physician who, on joining a clinic, was asked by his Chief to find out why so many healthy-looking, wide-awake persons in the community had a basal metabolic rate of —35 per cent. In all the cases the test had been carried out by a certain laboratory girl. On examining her closed circuit machine the physician found that the soda lime that removes the carbon dioxide was ancient and exhausted and useless. When asked why she hadn't noticed this and put in a new canister, the girl looked surprised and admitted that she had never known what the thing was there for, and could not remember ever having been told that from time to time it would have to be renewed! Doubtless many other girls all over the country are making the same mistake.

Incidentally, it is not widely enough known that many frail women have a basal metabolic rate around —17 which is normal for their weak bodies, and is not due to any disease of the thyroid gland; at least these patients will not be helped by the taking of thyroid substance.

Laboratory reports can be wrong. As I have been saying, I often marvel at the way in which even an able internist will accept the report of a test made by some perhaps unknown laboratory girl as if it were Holy Writ. The doctor may know that his own measurements and judgments are fallible; he knows that if he measures the blood pressure on each of several days he will get different figures; but it never occurs to him that if that unknown girl were to make several counts from drops, taken from one pipetteful of red blood, she would get different figures, ranging perhaps from 3,500,000 to 4,500,000 cells. The range of these figures would be due partly to the inherent error of the method and largely to the error of the girl.

Often such a girl, after leaving high school, goes into a laboratory and there picks up the several commonly used technics. If, thereafter, she does a certain limited type of work, if she does it all day long, and especially if she works under the supervision of a good clinical pathologist who can straighten her out when she gets into difficulties, all may go well. If daily she does many estimates of, let us say, blood calcium, her results will probably be accurate, but if, without supervision, she works in a small city for one or two physicians, and is called on to estimate a blood calcium only a few times a month, her error may be so large as to make her results of no value.

Worse yet, if, while working alone, she runs into difficulties, she may not be able to straighten herself out. For years she follows a routine long after she has forgotten why she goes through the several steps. I had this shown me clearly one day years ago when my laboratory girl,

almost in tears, begged me to help her with her Wassermann tests: For
days they had not come out right. A glance at her controls showed that
her salt solution was laking the blood cells. The roentgenologic
technician next door had borrowed her liter graduate and had left
developer in it. The astounding fact was that the laboratory girl did
not seem to know what her controls were there for, or at any rate,
what they showed did not register in her brain. Evidently she set up
controls, not to control her work but because she had been taught to
do Wassermanns that way!

Some forty years ago, when I was teaching clinical pathology, I
used to be asked sometimes to check up on some physician's laboratory
girl who had been reporting the finding of, let us say, malarial plasmodia in the blood of a man who had a big leucocytosis and evidently
an abscess somewhere. I would find that what she had thought were
plasmodia were granules of dirt. Similarly, her "amebas" in the stools
proved to be globules of oil or bits of vegetable tissue. She had not
been trained well enough to work alone.

Mistakes due to copying records wrongly. As I said, a few pages
back, every so often I see a patient who has been scared "half to death"
and caused to spend large sums of money on re-examinations simply
because some girl *copied* a laboratory report wrongly. For instance, I
recently saw an apparently healthy man frantic with fear because, after
an extensive overhauling, his physician had told him that with a blood
sedimentation rate of 118 mm. in a hour, he must have cancer scattered
all over his body. When I found a sedimentation rate of 9 mm. I asked
the home doctor to look up the original report. To his disgust he
found that in copying the figures onto the history sheet, a girl had
inadvertently put the one for the blood sugar in the space reserved for
the blood sedimentation rate! If the physician had only thought a bit
he might have suspected that there was something wrong, and checked
to find what it was. The thing that keeps worrying me is that today so
many men do not question the incongruous report enough to have it
repeated. They accept it, no matter how improbable and out of line
it may be.

Another patient came in terribly upset over a diagnosis of "potential
diabetes," made because, in copying the report of her blood sugar
reading onto the history sheet, a girl had reversed the figures and had
turned 117 mg. into 171 mg. One would have thought that, especially
with a woman who had a normal urine and no symptoms of diabetes,
her nationally eminent internist would have checked the finding before
saying anything about it; but he did not. He did not offer to check it
even after he saw that his diagnosis had horrified her.

It is not pleasant to have to record such happenings, but if the consultants who hear of them every little while do not raise a warning voice, who is going to?

The first reports after the patient comes may be affected by emotion. Occasionally I see a patient who, when she first came in, had albumin grade II in the urine. Next day it was gone. On the first day, also, she may have had a systolic blood pressure of 165 mm. of mercury. Next day it had dropped to 130 mm. Also, on the first day the pulse rate was 120 beats a minute and the leucocyte count was around 15,000 per cu. mm. Next day the figures were normal. The first day, under the influence of excitement, the woman had a temperature of 99.6° F. I have seen such temperatures as high as 102° F., purely because of anxiety. All these transitory effects of emotion should be recognized for what they are, so that they will not be looked on with alarm. They mean only that the doctor is dealing with a certain type of highly reactive patient.

Confusing reports on tests for syphilis. The test for syphilis will occasionally be confusing, due to anticomplementary bloods or recent vaccination for smallpox or something else. Then it is well, if possible, to get a set of tests. At the Mayo Clinic in puzzling cases the syphilologists order a Kline, a Kahn, a Hinton, and a Kolmer-Wassermann test.

Naturally, in doubtful cases the kindly physician will try to settle the question with the help of a syphilologist before saying anything to worry the patient. It may be a terrible thing to tell a worrisome young woman that the laboratory has reported a positive Wassermann test. After this, no amount of reassurance may ever make her feel clean again.

Disastrous consequences from a too ready acceptance of a laboratory report. Occasionally one sees a patient who is going to lose his or her life because a physician thoughtlessly accepted a laboratory report. For instance, I remember a woman with a cancer of the rectum who was treated too long for a laboratory diagnosis of amebiasis. A man with a cancer of the rectum was treated too long for a roentgenologic diagnosis of duodenal ulcer.

Whenever specific treatment for amebiasis or a Sippy type of treatment for supposed ulcer fails to do any good, the physician should immediately repeat his tests and take a better history; it is probable that his first diagnosis was wrong.

The poor interpretation of roentgenologic reports. Wrong diagnoses are based sometimes on poor interpretations of roentgenograms by men who are handicapped either by an inadequate training and experience, or else by a fear of losing the good will and referred business of physicians if they often fail to make positive diagnoses. They are afraid to keep reporting "negative thorax," "normally functioning gallbladder," and "normal stomach, duodenum, terminal ileum, and colon." They fear that if they do this the doctor will think that they haven't looked hard enough, or that they are not helpful enough, and hence most roentgenologists write a couple of pages about minor variations from normal which, if the referring physician wishes, can be used as diagnoses, and especially as a basis for ordering an operation. Instead of saying simply, "Normally functioning gallbladder," the roentgenologist writes something like this: "Large gallbladder that fills with the dye. No stones seen but there are suggestive shadows. There probably are adhesions to the duodenum. The organ empties slowly and not as completely as it should. Possible cholecystitis."

Reports of a slowly emptying gallbladder are unwise and unfortunate because usually all that happened was that the dye went out of the gallbladder and down into the jejunum whence much of it was reabsorbed and sent back through the liver and into the gallbladder. This phenomenon is normal and to be expected, and it is not a sign of disease. Even when a nonfunctioning gallbladder with stones is reported it may have to be disregarded if the patient's symptoms are all those of a neurosis or psychosis.

Reports of duodenal stasis, or of a filling or nonfilling or slowly emptying or retrocecal appendix are bad because they often are used to impress a psychotic patient with the need for an appendectomy. Reports of adhesions, ptosis, or a spastic colon similarly are unwise and often harmful.

Roentgenologists, I think, are unwise in reporting as a duodenal ulcer some spasm or deformity in the cap. When no crater is seen, the roentgenologist might do well to report only "deformity of the cap," which is really all he saw. In many a case, if there is no history of ulcer the physician had better disregard the roentgenologist's report and keep on trying to make a diagnosis.

A small hernia through the diaphragm should commonly be disregarded unless the patient's symptoms are typical of such a lesion. Often the doctor should be able to see that a small hernia cannot produce a neurosis with distresses spread widely throughout the body. Diverticula of the duodenum are common and usually symptomless. They should practically never be operated on. In the course of thirty years I picked one for operation because it retained food for so long a time, but its removal did not help the woman's diarrhea. This was probably due to some neurosis. Diverticulosis of the colon should be ignored, and certainly this condition should never be confused with diverticulitis. Even writers of textbooks sometimes get the two conditions confused. One is a common and harmless accompaniment of age, and the other is a rare and serious inflammatory condition.

Many a patient brings me a report of a wide aortic arch or "beginning aneurysm." This was needlessly alarming because subsequent examinations show only a harmless torsion of the aorta. Calcification of the thoracic and abdominal aorta does not seem to produce symptoms.

Achlorhydria. Even in the case of a patient with indigestion or diarrhea, the discovery of achlorhydria is seldom helpful, and rarely can one ascribe the presenting symptoms to this failure of secretion. One in four persons past sixty years of age has no acid, and most of them have a good or a fair digestion. I often tell a man that the atrophic and senescent changes in his stomach are probably just as injurious to his health as are the similar changes in his scalp which resulted in the loss of much of his hair!

Gastritis. Now that the gastroscope is being used so widely, and changes are being found in the gastric mucosa of many persons, the physician will often be tempted to ascribe all the patient's indigestion to a diagnosed gastritis. But especially when the changes are slight, it is doubtful if they are producing symptoms, and the physician had better not wash his hands of further responsibility for the diagnosis. Further study may reveal a much better diagnosis than gastritis.

A poor interpretation of an electrocardiogram. As I point out in the chapter on cardiac neuroses, many bad mistakes are being made today because of an effort to read serious disease into almost every electrocardiogram made. Many doctors do not seem to know how many variations from the textbook type of record can be due to the shape of the body, or to hypertension, or to the taking of digitalis.

No one but a cardiologist can hope to know all the fine points of diagnosis from electrocardiograms, but everyone should learn enough so as not to scare the patients with his readings of their records. In cases of doubt, he will do well to base most of his opinion, as the cardiologist does, on a history that shows how good or bad a cardiac reserve the man has. In other words, the important point is that the patient can or cannot exercise without getting pain.

Heart murmurs. As every physician should know, many of the heart murmurs that are heard, especially at the first visit when the patient is nervous and excited, are functional in nature. When the cardiac reserve is obviously good, so that the person can exercise vigorously without distress, it is best not to say anything about a slight murmur. To do so may be only to give the patient a troublesome neurosis.

A low blood pressure. In most cases a low blood pressure should be ignored and not treated. If it had any significance one would expect the patient to feel some dizziness or faintness on long standing, or on changing suddenly from a stooping or supine position to a standing one. The points to remember are (1) that many healthy persons have a pressure as low as 90 mm., and (2) that a pressure of 100 mm. is excellent and often indicative of a long life to come.

A low blood sugar. For a while it was fashionable to blame feelings of fatigue or faintness on a low blood sugar of perhaps 75 mg. per 100 cc., but experts today who have seen and treated persons with cancer of the islands of Langerhans assure me that all but a very few of these so-called low blood sugars are without significance; they are not due to disease of the islets; they do not account for the patient's symptoms, and they should be ignored. The measurement of blood sugar should be repeated before anything is said to the patient about the first low reading.

The symptoms of true hyperinsulinism are generally definite and severe: The patient is in a serious condition, and his wife may have to sit by him all night to give him sugar. Experiments on man have shown that symptoms of wooziness usually do not appear until the blood sugar has been lowered to 50 mg. or so. In most cases one can tell from the history that the patient hasn't hyperinsulinism because he does not get his distress in the early morning when his blood sugar is at its lowest, and he often feels bad within an hour or two after a meal when the blood sugar is up. Furthermore, he may get perfect relief from a cup of black coffee or a tablet of aspirin, and this tends to rule out hyperinsulinism.

A low blood calcium. Only rarely does the commonly made diagnosis of a low blood calcium stand up under investigation. Usually two or three estimates made in a good laboratory show that the first report was probably erroneous. But even when the report is a little low, this finding usually has nothing to do with the patient's illness, and it can be ignored. Figures as low as 8.6 mg. may be normal.

A myomatous uterus. As I point out in the chapter on gynecology, myomas of the uterus are so commonly found, and are so often unassociated with symptoms, that only occasionally, as when they cause flooding and anemia, or when they are growing rapidly or to a large size, need they be removed.

Retroversion of the uterus. As time passes, less and less attention is being paid to the position of the uterus in the pelvis, and fewer and fewer suspension operations are being done. Hence it is that a retroversion should probably never be used as an explanation for all the pelvic and other distresses of a frail woman who menstruates with difficulty or fails to conceive as she would like to do.

The wisest clinician knows what can and should be ignored. One of the surest signs of maturity and wisdom in a clinician is his ability in many cases to disregard the organic disease that has been found during an examination and to continue looking for something more important. I remember an unhappy, weepy woman who was full of organic diseases, none of which accounted for her symptoms. She had a moderate hypertension without symptoms. She had gallstones in a well-functioning gallbladder and no symptoms. She had some kidney stones but they were embedded in the kidney tissue and were not producing symptoms. She had a slightly increased basal metabolic rate, but since the removal of much of her thyroid gland by her home surgeon had not helped any, my assumption was that the elevated rate was due to nervousness and hypertension. She had some myomas in the uterus but they were silent. She had a chronic urethritis grade 1 but since this was likely only to get worse with treatment the urologists said it should be ignored.

Why, then, did the woman suffer from much nervousness, aches all over her body, insomnia, and great feelings of weakness? Because her husband, having become fed up with her complaining, had decamped with a younger and merrier woman! I did not know of any medicine that could be given to the patient to cure this sort of trouble, so I gave none.

What an abnormality cannot produce. The wise physician should know not only what symptoms a certain disease can produce but also what it cannot produce or is most unlikely to produce. As I look back on the mistakes of my medical youth I am appalled to think how, when recently out of college, I would try to ascribe all of a woman's many neurotic symptoms to a little ventral hernia, a torn cervix, a myomatous or retroverted uterus, ptosis of her stomach, or colon, or kidney, a few diverticula of the colon, a "mucous colitis," "achlorhydria," a few amebas in the stools, a sacralized fifth lumbar vertebra, or a slight "anemia." I am so glad that gradually I came to see how healthy some persons could be with these "diseases," and hence how reluctant I should be in using them as diagnoses. I can remember how impressed I was one day when a woman with bleeding hemorrhoids was found to have a hemoglobin reading of 50 per cent. I asked repeatedly if she did not feel weak or tired or dizzy, but she said, "No, absolutely not. I do all my own housework and washing, and I could not feel better!" That day I learned that I could not safely blame all of a woman's distresses on a hemoglobin reading of, let us say, 75 per cent as so many doctors do today.

Unfortunately, in college no one had ever taught me what certain abnormalities would not do, or how commonly they are found in the case of persons who have no symptoms, or how futile often it is to treat them. Gradually I had to learn these things by observing persons who had certain "defects" but not a symptom to go with them.

Sometimes when I get a letter from a physician who is satisfied that he has explained all of the many nervous complaints of a psychopathic woman by finding a few amebas in her stools, I wish I could show him the husky Mexican rancher, never sick a day of his life, who went through an examination just to please his wife. When, in his stools, there were found enormous numbers of amebas of all kinds, together with many eggs of hookworms, round worms, Strongyloides, and whipworms, I quizzed him again and again but could get no history of his ever having had indigestion, diarrhea, abdominal discomfort, or poor health. Such cases should be well remembered because they show (1) how much "disease" a man can have without ever getting symptoms, and (2) how unwise it is to try to blame all of a person's constitutional inadequacy on a few parasites in the bowel.

Many persons with marked abnormalities have no symptoms. Often when I see a neurotic or psychopathic patient whose illness and discomforts are all supposed to be due to a disturbance in the function of the glands of internal secretion, to intestinal autointoxication, a disturbance in hepatic function, a mild anemia, hypertension, or poor pelvic organs, I hesitate, and I look further, because I remember the hundreds of persons I have seen who had marked disturbances in the glands of internal secretion, or severe constipation, or a big hypertension, and still no distress of any kind. I can remember persons with acromegaly, Fröhlich's syndrome, eunuchoidism, early complete hysterectomy, a big rubbery goiter, parathyroid disease, slight Addison's disease, and diabetes who felt well and kept at work. Evidently, disease of the glands of internal secretion does not always produce feelings of ill health. I have known strong healthy women whose bowels moved only once in ten days; and I have known men with an old healed cirrhosis of the liver and a dye retention grade III who, for years, had no indigestion or feelings of illness.

Slight abnormalities that may not be producing the local symptoms. Sometimes a specialist will report a slight abnormality but he may warn that it is probably of no significance or not worth treating. For instance, a fretty, fussy woman of fifty often complains of some frequency of urination and some burning, and the cystoscopist reports a chronic urethritis grade I. He tells the woman to leave it alone. I remember an athletic strongly built woman who had cystoscopy performed because of a few red blood cells in her urine. She was found to have a chronic urethritis grade II. Although her urethra was twice as red and granular as it is in most of the fussy complaining women, she had no symptoms from it, probably because she was not hypersensitive.

It is a case like this that the wise clinician makes special note of and tries never to forget because it can teach him so much.

Part III

Causes of Neuroses and Psychoses

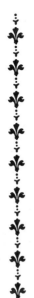

CHAPTER 8

*Common Causes of Neuroses
and Minor Psychoses*

THE MAIN PREDISPOSING CAUSE of neuroses and minor psychoses seems to be a hereditary and inborn tendency to get nervous, to worry, and to adjust poorly to life. On top of this predisposition come such things as strain, overwork, unhappiness, anxiety, grief, dissatisfactions, and physical illness, all of which can bring out the latent tendency. The type of reaction that comes with strain depends much on the type of man or woman that was there to begin with. One must remember that it is the poorly welded ship that breaks up and founders in a storm. In the Armies it was found that the recruits with poor nervous systems broke down at the induction centers while those with strong nervous systems broke only after much battle fatigue.

William Barrow found that worry over business, or dissatisfaction with it, seemed to account for the nervous troubles of some 25 per cent of his men patients. Some did not have a good enough nervous system to carry much responsibility, and some could not stand taking risks and losses, as many businessmen have to do.

A man's uncertainty about his status in his company. A frequent source of distress among the millions of men who work for others is uncertainty as to their status. They are not sure that they are getting by, or that their work is satisfactory, or that their job is secure. Most men would be much happier if occasionally the boss would give a pat on the back and say, "You're doing fine and I'm pleased with you and your work. You are of value to the firm." As it is, often a man's only contacts with the "old man" come when he is "called on the carpet" to be scolded for something. This is bad enough for the smaller men in an organization, but even executives are often made to feel insecure and unhappy, especially when a new president or general manager has just come in—some Pharaoh who knows not Joseph. The new manager is likely to have his own friends whom he wants to advance, and then a man who sees his chances of promotion lost may sit down and quit, or may worry himself into an illness.

Many an executive is unhappy and inclined to get neurotic because never in his years of service in his company was he ever made to feel that he "belonged." Perhaps his associates never forgave him for having been brought in from another company and placed over them or alongside of them. He never knew what day some of these men would gang up on him and either ease him out or force him out, or make him so unhappy he'd have to quit. For instance, an able professor was imported to head and strengthen a weak department in a university. Although he was a kind and generous man who tried hard to make friends of his new associates, they quietly thwarted him in so many ways that he eventually lost his health and resigned.

Frustrations in business. Occasionally, the neurosis of an able executive is due to the fact that, although his technical skill has done much to build up his company, he has constantly to struggle for survival with a few old big stockholders who have little sympathy with his research laboratories and his new products. They want dividends. Other managers of businesses have admitted that their insomnia, their fatigue, and their habit of waking at 2 A.M. with a panic of extrasystoles and loud belchings were due to the fact that they were being constantly harried, thwarted, and told what to do by some stupid man or woman who happened to have inherited the business. In many cases the offender was the widow of the man who built up the company. Knowing little about the industry, she kept coming in to tell the manager what to buy and not to buy until he was nearly crazy. Or, all the annoyance was coming from the woman's good-for-nothing playboy of a son who occasionally came in to raise Cain about things which he did not understand.

Many businessmen are much worn down by lawsuits, labor troubles, government regulations, and government interference in their business. As the president of a great company once said to me, "I hardly work at manufacturing any more; I just struggle with officials for the bare privilege of staying in business. Because my company used to make big money they look on me as a malefactor."

The causes of disease that interest many psychiatrists. Many a patient who has been to a psychiatrist in the last few years has told me that the doctor immediately began asking about psychic and sexual traumas in childhood. Sometimes he kept this up for days, showing that his main hope of explaining the person's psychic troubles lay in uncovering early sexual fantasies and perhaps an Oedipus complex. As one woman said, "I didn't see much sense in that: I could have told him in two minutes that if only my husband would quit drinking I could soon get my grip again." Another woman who went to a psychiatrist wrote that for weeks he had asked her about her earliest memories of sex. "But finally he gave up and accepted the obvious fact, which you know, namely that I get my diarrhea when my unloved husband comes home from a trip and makes me all upset."

There is no doubt that a trying and unhappy childhood with poor training in fortitude, self-control, and unselfishness has done much harm to millions of persons. But we must always remember that some of the children in a bad home can have inherited those tendencies to psychic disease which, in one or both parents, caused the home to be a hell.

Some highly possessive and foolish mothers bring up their sons with the hope that they will never marry but will stay on in the home as gigolos, with all their affections fixed on "Mom." When the young man begins to show an interest in some girl the mother tries to break up the affair, and if she fails in this she tries later to break up the marriage. She goes often into the boy's home and does everything she can to keep him more deferent to her and her wishes and needs than to those of his wife.

Similarly, she may cling to her daughters, trying to keep them like little girls, dependent on her. She will keep buying all their clothes and directing their lives, and often she will break up one love affair after another until the girls are left, hopeless, on the matrimonial counter.

However, as I note in the chapter on heredity, often in a family of such a matriarch one finds one son or daughter who refused to be dominated, and did not become neurotic. Everything depends on the size of the individual's share of the bad nervous inheritance. The child who is much like the psychopathic mother may go under and develop a neurosis, while the one who much resembles a stable father lets his mother's demands and injunctions go in one ear and out the other, until eventually he leaves the home, unscathed.

The great importance of recent strains. Doubtless, if psychiatrists cared to glance through this book, many would feel that I have been too superficial in blaming most neuroses on *recent* strains, and in paying little attention to childhood traumas, old resentments, and aggressive feelings. I have not gone into these modern psychiatric theories, partly because I am not so impressed with their importance as with the importance of recent or constant strains, and largely because I doubt if the physicians for whom I am writing would be much interested in the theories that now interest so many psychiatrists. I do not doubt that many of the studies they are making will in time bear fruit. I do not question that many Freudian theories have a basis and some usefulness. The point I would make is that as yet these things cannot much interest the non-psychiatrist, and to him they do not seem to be responsible for most of the nervous troubles which he sees. He can never be expected to go deeply into the psychic processes of the fairly sane patients whom he sees every day, and he will never go deeply into the mental processes of the psychotic type of person whom the psychiatrist has to treat.

I was interested recently in reading a psychiatric study of the personality of patients suffering from ulcerative colitis to see how several good psychiatrists went at the problem. They investigated at length each patient's personality, apparently ignoring the problems that had overwhelmed the poor fellow from time to time during the course of his illness. Personally, I would be more interested in recent strains such as the public Ph.D. examination or the campaign for senatorship which sent to their deaths two of my patients who previously had recovered well, one from sprue and the other from chronic ulcerative colitis.

Neuroses dependent on the person's attitude toward health. Most important in producing neuroses seems often to be the individual's attitude toward his health and that of members of his family. Some persons are not much concerned about health and are not fearful when they fall ill; others, with even a little cold, would like to call several physicians and perhaps go into a hospital and get penicillin. Some have a great fear of death and a great and almost constant presentiment of disaster. Some never take medicine while others take several kinds of pills every day of their lives.

That feelings of good health or ill health reside in the core of the personality was called to my attention years ago by that keen clinician, Emanuel Libman. He told of an old woman who, after telling him that she had a headache, a backache, palpitation, missing beats, heartburn, a pain in her stomach, belching, biliousness, hot flushes, a soreness in her bladder, piles, and varicose veins, said, "And I, myself, I don't feel so good either!" She evidently had sensed that there is a difference between the external aches and pains and discomforts and pinpricks of life, and the feelings of health or ill health that reside in the very core of a person's being.

The intensity of some persons' fears. Those of us physicians who have not inherited the tendency to go into panics of fear about disease or death can have no idea of the intensity of the storms of worry that often go sweeping through the minds of many of our patients. Daily these persons see themselves dying a horrible death from cancer or heart disease, such as some close relative or business associate has recently had. Others live in constant expectation of dropping dead with a stroke or a coronary attack. Others are just vaguely but painfully apprehensive. Thus, I remember an excitable and temperamental man, about to be operated on for a simple hernia, whose surgeon was called out of town. Because of this the patient was put on the list of one of the surgeon's colleagues. Although, again and again, the reason for this change was explained to the man, he went from one panic into another, feeling sure that the real reason for the switch must have been that such an awful cancer had been found in him that only the oldest surgeon in the group dared tackle the job. To persons with such a temperament every little contretemps like this will assume the proportions of a major tragedy. As a very excitable Latin woman said to me after having been around Rochester for a week, "How wonderful it would be if we, in my country and my family, could live unemotionally and peacefully as you North Americans do. In my family we are all violent persons who, with any little annoyance, start screaming and cursing and tearing our hair." And yet they were charming people to meet.

Different reactions to the threat of death. The difference between the reactions of individuals when they face death was impressed on me once as I watched how two physicians faced the conviction that they must soon die with cancer. The first one, who had good reason to believe that he had a sarcoma in his mediastinum, quietly put his affairs in order and went about his work as if nothing had happened. The only two persons to whom he spoke of his expected early demise were his lawyer and his physician. He did not lose an hour out of his night's sleep, and he paid little attention to his pain. He remained the same cheery fellow he had always been. The other man, suspecting wrongly that he had a cancer of his stomach, went to pieces nervously; he was unable to sleep, he gave up his practice, and for a year lived in an agony of fear, weeping on the shoulders of any and all who would stop and listen.

The effects of suggestion. A high percentage of the illnesses seen, especially in members of certain racial groups, are due to suggestion. Usually what happens is that a relative or business associate dies rather suddenly from heart disease or cancer. Then the person starts going from one physician to another, terribly frightened and anxious, often with a distress localized about the spot where the relative or friend had his pain.

For instance, and this is a common story, a big strong man was well enough until one day a friend dropped dead on the golf course. This upset him so that thereafter he could not go to this club without getting an attack of what he thought was angina pectoris. The world is full of such persons who are constantly suffering because of suggestions they get from the daily paper or the movies or some radio program or from a physician.

Hypersensitiveness, over-reactivity, and lack of stoicism. Much of the nervous suffering of many persons appears to be due to hypersensitiveness and over-reactivity, perhaps with a lack of stoicism (see Chapter 13). Some of the persons who suffer from hypersensitiveness complain little because they have in their character a valuable element of stoicism. They do not fuss or complain; they acquiesce, and hence do not develop a neurosis. Others who have no stoicism complain bitterly and become ill. Others become ill because of a great fear of pain and its possible late results. Those who do not fear pain can stand an immense amount of it without becoming neurotic. Like Robert Louis Stevenson, they can take a lifetime of it and every day keep at work.

Inner conflicts. Often a person breaks down nervously because of secret inner conflicts; he is like a house divided against itself. He may have conflicts between a spiritual and a carnal nature, or between inheritances derived from two different human strains or cultures. Thus, a man may be unhappy because the strongly religious tendency inherited from one fine ancestor is in constant conflict with a strongly sensual and animal nature derived from another ancestor. Perhaps all men and women at times feel some conflict between the saint and the anthropoid within them. Fortunate is the person whose four grandparents were pretty much alike in goodness and sanity and mental trends! Such a man may be spared many of the inner conflicts that rack and wear down the son of, perhaps, a merry playful Irish girl and a dour, silent, and deeply religious Scot.

Gamaliel Bradford said of John Randolph, of Roanoke, "He was perpetually at odds with his own soul." He was a maze of contradictions; a slaveholder who loved liberty, an aristocrat who loved democracy. He "kept up a constant exhausting devouring quarrel even with himself." He liked to take long walks hoping "to tire out thought, if he could not get rid of it." He longed to escape, anywhere from the incubus that weighed him down.

Many persons are torn by feelings of inferiority or inadequacy. They fear failure and are afraid to tackle things. They fear to accept responsibility or to make decisions. Others are racked by a bad temper that can be controlled only with the greatest effort, or they are torn by violent likes and dislikes. Many are hurt and bitter all their days because of the feeling of racial discrimination, or early poverty, social inferiority, or a lack of opportunity to rise and get ahead.

Many are poisoned by frustrations, animosities, hatreds, resentments, and desires for revenge. Others are sad and ill because life has treated them so shabbily. Many are bitter against those who they feel have thwarted or cheated or robbed them, or stood in their way, or they are bitter against the upper classes or against men and women who had a college education.

Needless conflict with others. The wise person avoids conflict with others and avoids blowing up at them. Many persons ask the doctor if he doesn't think it is a good thing to blow up and in this way get anger and resentment out of the system. I always say, "No, don't blow up and don't lose your temper. You can easily get in the habit of doing this, and it is a bad form of selfishness. It is childish behavior. When you blow up and abuse, insult, and humiliate someone, you injure that person, perhaps a loved one, and this hurt reacts on you, the offender." I often marvel how a wife can retain much of her affection for a choleric husband who for years has been exploding violently and profanely at her every time she annoys him.

In my own case, I know that I can work all day without any feelings of fatigue if, as usually happens, I have no unpleasantness with anyone. If, however, someone does become offensive and manages to annoy me or hurt me, that afternoon I am very tired. It seems to me that a man would have to be extremely thick skinned and brutal to be able to bawl out several employees a day and not be hurt by it himself. One would think that the sullenness or dislike or hurt or enmity in the eyes of the injured employees should produce some distress in the man, and thereby add much to the strain of his day's work. Sometimes I can get a man to make an effort to stop bawling out his employees by getting him to see that this shoots his blood pressure up or makes a peptic ulcer much worse. I have seen many a patient whose blood pressure shot up 60 points after a tantrum.

How much a choleric man or woman adds to the strain of others! I will never forget one day, during World War II, when stocks of many things were low, listening in a store to a well-dressed middle-aged woman who was brow-beating a nice-looking saleswoman because she could not supply some item of merchandise. The saleswoman remained courteous throughout the tirade, as she had to, but this seemed only to further enrage the sadistic woman, until she left, saying she would see the manager and complain of poor service. As the saleswoman turned to wait on me, I saw tears in her eyes, and said a few words of sympathy. She said, "As it happens, it is especially hard to take today; I am a widow with three children; this morning when I left home one had a temperature of 104°. I left her with a neighbor who was to call a doctor and phone me his report. I have not heard yet and you can imagine how frantic I am." Whenever people ask me if it wouldn't be a good idea to spit out quickly the nasty ideas that come into their minds, I tell them this story.

Jealousy. Occasionally I see a woman with a neurosis due, in large part, to jealousy. Perhaps she is racked by jealousy of her husband's relatives or his friends, male and female, or even of her own children who, she thinks, compete with her for her husband's love. Often an older woman is jealous of her daughters-in-law and their places in the affections of her sons. Or a woman may be reduced to a nervous state by the constant jealousy, espionage, suspicion, and baseless accusations of a paranoid husband. Jealousy and envy of the honors that come to business associates rack the nerves of many a man, and add to the strain of his day's work. Jealousy also racks children as they compete for the love of a mother or father, or teacher; and later, it can nearly wreck adolescents as they come up against the problems of getting and holding a "steady."

Curiously, many a husband or wife who raises Cain because of jealousy, and perhaps is wrecking the marriage, will admit that his or her suspicions are practically without foundation, and are not really believed in. Some of these persons appear to be paranoid. In his book, *The Confessions of a Fool,* Strindberg tells how he drove his loving wife from him by insane and unfounded jealousy. In the cases of many persons jealousy is a fairly incurable disease. More fortunate persons are largely free of this curse, and suffer only occasional twinges.

Some persons are also much more envious than others are. Envy is such a common human trait that no one need feel ashamed if sometimes he feels a twinge, but he should feel ashamed of acting on it and trying to injure the person envied. Many businesses are wrecked by the feuds of executives who block each other from doing anything that might bring credit or a promotion to one of them.

Even a big executive will oftentimes be found squelching his ablest subordinate and pigeon-holing the good suggestions he makes, all for fear that the young man will get ahead and be promoted over him. Such efforts of mediocre men to hold their abler subordinates down are to be noted in many a business, in many a government office, and in many a university department. They account for much unhappiness, much loss in accomplishment, and much wastage of money and opportunity. Blessed is the department in which the Chief is such a fine and able and generous man that, instead of fearing his assistants, he keeps constantly giving them opportunities and praise, and building them up for promotion as if they were his own sons. Cursed is the department run by an incompetent nephew of someone whose main concern is not to be outdone by the men under him. Cursed is the idea of many labor bosses that no man must do more work in a day than is done by the most incompetent man in the group.

Strains due to the tension produced by certain types of work. Many tensions arise in trying types of work, especially those in which there is a constant need for watchfulness, as in banking or accounting. Men break down sometimes when life is speeded up, especially in the presence of turmoil, as in a stock exchange. There are turbulent occupations which certain persons should not attempt to follow, because they haven't the requisite type of nervous system.

Often a man's feelings of fatigue, or his tendencies to loaf, or to drink to excess, or his inability to learn the technics of his job, or his unhappiness and ill health are all due to his lack of interest in what he is doing, and his lack of joy or satisfaction in it. Fortunately, at last, personnel managers are now being trained to study these problems and to fit men into the right place for them. They also are trying to correct the evils that arise from the irritabilities, personal animosities, and stupidities of bosses and superintendents and supervisors.

Hard work alone will rarely make a neurosis or bring on a psychosis. That hard work alone rarely makes a neurosis has been proved by many a busy obstetrician or general practitioner or surgeon who, for years, has worked day and night without breaking down. Such a man, to do what he does, requires, first, an iron constitution, second, an ability to snatch a short nap at intervals during the day and night, and third, an ability to work without tension or anxiety or annoyance, taking up only one problem at a time and dropping it as soon as it is attended to.

Sadler has said that some persons appear to have been born nervously bankrupt: They are the constitutional inadequates who have slender margins of nervous safety. In them the slightest overdraft in the way of mental strain or overwork is likely to bring prostration. On the other hand, we see occasionally a man like Henry Kaiser who is born nervously rich, with such enormous energy that he can run several big businesses at a time.

There are certain types of work which, after some years, may bring a neurosis. They are occupations which keep a man on the job for long hours. I have already mentioned the general practice of medicine. The druggist with a store so small that he cannot afford a partner may work every day of the week from 7 in the morning until 10 at night. Another man who, at certain times of the year, does not take off his clothes for a week or more is the village mechanic who repairs tractors for the farmers who are in a hurry to plow or reap. Other hard workers are the men who run delicatessen shops or small grocery stores or shoe-repair shops, or corner tobacco shops. After years of overwork such men will come in with curious paresthesias, nausea, cardiospasm, or a numbness somewhere.

The human brain was not built to stand the strains of modern life. After having lived alongside primitive Kanakas in Polynesia and Indians in the mountains of Mexico, and after having observed their lazy ways of life, their joyous loafing, their utter unconcern for time, and their habit of going to bed at sunset, I marvel that we Americans, with much the same nervous system as the primitive person has, can drive at our work all day and late into the night. I doubt if the Great Designer ever intended the human brain to work so constantly or at such high pressure, and I marvel that so many persons can stand the grind as long as they do. I marvel that many a frail little woman can stand typing all day, or punching a comptometer, or making change in a store. I doubt if my brain could stand half a day of it. I used to wonder, also, how an old-fashioned cobbler could repair shoes all day and then work on far into the night.

It is the unusual event or task that upsets nervous persons. Most nervous persons have learned that they can get along fairly well with routine tasks and routine contacts; it is the unusual task, the unusual problem, and the unusual human contact that causes trouble. In the case of many a nervous woman, a guest in for dinner, a shopping trip, an automobile ride, a little sightseeing, or the very thought of starting on a journey is likely to bring a sick headache, a mucous colic, an attack of regurgitation, or a spell of insomnia.

I remember a tense nervous consultant who could have made much money going out into the suburbs on consultations, but he would not accept these calls because he had learned that such a trip always took much more out of him than a whole afternoon of routine work in his office. Darwin spoke often of the fact that he could stand a little work done quietly in his study or his garden, but a chat with visitors or a short trip to London would leave him a shivering, vomiting wreck.

Ways in which a person's nerves can break. Ross felt that there are three ways in which a person can respond to strain: one, by over-reaction; two, by under-reaction, or by failure to react at all; and three, by pretending, like a Christian Scientist, that the difficulty does not exist. Over-reaction gives rise to those symptoms which are commonly called neurasthenic; the patient is too anxious and fussy about his troubles. Under-reaction may be represented by hysteria. In this disease the patient seems to lie down and quit; he accepts his paralysis and does not worry about it or want to do anything to cure it.

Why nervous strain does not alway produce the expected disease. It has interested me that in hundreds of cases a bad psychic situation which might well have produced a peptic ulcer did not cause any such illness. A much-harried man may be found to have a free acidity of 90 units, he may have hunger pain in spells, he may have a typical intense, worrisome nature, and a trying administrative job, and he never develops an ulcer. Why doesn't he develop it? Probably because some gene was lacking in his inheritance.

Another man may be a short, stocky, thick-necked, red-faced, choleric master of industry who overworks, smokes too much, and loses his temper often, and yet he never gets the expected high blood pressure or apoplexy. Why not? Apparently because he did not get the necessary gene or genes. Or here is a highly temperamental and brilliant musician, a friend of mine, who saw most of his relatives beaten and abused and done away with by the Nazis. He himself was beaten and left for dead with a fractured skull, but somehow survived and later got away, going through many hairbreadth escapes until he reached safety. He might well have gone insane, or developed a bad neurosis, but he didn't. Why not? He must have lacked some of the necessary genes. He remains a strong-minded and able person. Or, here is a fine normal woman, happy in her life with her husband. As a little girl she was sexually attacked and injured and terribly frightened by a criminal. Today she ought, perhaps, to be highly neurotic and sexually frigid, but she isn't. Why not? Apparently she lacked the genes to become neurotic.

Why certain patients choose certain diseases for worry. Often a little questioning will show why an overly worrisome patient thinks he has heart disease rather than cancer of the stomach or a brain tumor. As every physician knows who talks with his patients, many a man has good reason to fear disease of a certain type or in a certain organ: The weakness runs through the family, and the patient may have been shocked at seeing one relative after another die of it.

I remember a man who for years had suffered from a nervous breakdown. Physically, he seemed well, and nothing wrong could be found. He had been healthy until one day he was called to the telephone and told that his son, playing football, had been kicked in the head and was bleeding from a small scalp wound. On reaching the field he found the boy patched up and back in the game again, but, in spite of this reassurance, he went to pieces nervously, he fainted, and he never got back to work again. Now why was he so upset by this little accident which did not bother the boy? The answer appeared to be that years before, this man's younger brother had become epileptic after a blow on the head. For years my patient had slept in the same room with the boy, jumping up to hold him every time he woke with a convulsion. During those years the youth had come to feel such a horror of epilepsy and of blows on the head that when as a man he heard that his boy had been

hurt in this way he was overwhelmed with the conviction that here was
the eventuality that he had long feared. Curiously, after this shock, he
couldn't get his grip again, and I was unable to get him back to work.

Neurosis due to a sudden psychic shock. Other sudden psychic
shocks will sometimes produce a neurosis. For instance, a girl of nineteen complained of a poorly localized pain in the face which had defied
treatment by a number of specialists. Questioning revealed the fact that
the pain had come suddenly on a day when, coming home early from
school, she had burst into her mother's room and had found her in
bed with a man not her father. Dumbfounded and shocked and almost
hysterical, she sought out her father and received another shock when
he didn't seem to be concerned.

I soon found that the parents, cousins, had in their youth been talked
into a loveless marriage designed to keep much wealth in the family.
When they could no longer stand living together, they agreed to go
their separate ways sexually, but to keep the home going for appear-
ances' sake and for the sake of the girl who had been born to them.
When the girl saw that her parents were more to be pitied than censured,
she immediately got well. Another girl with a similar facial pain got
it when, at boarding school, she burst unannounced into the room of
a woman teacher on whom she had a crush, and found her in the arms
of a man.

Puzzlement over the morality of things done. Religiously well-
trained young persons, in their youth, are likely to feel that they can
easily tell right from wrong. To them, white is white and black is black.
They fail to note that commonly even the Supreme Court of the United
States divides 5 to 4 in attempting to decide certain matters of morality
and ethics.

Occasionally I see a woman who is upset because she cannot figure
out whether she is culpably immoral because of something she once did.
For instance, an attractive, highly intelligent woman was in a distressing
quandary because, although she had a wedding ring, she said she
realized she was a prostitute. What she had done was to marry a
wealthy drunk in order to get enough money to put her boy through
college. Many a minister would probably have told her that since she
had been married in church she was all right, but she knew better, and
this bothered her. Another woman was upset because, in order to put
her daughter through college, for several years she had helped to run
a fancy house of prostitution.

Compulsions. Some psychiatrists state that a compulsion neurosis
is due to some hostility. Actually, so far as I can learn, many of the
women with this trouble appear to be troubled because of an overconscientiousness and a great fear that they will do something that will

injure a loved husband or children. In some cases the trouble seems to stem from a tremendous feeling of responsibility, and in other cases it is probably just an expression of the family tendency to neurosis, or to strong feelings of religious duty.

Maladjustment due to inheritance of narrow religious ideas. After living as a boy in Polynesia, it has always interested me to see how the psychic traits, which in the early nineteenth century caused a man and his wife to leave the comforts of civilization and go to the South Seas for missionary work, have cropped out and distressed some of the members of the second, third, and fourth generations. Many persons do not realize that these things are inherited, but they are, just like any other trait. Once I took care of a great-grandson of one of these missionaries and was interested to note that the young man was being divorced by his wife because he rarely would have sexual intercourse with her. He thought the act was sinful if it gave any pleasure! It would seem more than a coincidence that his ancestors were reputed to have similar ideas.

The possible effect of chemical substances acting on the brain. As I mention elsewhere in this book, it is possible that some of the troubles that seem to arise in the nervous system are really due to chemical substances circulating in the blood. A number of biochemists have been searching for such substances, and it may be that some day a number will be found. Rather against the idea that they will be found is the fact, noted elsewhere in this book, that a nervous defect which shows up in one brother as manic-depressive insanity can show up in others as schizophrenia, feeble-mindedness, or epilepsy. It would seem that if in these families a specific toxin were affecting the brain, it ought usually to have a certain characteristic effect, such as one expects to see after the giving of alcohol, or opium, or marihuana, or an extract of the mescal button.

But then again, it must be admitted that alcohol makes one man gay and happy and talkative, another man sleepy and quiet, another one weepy, another violent and murderous, another surly and insulting and another overly generous. Perhaps, then, a metabolic toxin that makes one man depressed can make another shy or suspicious or violent.

That metabolic products from the suprarenal glands or other parts of the body may affect the brain was shown recently in the case of one of my depressed patients who, because of some arthritis, was given cortisone. In a few days she was out of her depression and feeling wonderfully well and gay.

That the chemistry of the brain can determine the behavior of living creatures is demonstrated not only by every drunken man in the gutter, but by those insects like the mud wasps, whose parents die before they are born. Because of this, all of their complicated life-behavior must be dependent on the many chemical ferments that make up their tiny genes: the genes which determine what they do, how they live, and how they prepare the food for the infant wasps which they will never live to see.

Neuroses due to living in an atmosphere of tension. Many a person has told me of a nerve-breaking strain due to living in an atmosphere of great tension between two other persons, such as husband and father-in-law. A woman patient of mine quickly became a wreck trying to live in the home of her sister. What distressed her was the feeling of tension between the sister and her mother-in-law. It was so great that no maid would stay in the house. Another old patient of mine wrote, "Mother came, and the efforts she and my brother-in-law make just trying to stay civil, can be sort of heard bumping all around the room! My head aches from the moment they greet each other until they part. I expect war to break out any moment, and will it be a war!"

NEUROSES PRODUCED BY PHYSICIANS WHO SAY
FRIGHTENING THINGS

Unless a physician is an optimist, usually accurate in his diagnoses and prognoses, always willing to assume the full responsibility that goes with telling a patient he is well and safe, and always guarded in his speech, he will often frighten his patients and cause them mental distress. He may even throw them into illness or fasten on them a neurosis. I know that, after forty years of trying to guard my tongue and to avoid saying things that will needlessly worry my patients, every so often I learn that I have badly frightened one of them.

If all people were sensible, and able to grasp and understand and accept what is told them it would not be so bad, but so many persons ignore all the cheerful words a physician says and pick up and cling to some little thing he said that could be twisted into something alarming.

Patients often misunderstand what is told them. We physicians need to watch what we say and how we say it because in spite of all the care we may take, some patients will misunderstand us. Thus, I remember an intense, intelligent woman who came years ago with what appeared to be a functional paralysis of one leg. I immediately got her out of her wheel chair and walking again, and during the days that followed, I tried to get her to see how, after years of overwork, strain, and undisciplined and unhygienic living, her nerves had started playing tricks on her. Neurologists, after a careful study, agreed with me that there was no organic disease of the spinal cord or the nerves, and they also reassured her. Evidently, we did not speak clearly enough because recently she told me that for years she has lived in terror because I left her with the impression that I thought she would soon become hopelessly paralyzed!

Patients black out during important interviews. At the last interview, when the doctor hands out the verdict, he must be particularly careful in his speech because at this time many anxious persons are so upset and fearful of bad news that they are in a confused mental state in which they do not appear to hear or understand much of what is said. Certainly they get things all mixed up. One would think that when told repeatedly that nothing wrong was found, and when shown the "negative" reports from the laboratories, they would be perfectly reassured; but often they are not. Many a time, after telling a woman with a sore colon that all she had was a lot of nervousness, I have had a relative come back to ask, "Why did you frighten my sister (or mother) half to death?" or, "Since you have now found a cancer, why are you not going ahead to try to get it out?"

As I said at the beginning of this chapter, a miserable habit these frightened, flustered, and abnormally worrisome patients have is that of disregarding the encouraging things the physician told them, and clinging to some sentence which they thought contradicted the others, and into which they could read the threat of death. Many seem to love to do this, and when we find them reacting in this way we can make the diagnosis of a certain type of psychopathy. A really normal person would not behave in this way.

As a physician grows older and more experienced he should become ever more skillful in avoiding the saying of things that the patient can twist into a threat of disaster. In his efforts to avoid such trouble many a physician becomes more and more taciturn and close-mouthed; when asked a question he ignores it or grunts, or walks away, and he tells his patients almost nothing. Unfortunately, this practice is far from satisfactory to patients, and it deprives them of all that information about their illness which they must have if they are to help themselves to get well and stay well.

As I point out in the chapter on handling patients, it is highly important that we physicians learn to talk to them in simple speech that they can understand. Then we are less likely to confuse them.

The problem of what not to tell a patient. As I say in Chapter 19, daily we physicians are faced with the problem of whether to tell a patient that he has a murmur, slurrings in his electrocardiogram, or some other little deviation from normal which might cause him to worry himself sick. If we knew that the thing would never be discovered or commented on in the future, most of us would never think of saying a word about it, but, today, many patients go again and again for complete examinations, and sooner or later, some man is likely to look with concern on what we thought so harmless that we failed to mention it. Then the patient will be all upset, with his faith in us gone. Commonly I do not mention to patients unimportant details that might cause worry. Instead of telling of a left ventricular preponderance and an inverted T in lead III I will say, "Your electrocardiogram is normal for your age," or "It looks good to me."

The writing of reports for patients. The question of what to say and not to say becomes more acute when, as commonly happens, we consultants have to write a report to the patient or to the home physician. In the report we may say that we do not believe that the few slight abnormalities found are producing any symptoms or that they have any significance; but the question is, will the patient or his physician agree to this? Sometimes they will not, and later, we may learn that the report caused much worry, much expense, much futile treatment, and even a useless operation.

Recently I heard from a woman who has long been treated by her doctor for a supposed myxedema and made toxic by the taking of much unneeded thyroid substance. I am somewhat responsible for her troubles because, years ago, I reported a basal metabolic rate of —12 per cent. I added that this was normal and to be ignored, but to the patient's way of thinking such a divergence from "normal" just had to represent disease. She worried about it, and she lost faith in my good sense and in the value of the examination I had given her; she thought I was careless and slipshod to disregard such a finding. As she said, she had to go elsewhere to get decent care, and, as a result, she felt I had treated her badly.

What a consultant often forgets is that commonly the home physician hands over to the patient the letter which was written with only the doctor's needs and understanding in mind. Because of this habit, the wise consultant will avoid writing anything that might hurt or anger or confuse or greatly worry a patient. If the doctor feels he must report harmless slurrings and notchings in an electrocardiogram he should add that these variations do not mean that the heart is diseased. In many cases it is kinder and safer to say simply that the heart was in good shape for the man's age and weight and amount of physical activity.

Often, when I see the distress I have caused a patient by reporting some slight deviation from the norm, I wonder if I should not vow never to mention such things again, and to accept the risk of someday being blamed. It doubtless would be kinder to let my reputation take care of itself, and to think first of the need for not scaring patients; but often it is hard to know what is best to do. I have, also, to guard the reputation of the institution in which I work.

The bad psychic results of disagreements as to diagnosis. One difficulty about medical opinions is that so many persons think the diagnosis of an Osler and that of a chiropractor can be balanced one against the other; the opinions are assumed to have about equal value. Or a patient will assume that the opinions of three chiropractors must outweigh that of one Osler. They say that seven students were being given a practical examination in a city hospital. After they had examined a patient the professor asked them how they would treat him. All said they would not operate. "That shows how wrong you are," said the professor, "I am operating on him tomorrow." "No, you are not," said the patient; "get me my clothes; 7 to 1 is enough for me!"

Oftentimes a worrisome patient will be all upset, and will be led to lose faith in the medical profession because one doctor will have nothing to do with the diagnosis made by another, or one will say, "You must be operated on immediately," while another will say, "You do not need an operation any more than I do."

For instance, one day a psychopathically worrisome woman of fifty years, having heard a popular lecture on cancer, went to the best-trained surgeon in her large city for a pelvic examination. He told her she had a tumor of the uterus which he was going to remove next morning because any day it might become cancerous. Frantic with worry, she started going from one physician to another. What upset her still more was that some of the men she saw told her indignantly that she had no tumor; others said she had a tumor of no significance, which needed no treatment, while others agreed that she had a tumor which should be operated on.

I tried to straighten her out by explaining that all the men who had given her the differing opinions were right according to their lights. What she had was the commonly seen hard fibrous uterus half a size too big, with a nubbin of muscle about 2 cm. in diameter near one cornua. As I said, some men might call this a tumor while others would not; some men might fear cancer while others would say that myomas so seldom become sarcomatous that the danger of leaving them in is much less than the danger of taking them out; some would believe in operating, while others would wait for the approaching menopause to shrink the uterus and put an end to the so-called tumor. My advice was to wait and stop worrying. The chances are that she did not take it. I imagine that some good salesman soon got her up on his operating table. Doubtless he cleared his conscience by saying, what was true, that that type of woman would never have any peace of mind again until the uterus was out.

The dangers of talking to an unrecognized psychotic. I remember a manic-depressive veterinarian whom I had turned over to a

psychiatrist in his home city. Because the veterinarian took an occasional glass of wine with his meals he one day was staggered by the
awful thought that he might have produced in himself an alcoholic
gastritis! Accordingly, he went to a prominent gastroscopist for an
examination. Unfortunately, the gastroscopist, all unconscious of the
fact that he was dealing with a mentally disturbed man, examined him
and told him that he had a superficial gastritis with one tiny bleeding
point. The words "bleeding point" sent the patient into a panic of
fear. He saw himself soon vomiting quarts of blood. He immediately
placed himself on a diet of nothing but milk, and soon he was almost
too weak to walk. When I saw him again he was in bad shape, and I
had to labor hard to get him straightened out. Interestingly, I could
do this better than could my friend the psychiatrist, because the veterinarian respected my opinion as to *stomachs*.

**Unwise and uncalled-for remarks made by interns, nurses, and
even physicians.** I remember a man who once traveled 2,000 miles
for an examination simply because one evening at a friend's house he
had a slight nosebleed. A young intern in the party, proud to show
off his new-gotten knowledge, said that he had recently seen a case of
nosebleed. The cause was an acute leukemia from which the patient
soon succumbed with a hemorrhage in his brain! With this information
the man was thrown into such a panic that I fear, with all my efforts
at reassurance, he is still going the rounds of internists and hematologists, getting his blood examined.

Much disease is produced by the incurable tendency of some nurses
to chatter, telling of all the patients they had who died, some "in this
very room," or "in that very bed, just before you came in!"

Sometimes, a physician, with a thoughtless remark, can wreck a
person's life. For instance, a fine woman was told by her garrulous
druggist that her dead husband had taken iodides that could have been
prescribed for syphilis. This upset her terribly, and caused her to start
going from one physician to another getting Wassermann tests. All
were negative, but still, after she had calmed down and become pretty
well reassured, she went to get "just one more." When it was reported
negative, the physician said, "Yes, but you know that a negative Wassermann is not positive proof that you haven't syphilis." This was the
cruelest thing he could have said, and after that the poor woman never
had a happy or carefree day.

The dangers in medical fads. Some of us physicians get patients
mixed up because we tag them with some favorite diagnosis with
which we are obsessed. A few of us are likely to find amebas in almost
every patient who comes in, while others of us find brucellosis, hyperinsulinism, allergy, or glandular deficiencies. I have known kindly, well-

intentioned men who built huge practices doing this sort of thing. Chronic complainers flocked to them when it got noised about that here was a doctor who quickly "found what was wrong after everyone else had failed or had diagnosed nervousness." The only trouble with this type of practice is that it does not permanently help neurotic or psychotic persons. Often it puts an idea into their heads that does harm, and is later very hard to get out. This sort of practice can make a man wealthy, but it ruins him intellectually and it makes him a laughing-stock among his fellows.

The terrible results of trying to play safe. Too many doctors hurt their patients by failing to give positive reassurance. They want to play safe. Following is an example of what an occasional physician does to a patient when he is too pessimistic, or too fearful of saying that a heart is normal, or too anxious to play safe. A fine musician, after years of practicing by day and working by night, one day got to the end of his rope, and felt as if he were going to collapse. Because, with this distress, he had a little feeling of oppression in his chest, his doctor decided it was a heart attack and rushed him to a hospital. There all the usual tests were negative. The electrocardiograms were normal, and everyone agreed that there had been no injury to the heart. But then a common mistake was made. The well-meaning family doctor, still influenced by his original hunch, decided to "play safe." Accordingly, he told the patient to stop work, to stop walking upstairs, and to give up all exercise, sexual intercourse, driving of his car, eating of meat, smoking, and drinking of the before-dinner cocktail. He told the patient, also, to move out of his home and into a one-floor apartment!

The impact of this discouraging regimen, with all its implications of serious disease, on the mind of a very tired and temperamental musician can be imagined. The man became depressed, and afraid almost to move. He lost all confidence in himself, and all hope for the future. When I saw him I had a hard time to get him back to work. It took a year and more of reassurance to give him back his confidence, his courage, and his old happy disposition. Fortunately, he eventually recovered, but still he is distressed at times, wondering why, if he did not have a coronary attack, he was told to be so careful.

The physician must guard his tongue. Obviously, every good and kindly physician must constantly be guarding his tongue, especially when dealing with a certain type of patient who seems to crave bad news. The physician should always guard his tongue if only to save himself from endless trouble and annoyance later. Just let him put a worrisome idea into a person's head and it may be years before he can get it out again. Thus, once, in a misguided moment, I let an anxious school superintendent with a little diarrhea know that Bargen's streptococcus had been found in his stools. He looked this up in a book and then had the horrors, being sure that he was soon going to die from chronic ulcerative colitis. That was fifteen years ago, and still, twice a year or oftener, I have to examine him and then spend a half-hour trying to reassure him.

All of us physicians should try to become optimists. We should keep noting that many persons refuse to die of the serious diseases they have or are supposed to have. Sometimes, even with much dissipation, they keep going for years. We should cheer many patients by telling them of the many cases we know of in which a bad prognosis turned out to have been all wrong.

Thinking aloud before a patient as we make the differential diagnosis and telling of all the awful diseases he or she could have is a pernicious habit. It is terribly hard on the nerves of the victim. We physicians must not always tell all we know. Thus, in a case of chronic cough in an oldish person, as we order tests to rule out carcinoma of the lung, why tell the man of what we fear? If the trouble turns out to be all due to smoking, then the man is spared much worry, and we do not have to spend time on explanations and reassurance.

The need for being positive. As I point out elsewhere in this book, the physician needs to be positive in his statements—whenever the facts permit. The doctor who often wavers and hedges and keeps open a line of retreat can upset his patients badly, and the one who is not clear in his diagnostic vision is more likely to upset a patient than to help him. Thus, let us say that a thin young man comes complaining of a cough and loss of weight. The doctor who cannot be sure of what is wrong is likely to upset the fellow by communicating his doubts. He may talk vaguely about "weak lungs" and a need for being careful. With this the patient may be more alarmed than if he had been told definitely that he had a small tuberculous lesion. When puzzled in such cases, the physician will do well to call in a man who is expert enough in the field of tuberculosis to make a clear-cut diagnosis, one way or the other. This is the only fair thing to do for the patient.

QUIRKS OF HUMAN THINKING

Some psychiatrists, in trying to explain the production of neuroses, place such importance on certain quirks of human behavior that I will briefly mention them here.

Conversion. By means of conversion, anxieties can be transformed into physical symptoms, and the person can then get a hysterical paralysis or an anesthesia.

Evasion or an escape mechanism. A neurotic person can evade life's responsibilities by day-dreaming, by taking alcohol, by entering a monastery, by dropping out of sight, by becoming a vagrant, or by going insane. The day-dreamer keeps happy by living part of his time in a world of fantasy in which he is a great success and does things which make him the center of all eyes.

Many persons escape from an unpleasant predicament by flight into some situation. Many flee into illness, and thereby escape duties and responsibilities and punishments. Others obtain forgetfulness of their duties and their failures and their inadequacy by taking some sedative drug such as alcohol or morphine. A few escape into constant excitement and conviviality, others into travel, and others into solitude. Many wish they could go to the South Seas and "go native."

The flight from an unpleasant situation to the use of a drug was well shown me in 1906, on the morning of the great earthquake in San Francisco. A man whom I had apparently cured of morphinism and who had gone for months without asking for the drug, promptly came whining and begging for it; he could not stand the excitement and confusion that went with the earthquake.

Regression. Regression is a turning backward or a withdrawal from an unpleasant situation. It may mean that the person does not react to his problems as does a mature person. He may regress or try to regress to the status of a child who has no responsibilities. The person may also draw into himself and become apathetic and uncommunicative.

Devaluation and denial. A person's anxiety can be lessened by minimizing unpleasant things in the environment, or even by denying their reality, as is done by Christian Scientists. One is reminded of Pollyanna who always tried to make it appear that misfortunes were blessings in disguise. Religious people, when bereaved, say that God took the loved one for some good but inscrutable purpose. Another form of devaluation is the "sour grapes" one. The weakling says that success would be of little value and not worth the effort.

Postponement. Many weak personalities put off all unpleasant decisions. Some are always waiting for "something to turn up."

Repression. My feeling, after talking to a few thousand neurotic persons, is that repression is not as productive of neuroses and psychoses as Freud and others have thought. Psychiatrists seem to lose sight of the fact that the millions of "normal" persons who do not suffer from neuroses or psychoses all have had to submit to those same disciplines and repressions of home and society which are supposed to be so productive of trouble.

Many prohibitions and taboos are imposed upon every one of us men by the mores of the community, by the demands and expectations of, first, a mother and later, a wife, and by the demands of religion. In a hundred ways every man or woman on earth must conform to the rules or suffer. My feeling, therefore, is that a person with normal psychologic tendencies can be brought up somewhat unhappily by neurotic parents; he may have to submit to the tyranny of a narrow religious sect, or he may suffer many psychic traumas, and yet he may grow up a happy, normal, well-balanced man.

The Freudian makes much of repressed guilt, but my observation has been that many persons sin and sin again without worrying about it, without making any effort to reform, and without falling into any neurosis. The man who gets into serious trouble with feelings of guilt proves commonly to be a manic-depressive. He gets into trouble because he was psychopathic to begin with.

Sublimation. Sublimation is a process through which a person, thwarted in some way, tries to find happiness by filling his life with other activities. The homely woman who cannot get a husband may do good in the community. In this way she tries to forget her frustration, or she tries to buoy her self-respect. A childless or sex-starved woman who feels useless and neglected at home, may run a church or some clubs, and she may campaign for this or that.

Rationalization. By rationalization is meant an effort to invent convenient reasons for doing certain unwise things or for justifying certain condemned types of behavior. A slang term for this sort of thing is to get "an alibi." For instance, a selfish woman who neglects her husband's comfort and his needs can easily excuse herself by saying she is too ill to do her housework. She has to take care of her health. The very stout woman often says, "I must not reduce because if I do I get so irritable. My husband prefers me pleasant." The weaklings in this world are always explaining to themselves why they have failed. One reason "isms" gain so many converts is that there are so many "screwballs" and weaklings in the world who see that the only way they can succeed is through changing the rules of life and business and finance so they can always win.

Compulsion. In a compulsion neurosis, the victim feels compelled to do certain things, often for fear that if he doesn't do them some dire result may follow. Perhaps a loved one will sicken or die. Bothersome and time-consuming as the ritual may be, the patient finds it easier on his nerves to give in than to fight. Sometimes these people eventually become exhausted by the number of ritualistic acts which daily they must carry out.

Many fairly normal persons, of course, suffer from mild degrees of this sort of thing. We all know the woman who goes back into the house more than once to make sure that the gas jets are turned off and the doors locked. We also know the woman who washes her hands several times with soap and then perhaps disinfects them before preparing food for her husband. She fears that otherwise she might carry some infection to him. These people resemble the savage who, before starting on a hunting or fishing trip, has to go through many ritual acts. Similarly, his wife, while her husband is away, must follow certain rituals. She has been taught that if she forgets a taboo the man will return empty handed or he may even lose his life. Sometimes the ritualistic actions of a civilized person appear to represent an expiation for some supposed guilt.

Some persons are inclined to count things such as the number of steps in a staircase, or the number of squares in a pavement. Other persons feel compelled to touch certain things or to touch them a certain number of times. Others have to follow a certain ritual in dressing. Sometimes a person will be much annoyed because hour after hour he keeps repeating some one word that has come into his head.

Psychic orders. Some persons wreck their lives by imposing some taboo or vow or restriction upon themselves. Some promise never to marry so long as a mother or brother or sister lives, and some, after the death of a loved one, seem to vow that they never will be happy or social again.

Obsession. A person may be obsessed with an idea that annoys him, such as that he has a certain disease, or that he may commit suicide, or kill someone. Naturally, the diagnosis between a severe obsession neurosis and a dangerous psychosis is often hard to make, and the patient with such troubles had better be turned over promptly to an experienced psychiatrist.

Efforts to forget and erase. According to some psychiatrists, a neurosis can be due to the effort of the patient to erase and banish from his memory some unpleasant and disturbing idea. This idea may have come during childhood, and it may be associated with resentments and hostilities.

Projection. By projection, psychologists mean a tendency of a person to accuse others of having the unworthy traits or motives that he has. It is often the reaction of the paranoid person, and it is the typical behavior of a warlike dictator who is preparing to gobble up some harmless small neighbor country. He keeps accusing the people in the neighbor country of planning to attack him.

Displacement. By displacement is meant a partially conscious or unconscious shifting of, let us say, anger or hate from one person to another. For instance, a man who has been humiliated by someone against whom he dare not strike back may take it out on some weaker person standing near-by.

Overcompensation. Overcompensation is seen sometimes in persons with an inferiority complex who, perhaps, after taking a Dale

Carnegie course, make too big an effort to appear like strong, hail-fellows-well-met.

Introjection. Introjection is the habit some neurotic persons have of ascribing to someone all sorts of virtues which obviously he never had. Then they feel exalted by their close relationship to this heroic personage. Widows oftentimes do this sort of thing with the memory of a good-for-nothing husband, and nations commonly do it to the memory of some stupid general who stumbled into a victory, or of some stupid and brutal and strutting dictator who led them to disaster and ignominy.

Methods of exalting self. Many persons overcome their feelings of inferiority and get to feeling very superior by raving over the stupid writings of some person whose thoughts and mode of expression are so hopelessly muddled that no able man can make much sense out of them. The impression the neurotic person evidently enjoys giving is that he, with his superior wisdom, is able to understand and enjoy that which others cannot understand. This quirk of human nature has been the making of a lot of very stupid but now very famous people. It has been the making, also, of a lot of "artists" who could not draw a cat so that anyone could tell it from a dog!

Another way in which a man can unconsciously exalt his ego is by bitterly criticizing and demeaning some able or perhaps eminent person. Some politicians love this sort of thing. Other men exalt themselves by saying that they are very tolerant of things which others condemn, or they greatly disparage themselves, or they build a house much larger than they need, or they try to run the lives of all those about them, or they try to get themselves elected chairman of every committee.

WHAT CAN BE LEARNED FROM THE EXPERIMENTAL CAUSATION OF NEUROSES IN ANIMALS

Masserman has shown how several experimenters made nervous wrecks of animals. They accustomed the animal to get his food in a certain way and then changed the mechanism so as to get the poor rat or cat all mixed up, confused, and afraid to even try to get at the food. I am sure we must not conclude from this work that all the neuroses are produced by unpleasant or frustrating experiences, an unhappy childhood, a difficult environment or a psychic trauma. My impression is strong that in most of the cases of neurosis that I see, an inborn predisposition had most to do with producing the symptoms.

I can easily see why an animal would have to break down nervously when treated as the experimental animals are treated, and I imagine a cruel dictator .could quickly break the spirit of any man, and even a strong one, by jailing him and using a similar technic. We know that even well-balanced men eventually break under the stress of war, and we know from the accounts of those few men who have escaped from torture by secret police, that simple starvation plus solitary confinement in the dark will soon reduce a man to a state in which he will gladly confess to anything if only so that he can get quickly to his execution and have it over with.

Let anyone who would like to believe that the animal experiments show that human neuroses are made by psychic trauma remember that few of the patients he sees have ever been as mentally traumatized as the rats and cats are traumatized by a laboratory psychologist. Let all psychiatrists remember, also, that they see innumerable persons who are suffering from neuroses in spite of the fact that life has always been pleasant and easy enough for them. Some of them might even have been better for a little psychic trauma, gained while bucking against the world and learning how to earn a living.

NERVOUS ILLNESS DUE TO THE PATIENT'S FEELING OF BEING CAUGHT IN A TRAP

If a physician will only take the time to talk to patients about their problems of living he will find quite a few whose illness is due to their feeling of being caught in a miserable trap from which they can see no way of escape. Oftentimes the patient is reticent and it is hard to get the story. A man will hate to confess, let us say, that his nervousness is due to the presence in his home of an aged mother who fights with his wife and children and keeps everyone upset and unhappy. He may feel that there is nothing he can do about the situation and at the same time keep peace with his conscience. In most cases the patient fails to see that his illness came with his unhappiness and strain.

There are traps which could be escaped from if the patient only had money with which to pay for the care of a dependent; other traps could be escaped from if the victim could be selfish enough and tough enough to walk out and ignore duties or responsibilities or the great hurt that would be left in another's heart. Other traps would open up if only a wealthy uncle would die and leave the person an annuity that would enable him or her to care for a dependent or give up an exhausting and unliked job.

For instance, a sad-eyed Irish girl came complaining of headache, backache, stomach-ache, insomnia, and a great sense of fatigue for which no organic cause could be found by her home internist. What was wrong was that the girl was working long hours to support her mother and her good-for-nothing, hard-drinking father. Four months before, when her illness began, her fiance had decided that since, on his small salary, he could not hope ever to support four, and since the girl had made it clear that she would never abandon her mother, it was useless for him to hang around any longer. Accordingly, he had said good-by, and had departed to look for some other girl who would be free and willing to marry him. My poor patient was left then to stare into the dark, night after night, unhappy, sleepless, and hopeless; caught in a trap from which neither she nor I could see any way of escape. So long as she felt she could never respect herself again if she deserted her mother, all I could do was to express my sympathy. I knew of no medicine except a soporific that could help her to rest at night. There are many women so trapped by the need for caring for aged relatives that they cannot marry. Thus, a fine-looking woman was unable to marry because she had to support the two aunts who had brought her up and put her through college. She could not desert them.

Another college-trained, high-salaried woman had married a good-looking young clerk whom she thought she could educate and make something of. When she found that he was too slow-witted to learn she slipped into a nervous breakdown, and then he nursed her so devotedly that she could not bring herself to leave him.

Many other women patients, married to dipsomaniacs or men they did not like, would not leave them, either because of economic dependence, or a feeling of responsibility. They said, "If I leave him he'll go utterly to the dogs." Many were chained to the unloved or even much disliked husband by the financial needs of children. Many a one, with her health ruined and no training for business, did not dare leave and strike out on her own.

Another group consists of women trapped by marriage to a good kindly man whose only fault, perhaps, is that he is unattractive, prosaic, and without any of the skills of a lover. The trouble is that the wife did not love the man when she married, and later could not learn to love him. Now she has to stay on because she is too kind to hurt someone who has always been kind and good and generous to her.

Parents will sometimes trap a daughter and keep her from marrying simply because they are selfish and like to keep her around. Some school teachers in small towns are trapped by the lack of eligible men. Other women get trapped by uncongenial work.

A woman may become trapped at home by a mentally defective child. A young woman felt trapped by a mentally defective brother because beaus, when they saw the brother, shied away and did not come back. Other women are trapped by some defect, such as a polio leg, or a big port-wine mark. One nice woman I know is trapped by having had congenital syphilis, another by having a little Negro blood in her veins. Many are trapped by constitutional frailness, and many by a certain amount of psychopathy or perhaps excessive shyness, or a bad temper, or an occasional epileptic fit, or homosexualism.

Young widows may be trapped by the need for bringing up several children. Many married women feel trapped because they have to live in some very uncongenial or lonely place, such as a little mining camp in a foreign land.

Many a mother is caught in a trap because of a dipsomanic son or daughter. Her nervous system may crack under the strain of never knowing when she will hear of another escapade.

Some persons become trapped by their conscience when someone dies and they realize that they had been very unkind. For instance, a young woman "dressed down" her father for investing her money poorly and losing it. The father went to his room and shot himself. With great cruelty, he left a note saying, "Get your money back out of my insurance!"

Men also get caught in traps. I remember the fine handsome man who was ill because his lovely wife was a dipsomaniac who went on frequent "benders." Another man was all set to divorce a devil of a wife and marry again, when the woman became crippled in an auto accident. Then he hadn't the heart to leave her.

Many men are trapped in uncongenial or much disliked jobs. Because of heavy responsibilities or lack of courage or energy they stay and suffer. Some men feel trapped by a great family name which makes them feel that they must succeed in life and become eminent. This they cannot do. Others are trapped by a burden of debt or by the sorrow of an unfortunate marriage. Some youths in college feel trapped by what is expected of them by ambitious parents and often, then, they go into a sort of nervous breakdown. One sees this phenomenon in the case of divinity students who have lost their faith or their desire to go into the ministry, but who hate to disappoint a devout mother.

The important point in all these cases is that the physician should know that nervous illness is sometimes due to frustration caused by being "caught in a trap." The doctor should think of these possibilities and he should ask enough questions to uncover the unhappy situation. Then he will not go on wasting money on examinations, treatments, and operations. He will go over the situation with the patient to see if there is any honorable way out of the trap. Often an escape could be purchased with a comfortable income for the person or his dependents, but there is no one who can supply this.

Oftentimes it helps the patient to see clearly what the situation is and why he or she is ill. Sometimes the physician can help the patient to go free, as when he talks a lonely school teacher in a village into getting a position in a big city hotel, a place where she can meet eligible men.

A sad feature of this type of neurosis is that sometimes, when one tells a physician why his patient is ill, he is uninterested and goes on trying to cure her with injections of B_1, antihistaminics, or penicillin!

CHAPTER 9

Nervous Syndromes Due to
Physiologic Rather than
Psychic Storms

I THINK IT IMPORTANT that we physicians recognize the fact that in the cases of many nervous persons, flare-ups of distress are not due to painful thinking. Many appear to be due to storms coming down the autonomic nervous system from the brain: storms which may come out of what the patient maintains was a clear sky. He says he was not under any great strain at the time, and was not thinking any painful thoughts. Often, unless we accept this statement, we will antagonize the patient and destroy his confidence in our understanding of his disease. I always put such persons at their ease by telling them what is true, and that is, that often, with all my knowledge of physiology, I cannot guess why an attack of migraine or great tenseness hit me.

The mechanism of some spells appears often to be more a physiologic than a psychologic one. I am thinking of such troubles as the nervous attacks associated with migraine, dysrhythmia in the electroencephalogram, a premenstrual tension state, paroxysmal tachycardia, paroxysmal auricular fibrillation, mucous colics, nervous chills, showers of severe hot flushes, the jitters of hyperthyroidism, or sudden "storms" due to histaminic hypersensitiveness, or to a pheochromocytoma of a suprarenal gland. In these cases erratic autonomic nerves keep playing miserable tricks with a person's heart, lungs, kidneys, blood pressure, sweat glands, stomach, bowel, urinary bladder, arteries, or skin. For illustrative cases see Chapter 15.

In the many cases in which the person suffers in this way, first he probably has inherited a somewhat abnormal nervous system, and then, he probably has made matters worse for himself by living too intensely, or by worrying, "blowing up at people," or working too hard or for too long hours each day. The "storms" seem to get touched off, perhaps by triggers which get set too fine. When set fine enough, any slight stimulus may set one off, and this stimulus may come from some point beyond the control of the patient. It probably comes often from the hypothalamus, or from an upsurge in some tide in the chemistry of the body, or from the presence of a cold with a slight blood infection.

Certain intelligent patients may be right when they say that at times they feel as if some poison were accumulating in them until enough is present to bring a "spell."

Nervous states due to chemicals in the blood. In the case of a woman, a "storm" may come at a certain point in one of the chemical cycles of her body, and it is probable that other "nervous" spells are due to the accumulation in the blood of substances as yet unknown. It is said that in some women with a marked premenstrual tension state an excess of estrogen accumulates. Whatever the cause, a usually pleasant and loving wife and mother may be changed into a shrew, who abuses a kindly husband and shrieks at her children. Such a woman may be driven for a time to great activity, cleaning house, washing clothes, or putting up curtains. She then reminds me of the rats which, during oestrus, run for miles, driven by hormones in the blood.

Nervous tension and mental distress can be produced in young men by distention of the prostate gland and the seminal vesicles, or in women by a state of erethism due to lack of sexual intercourse. Under such conditions an orgasm can bring great relaxation of tension, and with this can come mental relief and peace.

After the menopause, a chemical rhythm may for a time continue, as evidenced by the fact that at regular intervals the flushes come in distressing showers.

McFarland and Goldstein (1937) reviewed much of what has been written about the biochemistry of the psychoneuroses but did not find much definitely known.

Occasionally, a person during a period of manic excitement has been found to have measurable changes in the titer of certain chemicals in the blood, but this might well have been secondary to the nervous storm. The great difficulty in such studies is that the chemist knows of so few things to look for. It may be that there are a thousand metabolites which can be harmful, but as yet their very names are unknown.

A woman suffering from exophthalmic goiter, with her blood full of thyroxin and perhaps some other toxic relatives of this drug, is often unreasonable and hypomanic. An angry man may be almost ill because of the presence in his blood of epinephrine and other hormones. A man with a tumor of the islets of Langerhans, causing hyperinsulinism and a very low blood sugar, may get spells in which he behaves as if insane or intoxicated. Toward the end of a severe nephritis, the accumulation in the blood of urea and other end-products of protein metabolism can dull the workings of the brain and can help to bring on the final coma.

There are a number of products of the glands of internal secretion which may well have effects good or bad on the brain, but as yet we do not know enough about them. We know that the lack of thyroxin in myxedematous states and cretinism can greatly injure the brain and leave it inefficient and slowed-up. An injection of a few milligrams of cortisone can make a person feel wonderfully well.

It is suggestive that in the case of chickens the injection of testosterone will change a submissive hen into something that acts like an aggressive cock, but such striking effects are not seen in the cases of men and women. An excessive dose of some suprarenal hormone, as in cases of Cushing's syndrome or of pheochromocytomas, can have decided effects on the brain.

Persons with an excess of porphyrins in their urine often suffer from nervousness and pain. Children born with an inability to metabolize and get rid of phenylpyruvic acid are always mentally defective. Unless the defects in metabolism and brain are linked and inherited together, we must conclude that the unmetabolized drug which accumulates in the body of the fetus must injure the brain.

That toxins of disease, or a metabolism speeded up by fever, can affect the functions of the brain is suggested by the fact that sometimes a person on the first day of a febrile illness will feel stimulated. Thus, one afternoon, Raymond Pearl, while suffering from a temperature of 102° F., felt so lit up that he sent for his secretary and dictated most of his charming and learned book, *To Begin With*. Another friend of mine, whom I have known for years as a sensible, friendly person, when coming down with pneumonia, developed delusions of persecution. Still another friend, a gifted biochemist, when attacked by influenza became decidedly paranoiac and turned on his best friend. Other persons with a little fever may get hallucinations, or they may become delirious. Some of the mental disturbance seen in cases of heart disease is often manifested by bad nightmares. The eating of chicken can make me feel dull and stupid all day, and a plate of chicken soup can give me weird hallucinations.

That the brain can be inhibited by some chemical is suggested by observations on patients who recovered suddenly after years of insanity. For instance, in an interesting article, Pickworth (1938) told of a patient who for sixteen years had led a mute vegetative existence in an asylum; it did not seem possible that there could be much of his brain left. But then the man got pneumonia and, with this, his mental clarity returned so completely that he called his relatives and conversed with them in a perfectly rational manner. This observation shows that for much of a lifetime a brain can be inhibited or thrown out of function in some way.

In 1929 Loevenhart discovered that if he almost asphyxiated some psychopathically mute and apathetic persons, they might for a while be rational. Then they lapsed again. Similar sudden improvements are now seen after shock treatments or after giving cortisone. Such a temporary improvement cannot, of course, be expected in those cases of dementia in which serious brain injury has taken place. Pickworth had the idea that many of the disturbances of brain action are really based on disturbances in its circulation. Royle felt that he had helped some persons with a pre-psychotic state by doing a cerebral sympathectomy. A serious closing-off of arteries has been found in the brains of deteriorated epileptics. The nervous storm of an attack of migraine is associated, first, with constriction of cerebral arteries, and, then, dilation of some of these arteries.

Nervous states due to lesions in the brain. There are many places in the brain in which a lesion can produce disturbances in a person's feelings of comfort or health or sanity. Such lesions must often be thought of, and every psychiatrist should have such training as will help him to recognize them before he wastes time and energy on psychotherapy. He must keep remembering that spells of nervousness and odd behavior can have an organic basis. He must think of brain tumors, cysts and abscesses, of mild encephalitis, and particularly of small strokes. A boy who had recovered from a severe mastoid infection would sometimes vomit and thus get out of going to school. Because a psychiatrist, with tests, found signs of psychic abnormality, the boy was disciplined and made to go to school. But the vomiting got worse and then an abscess in the temporal lobe was found and drained.

Richter and his associates found that in rats, cats, and monkeys the removal of a small part of the frontal poles of the brain produced a state of great overactivity. Some rats so operated on ran an estimated 48 miles in twenty-four hours, and some cats ran until they were completely exhausted. The removal of small bits of tissue from other parts of the frontal lobes had a calming effect.

As I shall point out later, lesions of the optic thalamus can produce hyperesthesia of one half of the body such as one sees in many nervous and unhappy women, and it may well be that some of the women who complain of a constant ache in one side have a small lesion of this sensory node.

Migrainous women, when in a state of high tension, may get burning areas on the skin. Doubtless there are many such cases in which a small brain lesion, produced by a tiny stroke, gives the patient a distress which is interpreted by his physicians as a sign of some silly anxiety. I will never forget a young man whose main symptom for months was an agonizing fear of death. Most of the physicians who saw him were disgusted with him, but one day he got much worse and soon he was dead. It appeared then that from the start, he had been suffering from a curious form of encephalitis.

Nervous disturbances arising in the hypothalamus. It seems probable today that many of the nervous storms which distress some persons arise in a hypothalamus which has temporarily escaped from the control of higher centers, or which has been injured by arteriosclerosis or encephalitis. This extremely important part of the body is to be found at the base of the brain, between the cerebral peduncles and the optic tracts. It constitutes the floor of the third ventricle. It is a small diamond-shaped button of tissue weighing only about 4 gm. Through its center goes the stalk of the hypophysis. This little part of the brain is now thought (1) to regulate endocrine functions and their interrelation; (2) to regulate the functions of the autonomic nerves and to integrate them with the functions of the endocrine glands; (3) to integrate body defensive reactions and emotional expressions (see Bard, 1934); (4) to influence the activity of the cerebral cortex so as to regulate the degree of wakefulness and excitation of the individual; (5) to house scores of little "thermostats" which regulate body temperature and many of the rhythms of the body, such as the menstrual ones, and which facilitate homeostasis, or the keeping of the chemical constitution of the several body fluids within certain limits. The hypothalamus is one of the centers of regulation, also, for visceral activities.

An important point is that the cortex damps or quiets the responses of the hypothalamus. It keeps them from swinging too widely in either direction. If it did not do this we might, like decorticate animals, be reacting reflexly and too violently to many stimuli which produce anger and fear.

Injuries to the hypothalamus, usually wrought by encephalitis, are now known to produce curious syndromes associated with too great sleepiness or too great wakefulness. They produce, also, sudden and sometimes large fluctuatious in body weight, and in women, marked disturbances in menstruation. I remember a young woman who had been going from gynecologist to endocrinologist to gynecologist getting endless injections of hormones because the year before she had stopped menstruating and had gained much weight. On meeting the girl I thought her face was a bit Parkinsonian, and I soon drew from the mother the typical story of an attack of encephalitis with somnolence and a little fever.

Such attacks of encephalitis are doubtless commoner than we physicians now think, and, as in the case just mentioned, they often pass unrecognized. When they produce obesity, amenorrhea, and lack of sexuality, we physicians usually think only of disease in the glands of internal secretion. Eunochoid syndromes have been observed in men following disease of the hypothalamus. I have seen a number of young women who, after a psychic shock, never menstruated again. In them the mechanism producing this amenorrhea would appear to have been a nervous one, and they remained feminine and attractive.

Possibly the person with a well-balanced and well-running nervous system has good "thermostats" which keep him comfortable and unaware of his body and its functions, while a person who inherited erratic and poorly controlled "thermostats" is always suffering because his autonomic nerves are playing tricks on him and causing him to feel uneasy about his body and his health.

It is suggestive that all of the research workers who, by operations on the brain of dogs and cats, have removed from the hypothalamus the calming effects of the cortical centers, have obtained animals which could be thrown easily into attacks either of rage or of cowering fear. According to Bard, these reactions are abolished by destruction of the hypothalamus. This makes me wonder if some of the irascibility of persons who have suffered from much arteriosclerotic destruction of the higher parts of the brain, or who are under the influence of a drug like alcohol or ether which depresses the higher centers, may not be due, at least in part, to a removal of control from the hypothalamus. I wonder, also, if some of the panicky fears, and the unreasoning anxieties and forebodings of certain nervous persons may not be due to the same mechanism. Certainly, the alcoholic in an attack of delirium tremens can present a picture of overpowering fear similar to that of the experimental animals.

In man, Grinker found that stimulation of the hypothalamus produced profound anxiety. In one case the person broke into uncontrollable sobbing. I have seen such cases in which, after a minor apoplexy, which perhaps severed tracts exerting a calming effect on the hypothalamus, the patient kept suffering unprovoked and very annoying attacks of weeping which were not associated with any feeling of sadness.

Stimulation of the hypothalamus can produce a rise in blood pressure, contraction of the arterioles, dilatation of the pupils, elevation of the hairs of the skin, an increase in the heart rate, contractions of the urinary bladder, the uterus and the gastro-intestinal tract, and an excessive secretion of tears and saliva.

Lesions made in the hypothalamus of guinea pigs will abolish mating reactions and may produce anatomic changes in the pelvis and vagina. Irritation of the posterior part of the hypothalamus can produce epileptiform attacks.

Penfield had a patient who had a ball-valve tumor in the third ventricle which gave rise to epileptiform seizures. They began with a sensation of fever; the body surfaces became flushed, respiration was slowed, perspiration became profuse, the saliva and tears flowed, the pupils enlarged, and the eyes became prominent. There was violent hiccupping and shivering, and the pulse varied in strength and rapidity. This case is most interesting because it shows how a nervous syndrome can be produced, not by emotion, but by irritation of a small spot in the brain. How many of us physicians, if we had seen this patient, would immediately have started trying to get a history of infantile sexual trauma, or recent psychic strain?

Foerster stimulated the anterior end of the hypothalamus and produced restlessness, excitement, euphoria, and some mania. According to Alpers (1940) changes in emotional states and in personality have been observed in men and women with lesions of the hypothalamus. Some of the patients became coarse and immoral in their behavior. They lost their inhibitions. A few developed hallucinations. Others were slowed up mentally, and some became psychotic. There were marked swings of mood, from excitement to depression. There was either apathy or negativism or irascibility. In some cases there came antisocial tendencies and the sort of poor grooming that sometimes follows a minor apoplexy.

Nervous symptoms due perhaps to an excess of neuromimetic chemicals in the blood. It now seems probable that some of the distresses of the persons whose emotions are violent or who suffer from storms coming down the autonomic nerves are due to an excess formation of those substances with neuromimetic activity that are constantly being produced through the action of the nerves. We physicians know that toxins coming out of a goiter can produce nervous storms with sweating, tachycardia, auricular fibrillation, flushing, and diarrhea. Similarly, the giving of too much thyroid substance can make the person jittery. An injection of epinephrine can cause trembling, tachycardia, shivering, apprehension, cardiac oppression, and the feeling that one has either been much frightened or made very angry. Pilocarpine can produce sweating, an urgent desire to urinate or defecate, and the secretion of much mucus from the bowel. Outpourings of histamine, acetylcholine, and sympathins or nor-epinephrine may well produce much distress in nervous persons. The injection of an acetylcholine type of drug has produced in the colon symptoms resembling those of a mucous colic.

Too much histamine in the blood can cause a number of distresses, such as giant hives or severe facial pain. The heart action is extremely sensitive to sympathins. A good example of the tremendous nervous storms that can be produced by circulating chemicals is that seen in cases of pheochromocytomas of the suprarenal gland. Here one sees a sudden rise in blood pressure with a number of distressing nervous symptoms.

An ancient sage once said, very wisely, that an angry man is a poisoned man. Myerson and Blackburn and others have told of women who, while nursing an infant, became very angry, and in this way upset the baby's digestive tract. There have been so many reports of this sort of thing that there can be little doubt that persons under violent emotion pour out some poison into the blood, a poison that can be excreted with the milk. Elsewhere in this book I tell of a man so enraged by family litigation that he became like a man severely poisoned; he went down hill and died a cardiorenal death.

Vagotonia and sympatheticotonia. Some readers may wonder why I do not discuss the long-popular ideas about the antagonism between the sympathetic and parasympathetic nerves and between adrenergic and cholinergic hormones. I will not go into that because, after thirty years of reading the research literature on the subject and many years of studying laboratory animals with first one and then the other set of nerves cut and degenerated, I have no patience with much of the clinical literature on the subject. Hundreds of clinical articles would never have seen the light if the writers had known well the experimental literature, or had worked for a few months in a pharmacologic laboratory. Although for nearly forty years the ideas of Eppinger and Hess have fascinated physicians, they were based on a lot of wrong information, and I doubt if they have had any clinical value.

Transitory mental disturbances due to slight infections. There are many persons who would probably have perfect health and a constant feeling of splendid energy if it were not for recurrent mild infections with some virus or bacterium. Oftentimes this infection appears to be that of a cold. In many other cases, perhaps after a slight cold, a fibrositis will flare up, with aches in joints and muscles. In other cases little boil-like lesions will appear in the skin, perhaps around the nose, on the upper lip, in the axilla, or on the buttocks. With these there may be malaise, mental depression, and a feeling of fatigue. The lesions usually dry up in a few hours or days. Evidently there was a shower of bacteria into the blood.

In other cases there will appear a herpetic blister on the lip, or little petechiae in the skin. Lymph nodes may swell, and the patient's blood may show a lymphocytosis. There may be a slight fever for a few days. Such infections may appear in some of the adults in a family at a time when a child is down with some exanthem. Physicians with an inquiring mind ought to study these coincidences.

Children's infections and exanthems somewhat injure the nervous system in a small percentage of cases. The virus circulates through the brain and cord and nerves and can have serious effects. Brown, Kirkland, and Hein (1948) presented evidence to show that if more often physicians were to study the spinal fluid of persons suffering from severe attacks of mumps, measles, and other types of febrile illness they would find signs of meningitis. In cases with extra cells in the spinal fluid the patient usually shows more than the usual amount of mental confusion, vomiting, headache, stiff neck, and aching in the muscles.

Epidemiologic studies have shown that the viruses of poliomyelitis can go through a community, making hundreds of children ill, but producing paralysis in only a few. During the last epidemic I saw necropsies on two persons who died of poliomyelitis. In both of these cases considerable injury had been done to the brain as well as to the spinal cord. According, however, to some recent studies, the mind of patients with poliomyelitis is rarely affected.

Bacteria and viruses slumber in many organs of the body. Infectious agents often slumber in certain organs of the body such as the spleen. Few physicians know that many years ago Ford and others showed that the organs of apparently normal animals contain viable bacteria, characteristic for the animal and the organ. Thus, the liver of the dog is normally full of gas bacilli. Recently McVay, Guthrie, Michelson, and Sprunt reported that they had cultured *Brucella abortus* from bits of prostate gland and from fallopian tubes removed at operations on men and women who were not very ill. At many a necropsy on an old person who died, perhaps of cancer, active tuberculosis is found. It may be, therefore, that the poor nervous health of some people is due, as they suppose, to an occult and smoldering infection somewhere. Somewhat against this idea often is their low blood sedimentation rate.

Mild forms of encephalitis may be more frequent than we think. Many persons are probably carriers of neurotropic viruses just as animals are. Years ago, men studying encephalitic viruses were much confused until they learned that a high percentage of their experimental animals were carriers of such viruses. I think we physicians have reason to believe that some transient and poorly explained nervous breakdowns are due to mild attacks of unrecognized encephalitis, or to flare-ups in a very mild smoldering infection. How can we recognize such things if we never think of them?

According to T. M. Rivers (J.A.M.A. *132*) some fifteen viruses are known to cause encephalitis of various types in man. On a number of occasions I have been impressed by the fact that a person who almost certainly was suffering from the effect of a mild attack of encephalitis had long been going from physician to physician without anyone's suspecting what really was wrong. All one had to do was to note that the man was slowed up mentally and physically, and then to draw forth from the wife the story that the loss of health dated from an attack of what, at the time, was assumed to be influenza but which evidently was encephalitis. Usually, when questioned, the wife said, "He went into that spell a youngish man with a quick step and a twinkle in his eye, and he came out an oldish man with a face that seldom smiles."

The fact that most of the patients I have seen with a mild encephalitis have, for years, been treated for supposed ulcers, indigestion, or heart disease shows that today there must be thousands of such sufferers going about with wrong medical labels on them. What is needed is that more often we physicians note that the patient is not wide-awake enough and quick enough for the job that he used to have. For one case in which one can be sure that a breakdown was caused by a mild encephalitis there are several in which one can only suspect it. Oftentimes one cannot be sure until a few years later when the patient returns with more definite symptoms. The difficulty in some cases is that the injury to the brain could just as easily have been produced by a poor nervous heredity or a little stroke.

Endocrine disturbances. The psychiatrist must sometimes suspect that a mental disturbance was due to a change in function of some gland of internal secretion. Often at necropsies small adenomas are found in the pituitary gland or in the cortex of the adrenal glands, or changes will be found in the thyroid, parathyroid, or thymus glands. Unfortunately, often, it is hard to know how much significance to place on the disease found. One must remember that many persons with frank disease in the glands of internal secretion have little trouble with their brain or their nerves. Always there is the possibility that the nervous or mental troubles present are due to a poor psychic inheritance or some other common cause for nervousness.

Distresses due to the influencing of the brain by certain rhythmic stimuli. Recent studies have shown that the imposition of abnormal rhythms on the brain, with a rate of 6 cycles a second, like that noted in the electroencephalograms of some bad-tempered people, can produce in the person emotional discomfort and irritability. It appears probable from this and other electroencephalographic studies that our good and bad moods may depend partly on certain rhythmic activities in the brain, activities which may perhaps be induced at times by factors outside the brain. For instance, certain migrainous persons can in a few moments be thrown into a spell by flickering lights, or by looking at a tessellated floor with light slanting on it. Others are terribly upset by someone brushing a bedspread, and a good musician can be physically hurt by a soprano who is flatting.

Storms due to epilepsy equivalents. An epileptic inheritance can cause many a person to suffer from stormy crises of one kind or another. These are described in this book under the heading of "equivalents of epilepsy." A description of migrainous equivalents will also be found elsewhere in this book (see Chapter 17).

Mental storms due to the ingestion of an allergen. In susceptible persons nervous storms, migrainous attacks, and perhaps epileptiform spells can be produced by some allergen. (See the section on allergy.) On many occasions I have been much impressed with the amount of mental hebetude that can be produced by eating some food to which the person is sensitive. The head will ache and the man will feel stupid, and in rare cases he will suffer from some meningism and even a feeling of being in a curious hallucinatory state intermediate between waking and sleeping.

Distress produced by an approaching storm. As every physician knows, there are arthritics who get pains in their joints the day before a rainstorm arrives. Few realize that there are other persons who, with the same stimulus, get feelings of fatigue and illness or abdominal distress. A migrainous banker told me once that when a storm is approaching his eyes will pull and seem to get out of focus, and he will feel mentally slowed-up. Such phenomena need more study by physicians. Their mechanism is not yet known.

Poisoning by toxins of intestinal origin. It used to be thought that toxins being absorbed from the bowel can affect the brain deleteriously, but the best evidence is against this view. The mental distress and headache disappear so quickly after emptying the rectum that they must be produced mechanically by irritation of the rectal nerves. This can happen only in a specially sensitive person. In such persons similar disturbing effects on the brain can be produced by a full bladder or a large tampon in the vagina.

Summary. The point to remember is that there are many nervous crises and storms which are beyond the person's control. Any time of the day or night such a storm can come out of some center in the nervous system and can perhaps flood the body with a neuromimetic substance. The physician must know that there are such happenings, and he must try to recognize them. He must not try to blame all of a nervous person's difficulties on wrong thinking.

CHAPTER 10

A Poor Nervous Heredity
the Cause of Many Neuroses

TODAY, IN MOST BOOKS and articles on psychiatry, the great subject of the inheritance of neuroses is either ignored or hooted at. All neuroses and psychoses are supposed to be due to psychic traumas in early life. Fortunately, here and there, a few men like Kallmann are showing how tremendously important heredity is in the production of mental illness.

Sir James Purves-Stewart, Britain's great neurologist, writing on the causation of psychoneurosis said, "Heredity is by far the most important factor. As the clinician progressively gains experience he becomes impressed by the fact that the vast majority of psychoneuroses occur in individuals who started life with an inborn neuropathic or psychopathic tendency."

The minor manifestations of a poor nervous inheritance. To my way of thinking, the big mistake that many students of the heredity of mental disease have made has been to divide the members of each family studied into only two categories, the sane and the insane. If the investigators had only taken the time to get well acquainted with each family I think they would have seen the need for listing the relatives in at least six categories: (1) the psychotic; (2) the eminently sane, intelligent, and well-adjusted; (3) the slightly "touched" persons with a cycloid, schizoid, paranoid, or psychopathic personality; (4) the persons with gross equivalents of psychosis, such as feeble-mindedness, epilepsy, dipsomania, vagabondism, criminality, deaf-mutism, bad stuttering, severe hysteria, defects of vision, and paralysis; (5) the persons with minor equivalents, such as I describe in this chapter; and (6) the persons with ordinary nervousness and worry due mainly to the strain of life and only slightly to a family tendency to neurosis.

The persons with a small dose of a mental defect. My hunch has long been that some of the curious syndromes of the relatives of the psychotic represent a small dose of an ancestor's psychosis, while others represent perhaps a shifting of the localization of the hereditary defect to some part of the brain or nervous system which is not essential to sanity. Thus, the defect may involve perhaps the thalamus, or hypothalamus, or the autonomic nervous system, or a part of the spinal cord, or the eyes or the ears, or some part of the muscular system.

If we assume that it takes perhaps 300 good genes to make a fine, sane, normal brain (actually no one knows how many it takes), a child born with, let us say, 200 such genes might well be imbecilic or insane or epileptic. A person born with 250 good genes might be just eccentric, pathologically worrisome, jittery, or constitutionally inadequate; and one with perhaps 275 good genes might be just nervous. This, of course, is only a way of thinking about the problem. We know that the lack of even one highly important gene can result in phenylpyruvic idiocy. E. B. Ford thought that retinitis pigmentosa could result from the working of five poor genes. In a banana fly, if I remember correctly, it takes a combination of a dozen genes to produce so simple a feature as a certain color of the eyes. Doubtless, with time, geneticists will supply more explanations for the facts as they are commonly observed.

An interesting observation which I think strengthens my hunch that a few poor genes or the lack of some good ones can produce a bad neurosis is that a slight tendency to a certain nervous disease carried by a husband can be reinforced by a slight tendency to the same or another nervous disease in the wife, and with disastrous results. For instance, two slightly schizoid, shy persons had a daughter who, while always rational, was so highly schizoid that she had to spend part of her life in institutions, away from the hurly-burly of the world. Another patient of mine, a fine able man, had an epileptic uncle. If he had married a girl from a normal family he might perhaps have had all normal children, but unfortunately, he married a woman whose aunt was depressed, and I suspect this reinforcement made it easier for one of his children to become an epileptic imbecile. There are many similar cases in the literature to support this hunch.

A good precedent for thinking of nervous persons as inheriting only a part of the mental disease that struck down an ancestor is to be found in the experiences of the hematologist who learned long ago that some of the apparently normal relatives of a person with primary anemia have an achylia gastrica or early graying of the hair or (rarely) cord changes, *without the anemia*. Similarly, many relatives of an epileptic inherit the explosive temper or a sullen disposition or the dysrhythmia, *but never a fit!*

As J. V. Neel has pointed out, the world is full of "carriers" of chronic inherited disease, and their presence makes more difficult the problems of the geneticist. To illustrate: A sensitive little girl of eight began to come home from school with spells of migrainous vomiting. The pediatrician, asking about migraine in the family, was told that none was known in the preceding two generations. A physician friend then remarked that he happened to know that the father and the grandfather had marked scintillating scotomas without headache or nausea and the great-grandmother suffered frequent spells of atypical migraine. Almost certainly, then, the father and the grandfather were carriers of migraine.

Psychoses do not breed true. There is another interesting feature about the genetics of mental disease and that is that the different types of trouble do not necessarily breed true. By this I mean that although the descendants of a sufferer from manic-depressive psychosis, when they go insane, tend to be manic-depressives, an occasional one is likely to be a schizophrenic or a paranoiac, and a few will be epileptics, imbeciles, alcoholics, stutterers, enuretics, paralytics, or deaf mutes.

This failure of a nervous defect always to produce the same disease can be seen strikingly in the reports of Androp, Penrose, Dugdale, Goddard, Henry, and others. For instance, in Androp's "S" family, a brother of an epileptic married an apparently normal woman. In the next three generations there were five epileptics, which is understandable; but in addition there were nine feeble-minded persons, one congenitally deaf person, four criminals, two insane persons, and · one suicide. Besides these there doubtless were others who were simpletons, or nervous ne'er-do-wells, or chronic invalids, but unfortunately Androp did not list the minor equivalents.

In 1906 Woods showed that among the descendants of the Spanish queen, "Joanna the mad," there were such persons as "Luis the weak," "Luis the foolish," "Maria the licentious," "Philip the imbecile," "Maria Luisa the stupid," "Francis the bigoted," "Carlotta the violent," "Ferdinand the brutal," "Balthasar the degenerate," and "Philip the lazy."

Physical defects of the "relatives." Studies made of the relatives of the psychotic have strengthened my hunch that, in many, the inherited defect shows up not in the cerebrum but lower down perhaps in some part of the nervous system that is not concerned with sanity. For instance, in the descendants of the insane there may be defects in vision or in attaining binocular vision, or in hearing, or there may be paralyses of a group of muscles, or disturbances in the functions of the spinal cord. In many "relatives" there is an erratic hypothalamus, and, as I shall show in this chapter, commonly there are poorly controlled autonomic nerves.

I suspect, also, that "relatives" are more than ordinarily subject to disease of the glands of internal secretion. For instance, I think it more than a coincidence that when one of my patients, who had a bad nervous inheritance, had three daughters, two were insane, and the third died young of Addison's disease. One suspects that her suprarenal glands had not developed normally. Such strange "coincidences" should more often be recorded and studied. In other families I have seen an apparent association between psychosis in some individuals, and in others, defective ovaries, a diseased thyroid gland, or abnormal islands of Langerhans.

Another well-known fact emphasized by Kretschmer and now by Sheldon and others is that the body of a schizophrenic or a feeble-minded person is often a bit botched. It is not well proportioned, and the person has poor control over his muscles. He or she is often a bit of a "slob," and hearing and vision may be poor. In a gymnasium or a dancing class such a person cannot be taught to do anything gracefully. Commonly the skin is dry or greasy or unpleasant or malodorous. On the other hand, one finds the mentally alert and highly intelligent migrainous woman with almost always a trim, nicely proportioned body, perhaps perfect vision, a nice skin, and muscles that respond well to her will. As Hrdlicka found when he studied the members of the National Academy of Sciences, a man with an unusually good brain usually has a fine body.

Hopefulness that can be derived from a study of heredity. Those psychiatrists who are now closing their eyes to the tremendous influence of heredity in producing neuroses are losing sight of a most encouraging aspect of the genetics of sanity and insanity. They are forgetting that when a fine intelligent couple with good nervous heredity are getting married, they can almost count on any children they may have being fine and sane and intelligent like themselves. Barring the coming in utero of some nonhereditary disease of the brain, or an accidental injury to it in the womb or at birth or shortly after, the children will probably all have more than average ability, energy, good sense, and charm. How good it is that the parents can be sure of this!

But if a physician is going to accept this happy half of the picture and rejoice in it, he cannot reject the other discouraging half, and tell two young people with schizophrenic or epileptic ancestry or a dysrhythmic electroencephalogram that they can marry without concern over what is likely to happen to some of the children they may have. He must not hide a chart like Androp's No. 48 which shows that when a feeble-minded man married an epileptic woman seven of their eight children were feeble-minded and the eighth was epileptic!

A nervous patient's knowledge that he has good heredity back of him can give him great comfort, also, when, after much overwork, he has become tired out and depressed. In that case, with a little rest he can expect to be well again. On the other hand, if several of his ancestors have had bad spells of depression, the outlook for him will not be so good.

The probability that a person will inherit a tendency to psychosis. We physicians must study the genetics of psychoses, epilepsy, and feeble-mindedness if only because one of these days many young men and women of intelligence and education are going to come to us to ask if, with their poor nervous heredity, they dare marry and have children. Already some of them are refusing to marry or to have children. Surely, when these persons come to us for advice, we should know what is the truth and we should tell it to them. Fortunately, figures expressing the probabilities of the inheritance of mental disease are now becoming available. For instance, Kallmann (1946) has reported the incidence of schizophrenia and schizoid states in a large group of relatives of the schizophrenic. He found the morbidity for the relatives of schizophrenics, expressed in numbers of affected per 100 persons, was

0.9 for children born of two normal parents; plus 2.9 schizoid.
16.4 for children born of one schizophrenic parent; plus 32.6 schizoid.
68.1 for children born of two schizophrenic parents; plus 17.1 schizoid.
 1.8 for step-siblings.
 7.0 for half-siblings; plus 12.5 schizoid.
14.3 for full-siblings; plus 31.5 schizoid.
14.7 for dizygotic or unlike twins.
91.5 for monozygotic or alike twins from one ovum who were reared together. An extra 8.5 were schizoid.
77.6 for monozygotic twins who were reared in separate environments. An extra 20.7 were schizoid.

With figures like this available, a psychiatrist can no longer take refuge, as some are now doing, in the position that he does not have to believe in the heredity of mental disease until every last detail is known about it. It is true that today no one can predict *exactly* how the children of a given couple, each with a poor nervous inheritance, will come out. If the couple should have only one child he or she might well escape, but if they should have many children, one or two would probably be abnormal. Always the estimated probabilities can be altered by German measles early in the mother's pregnancy, or a birth trauma to the brain, or an attack of encephalitis during the child's infancy.

One thing we doctors can tell people from a highly neurotic family is that a man does not necessarily inherit a psychosis full blown: *He usually inherits a tendency to it,* and if he keeps physically fit, if he observes good mental hygiene, and if during his lifetime he does not run into too much sorrow and disaster and strain, he may stay sane and never break down. (See Kallmann.) Many persons with a tendency to psychosis do not break down until they are old, or until overwork or discouragement or cerebral arteriosclerosis or a little stroke has come to pull them down or to weaken their self-control.

It is hard to understand how some psychiatrists can question the idea that the commonest cause of psychosis is heredity. All they would have to do to get convinced would be to go into a state asylum and see how many of the inmates belong to a few families. Or they could look at some of the diagrams showing the family trees of the insane, diagrams full of black squares and circles showing the frequent incidence of psychosis, epilepsy, alcoholism, feeble-mindedness, and other mental defects.

THE RELATIVE IMPORTANCE OF HEREDITY AND ENVIRONMENT

Many psychiatrists today feel that enviroment has everything to do with producing intelligence and sanity, but in doing this they are not facing abundant facts, well gathered for many years by many workers. No one can read Galton and not be impressed with the hereditary nature of decided ability. Teachers have learned to their sorrow that environment can bring out only the mental faculties that are in the child to begin with. Worse yet, a good environment cannot always subdue or eradicate bad qualities and traits and tendencies. Even with much devoted coaching, a teacher cannot greatly increase a child's I.Q., and she can never put good judgment or any reasoning power into a moron. No matter how hard teachers may try, they can never make a research physicist or a fine physician or mathematician or musician out of *any* boy. A distinguished scientist can be made only out of a very unusual boy, the sort who can be found in a large high school only once in several years. Incidentally, when such a boy comes along he will usually be found to be the son of gifted and able and perhaps distinguished parents. (See Terman.)

Much research has been done to find out what part of a person's good sense is due to heredity and what to environment. One technic has been to see what happens to children from unintelligent couples when they are adopted by intelligent and well-to-do people. Several such studies have been made, and the impression I get from them is that the influence of heredity is much stronger than that of environment. Even when brought up in a fine home by cultured people, the son of a day-laborer is usually unable to get past the eighth grade in school. His intelligence does not rise much because of the good environment about him, and without a fair I.Q. he cannot get through high school.

The most convincing work has been done with like twins (derived from one ovum) who were separated early in life and reared in dissimilar homes. It appears from several such studies that the culture of one twin can be considerably improved over that of the other, and the I.Q. can be raised a little, but the temperaments and characters of the two twins are likely to remain much the same. For instance, two like-twin boys were separated at birth. One was brought up in New York and the other in Utah. Although for years they did not know of each other's existence, when a research worker studied them he found them remarkably alike in interests and activities. They both loved boxing, and they both had gone to the top in championship contests.

To me one of the most convincing bits of evidence against the value of environment has been the failure of some of my more intelligent patients to much improve the culture of children whom they adopted from the homes of ignorant parents. In spite of all the advantages these well-to-do foster parents gave, the children grew up without much refinement. Some remained the stupid hoydens, criminals, or hooligans that they were born to be.

Another fact that has impressed me tremendously, just as years ago it impressed Galton, is that the several sibs in a family, all brought up in the same home environment with the same mother and the same teachers, are often remarkably different from birth, and then they stay different all their days. Evidently, during the maturation of the ovum and the spermatozoon, when half of the chromatin with its genes was thrown away, one child lost certain attributes available in the two parental stirpes, while his brother lost others. As a result, the brother of an eminent electrical inventor may be unable to hook up a doorbell; the brother of an eminent scientist may think only of stocks and bonds; and the brother of a great musician may be unable to hum a tune. The experience of such sets of brothers proves to me the inability of environment to do much in the way of producing or changing interests and abilities. A good environment can only help a man to follow his bent and to develop the gifts with which he was born.

One day, going up in a Mayo Clinic elevator, I was so impressed by the very different behavior of two sisters, six and eight years old. One stood by herself, evidently greatly interested in the sensations she was getting from the moving car. Her face was merry and eager, and she was enjoying her new experiences. The older sister, with each move of the elevator, shuddered and trembled; she cried out, she clutched her mother, and she buried her face in the mother's skirts. The mother kept trying to comfort and reassure her.

As I watched I marveled at the tremendous difference between the two children born of a lovely sensible mother. I could look into the future and see one child growing up happy, athletic, and merry, surrounded by friends and beaus; I could see the other, always sickly, complaining, solitary, and full of fears.

One day a patient greatly impressed me with the comment that as soon as her first child was able to talk it was evident that he was "a little hypochondriac just like several of his uncles and aunts." With the least scratch or bump he would set up a howl, and he would be so worried about it that he would insist that his mother put on a disinfectant and a band-aid. The second child was entirely different, showing no concern over even a painful fall or a badly skinned knee. When his mother would want to apply some first aid, he'd say, "No, it's all right."

A point which many psychiatrists of late seem to be missing entirely and never thinking of is that the child who is brought up in a miserable home by a slattern mother and a drunken father can owe his later psychosis, if it comes, not only to the traumas of his childhood but to the fact that his brain was made from the poor genes which he got from that defective father and mother.

Very interesting is Kallmann's account of two women, identical twins, who were separated at birth. One was brought up in a poor home. At fifteen she was seduced. With the mental trauma of giving birth to an illegitimate child, she went insane. Some might say, "See what a bad environment and sexual trauma will do." But wait; the other sister, brought up happy and carefree in a good home, went insane about the same time and joined her sister in the asylum!

A remarkable fact which must not be ignored is that some of the children from a miserable home, when they fail to inherit any of the bad genes, grow up to be good sensible citizens. This point has been emphasized by Ross, Myerson, Riggs, and other able psychiatrists. As they have said, out of the worst type of home there sometimes comes a good, fine, hard-working and sensible man or woman. Because this person failed to get enough bad genes to produce a psychosis, he or she was so sane and sensible and well-intentioned that even the awful environment in which he grew up could not work much injury. Woods, in his splendid book, *Heredity and Royalty,* commented on the same phenomenon. As he said, when a young prince inherited good genes, even the many temptations of a dissolute court did not succeed in pulling him down and making a good-for-nothing roué out of him. Woods proved abundantly that a man's morality is determined more by his inheritance than by his environment and his training. Some of the worst kings of history had excellent teachers and were steeped in religion every day of their lives.

A neurotic person is most likely to suffer a breakdown. Investigators who have succeeded in producing neuroses in animals have noticed that those with signs of a neurotic disposition to begin with are the ones that can most easily be thrown into a nervous breakdown. Maier succeeded in breeding strains of white rats almost all of which were highly nervous. He did this by mating those nervous and apprehensive animals which urinated and defecated under excitement. The neurotic rats so produced remind me of some of the frail children that I have seen, born perhaps to a thin neurotic university instructor and a jittery ex-music teacher. Such children are likely to be highly nervous, oversensitive, and asthmatic, and given to such troubles as night terrors, late bed-wetting, severe hay fever, frequent infections, or "bilious vomiting."

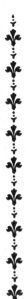

CHAPTER 11

Marriage as a Cause
of Neuroses

NEUROSES THAT ARISE FROM UNHAPPINESS IN MARRIAGE. As Myerson showed so well in his book, *The Nervous Housewife,* many of the nervous and psychic troubles of men and women arise in the home, and in the problems of finding there peace, love, happiness, and security. It would be difficult enough for two persons to adjust happily to living together if both were sane, sensible, and always self-controlled adults, but when both are often somewhat childish and uncontrolled, it is a wonder that they ever stick together, or ever have any love or nerves left after their many conflicts. Worse yet, many an unfortunate man or woman discovers soon after marriage that the spouse is somewhat psychotic and at times impossible to get along with.

In this chapter there is much that will be "old stuff" to the wise physician of years of practice. He knows well these common sorrows and mistakes and worries and neurosis-breeders, but the young physician, or even the young psychiatrist starting his practice, may not yet know them all, and hence I will mention some of them. The young physician can profit from hearing about them because if he knows what to ask patients about, he can the more quickly uncover a story of unhappiness, strain, or incompatibility.

When marriage starts without love or much acquaintance. Adjustments to living in the same room and bed with another person would be hard enough to make if both started out much in love, but commonly the couple start without love and without even much acquaintance. A young man, after being turned down by a girl, is often engaged to another a few weeks later. In such a case it is obvious that the two cannot be much in love, and it is highly probable that the girl said, "Yes," only because she was asked, and because she much preferred marriage with almost anyone to the chance of staying single. Many women have admitted to me that they married without any love.

Many a woman has said, "How I wish I had backed out the day before the wedding; and I would have done it if my mother or my sister had not insisted that the invitations were out and it would be very embarrassing for them if I refused to go on. They said I'd learn to love him. But I didn't. The first night I should have gotten right out of that bed and gone home because I knew then that I could never like any physical contact with him." In a study once made of dissatisfactions in marriage it was found that in a high percentage of cases the man or the woman or both were dissatisfied before the marriage or during the honeymoon, and would have liked then to go separate ways.

Often a woman is willing to marry almost anyone to avoid the stigma of remaining single during the years when her sisters are getting their own homes. Other girls are frantic to leave home because of friction with a domineering mother, or a hated father or step-mother. Perhaps the girl elopes only to find, in a few days, that she has married a good-for-nothing fellow who will not support her. Often, all she gets out of her marriage is a child whom later she has to support.

Love is a precious plant that should be tended. It would be wonderful if all young married couples could be taught that love is a precious plant that must be handled with reverence and carefully nurtured. Often a kindly physician should warn the two that nothing must ever be done carelessly to break down love and mar its beauty. Efforts should constantly be made by both partners to make it stronger and more lovely. Never should either person wantonly injure love by silly jealousy, selfishness, childish behavior, temper tantrums, or "lovers' quarrels."

Many persons get into trouble *demanding* love, and trying to punish the other for not giving enough. They need to be told that love cannot be *forced;* it can only be *earned* by constant loving thoughtfulness and sweet little services and kindnesses. With sensible persons words do not count half so much as do little thought-taking and trouble-taking unselfish deeds. To paraphrase a Russian proverb, "What you say is drowned out by what you do not do." Many a man who says he loves a woman is so unkind to her in so many ways it is hard to believe that he has any love for her.

On efforts to keep romance in marriage. Perhaps the greatest cause of complaint against marriage among refined, educated women is that, especially as the husband becomes "successful," well-to-do, and engrossed in business, he loses interest in all the little niceties of life with a spouse. He forgets his wife's birthday and their wedding anniversary; he never sends flowers; if he ever gives a present it is in the form of a soulless check; he seldom gives her any time or anything of himself; they never go on a merry trip together, and they never have any fun. Many an intelligent woman gets more and more resentful because she feels that she is little more than an unpaid housekeeper —a convenience to the husband and one who is taken for granted by him.

It never occurs to many a husband that he should keep on making love to his wife and trying to make her happy, and it never occurs to the wife that she should continue to keep herself clean, neat, trim, well-dressed, and attractive. If remonstrated with, the man may say, "When you have caught a street-car why keep running after it?"

The need for fun, good humor, and playfulness. Often a wife's main complaint about her husband is that there is no fun or playfulness in him. When she feels merry, he is serious or moody or silent. For a whole evening he may not speak to her, and then she wonders if it's because he is angry about something, or has heard something unpleasant about her. Many a woman says, especially when the husband is many years older than she, "I wanted a lover and a playfellow and all I have is a sort of father." Two people who can play together are fairly safe from unhappiness and neuroses.

The sorrow of the refined, artistic, idealistic, and highly intelligent woman is that, because she can imagine an ideal type of marriage with a fine, sensitive, loving man, she is dissatisfied with the sort of stodgy "good provider" who has fallen to her lot. Many a woman has said to me, "My husband is a good man and a fine man, but although married to me he is still at heart a bachelor. He never loved me or anyone deeply; he never saw much need for trying to make me happy, and after marriage he went his own way and lived pretty much his old life."

A woman's need for pride in her husband. To be happy and well a woman needs to be proud of her husband as a useful and honored member of the community. I have known a number of spirited women who either wanted to leave a nice husband or who at last did leave him, not because he had any unpleasant habits, but just because all he did was to cut coupons and play golf. The wife felt ashamed of him. Especially when it was her money on which they lived, she felt he was a gigolo.

I have known marriages that were going on the rocks, and then the man found himself: He won a promotion, or he succeeded in business, and then, with her renewed pride in him, the wife was happy and stable and much more affectionate. Few realize how much importance a woman places in her husband's status in the eyes of his fellows.

Persons who are ashamed of the spouse. A marriage is not safe when one spouse is a bit ashamed of the other, perhaps because of a poor physical appearance, a lack of education, poor manners, ill-breeding, or some deformity such as a squint or a clubfoot or a polio leg. Before marriage a girl may have hoped that love would conquer her distress over her fiancé's limp, but with the passage of time the embarrassment grew until it produced a neurosis. A bad feature of this sort of trouble is that when a woman of nice feelings realizes that she is being badly upset by her husband's handicap, she is ashamed because she feels that she is welshing on her bargain. Since she accepted him that way she should not be complaining now; and so she fights all the harder to overcome her distress. Perhaps she tries to do penance, and with this she becomes still more upset.

Oftentimes it is the husband who is ashamed of the wife, and so critical of her that he makes her frightened and ill. When friends are around she says little because if she opens her mouth she is likely to be told then or later that she has talked stupidly and exposed her ignorance. But when she keeps quiet, he scolds her for being a "dummy." Naturally, a situation like this grows worse with time. Often it develops during the engagement. In not a few cases it is the wife who is critical of the man, and always ready to jump on him if he says anything that conflicts with her many religious and other prejudices. Then it is he who becomes silent and on his guard, and "a different person" when she is around.

Troubles with religion. Many married couples split up because of religion. They would not have to do this if only one spouse would not insist on converting the other. The overly religious one would be wise to let the other go to the church of his or her choice. The worst troubles are likely to come when the couples' parents with rigid ideas start insisting that their grandchildren be brought up strictly in some faith. It probably will not do any good, but the physician can tease a trouble-making old mother by reminding her that if she, who is now such a devout and rigid, let us say, Baptist, had only been adopted in infancy into a Holy Roller family she most certainly would today be a devout Holy Roller!

Troubles due to rigidities in thinking. Many married couples stop talking to each other because so often the man or the wife jeers or rails at things the other says. As a result, there are more and more topics that one of the spouses must never mention or ever attempt to discuss. Some persons, as they grow older, become so angry at the President or the government or some "pet peeve" that with the least provocation they launch into a violent denunciation which may last for the rest of the evening. After the wife has heard this tirade a hundred times she dreads a repetition. Similarly, after a man has heard his relatives or some woman whom he is supposed to like thoroughly denounced many times he gets highly annoyed the minute the tirade starts.

The need for making adjustments. In marriage there are many adjustments to make. Even two loving persons may have to learn that what is acceptable loving to one is not acceptable to the other. One person may love to touch the beloved while the other may hate to be touched. She may be ticklish or slightly schizoid.

The two must learn not only to be lovers, but good friends. They have to learn to share a house and perhaps the same room and even the same bed. They may have to learn to play together and perhaps to share a hobby. Often, if a wife is not to become a week-end widow she must learn to hunt or fish, sail a boat, work in a basement shop, play golf, or go to baseball games.

The two must learn to live out of one bank account, and often this causes trouble. One may be a spendthrift while the other may be frugal or even a bit miserly. In many cases the wife must learn to work alongside her husband in a store, and this may bring many arguments and even fights. Often the husband and wife must learn to be good co-parents, backing up each other's authority with the children.

So often people fail in these adjustments because of childishness, selfishness, uncontrolled behavior, evil temper, sulking, efforts to have each his or her own way, and an inability to be a sport and to play the game. Often the man or wife is a bit psychopathic, perhaps constantly worrying and fretting or prophesying disaster.

Fretting. Much of the trouble of women in the home is due to their tendency to worry and fret too much over their loved ones when they are slightly ill or when they come home late. Many persons are too apprehensive over everything. Then they are inclined to tyrannize and fuss over the loved one until he or she can hardly stand it. As a good writer once put it, for years he had endured "that constant persecution that went under the name of love."

One of the worst, if only the mildest of the domestic tyrannies, is the constant effort of a wife to make her husband and her children put on rubbers and mufflers and overcoats at the slightest sign of cold or rain or snow. A woman may know that such efforts enrage the husband whose love she craves, but she just can't leave him alone. He may keep longing for a day, perhaps when he is seventy, when his wife will at last grant that he is grown-up enough to decide for himself whether or not to go out when it is raining!

Many women who haven't children and who live in apartments haven't enough to do. When the dishes are done and the rooms are dusted, the woman is bored. A woman of this type in summer may spend her whole day in her garden. This is her salvation. Some women spend too much time on bridge or canasta, and some get into trouble because they lose too much money at these games.

Finances. Much trouble in marriage is due to clashes over money. Some men make too little, others make enough, but waste it on liquor, gambling or women. A woman who has to skimp to make ends meet resents it when the man comes home with an expensive radio or television set or a custom-built shotgun. Similarly, the man will resent it if the woman takes advantage of her charge accounts and runs up big bills. Many a woman spends all a man can earn on clothes or on doctors' bills and medicines. In some cases she gets to gambling or drinking, and then the money goes fast.

Some men regularly turn over their whole pay check to the wife because she is the more methodical one of the pair and a better saver; others are stingy and make the wife wheedle for even necessary house money. The happiest situation is one in which the wife has two allowances: one for the house and one for "play money," all her own. It is sad when a man does not or dare not trust his wife with a few hundred dollars with which to pay the monthly bills. Often a husband complains that if his wife loved him she would not spend so much and run him into debt; she counters with, "If you loved me you'd work harder and make more money."

Many a woman with an undesirable husband is torn between the remnants of her old love for him and her deep resentments against him, produced perhaps by many unkindnesses or cruelties, or by his inability to earn a decent or steady living for her and her children. Because of his failures in business she may have to be ashamed of him before her relatives and friends. She must always be making excuses for him. He may distress her by being moody or silent or unfriendly when her relatives or old friends drop in. He may distress her much because of his lack of courtesy to her in public. More rarely, an essentially good husband will distress his wife because he is so boisterous and full of fun that she thinks he is rowdy. He embarrasses her.

Many a woman resents being brighter and abler than her husband. Soon after marriage she will be making all the important decisions in the man's business, and she may even have to supply him with ambition and backbone. The normal woman much prefers that her husband be the leader in the family. Often the man also comes to resent the situation, and hence the woman has to try constantly to make him think that he is head of the household. I remember a woman who ran a big business, but she made her husband sign all the checks.

A hard thing about women's work is that it is lonely work. Two or more persons working together can make fun out of a job, but one alone may feel that it is drudgery. Another trouble is that when there is a large house and a large family, the wife's work is never done. Another bad feature of a woman's life is that she meets too few persons in a day. She lacks the intellectual contacts that keep her husband happy and on his toes.

Lack of common interests and of growing together through the years. If only a physician would ask he would often find that for years there had been little community of interest between a man and his wife. The man often is interested in only two things: what he sells or makes, and his hobby or favorite sport. Usually the wife has few interests outside of the care of the home and the children. In later years if she is educated, she may become interested in the beautiful things of life; she may read, she may go to concerts and lectures, she may go back to the study of music, or she may collect antiques. Then it may bother her that her husband does not share her interest in these things and cannot enjoy them with her; perhaps he even resents the time and money she spends on them.

In other homes it is the other way around. A prominent physician, lawyer, architect, or businessman, especially in the first forty years of his life, has to keep learning so many things, and he keeps meeting so many interesting men and women that he keeps growing in education and character, much as if he were in college. If, during these years the wife stagnates mentally, perhaps just taking care of the house and children, reading only "the funnies" and poor novels, she falls out of step with her husband, and soon she has little to talk about that will ever interest him. Worse yet, she may resent his friends and may sneer at them, and then some day she will wake to find that she is married to a stranger who does not like her very well and who has little that he cares to discuss with her. Through kindness and a sense of responsibility he may continue to live with her, but she will have little happiness out of the association, and as a result she may develop a neurosis. In the upper classes a high percentage of American marriages end up in this way. Other marriages soon are boresome but the wife does not get a neurosis because she did not expect much. She, perhaps, was not intelligent or bright or interesting enough to bring much to the marriage, and so she is only vaguely disappointed with it.

Persons who would fail in any marriage. As I have said, most of us humans are not well enough controlled always to work out a happy marriage with anyone. Many of us are not sane enough, adult enough, or sufficiently tolerant and clear visioned. We are not good enough at making all the compromises and adjustments that are necessary in marriage. We are not always good natured and reasonable. A man may act like a madman when angry, or a woman, usually lovely, may be a nagging devil when menstruating. Other men and women can find little happiness in marriage or anywhere in life because they are so colorless, dull, quiet, uninteresting, and unenthusiastic. Others are too selfish to love anyone deeply, and others are too undemonstrative to show much love. I remember the fine, able, but unemotional Vermonter who, when asked by his lovely temperamental Irish wife why he never would say that he loved her, answered quietly, "I said that thirty years ago when I asked you to marry me. Since then I have not changed."

Oftentimes when a man or woman talks to me of divorce I remind him or her that the inadequacies and sins which wrecked the marriage that is now to be broken will probably wreck the second one and the third. So often in the newspapers, especially of Hollywood, one reads about a certain couple, "This is his fourth marriage and her third." That tells a lot about the two contracting parties.

Illness due to living with a psychopathic or insane man who is, at times, dangerous and brutal. It is terrible the suffering some women and children have to endure, living with a dangerously brutal, violent, abusive, insane, or alcoholic man. Not only has the wife her problems of danger, sorrow, and humiliation, but often she has to stand by and see a child abused or beaten. Few know the cruelties that are constantly being practised in many a home.

Causes for divorce. Most enlightening is the analysis of the troubles of 425 divorced women reported in five of the January and February, 1950, issues of the *Saturday Evening Post*. It tells what caused the divorces, and what the separation did to the lives of the women and children concerned. From this study, David G. Wittels and Professor Goode concluded that the commonest causes of trouble in marriage are:

1. The emotional immaturity and childishness of the contracting parties. As I have said, innumerable persons are too childish, uncontrolled, or psychopathic to live happily with any mate.

2. Our modern industrial civilization which has wiped out many of the material reasons for family life. Years ago a man could hardly run a farm without a wife, and most women got married because there was little else for them to do. Now most of the things a wife used to make are made for her. Now, so many women can earn as much as a man does that they feel that they do not have to get married or stay married unless the man is just what they want.

In the old days the more children a farmer had, the better; they all helped with the work. Today in many families, each child who will want to go through high school, college, and perhaps a professional school, represents a need for the expenditure of many thousands of dollars. A boy who is to be a physician and a specialist is not likely to earn anything until he is twenty-eight. Hence it is that many couples just must restrict the size of their families.

3. The idea that romantic love is a sufficient basis for marriage. Young people forget that marriage means also running a home together and perhaps raising and educating a family together.

4. Parental disapproval of the new son- or daughter-in-law. This is commonly met with, and often it leads to the destruction of the marriage. As everyone knows, mother-in-law trouble is common, and often it puts an end to the happiness of the young people.

5. Differences in the social, religious, and educational backgrounds of the spouses are great handicaps.

6. Insufficient income wrecks many a marriage in its first year or two. Sometimes the wife, previously spoiled by a wealthy and indulgent father, expects too much of her young husband who is starting out as a clerk.

7. Jobs for women enable many a dissatisfied woman to walk out or to defy the husband.

8. The ambition of a wife to go into a career wrecks some marriages.

9. Professor Goode placed infidelity last as a cause of broken homes. He found that in most cases it was only a sign of the final break-up of a marriage and not the cause. Alcoholism, also, is sometimes only the result of the unhappiness of one of the spouses.

In some cases trouble seems to start when the wife or husband meets again an old flame, or meets the person that she or he should originally have married. But, actually, in these cases the marriage was unstable to begin with because it started with one or both of the spouses accepting a "second best."

Should the couple separate? Not infrequently the physician has to talk over with a woman the question of whether she should leave a brutal, alcoholic, unfaithful, or good-for-nothing husband. Obviously, in such a discussion the doctor must not let himself be influenced by any religious ideas he may have. He must be like the good and wise priest who advised his sister to leave a drunken brute because, as he said, to live longer with him could result only in her demoralization and degradation, and in injury to the children.

Always the fine physician will keep thinking only of what is best or necessary for the salvaging of the health of the woman and for the care of her children. Sometimes, as Weiss and English say, better for children are one parent and peace than two parents and life lived in an atmosphere of daily hostility, unhappiness, and uncertainty as to the future. In other cases the physician will agree with the woman that if she can stand the situation she had better stick it out until the children are educated. So commonly, when a couple are divorced, the husband either disappears or slides out of caring for or educating his children; the poor wife usually carries the burden alone. One suspects that in this country it is only the childless gold digger who gets her alimony regularly.

If a couple are obviously incompatible, without love, and without children, I see no reason why they should go on living a cat-and-dog existence. If eventually they are going to get a divorce it would seem logical to get it early while the wife is young and likely to find another husband. Also, if they are fighting, and very doubtful about their ability ever to learn to live together in peace, it would seem that they should delay starting a family until they know what they want to do. Once a lovely curly-haired child is born to them they may be hand-cuffed together for life.

When a woman tells me of years of thinking and talking about divorce I say to her, "See this imaginary button on my desk; just press it and you'll be back from Reno with your little decree in your hand; come on now and press it." And she will not touch it. Then I get her to tell me her reasons for staying with her husband, and I point out that since apparently she is never going to institute divorce proceedings, she must stop thinking of the separation, and debating the question with herself night after night.

When a woman's marriage has been disappointing and unsatisfying she is likely to keep wishing for another chance. Hence, when she approaches forty she may get very unhappy and restless, realizing that her chances of a new deal are fading away.

What can be done to help? Often, when a physician thinks a reconciliation is desirable, he can say a few helpful words. He can find out from each one what the main complaints and annoyances are, and sometimes he can talk the two into trying to behave better and more sensibly. Sometimes he can take sides with wife or husband to help settle some argument. For instance, the wife may be distressed because she never gets a chance to eat out or go to a movie or a dance or for a little vacation. Perhaps the physician can get the husband to see that his wife ought to have at least one night out, like the maids whom we once used to have. Sometimes I try to get the husband to see how silly it is to keep spending thousands of dollars trying to cure his wife's illness when he could so quickly cure it himself by stopping some behavior which is making her upset.

Obviously, the physician will not want to urge a man or woman to get a divorce; that should be for him or her to decide, but, as I have said, often the doctor can stop the couple from constantly talking about it by getting them to see clearly that neither of them will ever take the step. Then he may get them to admit, seeing that they have decided to stay together, they had better turn to and learn to live more pleasantly.

Sometimes the doctor can induce the couple more often to say, and say more quickly, those wonderfully helpful words, "I am sorry, dear; forgive me." All of us humans are likely at times to be tired or uncomfortable, and hence irritable, complaining, impatient, or snappy. To snap is forgivable, but not to repent and apologize quickly is bad; sulking is one of the curses of marriage.

Some troubles of the divorced woman. The divorced woman often is worn down, working and supporting a few children. It is hard to work all day in an office and then to keep up a home at night. Oftentimes it can be done only with the help of the woman's mother.

According to Professor Goode, some nine in ten divorcées with children had to work to supplement what the court had ordered the husband to pay, and which often he slid out of paying. Unfortunately, the needs of the children often keep the woman from getting a job, they keep her from getting a new husband, and they keep her from having any social life.

Besides overwork the woman may have the strains of loneliness and perhaps some sex-hunger. Then there may come the problem of what to do about the man who proposes marriage but who does not want to assume the burden of supporting children, or who cannot earn enough to support more than a wife and himself. Or there are the hard problems of having children cared for all day by some ignorant woman. There are annoyances due to the tendency of many men to assume that the divorcée will promptly accept any indecent proposal, and there are problems due to the lack of acceptance of the divorcée in many social circles. She is not invited to the homes of her old friends as she used to be when she had a husband and was one of a pair. Now she is an extra who would unbalance the dining table or the card table.

Often a woman suffers from shame, realizing that she failed to hold her man and to make him happy. That was the biggest job she had in the world and she failed at it. She may blame her husband or another woman for the final break-up, but in moments of frankness, she will say, "It was my fault, too; if only I had known then what I know now, I would have kept him happy; I would have kept him so happy at home that he would never have gone out to drink and chase women. If only someone had made me see that making a happy home was my most important job on earth, I wouldn't be the lonely, bitter woman I am today."

Many divorced persons suffer because of estrangement from their church, and later, perhaps, because of their church's refusal to countenance a second marriage. Other divorced persons suffer because of their parents' strong disapproval of their action in terminating their marriage.

Sometimes a divorced person suffers because he or she is still in love with the spouse and still concerned over where she or he is and what she or he is doing. In such cases there may be a legal separation but not an emotional one. Some divorced couples keep seeing each other, dining occasionally together, running a business together, or even living near each other. They say they get along well enough if they do not have to live too closely together. Many divorcées say they miss having the man around even if he was a stinker.

Divorcées Anonymous. In Chicago there is a helpful society called Divorcées Anonymous. The idea is like that of Alcoholics Anonymous: In other words, women who have been divorced, who have learned their lesson, and have come to see why they lost out, will go to the aid of women who are much distressed at the sight of their marriage going on the rocks. Often only a divorcée can talk the troubled woman and her husband into making a new try, with a little more sense and a better knowledge of why things have gone wrong.

If a couple has been quarreling mainly about finances, a member of Divorcées Anonymous (called DA) whose marriage was broken up by money troubles comes in to help them to make a budget and to live by it. Or, if a marriage is being broken up by in-laws, the unhappy wife is helped and advised by a member of DA whose marriage was wrecked by a mother-in-law.

The troubles of the divorced man. The divorced man often marries again, sometimes for better and sometimes for worse. Oftentimes he is troubled by the criticism or ostracism of his friends; sometimes he is hurt through loss of business good will; often if he pays alimony faithfully he is pinched by the need for money. If he marries again, he has to pay for two families, and this is a strain. Sometimes he gets restless and wants to go to another community to start again with a new set of neighbors. A divorcée usually has the same desire to flee and hide. Sometimes the new wife fusses because she has to live in the old wife's house, and she may fuss and get bitter over the fact that she has to go without many things so that the first wife can get her alimony.

As many divorced men have discovered, the securing of transient sexual outlets outside of marriage is easy enough, but the finding of a fine lasting lovelife outside of marriage is not always easy. Often a mature man with considerable means will hesitate to marry again, knowing that if the new venture should also go on the rocks he will find himself stripped of half of what is left of his property, and his children stripped of most of their inheritance.

The woman who gets distressed at five-thirty. There are quite a few women who get distressed about 5:30 in the afternoon when they begin to brace themselves for the strain of welcoming home a husband who is not congenial, or not loved, or is just gloomy, or unpleasant, or desirous of being entertained all evening, or so strenuous that he blows in through the front door like a whirlwind. I have known women who, when they heard the car coming into the driveway, or heard the key in the lock of the front door, became nauseated, trembly, faint, or ill. In the worst cases the maid and the children, also, got tense and afraid.

The woman may say that her husband is good and generous and means to be kind, but in one way or another, he succeeds in making her tense. She is a different, happier person when he is not at home. Then she loses her abdominal distress, her headache, or her diarrhea. Often her intimates will say, "You are a different person when your husband is away. When he is around you are quiet and guarded in your speech, you say little and there is no sparkle in you. When he is away you are fun." The wife in such a situation dreads week ends and especially vacation trips when she must be cooped up with the man in a hotel room, and must make a more prolonged effort to entertain him and keep him from getting too restless. Often the man is a person without inner resources or a hobby or much interest in anything outside his business.

Sometimes he is a gloomy fellow who, each evening, says his health is failing or his business is going on the rocks. Perhaps he describes in detail his dyspepsia and the day's unpleasantnesses. Then it is up to the wife to sympathize and to reassure. And she has to be skillful at this because if she dismisses his worries too lightly he will be hurt and will feel she is unsympathetic, flippant, or heartless, while if she is too sympathetic he will get alarmed, fearing that things must be even worse than he thought they were.

The wife who makes her husband tense and nervous. There are some cases, also, in which a bossy and critical or socially superior wife makes her husband feel tense and on his guard. I have even seen cases in which the tension caused abdominal pain.

Hostilities and resentments. Between many married partners there is much resentment and hostility alongside of some love. Often this is apparent from the unpleasant way in which a man or woman "kids" the spouse, says mean things, tells embarrassing stories about the other, or appeals for sympathy to the people in the room. This sort of thing is embarrassing to the people who have to listen to it.

Disagreements over child bearing and contraception. Many married persons have much trouble because of disagreement over the question of having a child or several children. Sometimes one of the spouses loves children and the other does not. There often are conflicts, also, over the use of contraceptive measures. One spouse may insist on them while the other may feel that their use is sinful. Only rarely are these things discussed with the physician, but often they should be, as when they are tending to disrupt a woman's marriage or to wreck her nerves.

The rolling-up of annoyances until an explosion comes. One of the difficulties in marriage is the tendency for little annoyances to add up until some day there is an explosion. A woman will get more and more distressed over her husband's poor table manners, or his love of eating too much, or his tendency to stay too long in the bathroom, or his habit of hawking and spitting for a half-hour in the morning, or his fondness for starting late for everything, or his liking to tease her uproariously. Perhaps these things irritate her until she fears she will scream. Then, some day, after some slight annoyance, she will explode so violently that the man will be astounded and puzzled. He will not be able to guess what he did that deserved such a dressing-down. I remember a couple who, after years of making one another tense, exploded violently and got a divorce over the question of drowning or not drowning a kitten that had strayed into the house!

Sexual deficiencies. Although many women admit that they get little satisfaction from sexual intercourse and rarely if ever achieve an orgasm, few seem to drift into a neurosis because of this. Many say they wish the husband would "bother them" less often. Only a few well-sexed women say they wish the man would come to their bed more often. Many a woman who says she has little sexual feeling still wants to have regular intercourse, perhaps because it brings her some little sign of affection on the part of the husband. It is a bond between them which she will miss when it is gone.

Many a woman who admits that she is a very poor sexual partner will say that her husband has been kind and "understanding." She says he seldom bothers her, or he hasn't been to her bed for years. Often when I see the husband I find that he seems still to be in love with his wife, and he is kind and devoted. Husbands rarely complain to a physician of frigidity in the wife; they seem either to accept it, or else they leave the woman, or they find help elsewhere.

Wives occasionally will complain that the husband is a poor sexual partner, usually because he ejaculates prematurely or withdraws or uses a condom. This leaves the woman nervous and upset. Other husbands are unsatisfactory because they are not much interested in sex, or are prudish, or merely animal-like about it, or they lose interest entirely by the age of forty. A few are annoying because they demand intercourse twice a day or at a time when the woman cannot get interested. Some of the trouble in many marriages is that there is seldom a time, morning or evening, when husband and wife are both wide awake and rested enough so that they can enjoy intercourse. There is often need for the husband's taking thought to have intercourse when the wife is not tired or sleepy or otherwise indisposed and not in the mood. A wife, if wise, will want to give her husband pleasure at those times when he is most inclined to be affectionate. The couple will be fortunate if they can agree on an amount of intercourse which is fairly satisfactory to both. They are exceedingly fortunate, also, if they can usually achieve orgasm at the same time. It is unfortunate when a sexual athlete marries a sexual weakling.

Most women are not inclined to fuss much about a man's defects as a sexual partner. The wife may ask her husband to see a urologist but almost always he refuses. If he is friendly, kind, and a good provider, and if the wife likes and respects him, she will usually take him as he is and will soon stop complaining.

Many sexual dissatisfactions, disgusts, and conflicts begin the first night when the spouses find that one or the other is a poor partner, or one of them feels disgust at the touch of the other, or the woman learns that intercourse is something she will never be able to enjoy or perhaps even tolerate. Naturally, it can be a shock to both the partners to find that the woman is frigid. In many cases during the first night the husband becomes dissatisfied with his wife's appearance, and then, especially if he complains, trouble begins. One wonders if many marriages ought not to be annulled the day after the wedding. Certainly this would save much more suffering later when divorce has to come, and perhaps children have to be hurt.

In later life, when many women become fat, misshapen, and perhaps somewhat malodorous because of the growth of molds in the vagina and under heavy breasts, and when they lose what little sexual desire they had, the husband's small remainder of libido may not be sufficient to overcome these handicaps. If then he leaves his wife alone, she may get the idea that he is getting satisfaction elsewhere, and then come reproaches.

On a better approach to the sexual act. Much has been written on the desirability of a husband's learning a better approach to sex, and there is no doubt that in some cases there is need for such instruction, especially before the honeymoon.

The greatest need for the husband's learning to adjust well to intercourse comes usually when the wife is very slow to achieve orgasm. Women who achieve orgasm quickly say that they do not need any prolonged approach to the act, in fact, many prefer not to have any.

Men usually stand an unhappy marriage without breaking nervously. Interestingly, few of the men caught in an unhappy marriage ever complain about it, and few seem to get neurotic enough over it to consult a physician. They escape neurosis perhaps because marriage does not mean so much to a man as it does to a woman; it is only a part of his life. Furthermore, he is not tied so firmly to the home as the woman is. He has his business, his work, his sport, and his companionships outside the home. To a woman, home and marriage and husband often mean everything.

When a man with a strong sense of responsibility finds himself with an unsatisfactory wife he generally accepts the situation and makes the best of it. Many a man uncomplainingly accepts marriage with an unattractive woman who never loved him, who is a poor bed-fellow, who shows no affection, who is always sick and complaining and running up doctors' bills, who cannot cook a decent meal, and who cannot care properly for home and children.

The man who does go to pieces nervously because of a poor marriage is usually a young fellow who, after marrying a woman with whom he was infatuated, finds that she does not love him, and that he cannot win her or even hold her. Perhaps a former beau has come back to hang around, and then to the husband's unhappiness there is added jealousy and distrust and some hatred.

Unfaithfulness. As everyone knows, a disruptive influence in many marriages is unfaithfulness, and usually one thinks of this fault as lying with the man. One forgets that often the man starts stepping out only after the wife, by her unpleasant behavior, lack of affection, selfishness, or incompetency as a sexual partner, has driven him from her. Only after he has lost his love for his wife will he start looking for love elsewhere. Similarly, the wife, so long as she loves, is not likely ever to "step out."

Curiously, many a man who shows signs of being really in love with his wife, and who certainly is generous with her and does not want to lose her, will occasionally spend a night with some woman who does not mean a thing to him. If caught, he will say that the adventure was of no consequence, it was purely a matter of curiosity or of animal sex, and that it had no effect on his love for his wife. His subsequent behavior commonly shows that this is true, but the wife may not be satisfied with the explanation, and often her nerves will go to pieces under the impact, first, of her suspicions, and later, of her certainty. Often, in spite of many promises the husband will fall from grace again, apparently following the custom of many polygamous men the world over.

As I said above, in many cases the fault is primarily the wife's. After years of putting up with her childish or psychopathic behavior what love he had for her is gone, and then he may find a deep and permanent attachment elsewhere. After that he may live on in his home only from a sense of duty. Many other men, of course, are entirely at fault because they are naturally promiscuous and always "hunting."

The wife who feels that she is no longer needed. Many women around fifty who complain of a lot of vague symptoms have recently joined the "nobody-loves-me" club. So long as there was a child in the home to be cared for the woman felt needed and useful, but the minute the last child left she had the feeling that the husband would hardly notice it if she, too, were to leave.

Often in these cases the woman has her own foolishness to thank for her unhappy state. Perhaps when her first son came she practically moved into the nursery with him, and largely cut herself off from the husband. Sexually she deserted him. Now she would like to get him back but she cannot. In many a case the woman will admit that years before, the wise old family physician said, "Remember that some day the children will marry and go away. Then you will want to fall back on your husband. Better, then, cling to him now; love him and be good to him, and keep him always first in your heart."

The unwisdom of advising an unhappy wife to get herself a lover. Some physicians will advise an unhappily married or sex-starved woman to go and get herself a lover, but they are most unwise; they do not know women or the needs of their hearts. It is not sexual intercourse that the woman wants so much as a beautiful companionship and the ideal sort of marriage that she has always dreamed of. She wants a friendly, interesting, affectionate, attractive, and well-to-do man who will take her out and be her companion and escort wherever she wants to go. She wants someone in whom she will find strength in times of trouble. She wants a man who will remember birthdays and little anniversaries. She wants a home and a fine position in society, and she wants security.

Troubles due to a wife's having to work. Many a wife has to go on working because the husband does not make enough for two, or for two plus some children. Most women seem to be able to accept this philosophically, and I cannot remember when I heard one complain of it, but I suspect that a few resent the inability or unwillingness of the husband to set them free from the burden of earning a living. A few may wish to try another marriage so as perhaps to join the ranks of those women who are supported entirely by the man.

In some cases a wife will want to work for the joy and satisfaction of it, or to avoid boredom, or to get more money, and then the husband may object. He may want his wife to be at home, or he may feel ashamed to have her working, or he may prefer having her dependent on him. Women who supply all the money for the household are sometimes unhappy about it. I remember a wealthy woman like that who complained bitterly that her husband had never given her even a little present! Another such woman gave her husband a special allowance so that he could send her flowers several times a month!

Troubles due to a lack of liberty in marriage. One of the great needs in marriage is for the respecting by each spouse of the rights and liberties and personality of the other. Thus, when the husband wants to go fishing or hunting or golfing with his cronies, the wife should not raise Cain, and when the wife wants to continue her education in music or interior decorating the husband must not storm.

Often there is unhappiness in marriage because one of the spouses tries so hard to make the other over. Often I say to a woman, "If you could make your husband over into what he is not and does not care to be, you might not like him, and you might look down on him for having let you boss him."

I can remember several mannish women, each of whom married a Caspar Milquetoast, and then became disgusted with him because he did not stand up for his rights and refuse to be led around by the nose! They wanted to weep on my shoulder about it, but I was not sympathetic. As I said, if they had married a strong, able man who could and would have dominated, they would have fought with him, and their life would then have been a mixture of love and resentment. The women appeared to have too large an element of masculinity mixed up with their femininity, and until too late, they apparently had not decided whether to be clinging, feminine, and dependent, or independent, strong, and mannish and inclined to wear the pants.

No matter how loving a couple are, each should respect the other's rights of personality and privacy. For instance, neither should ever open the other's mail or ever go through the other's personal possessions. Neither should ask prying and personal questions, especially if the other does not appear to want to discuss a matter.

Disagreements over the discipline and education of children. Especially when the two spouses are very different in temperament, or upbringing, or religious faith, there are likely to be conflicts over the discipline and the education of children. The physician may then be able to help more than any one else in showing the two that quickly they should reach some compromise and then stick to it so that the children will not be upset by the quarreling of their parents and the countermanding of orders.

The wreckage of families by impossible living conditions. Many a couple get divorced largely because when first married they had to live with the parents of either the bride or the groom. The Chinese "character" for trouble began as a picture of two women under one roof. Even a girl and her mother are likely to have trouble if they have to use the same kitchen. Young people would be wise not to marry until they can afford to get a little apartment of their own.

Many couples are pried apart by some older relative who has to come and live with them. Often this is the husband's mother but it may be the wife's mother, or even a father of one of the spouses. One difficulty that arises when there are children is that the grandparent demands quiet, and this is hard to get and to keep when the children are healthy and naturally boisterous. Another difficulty is that the husband and wife, deprived of privacy and intimate companionship, drift apart. As one woman said, she and her husband could not even have a quarrel to themselves!

The wreckage of marriage by parents and in-laws. Perhaps when a young husband is not able to buy all the things his wife was used to and wants, the mother keeps saying to her, "If you had only taken my advice and married that man you wouldn't look at, you would now have a mink coat and perhaps your own car." The mother may also come around often to take her daughter's side and back her up in her quarrels with the husband. Worse yet, the mother may set out deliberately to break up the marriage. Often she starts in by refusing to admit her daughter-in-law or son-in-law into the circle of the family. If she writes a letter it is only to her child, or if she invites her child to dinner she does not include the spouse. Such feuds are especially bitter if the parent is very critical of a difference in religion.

One marriage in three is unhappy. Today about one marriage in three appears to be unhappy, and perhaps one in five ends in divorce. In a Gallup poll, some 56 per cent of the men and women questioned said that, if set free, they would not remarry the partner they then had. As Myerson once said, few of us realize the amount of bitter quarreling that goes on in the apartments and houses on all sides of us.

Many very unhappy marriages do not break up, simply because the couple cannot afford a divorce; they cannot afford to live separately, or they cannot afford to live separately and take care of their children, or one of them is reluctant to take the plunge and face the criticism of parents and friends. Often, after having listened to the complaints of a childless woman who, from her account, was married to a beast, I have said, "Why don't you leave him?" And her answer has been, "I am afraid to go out in the world alone; I am not qualified to hold any job, and I am appalled at the thought of living and eating alone."

CHAPTER 12

Little Strokes, A Common Cause of Nervous Syndromes

THE CONSULTING INTERNIST sees many patients past middle age who are miserable and unhappy and perhaps unable to work. Usually the doctor is treating what he thinks is indigestion, heart disease, Ménière's disease, or a fatigue state. Yet often the correct diagnosis would have been obvious to anyone, even a layman, *if only the significant story had been elicited*. Probably the patient had kept talking to his doctors only about a distress in his chest or abdomen, when he should have been telling of the bad dizzy spell which in a minute, had made a wreck out of him.

I fear though that, even if he had told his story properly, mentioning the marked mental changes that had come, or the inability to work or to use the right hand well, his physician might have missed the diagnosis, partly because in college he was never taught to think of the brain as a common seat of disease, and partly because he would have so hated to speak of a little stroke.

The stigma of having a stroke. There is so much stigma attached to the idea of having a stroke that few physicians will use the word or make the diagnosis. They fear to antagonize the patient and his family and perhaps to discourage them. From an impartial scientific point of view there should, of course, be no disgrace in having a little blood vessel thrombose in the brain. There is not the slightest stigma felt when a vessel thromboses in the heart; people are even rather proud of that, but they do not like the idea of having a vessel thrombose in the brain! The reason for this is wrapped up in that word "stroke." In this twentieth century, even college graduates vaguely accept the idea that at times an angry God strikes a man down. Naturally, then, they must suspect that He had some reason for doing this, and the man must have done something reprehensible. As a fine lovely minister's wife and former missionary kept saying to me over and over again after a big stroke: "What did I do to so anger my God? So far as I could, I served Him devotedly all my days; wherein did I fail? Why did He strike me down so cruelly?"

Seeing that people feel this way, it is not surprising that many conceal the fact of a stroke, much as they would conceal the fact of having contracted syphilis. All one has to do is to turn to the daily newspaper to see the number of notices of persons who suddenly "collapsed" and, after two or three days of coma, died. The paper says they suffered a heart attack, or acute indigestion, or, as in the case of Judge Rutledge of the Supreme Court, who was dying as I wrote this, they had "a vascular disorder." Physicians will sometimes put down as the diagnosis. cerebral arteriosclerosis, or Ménière's syndrome, or a heart attack, or a vascular accident, but rarely cerebral thrombosis, or apoplexy, and practically never, "a little stroke."

It is true that in some cases the disease of the person's arteries, and the tendency to thrombosis in them, affects *both* the heart muscle and the brain. Then it is that a physician can be somewhat pardoned for noting only the cardiac injury, but if he were to take a good history, he would see that perhaps long before the coronary arteries had narrowed down enough to cause trouble, the man's brain had been badly injured. For instance, a man who died from a stroke in his fifties, had been treated through his forties for coronary thrombosis. But careful questioning of the family showed that already in his thirties he was having little strokes which weakened some ocular muscles and so damaged his brain that he could no longer handle his business; his wife had to take over. At necropsy both his brain and heart were found to be full of little infarcts.

The reluctance of physicians to mention a stroke. As I was writing this, I received a letter from a man of fifty who described a series of little strokes, the first of which, some two years ago, had hit him hard with a bad dizzy spell. This came at 7:30 one morning, and left him full of discomforts and distresses on one side of his body. They left him utterly miserable, with ear noises, inability to work, and with some difficulty in balancing. With this story it was hard to imagine any physician not recognizing the nature of the trouble, and yet the man said that he had seen many diagnosticians and had spent thousands of dollars on tests and roentgenologic studies, "none of which had shown what was wrong." He said that his doctors were still trying to find the seat of the disease in his heart or liver or bowel!

One wonders why someone had not had the good sense or the kindness to tell him the truth, if only to stop his great wastage of effort and of a lifetime's savings!

I think physicians are usually wrong when they are afraid to mention a stroke to the patient who has had one. Many a time I have found a man most grateful for my having talked to him about the subject. Often I ask, "Did it occur to you at the time that you might be having a stroke?" and the man answers, "Yes, I was practically certain I was having a stroke; in fact I felt so queer I feared I was dying." Then he went on to say that when his physicians did not even mention the possibility of a stroke he was left wondering if either they were not keen enough to suspect what had gone wrong, or not honest enough to be frank with him.

I can remember only one patient who reacted badly to being told that she had had a little stroke. Later she wrote asking me "to take it back," but the rest of my patients with little strokes seemed relieved to know the worst, or at last to find a physician with whom they could talk over the situation. It was some comfort to them to know that there was nothing wrong in the heart or the abdomen. In many cases it greatly helped the morale of the patient and his family to know that there was no heart disease and no need for mantaining a strict regimen of bed rest and saltless food.

The difficulties in getting consultants to accept the diagnosis of a stroke. I am sorry to say that my unpleasant experiences in trying to get fellow-consultants to accept the diagnosis of a little stroke have made me somewhat reluctant to mention the subject; I always feel on the defensive. Time and again, when I have told the home internist that I thought his patient's trouble was all due to a stroke, he has appeared incredulous or annoyed, or even a bit disgusted. Some men, when they heard of my diagnosis, re-examined the patient and then wrote that I must be wrong because the fellow had none of the usual neurologic signs of a brain injury. His muscle strengths, his skin sensations, and his reflexes were all all right! Unfortunately, they had failed to note that the man's brain as a whole had been injured so severely that he was a wreck and a changeling, and almost a stranger to his wife and his business associates!

Such a tremendous change in character may not be a neurologic finding to some men, but it is to me. It may not be mentioned in the books, but if not, it should be. Many a neurologist will report that a man's facial muscles are all right because he does well enough at show-ing his teeth and raising his eyebrows. What the doctor failed to note was that as the fellow was talking he was using one side of his mouth a little more than the other. Many a time this fact alone has given me the hunch I needed to go on and get the story of a little stroke.

Many a time an assistant, after checking muscle strengths, will report that a man's hand and arm were all right. What he missed was that to the patient the hand did not feel right; it often felt numb or clumsy, or shaky, or the handwriting had changed. Several of my patients with little strokes, when asked, have told me that they had to learn to write with the left hand or with a typewriter, and this fact, almost alone, made the diagnosis. Unfortunately, the home internists who had seen these persons had not asked and so had not learned of this striking symptom. Several of the women patients, when asked about changes in handwriting, said, "Why, yes, after that dizzy spell my children com-plained that they had trouble reading my letters." Many a patient, when I questioned him, admitted that he had been called to his bank to give a new signature for his checks. And all the time some eminent internist was treating him for "colitis" or coronary heart disease!

I am happy to say that often I have no trouble selling my diagnosis to the old family physician. He says, "That's right; I suspected that," or "Why didn't I see that?", or "Come to think of it, now, that diagnosis would fit a dozen of my older patients about town, whose discomforts have been puzzling me."

Some common symptoms. In the case of a typical small stroke a person suddenly feels dizzy, with a sensation as if he were going to fall over or faint or collapse. Perhaps for a few seconds vision will black out, or there will be some mental confusion or fear of death, or the person may become nauseated, or may vomit. Sometimes after such a spell the person will feel miserable for a time, and in rare cases he or she will spend a few weeks in the hospital.

Often, later, when the internist's assistant takes the history, he will put down that the patient had vertigo, and he will diagnose Ménière's disease. But actually things did not spin around as they might have done if there had been an injury to the inner ear, the eighth nerve, or the cerebellum. All the patient felt was a sense of insecurity, or of top-heaviness, or a feeling as he turned a corner quickly, that if he had not been looking at the ground he might have lost his balance and fallen. Sometimes, of course, there is injury to the balancing mechanism in ear and brain, and then the patient will complain of true vertigo or ear noises or unilateral deafness.

Sometimes a nervous storm shoots down the vagus nerves into the thorax or abdomen, there to produce curious pains or rending feelings or distresses. This storm may make the stomach or bowel spastic so that the taking of food will promptly cause spasm and pain. The fact that nothing can be found locally to explain this discomfort should suggest that it was referred out from the brain.

Commonly after a little stroke there is some failure of memory for recent events. There may be some tingling or numbness in a spot on the face or in a hand or a foot. The legs may get distressingly restless at night, or they may work poorly and become a bit "rubbery."

With fairly extensive injury to the brain the patient will age suddenly; his face may look haggard, expression may go out of it, the springiness will go out of his step, and he may shuffle a bit. He will walk slowly and cautiously like an old man. Often the speech will become a bit thick, and there may be a little drooling at one corner of the mouth. These changes can establish the diagnosis.

In some cases the little stroke causes great moral deterioration, and then a man may get into scrapes with prostitutes or young girls or designing women. Some men lose their business judgment and start running through their fortune. Some have to be declared incompetent. Many can never work again.

Because of these changes in character many of the patients become terrible problems to their relatives. At home they may be irascible and hard to handle. At the office they not only are useless, but they obstruct the work of others. They may be too testy to get along well with their associates and employees. The president of the company will want to retire an executive who has slipped into this state, but usually he will want first to get from some physician a diagnosis of organic illness. He will send the fellow to one internist after another but the report will always come back that the man's essential organs are sound. Because of present-day medical habits no one will think of looking for the disease in the brain. (See Chapter 1.)

No note is made of the fact that the man has lost all his old interest in life. In bad cases, he will no longer care to hear about his children and grandchildren, and he will no longer care to see his old cronies or to hear of their hunting or fishing adventures.

Highly diagnostic is the fact, when elicited, that a man who, before his dizzy spell had never known fear, is now afraid to be alone. He is expecting another stroke, and he fears that when it comes he may be so crippled by it that he will be unable to reach the telephone to call for help.

Some of these patients drift on into a Parkinson's syndrome, and a few go into an agitated depression. Occasionally one will go blind in one eye because of a thrombus in the main artery or vein. A few persons get a trophic arthritis in the wrist or hand or hip on the side of the body that was weakened by the little stroke. Others who have always slept perfectly will suddenly find themselves suffering from insomnia. Others may suffer a decided weakening of the muscles on one side of the face. A few, after suffering injury to the brain stem, will have much trouble eating. Food will go down the wrong way to cause violent coughing. The throat may also be full of sticky mucus. Quite a few, particularly of the women, get a burning, or a foul or metallic taste in the mouth. The fact that often it is on only one side of the mouth shows that it is of nervous origin. Rarely the center for an ocular muscle will be involved, and then for a time the patient will see double. The head or a hand may begin to shake with a slow, coarse tremor.

Oftentimes the patient will suddenly lose 30 or 40 pounds in weight, and this may be the only symptom complained of. I suspect it is due to a change in the setting of some regulator in the hypothalamus. A similar change in the setting of the thermostat for the body will sometimes cause a nervous hyperthermia which will last for a few months.

Someone may ask, "Do these persons have to have hypertension?" No; a thrombosis can occur just as easily or perhaps even more easily if the blood pressure is low. It is highly significant of a little stroke if, after a puzzling spell, the pressure of a hypertensive person drops to normal and stays there, either for a while or permanently. Another question may be, "Do women suffer from this disease?" They certainly do, and possibly more often than men do.

What determines the nature of the syndrome? The nature of the syndrome that results must depend partly on the amount of brain tissue put out of action, and largely on the location of this dead tissue in the brain. For instance, a man in his eighties had had so much of his brain destroyed that he had practically no memory left of what he had done ten seconds before. He could not count up to ten because he would lose count after saying 5 or 6 or 7. But his judgment remained good; his original kindly, calm temperament remained unchanged, and he kept clean and well-groomed. Another man with one little stroke lost most of his memory but otherwise seemed unchanged. Another man with the first strokelet became inefficient and fearful and unable to do his work; another changed from a kindly man to an irascible one; another changed from a fine banker and head deacon to a dissolute person who went to live with a common prostitute. Another patient, a woman, after the first shock lay in a stupor for fifteen years.

Many thromboses are not noted because they occur during sleep, or they come by day and occasion no discomfort. In many cases in which an older patient has evidently suffered an injury to the brain, no matter how carefully one questions him and the family one cannot get a history of an acute episode. I think this is usually because the injury came at night when the blood pressure was lowest. Perhaps most of the small thromboses in the brain occur at night. The patient may wake feeling all right, or he may wake feeling stupid and dull, or suffering from a bad headache, or he may discover that he has lost some of his memory.

In many cases the small strokes probably come during the day but are not sensed by the patient. This must be so because a man can have a big stroke, with half his body paralyzed, without feeling any pain or shock or distress. I remember a physician whom I saw shortly after he had suffered a big stroke. He said he felt fine, and at the moment of the paralysis he had felt no mental distress, pain, dizziness, nausea, or confusion. If this can happen with a big stroke, how easily it can happen with a small one that destroys only a few cubic millimeters of tissue in a silent area of the brain.

At necropsy, although a man's brain may be found full of the little brown scars of thromboses, the wife may be unable to recall more than one or two episodes which could have represented a stroke. Sometimes the patient says that he fell or slipped or stumbled or miscalculated the height of a step, but the fact that for weeks or months afterward he was miserable and unable to work makes it probable that the fall was the result of a slight stroke. In some cases the patient, if encouraged to talk, will say, "I know I blacked out *before* I fell down those steps. That is why I fell, but my doctor wouldn't listen to me."

Occasionally the story is that the patient fell out of a chair; he quickly picked himself up, but after that he was never well again. I remember a station master who, while standing watching a train come in, fell to the ground. In a moment he picked himself up but after that his brain never worked comfortably or efficiently. Sometimes the little shocks are over in a minute. Thus, an elderly physician who had had several of these episodes, one night while lying on his bed reading, felt for perhaps thirty seconds, a complete loss of his sense of position in space. Later, he had a spell lasting a few seconds in which he feared he would fall, and still later, one in which marked vertigo lasted perhaps ten minutes. Fortunately for him, the vessels thrombosed were so small that his general health and his mental health remained excellent.

One cannot always be sure of the nature of the first suspicious episode; it might have been anything; but after the man has had several little shocks, and perhaps eventually a big one, one can be almost certain about the nature of the first one.

Are the attacks ever due to angiospasm? With very short spells in which there is a brief aphasia or hemiplegia, most physicians believe that the trouble in the brain was a momentary spasm of a small artery. This, of course, is possible, but Dr. James Kernohan, the brain pathologist of the Mayo Clinic, thinks it far more probable that most, even of these transient spells, represent thromboses. I feel the same way, because even when persons have the very transitory spells, they generally go on to peter out with the usual signs of cerebral arteriosclerosis. Osler also commented on this fact. For instance, an able lawyer of seventy, in the course of a few weeks, suffered several attacks of aphasia and hemiplegia lasting only a matter of minutes. His physicians felt that each time there could hardly have been more than a brief spasm in some artery of the brain, but to me the significant fact is that with these spells the man's legs became progressively weaker and uncertain in their behavior, so that soon he could barely walk even with the help of crutches. And through the years he did not get any better.

The one good thing about this idea of spasm in blood vessels is that oftentimes it serves to soften the blow for some timid patient and also for his physicians, who cannot bring themselves to accept the idea of a thrombosis.

A series of strokes commonly take from ten to twenty years to kill a man. In many cases a long series of little strokes all serve one purpose and are part of one process, the process that slowly kills the victim. Thus, a friend of mine, an able man with a large business, came in one day to tell me that after forty-five years of perfect health and great energy he had suddenly found himself so weak and tired that it was hard to push himself to work. With this he began to have distress in his abdomen. I went over him carefully and could find nothing wrong. At that time I had no idea what had happened to him, and like other physicians, I looked for disease only below the neck.

I then left California and my friend went to another physician who promptly had his appendix removed. When this did not do any good, another physician diagnosed coronary heart disease. It is doubtful if he ever had this because in the many years that remained to him he did not suffer from angina or dyspnea. His powers just failed. He did not go out much because he was afraid to be on the street alone. After a while he could no longer force himself to do much work. Then his feet began to shuffle, and soon it was apparent that he had a Parkinson's syndrome. Gradually he slid down hill until he became paralyzed. Almost to the end his mind remained clear, and his pleasant character remained unchanged. In many ways his brain was still keen, and he was interested in receiving letters from his family and friends. The interesting point is that it took him just twenty-one years to die. He started dying with a shock which apparently came at night and left him feeling tired out.

The reader who would like to learn more about the life stories of these many persons who die by inches over the course of years can

202   *Causes of Neuroses and Psychoses*

turn to my article in Geriatrics (*1*: 189, 1946) or in Oxford Medicine, Vol. 6: chapter II-A, p. 68. There I tell of the sweet old lady who
after several little strokes said, "Death is taking little bites of me."

Diagnosis. As I have said, the most important point in the diagnosis,
when it can be established, is that at a certain moment of a certain day
the person had a dizzy or faint or confused spell, or fell for a moment,
or vomited, or "blacked out." So-called nervous breakdowns in older
persons, especially if they come suddenly out of a clear sky and without any history of extra strain or overwork, are likely to be due to
thrombosis of some vessel in the brain. I say, "older persons," although
in World War II many soldiers under the age of thirty-five years were
seen to suffer strokes with hemiplegia. Every so often I see a young
person in his thirties who has suffered what could easily have been a
stroke, perhaps due to the rupture of a tiny aneurism of the circle of
Willis, but no one can ever be sure of what happened.

One of the most important points in the diagnosis of this common
disease is to learn from the family that after a little spell the patient's
character changed. Often, if questioned on this point, the wife will say,
"Yes, on that morning when my husband fell down, he suddenly aged
ten years and became a sort of stranger to me. He no longer was my
old lover and chum. After that all he would talk about was his bowels
or his misery; he became irascible and unreasonable, and he would cry
without reason. No longer did he want to keep clean and neat the way
he used to do. He didn't want to take a bath or change his clothes." One
of the most obvious signs of a small stroke is the presence of stains of
soup or gravy on the coat or vest of a man who always before was well
groomed and careful of his appearance. Perhaps, also, there comes a
stain of urine on the trousers, and the remarkable fact is that the man is
not ashamed of it.

Commonly, when an older person has a "dizzy spell" and vomits, the
diagnosis is made of Ménière's disease, and the patient is treated for
this. But, often a few questions will show that there were no losses of
hearing, no ear noises, and no true vertigo. Perhaps a good aurist will
report that to all the usual tests the internal ear is normal.

But even when there is some sign of injury to the inner ear or the
tracts of the eighth nerve, a wise internist will say, "Yes, but this man
has obviously suffered serious changes in his mind and character, and
hence there must be injury, also, in the upper part of the brain"; or the
doctor may note failures in the functions of other nerves besides the
eighth, and hence the injury must be in the bulb and not in the ear.

As I said at the beginning, the commonest diagnosis after a stroke is
a "heart attack." But usually this can be excluded in a number of ways.
Often a good history will show that the main symptoms were such as

could arise only in the brain. Often it will be found that the patient still has a good "wind" and never an anginal pain or even any dyspnea. The electrocardiograms will probably show a few changes but these can often be ascribed to age or fat or hypertension.

Occasionally, if the doctor will order stereoscopic roentgenograms of the skull he will see, at the base of the brain, calcified carotid arteries, and this may have some significance.

In a few cases it is helpful to find that some of the patient's ancestors were manic-depressives. Many a time I have seen a patient develop a mild psychosis after what looked like a little stroke, and then it was hard to say how much was due to the stroke and how much to an uncovering of an inherited tendency to depression.

Many physicians think that the coming of vertigo points to disease of the liver or of the gallbladder, but in my experience these troubles rarely cause dizziness, and they certainly do not cause a sudden big change in character.

The great diagnostic significance of the symptoms that came at the start. Often the secret of diagnosis in these cases is to inquire carefully as to the symptoms felt in the first minute or hour of the trouble. So often the consulting physician does not get the story of the first acute spell. For instance, a woman of sixty-five was referred to me because of a supposed postcholecystectomy syndrome. I found that she had been perfectly well until one morning some months before when, while crossing a street, she had suddenly lost her sense of balance, had become confused, and had nearly fallen. A passer-by, noting her distress, had grabbed her and had helped her into a drug store. There she felt dizzy, nauseated, and ill. On reaching home she had her daughter call a doctor who said she had had a heart attack and sent her to the hospital. There, many electrocardiograms were made, but no definite abnormality was found.

On returning home the woman was no better. Because she had some pain and distress right after eating a surgeon removed a thin, stoneless gallbladder. Naturally, this did not help. Later, one day while standing at the head of the kitchen stairs, things began to black out, and after an agonizing moment, she fell. Following this her right hand was clumsy, with a shiny red skin over it. I noticed this the moment I saw her and suspected what had happened. She said her doctors had paid no attention to the hand, saying that it must have been injured in the fall. They stuck to this idea in spite of her certainty that the fall was due to a second stroke. No one paid any attention to this belief of hers, and so she finally stopped talking about it.

I thought she was perfectly right about the two strokes. She had noted a loss of memory, some temporary weakness of the right leg after the second spell, an increased irritability, a sudden loss of 50 pounds in weight, a drop in a previously high blood pressure, a loss of joy in life, a loss of interests, a loss of her old ability to sleep well, and a loss of her ability to write. When I took her son aside and asked if he had noticed any change in her character, he said, yes, that he had marveled at the fact that his previously adoring mother had become so suspicious that she would not trust him even with a little money that had to be deposited in the bank.

It seemed to me that with all these mental changes the woman's essential disease had to be in the brain. The suddenness of the transition from health to great illness also showed this. The only puzzling feature was that good physicians had failed to notice these things or to think of their significance. They had not drawn out any of the story that I have given here, and hence had spent all their time looking for disease in abdomen or thorax.

On the diagnostic value of noting a patient's occupation. In diagnosing this type of illness in a man it is very important to note the nature of his occupation and then to glance at the fellow to see whether he looks the part. Many a time I have said to myself, "That dull man sitting there couldn't possibly be the leading attorney in his state; obviously, then, he is not the man he was, and he must have failed terribly." Then, on talking to the relative or business associate who came with him, I have found this to be true. Other physicians who hadn't noticed the lack of correlation between the man's position in the business world and his appearance, and therefore hadn't asked questions about this, had not obtained even a glimpse of the most important part of the clinical picture. Sometimes a patient is able to conceal from his physicians the fact that he has become a bit childish, and then this must be learned from the family.

A neurologic examination often shows little. One would think that a neurologist ought to be able to make the diagnosis in a few minutes, but sometimes he hates to commit himself because he depends so much on his usual examining technics, and these show nothing. Because the little stroke came in a silent area, the neurologist's pin, his cotton, and his hammer showed no abnormality. Then, if the neurologist does not note that much of the man's brain is not functioning well, he will fail to make the correct diagnosis.

Prognosis. One reason for making the correct diagnosis in these cases is that, since the prognosis is often bad, the physician had better not promise a quick cure. Oftentimes he should tell a man's family that they must prepare for bad times ahead, since his days of work and usefulness and happiness are probably over. Often there is a remarkable clearing-up of some symptoms such as weakness of a hand or leg or a little aphasia, but changes in ability and character are likely to remain.

Fortunately, one can reassure many of these patients on one point that greatly concerns them, and this is their fear that any day soon they will get two more bigger strokes and die. This idea that the third stroke must be fatal is a folk idea which is not true. One can honestly assure the patient that it may be years before he gets another stroke. I remember a man of seventy who, after three strokes, each bad enough to drop him on the floor, lived for the next ten years in good health. I remember other men who lived fifteen years in good health, and I remember one who, after several mentally crippling little strokes at the age of fifty-six years, lived on for thirty years. In his case, however, the great extension of life was only a misfortune to him and his family.

What one must hope for is that with the clearing away of edema, and perhaps with the rerouting of impulses around the destroyed area, the person will be comfortable again. Every physician knows of patients who, after lying for a time unable to speak a word or to move an arm or leg, got up and talked and walked and enjoyed life again. The other hope must be that any more spells will be very slow in coming.

Treatment. Unfortunately, since there is no treatment that will remove a thrombosis from a little artery or remake destroyed tissue in the brain, one cannot promise to give the patient back his health. The big point is not to treat these people with a lot of onerous restrictions. They must not be kept in bed, and efforts must not be made to lower the blood pressure. A high blood pressure should be a factor of safety. They should not be annoyed by the taking away of their salt, red meat, alcohol, and tobacco. Such annoyances are far more likely to shorten the man's life than to lengthen it. They make him more irritable, and in some cases, even paranoid. He gets the idea that people are persecuting him. They are, of course, but he misses the point that they are doing it for what they think is his good.

Because of the present-day fear of cholesterol in the production of arterial disease, and the discovery that fats stay long in the blood of older persons, it might be permissible to cut down on the patient's ration of fat. The amount of exercise should not be restricted. Sometimes it is well to let a man sit in his office each day if he is not too great a nuisance there. Every so often I hear of some old patient who is still working and perhaps earning a living five or ten years after I insisted that he be taken off all restrictions and allowed to go back to his office. I hear, also, from women whom years ago I rescued from a bed to which they had been consigned because of supposed heart disease. They are still taking care of a house and husband, and they still have no symptoms of heart disease.

If the patient has suffered trophic changes and some weakness in a hand or foot, physiotherapy will help. Some persons need sedatives to help them sleep. Unfortunately, I know of no medicine that will combat the utter misery in which some of these persons have to live out their life. Their brain does not feel right; it may "feel awful," and because of this terrible distress, the person may even commit suicide.

I often give each day a tablet or two of lipoiodine because the family insists on some medicine and my old teachers felt so sure that iodine would keep arteries soft.

The physician can oftentimes help the patient most by getting his family to understand what the true situation is, and especially by keeping them from fretting at him and telling him to "snap out of it." He cannot snap out of it, and it is not his fault that he is irascible and a problem in the home. The family must remember that he is sick, mentally crippled, and prematurely aged, and not just "ornery."

A MILD THALAMIC SYNDROME

Each year I see a few persons, usually women, who complain of an ache or distress or misery in one loin or in one side of the abdomen. Sometimes they describe it as "something in there." They may say, "I'd like to reach in there and claw it out." Usually in these cases, by the time a consultant sees the woman, she has had one or two abdominal operations which gave her no relief.

To me the most significant point is that the patient's distress really extends along the whole affected side from the head to the foot. Usually the woman fails to mention this at first but, if asked about it, she will say, "Yes, that is my bad side. I have headache, backache, loin-ache, and leg-ache, all on that side." Perhaps, then, if one pinches the superficial tissues of the abdominal wall on that side, the woman will jump and cry out with pain, showing that the side is hyperesthetic.

Other significant points are that usually the misery has been present for many years, and usually it has been present constantly, by day and by night. Even when the appendix and the gallbladder have not yet been sacrificed, this constancy of the distress over many years is enough to give me the strong impression that the source of the misery is in the central nervous system. Certainly a distress due to disease in the abdomen would tend to come and go.

Usually one learns, and this is significant, that the distress has no relation to any part of the rhythm of the digestive tract; it is not made worse or better by eating or by emptying the colon. Sometimes it is relieved for a day by purgation with castor oil, but then I think the effect of the drug is a sedative one, because a thorough cleansing of the colon with enemas does not have the same effect.

Possible causes for the distress. Because I have no necropsy reports in these cases, I can only speculate as to the nature and location of the lesion. Several of the persons whom I have seen with this syndrome were nervous women with a poor nervous heredity; a few were slightly depressed at times; and a few, after many years, wound up in an institution, getting shock treatments for their depression. The fact that I have seen two highly nervous sisters suffering from the syndrome reinforces my idea that at times it has a hereditary substratum. In a few other cases the pain was associated with an unhappy situational neurosis, or what I call disease due to the feeling of being caught in a trap. (See Chapter 8.)

In still other cases the trouble came suddenly, and then I suspected a slight stroke. In one case it came suddenly right after an attack of what looked like influenza, and in another case the woman discovered the distress when she woke from an anesthetic. She almost certainly had suffered an arterial thrombosis in her brain. Years later, when I saw her, she had a weakness of the muscles of the mouth on the hypersensitive side but she was not sure when that had come. Very interesting was the fact that with the hypersensitiveness of the one side there had come a dyspareunia due to hyperesthesia of one side of the vagina. This condition reminds me much of that in cats from which one half of the pallium has been removed. These animals, while still fond of being petted and stroked on the normal side, will go into a rage the moment they are barely touched on the side operated on.

When I see one of these men or women with distress all along one side, I think of a mild thalamic syndrome. I realize that this idea may be abhorrent to many neurologists because commonly one cannot demonstrate a decided hypesthesia or hyperesthesia or any other sign of a stroke along the side of the body. But Henry Head, in his classic description of the thalamic syndrome, reported cases in which there was mighty little to show objectively on the affected side; the distress was all subjective. Head pointed out that the optic thalamus is the center of awareness through which pass all the stimuli that are capable of producing sensation. When something goes wrong with this region the person is likely to feel that something is hurting him on one side of his body. But even this is not always true, because I know a man who with a stroke got a decided anesthesia of all the tissues of one half of his body, but no pain.

I see so many patients with a brain badly injured by a stroke which produced neither paralyses nor anesthesias that I can see no objection to assuming that some, at least, of the persons with a miserable distress in half the body once suffered a vascular injury to a small bit of the optic thalamus.

Some physicians may say, "But some of these persons got their misery in their thirties." True, but this does not rule out a vascular accident: during World War II a large number of soldiers under thirty years of age suffered a stroke with hemiplegia. Surely, then, there must have been others who suffered a small thrombosis, almost unrecognizable because it came in some silent area of the brain. In other cases the injury could easily be due to a localized encephalitis. Most physicians will probably be satisfied to say that these women with a sensitive side are just a bunch of nerves or that they suffer from a form of hysteria. This could be true in some cases. What we need are some necropsies.

As I said, I have seen this syndrome in two sisters. One came to have her kidney removed after years of futile dilation of a "Hunner stricture." (See Chapter 22.) We could not find anything wrong with the kidney or ureter. The woman was a spinster of fifty who broke down and wept as she told her story, so it was obvious that there was a large emotional element in the causation of the exacerbations of the disease. She was a migrainous person, and this explained much of her lifelong illness. Then it was found that her whole right side from head to foot was hyper-esthetic. It was found, also, that the father and two brothers were dipso-maniacs. One of the brothers looked like an epileptic and had at times all of the epileptic's surliness and violence of temper. His escapades often brought on the sister's pain in an acute form.

Another sister, a widow, was a pleasant, migrainous person who also had a one-sided ache. This had come suddenly fifteen years before, as she was recovering from what was thought to be a bad cold, and it had been present ever since. Remembering the brother's appearance, I had an electroencephalogram made and found a decided dysrhythmia. I then found that she had fainted often in her youth. She did not have fever convulsions but often she "passed out," and once she had dropped so hard that she hit something and broke a tooth. She may have also an epileptic equivalent which takes the form of spells in which she gets a very bad taste in her mouth. With such spells her colon gets sore, and she gets a severe pain in the left loin (on her other side), followed by diarrhea. She also has unexplained jittery spells, when she is too trembly to write. She gets nausea at night as do many persons with a poor nervous inheritance. This nausea comes in spells lasting two weeks or so.

I have not yet been able to get an electroencephalogram of the first sister seen, but she, also, has always fainted easily. I put both of the women on dilantin and they have since reported good results in the way of improved health.

Another one of the "relatives of the psychotic or alcoholic" (see also Chapter 15) who was full of many queer hallucinations of feeling throughout his body, complained that his whole left side felt weaker than the right. Another patient, a man of forty with a sort of thalamic syndrome, told a story of what was probably a stroke, suffered five years before. Suddenly it left his whole left side from the neck to the toes feeling peculiar. From the moment of the apparent stroke, although he had lost nearly all the sense of touch in the left lower extremity, he felt as if the left leg and foot were very hot. His left arm became numb and remained that way. It and the hand also felt hot. In a few days his distresses were less intense. At no time was there any weakness of the muscles or any difficulty with the sphincters or with getting an erection. With time the loss of sensation in the leg and foot largely cleared, but the feeling of heat in the tibia remained. Five months before I saw the man, he had what appeared to be another little stroke in which he lost his sense of balance and nearly fell down.

The thalamus can give trouble not only because it is injured in some way but because it has been freed from inhibition and control by injury to higher centers in the cerebral cortex.

Summary. A number of cases are here described in which pain or an ache or a "misery" or a numbness all along one side of a patient's body may have been due to disease, perhaps arterial or hereditary, in the thalamic area of the brain, through which passes a large sensory tract.

As yet the clinical syndrome is a bit vague, but it should be an important one to clear up by careful study of many cases.

Part IV

Types of Personality and
Several Syndromes

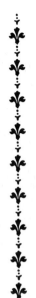

CHAPTER 13

Types of Nervous, Unhappy, and Frail Persons

I N THIS CHAPTER I describe a number of nervous, unhappy, or troubled persons so that the young physician may the more easily recognize them when he meets them, and so that he may know something
about their problems. With this knowledge he is more likely to take a
good history, more likely to make the correct diagnosis, and less likely
to get led astray by red herrings across the diagnostic trail.

Like Paulhon, I like the use of plain words in describing these persons.
Paulhon wrote about "Les Caractères." He called them the uneasy, the
contrary, the incoherent, the impulsive, the weak, the distracted, the
excitable, the passionate, the enterprising, the hesitant, the persistent,
the obstinate, the wide-awake, the dull, the impressionable, the cold and
phlegmatic, the sober, the ascetic, the highly sexual, the frigid, the affectionate and the deeply loving, the unfriendly, the solitary, the generous, the prodigal, the miserly, the vain, the proud, the ambitious, the
always climbing, the pushers, the hungry-for-power, the submissive, the
happy, the sad, the pessimistic, the over-religious, and the mystic.

Kraepelin, years ago, used to speak of the excitable, the unstable, the
impulsive, the egocentric, the liars and swindlers, the antisocials and
the quarrelsome.

Kahn mentioned the nervous, the anxious, the sensitive, the com-
pulsive, the excitable, the hyperthymic, the depressive, the moody, the

affectively cold, the weak-willed, the impulsive, the sexually perverse, the hysterical, the fantastic, the cranky, and the eccentric.

THE NERVOUS PERSON

The commonest complaint of many persons is nervousness. By this, different persons mean different things. Some mean that they feel tense and on edge, jittery, apprehensive, worrisome and full of fears, hyper-sensitive, perhaps overly irritable, easily annoyed, impatient, and too quick to respond to irritations. Sometimes a woman will say that she could jump out of her skin. The children and perhaps her husband annoy her unintentionally: They make too much noise for her, or they talk too much, or their mannerisms "drive her crazy." She cannot rest easily. The telephone makes her jump. Perhaps she has aches all over, or she is unpleasantly conscious of the movements of her heart or her intestines. Because of the outflow of excess energy from her brain, at times she may perspire to excess, or her heart may beat too rapidly, or she may urinate every twenty minutes. Usually she sleeps poorly, and often she suffers from headaches and premenstrual tension. She may wish that for a time she could live alone without anyone to disturb her.

Such a woman may often be overly emotional and a bit unreasonable. She may have moods in which she is inclined to pick on those about her, and to be hard to live with. She may scream at the children, and may punish them before she knows what she is doing. A woman may be pretty much this way all her days and may grow stout in spite of it.

There are, of course, many nervous *men* who are tense, irritable, jumpy, perhaps irascible, and hard to get along with. On a vacation they may lose most of their discomforts, and may become calm and easy-going. In the cases of both men and women, fatigue brings out and exaggerates these symptoms of nervousness.

Some children, also, are nervous and very different from their calm and easy-going brothers and sisters. They are inclined to have tics, to bite their nails, to be sickly, and to sleep poorly. Some families are made up of nervous persons.

As I point out, particularly in the chapters on the relatives of the psychotic, I think the experienced physician can quickly distinguish be-tween the person who has become nervous from strain and overwork, and the one who was born to be extremely jittery most of his or her life.

Treatment. Some of these persons cannot be helped much because they are nervous by nature and heredity. Others can be helped by a vaca-tion, and many can get relief at times with the help of ½ grain of pheno-barbital, taken after breakfast and luncheon, or an occasional 5-grain tablet of bromural. The old bromides are not good for steady use be-cause they accumulate in the blood. A nap after luncheon or in the late afternoon may be very helpful. Often a vacation or a month or two of mornings in bed is the best treatment. The person must be exhorted to avoid annoyances and all fretting and fussing. Much more on treatment will be found in the last few chapters of this book.

THE NEURASTHENIC

It is not clear just what neurasthenia is. Possibly this term and the commonly used "chronic nervous exhaustion" should be discarded. It was the American, Beard, who popularized the idea of neurasthenia. He included many conditions which today would be called by other names, such as nervousness, constitutional inadequacy, asthenia, troubles of the relatives of the psychotic, a mild depression, hypochondriasis, post-influenzal fatigue, neurocirculatory asthenia, cardiac neurosis, nervous indigestion, insomnia, headache, a mild Ménière's syndrome, hypersensitivity, chronic complaining, an anxiety state, phobias, backache, hysteria, or asthenopia.

In spite of anything that psychiatrists can ever do in the way of classifying these persons and their syndromes, individual physicians will doubtless go on with their habit of using some favorite label for almost all of them.

There are several types of "neurasthenic" persons, and the individual should be labeled accurately enough so that the prognosis and treatment will be satisfactory. It is well to recognize (1) those persons who can recover from their illness; (2) those who can adjust to it; (3) those who will probably always remain sickly and inadequate; (4) those who will always be more or less psychopathic; (5) those who are so stupid, hypochondriac, or otherwise psychopathic that for the non-psychiatrist or even the psychiatrist to spend time on them is foolish; (6) those who should promptly be placed in the hands of a good psychiatrist; (7) those who need a sojourn in an institution; and (8) those like the migrainous and the relatives of the epileptic who have special tendencies and who need special treatment.

Treatment. Weiss and English, in their book (1949), commented on the fact that the neurasthenic often comes to the physician with the idea that he will promptly be made over into a normal person. He seems to say, "There's my story, doctor; now you pat me and rub me and feed me medicine and take my pains away and give me inspiration and happiness, and tell me how to be successful, and, while you're about it, get my mother-in-law out of the house, and I'll pay you when I get a job!"

Obviously, the treatment of a "neurasthenic" must depend on what kind of a nervous person he is, how he got into difficulties, and what, if anything, can be done to make life easier for him.

THE ASTHENIC PERSON

There is one type of constitutionally inadequate person for whom I like to use the word "asthenic" because he tires so easily, he has so little strength, and he can do so little work. Darwin was an asthenic, grade IV. For forty years he never could do more than three hours of work a day, and he could never stand the least excitement. A trip to London, attendance at a meeting of the Geological Society, or even a quiet evening with friends, and he would go to pieces, unable to sleep that night, and shivering and vomiting all next day, or even for several days afterward. The fact that he lived on with this trouble unchanged until he was seventy-three, and then died after only a short illness, shows that his essential organs must have been sound. A careful study of biographies of the man and the four volumes of his letters left me with the impression that he was eminently sane. He was a kind, friendly man who took his great suffering without complaint.

I feel sure that his nervous weakness was his share of a psychopathic inheritance which showed up in a number of his relatives. His grandfather, Erasmus Darwin, was odd and a bad stammerer. Incidentally, Wendell Johnson says that the eminent Charles stammered. One of Erasmus' sons became depressed and committed suicide. Another son, Robert, the famous Charles' father, who was a good physician, was odd and reserved. Charles Darwin's mother was a Wedgwood, and unfortunately a tendency to psychosis ran in that otherwise very fine and able family. Charles' maternal grandfather had at least one "nervous breakdown," and one of Charles' maternal uncles, Tom Wedgwood, died in a depression. Tom's two sisters were apparently too odd and rigid in temperament ever to marry. One of Charles' brothers was a sickly odd person who never could do any work and who died in a melancholia. One of Charles' sisters had ill health and "poor spirits" and did not marry until she was fifty-three. One of Charles' children had ill health all his life, and one child failed to develop mentally.

It seems, then, that we have in this biography a beautiful example of what a poor nervous inheritance will do to some members of a family even when others are highly gifted and able; I shall describe this type of illness at length in Chapter 15 in the section on the relatives of the psychotic.

Treatment. The treatment of the asthenic is much the same as that for the constitutionally inadequate person. (See the end of this chapter.)

THE SICKLY, THE FRAIL, AND THE CONSTITUTIONALLY INADEQUATE

A large number of the "chronic patients" who are seen by internists are always ailing in one way or another. They seem to have been born with a tendency to be frail and sickly, and they are unable to stand up well to the strains of life. Many get operated on again and again, but if they get better at all they do not stay well. Many of the women get along well enough until some time in their early twenties when they tackle their first job or have their first baby. After that they are wrecks, dragging around, and barely able to do their housework. They keep going from doctor to doctor, hoping that eventually one localized cause will be found for their troubles, and perhaps cut out, but always they are disappointed. About all they get for their money are repeated examinations and hospitalizations.

To my way of thinking, most of these persons can best be classified as constitutionally inadequate, and it would be better for them and medical practice if more of us physicians would give up the hope of ever curing them quickly in any way. About the only way in which one might *cure* one of these frail sickly persons would be to start again with a different set of grandparents!

How to recognize the inadequates. Many of these patients can be recognized at a glance from their poor physical development. Many are small and thin and poorly put together. A woman may have small nodular breasts, a long thorax, a flat simian type of pelvis, a male type of thin legs, and an infantile uterus. As Osler used to say, the contractor put in poor materials.

Occasionally, one finds a constitutionally inadequate man who has a large well-built or stout body. But, then, one can recognize the fellow by his worrisome temperament, and his great concern about his health. He may react to the fear of disease just as his thin brothers and sisters do. As a sickly inadequate woman once said to me with much clarity of vision, "Dad may look big and strong, but let him get a pimple on his nose, and he'll be laid up for two weeks just as I would be."

The reverse of this picture is that there are many small, frail-looking, thin men and women who, although they look inadequate, are anything but that. They are tireless workers and highly efficient ones. What is the difference? I am sure the main difference is that the tireless ones inherited, along with their poor body, a fine brain which gives them much energy and drive, a feeling of good health, or an ability to stand much discomfort without complaint. As Robert Louis Stevenson once said, he could go on writing day after day, no matter how great his pain, his cough, or his fever.

Is there a need for the label of constitutional inadequacy? Sometimes when I see how many of the symptoms of inadequacy are those of neurosis, hypochondriasis, anxiety, hypersensitiveness, and minor psychoses, I wonder if we physicians need the extra term, "constitutional inadequacy," but then I think we do. I think it is good to have a label that will help us all to recognize the frail or the often-complaining type of person who probably will never be very well no matter what is done to him or her medically or surgically.

Today, one can find many inadequate women who have spent years going through university clinics: being sent from one department to another and costing the social service fund hundreds and thousands of dollars. In each department an effort is made to get the woman well, but she never stays well, and perhaps after years it begins to dawn on the doctors that from the beginning she was constitutionally inadequate, and perhaps in addition, feeble-minded, or a bit psychopathic. Much money and effort might have been saved if the true nature of the woman and her troubles had been recognized when she first came in.

One difficulty in handling such a patient is that even if a wise old clinician were to say at the start, "Don't waste time and money on that woman, you'll never cure her or satisfy her or make her see what the trouble is," some of the younger doctors would feel that this was not good medical practice. Never having heard much of inadequacy or neuroses or psychoses in college, they will expect to find organic disease in the woman, and to cure it. Years ago, when I wrote my first big article on the constitutionally inadequate (1942), I received a number of chiding letters from physicians who would not admit that there are innumerable persons whom medicine does not now cure and probably never will cure.

The common complaints of the inadequate. The commonest complaints of the inadequate are feelings of great fatigue, weakness, lack of energy and "pep," and joy in life. These persons have a hard time getting started in the morning and they may have to push themselves all day. If they do get going in the morning they "peter out" by noon. They are nervous, and they may have aches and pains everywhere, feelings of faintness or giddiness, indigestion, poor appetite, frequent losses of weight, palpitation, a sensitive colon, constipation, cold wet hands, poor resistance to infection, slow recovery from illnesses, weak eyes, an irritable bladder, cyanotic legs, and in women, shotty, painful breasts, dysmenorrhea, and sometimes painful intercourse.

Naturally, some inadequates have less trouble than others because life is made easier for them by a well-to-do father or a kindly, sympathetic husband who can supply a comfortable home with a servant to handle most of the work. It is a hard road that the inadequate woman has to travel when she marries a poor man and begets a houseful of children, most of them sickly like herself, and needing much care night after night. Then her home doctor will wonder how she ever keeps going year after year.

Treatment. The important point in handling constitutionally inadequate persons and asthenics is to get them to see what their problem is and to acquiesce somewhat in regard to it. They must learn to hoard their energies and to live within their means of strength. Some have to find a job that is not too hard for them. Some, like Darwin, may have to give up some of their ambitions. Darwin had to move to the country and live very quietly. He found that he could work only an hour and a half at a time or he would break down and start vomiting. He, of course, was fortunate in possessing private means.

Sometimes a physician will ask me, "Do you mean to say that you tell a man he is constitutionally inadequate? Is that not too discouraging?" Not necessarily. I often tell a patient that in a way I am inadequate too, because I could not earn my living as a prize-fighter or even as a day laborer. I had trouble even with the general practice of medicine because I could not stand the evening hours and the night work on top of a hard day. I had to limit my work in order to preserve my health, I also had to give up many activities that tended to tire me much. I was able to succeed in life only by finding a place in which I could work comfortably and always within my means of strength. It would have been very foolish of me to try, let us say, to run for governor of a state. Constant travel with four addresses a day would have flattened me.

What I try to get patients to see is that they must give thought to living in such a way as to earn a living with the least wastage of energy. Some jobs are out of the question because they would soon break the person down. The acceptance of a promotion might be unwise. To show what I mean: Sometimes a frail woman who could not endure typing all day can stand being a doctor's receptionist. In his office she need work hard for only two or three hours in the afternoon; the rest of the time she can be answering the telephone and keeping up the records.

It is highly important usually that the asthenic person get plenty of sleep. Usually it is best to advise inadequates to put up with a lot of aches and pains and indigestion. Strenuous treatments may be more trouble than they are worth.

THE PATIENT WHO IS ALWAYS TIRED OR WHO FATIGUES QUICKLY

So many of the patients seen by the physician every week complain bitterly of being always tired; they have no "pep" and they have lost their joy in life. A man will say that he is having to drive himself to work as he never had to before. A young woman will say, "I'd rather be dead than to go on this way. I haven't energy enough to go out with a beau." The married woman will say, "I am not a good mother; I am too tired to do my housework, or to be calm with my children, and I can't be a good pal to my husband. He wants me to go with him to a movie and I can't go; I'm too tired." In the worst cases the patient says to the doctor, "This isn't an ordinary fatigue; it is a terrible grueling sort of fatigue that makes me dread to get up in the morning and start the day."

Great efforts made to find a local cause. These patients say, "This time, spare no expense; give me the most complete overhauling possible. This time you are going to find the trouble somewhere in my body." They hope to find some focus of infection or some disease that can be cut out. Usually, when I see these patients, they have been well examined several times before, and nothing significant has been found. Some have had operations which did not reveal any disease and did not do any good. Most of these persons have been thoroughly dosed with vitamins, tonics, estrogens, and androgens, without effect. I hate to see them come in the office because I fear I must later disappoint them with a negative report. I know that in cases such as theirs I can rarely find any causative local disease.

Was there a precipitating cause? Always in these cases I want to find out when and how the fatigue came, and what, if anything, seemed to bring it on. Sometimes there was an attack of influenza which left the person weak and tired, or there was a sorrow, or an auto accident or a long spell of nursing a sick parent or child. The most puzzling cases are those in which there was no obvious precipitating cause for the trouble. Usually one cannot diagnose an "effort syndrome" because this is a fairly definite disease seen commonly in cases of neurocirculatory asthenia.

In normal persons fatigue is quickly relieved by rest. Ross used to say that some persons get tired when they have to keep doing someting they do not like, such as uncongenial work, and they do not get so tired when doing something which they enjoy, such as congenial work or play. Interesting, also, is Ross' statement that when a normal man is utterly exhausted after a short period of heavy strain, a little rest puts him back in good shape again.

It is worth noting that the laborer who works hard all day never goes to a doctor to complain of being tired. He sleeps heavily every night and gets rested. If he should start complaining of fatigue, one would suspect that he was ill.

Morning and afternoon fatigues. Always, when dealing with persons who complain of fatigue, it helps to know whether theirs is a morning or an afternoon distress. Persons with a poor nervous inheritance tend to get their fatigue in the morning, while normal persons who earn their fatigue tend to get it around four in the afternoon, when they begin to wish they could quit and go home.

Has a vacation been tried? It helps sometimes to know when a tired person last had a vacation. If he recently took a vacation it helps much to know (1) if it was a restful one; (2) if it was long enough, and (3) if it did any good. A normal person who earned his fatigue can usually be much helped by a vacation, unless it is too short or too strenuous; a depressed person is usually not helped at all. Another type of person who is not helped is the one who takes his or her troubles or worries along. Perhaps a wife has had to go with the husband who frets at her or bores her or makes her tense or nervous. A type of person who gets no help from a vacation is the one who works too hard at it, or stays up half the night playing cards or dancing or drinking. Others are so bored that a vacation does not help.

The age of the patient makes a difference. In thinking of what might be wrong with a tired man one must, of course, be influenced by his age. Thus, if a previously healthy boy in college has one or two intestinal upsets and then gets very tired so that he cannot study, the trouble may well be a smoldering appendicitis, and an operation may work a spectacular cure. In some cases the trouble may be due to over-work or to worry about finances, or to the strain of studying a subject in which the student has lost interest. In other cases one looks for a beginning tuberculosis, or an infectious mononucleosis, a mild encepha-litis, a brain tumor, a beginning multiple sclerosis, a chronic mesenteric lymphadenitis, a renal infection, an endocarditis, an infectious hepatitis, a beginning terminal ileitis, a beginning chronic ulcerative colitis, Hodgkin's disease, myasthenia gravis, Addison's disease, or a beginning psychosis. In the many cases in which a student has a poor nervous inheritance, the first schizophrenic or depressive breakdown may come while he or she is in the last year of college.

Breakdowns in older persons. In the cases of older persons one must think of carcinoma or cerebral arteriosclerosis. If the fatigue has been present for years, that tends to rule out carcinoma. To rule out ad-vanced carcinoma one should get a measurement of the blood sedi-mentation rate; one should get the roentgenologist to study the digestive tract from one end to the other; one should ask the proctologist to look into the sigmoid colon and rectum; and one should check the liver func-tion because metastasis so often involves that organ. In the case of men, one should search the prostate gland for hard nodules, and in the case of women one should examine the breasts and the pelvic organs.

The history may show that there have been previous episodes of thrombosis of small arteries in the brain, with a syndrome such as is described in Chapter 12 on small strokes. In a few cases one will suspect that an advancing hypertension is the cause of the fatigue. Thus I remember overly tired persons who came with a systolic blood pressure of perhaps only 160 but marked changes in the arterioles of the retinas. A year or two later they returned with a systolic blood pressure of perhaps 220.

In rare cases the tired patient will have had an attack of encephalitis which went unrecognized. The person may also be suffering from hypothyroidism or hyperthyroidism. In my experience, chronic brucellosis is a rare cause for fatigue states.

The migrainous and the constitutionally inadequate. Very common as a cause of fatigue in the cases of middle-aged women is migraine. Most women with this trouble tire easily and suddenly, and then they can hardly drag around. Many tired patients, also, are constitutionally inadequate or frail, and many have a neurocirculatory asthenia (see end of this chapter).

The undisciplined. Occasionally one will find that the tired patient is an undisciplined person who is dissipating or living most unhygienically. Under these circumstances, he *should* feel poorly.

The tired person who is worn out from working too long hours. There is a type of man in a small business who keeps his shop open from 7 in the morning until 10 or 11 at night, six days a week. Often, if remonstrated with, he will say that his business is not large enough so that he can take a partner or hire a clerk. One thinks of men like the old shoe-repairer, the druggist with a small store, or the man who repairs automobiles and tractors in a farming community who just before the plowing or reaping season is kept so busy that he does not take off his clothes for a week. The general practitioner oftentimes lives much this type of life.

It is interesting to see how these men eventually begin to crack and break down, some with one symptom, and some with another. They may get paresthesias, pains, nausea, difficulty in swallowing, headache, insomnia, or frequent infections.

It is a wonder how some women stand their years of overwork. I think of mothers with a large family or widows who must work all day and part of the night to take care of children. I marvel that they can keep going as long as they do, when they never have a minute's rest except, perhaps, in the hours from 1 to 7 A.M.

A breakdown which came suddenly but was due to years of overwork and fatigue. Occasionally one will see a youngish or middle-aged woman or man who tells a story of a sudden collapse, followed by a breakdown, all suggestive of a little stroke. But questioning of the patient and perhaps the spouse will bring out the fact that an unusually strong person overdid foolishly for years, working for long hours seven days a week. For months the spouse had noted signs of increasing fatigue and irritability and had feared that a break was coming. For long he or she had been begging the patient to let up a bit. Then came a day when the person apparently just got to the end of his or her rope and collapsed. Often I have wondered if there was a tiny stroke, but the youth of the patient made that assumption improbable. In such cases a good rest is likely to bring a cure.

The person who goes to pieces when a strain lets up. Many a woman for months will keep going bravely, so long as a child or a mother or a husband is very ill. During this time she may not mention pain or fatigue. But, then, the invalid recovers or dies, and with this the woman goes to pieces and starts complaining of many discomforts, all, apparently, of functional origin.

The manic-depressive. Quite a few persons who complain bitterly about fatigue are cyclothymic or mildly manic-depressive, moody persons. They are described in Chapter 14. Rarely, one of the first symptoms of a brain tumor or encephalitis is a sensation of great fatigue.

A number of abnormalities may be found which have nothing to do with the case. As I say in Chapter 7 on the art of disregarding inconsequential findings, in the cases of these tired people the physician must be careful not to accept as a cause for the trouble some little abnormality that could not possibly be responsible for it.

Diagnosis. In many cases one can tell in a moment from the history of long-standing fatigue that the cause is most probably constitutional in nature; because the person has had it so long it cannot be due to any disease which would kill or greatly injure the patient. If, then, in addition, the man has a normal blood and urine, a low blood sedimentation rate, and has not lost weight, the chances are that his trouble is a functional one.

Treatment. This will be taken up in Chapter 28.

THE WORRIER

It is said that in the mental hygiene departments of universities the counselors spend most of their time treating students with anxiety states and great worries.

The intensity of suffering in many cases. A normal person can have but little idea of the sufferings of the chronic worrier. For instance, I know a fine intelligent man with a well-running and long-established business whose wife tells me that almost every afternoon he comes home and says to her, "Things are looking bad, and I am terribly afraid. If our competitors cut in a little more we'll soon be ruined." Then it is up to her to reassure and encourage.

A patient told me once that whenever a little seborrheic patch on his face itches a bit he is sure it is turning into a cancer. With this, waves of fear begin to run all over him, and soon he feels "all shot to pieces." He shakes; he gets the jitters; his bowels become loose, and he runs to a physician for reassurance.

Some of the worst worriers suffer from a constant feeling of impending disaster which comes out of a disturbed brain of a type which does not give the possessor the normal feeling of comfort and good health. Other persons worry constantly over children or parents or finances. Others with a psychopathic inheritance go suddenly into panics *for no obvious cause,* and this is diagnostic. (See Chapters 14 and 15.)

It is interesting occasionally to see a child or a young person who already is a confirmed worrier. I remember a beautiful girl of twenty-one who could think of little but a supposed bad heart. She went from one physician to another having electrocardiograms made, and, as she admitted, she had no time to spare even for her nice husband.

The fear of illness and death that some persons have always with them must be almost unbearable. Worse yet, in the physician's office many seem reluctant to be reassured, and sometimes it looks as if they preferred bad news. They may even seem angry with the physician who says they have no sign of a fatal illness. They may leave him to go elsewhere to find someone who will be as pessimistic as they are.

Types of worriers. Naturally, there are several types of worriers. Some cannot be blamed because they have good reason to worry. With a business in the red and a sick wife or child, the man should be worried. Others worry too much and unnecessarily, and others worry unreasonably and pathologically. Some are not sure what they are anxious about or afraid of. They may have only a vague presentiment of disaster, and some know that there is no reason for their anxiety. Some say, "I know I am a 'worry wart.'"

Sometimes a worrier will realize that he ought to be ashamed of himself, but he will go ahead just the same, even when he sees that, by his folly, he is losing the respect and love of his wife and children. Often I have said to a man with a constant psychopathic type of apprehension over his health: "Why should you keep trying to change a loving and attractive wife into nothing but a bored, tired, psychiatric nurse?" The wise physician can often sense that these patients are not well balanced, and that they come of a psychotic family.

Sometimes, especially when a man knows that he has psychotic ancestry, he will be afraid that he is going insane, and then, every so often, he will get panicky with fear that he is about to slip. He will feel as if any moment he might find himself raving mad. Oftentimes the patient fears disease in some one particular organ, such as the heart, or of one particular type, such as cancer. Probably in these cases the symptoms are projected from the patient's mind out into the supposedly affected organ. Naturally, a fear of cancer is likely to be the more distressing when the person has a cancerous ancestry, or when he or she has watched some close relative die slowly with the disease.

Some persons are much afraid that anything eaten will make them sick. They may eat their food every day with a conviction that it is going to disagree with them. Some who have a fast pulse are afraid that it will overwork the heart, and thus wear it down.

An interesting story of needless worry is that of the Empress Eugenie at the celebration of the opening of the Suez Canal. She feared that the ship carrying the imperial party would run aground and those in charge would be disgraced. Actually, nothing happened, but the Empress was in such an agony of fear that she felt her head encircled by a band of fire. She was so suffocated by emotion that she could not eat, and she could be heard sobbing in her cabin.

Treatment. This will be discussed in Chapter 28.

SQUANDERERS OF EMOTION AND ENERGY

In the case of many a person a big cause of nervous illness would seem to be the squandering of large amounts of emotion on little things that do not count and are not worth fussing about, or not even worth noting or resenting. Many persons are constantly blowing in ten dollars' worth of energy on a ten-cent annoyance.

We all know the type of intense and fussy woman who is always getting into a stew over some little disappointment or irritation or "aggravation." There are too many things in life that can annoy and upset her. She gets into unnecessary arguments, and once in an argument, she keeps at it until either she or her opponent is angry or exhausted. A servant is never doing things exactly as she wanted her to do them, or at the exact time when she wanted them done. People do not show her the deference she feels they should, or she gets the idea that they are meddling in her affairs, and that makes her angry. Little slights upset her greatly, and cause her to retort angrily. Perhaps her grown son forgets her birthday and does not write, or the newspaper did not print a satisfactory account of her "At home."

If the woman is overly worrisome, as she usually is, she is likely to have horrors over all sorts of fears, some of them with but little basis in fact, and many without any basis. If she is addicted to "post mortems" or digging up old bones, she may get herself and her relatives all worked up by constantly talking over the harrowing details of old disasters, old unhappinesses, old wrongs, old family fights, and old illnesses. As a neurotic woman confessed one day, she had a photographic memory which enabled her to keep constantly recounting to her husband in exact detail all the unpleasant things he had ever said to her during their married life! Many women who have gotten into fights with their in-laws or their own children will keep talking of these things by the hour to anyone who cannot get away.

Some women have so vivid an imagination that they can see their husband or their children or parents dying, or actually stretched out on a slab at the morgue. They have horrors over these visions.

On the need for avoiding sources of annoyance. I will never forget one rainy morning when I saw a horse that had slipped and fallen in the street. The driver was beating the animal, trying to get it to rise, and there beside him, shrieking with excitement, was a woman, ordering him to stop, and threatening him with arrest if he went on hurting the animal. I could just see her later, after her debauch of emotion, ill and under the care of a physician. A wiser woman, on seeing the animal fall, would have turned the other way and gone about her business. Similarly, a man with a bad temper may eventually get himself under such control that he will walk away from an annoyance and not stay to "blow his top."

Someone once said so wisely that the greatness of a man can be estimated from the size of the annoyances that can get under his skin and upset him.

THE PERSON WHO IS OVEREMOTIONAL OR VIOLENT

It is hard for a calm, placid person to understand how violently and explosively some persons react to every mood and thought and happening, and how this racks and tires them. Some lose patience too easily, or they become too easily outraged at the stupid things some persons do. Or they get all upset over some little distress or disappointment. Every little contretemps becomes to them a tragedy. Some are too violently partisan, or they become outraged over the stupidities of men in government positions. When out in a car they flare in anger at every driver who cuts corners or who is slow in starting, or who almost grazes them. They rail at him like a fishwife. Because of this sort of thing, some persons live in a perpetual state of mental turmoil.

People of Mediterranean races are more addicted to this violent type of behavior than are Englishmen and Americans. The Latins often say of a certain man that he is particularly violent. One of my acquaintances, the leading consultant in his line in a Latin country, once confessed to me that if, in conversation, an old friend of his were to say that in some ways the premier was not such a bad fellow, before he knew what he was doing, he might have the friend by the throat and be choking him to death!

Another gifted Latin, in trying to show me what type of ancestry he had, said that one of his uncles, a famous writer, seldom left his house for fear he might kill a friend in a sudden fit of temper. Another uncle, similarly violent and unreasoning in his tantrums, was one day crossing a narrow suspension bridge over an Andean chasm when his mule objected to stepping over a loose plank. Enraged, the man drew his revolver and shot the mule through the head. The mule, in its death throes, jumped off the bridge and carried the man to his death on the rocks far below!

Often, as in the office I have talked to persons of this type, I have had them say, "How I wish I were like you Anglo-Saxons, calm and free from this constant violence of emotion." To get an idea of what a stormy person can be like, all physicians should read the autobiography of Benvenuto Cellini, the great Italian artist.

The person with a quick temper. I once worked with a man who, while usually kindly and good natured, was given to "blowing his top," usually because of some slight annoyance. As a result, the people about him would become upset, tense, hurt, and nervous. The women in the office might cry and go to pieces, while the men might get resentful and sullen. All this reacted on the Chief and made him uncomfortable. It added much to the strain of his day's work.

In many such cases the violent temper is inherited. In some it appears to be an equivalent of epilepsy, and an electroencephalogram will show some dysrhythmia. In other cases it appears to be part of a minor psychosis.

Treatment. Often a person with a quick temper thinks it is best to blow up and get things out of his system, but my belief is that it is immensely better to grow up, become an adult, and learn self-control. It is easier on the person's nervous system, and certainly it is easier on those who live in the same house or office.

THE PERSON WHOSE BRAIN GETS TOO ACTIVE

Many of the persons who suffer from distressing symptoms do so because the brain gets too active and too keyed-up over the day's work. Then energy flows out to the periphery, there to stimulate a number of organs until they overact and keep overacting long after they should have quieted down. I often think of such an overworked brain as a stove that has been kept so full of fuel that it gets red-hot and keeps radiating heat out into places in which it is not wanted.

A man with a brain of this type may be comfortable on a vacation. Then he will be unconscious of his bodily organs, and at night he will sleep like a baby. But after coming home and working a month, perhaps as a hard-driving sales manager, he may again be perspiring to excess, his heart may be racing, he may be urinating too often, he may be feeling too warm, and every night he may have to sit up for an hour or two, too wide-awake to sleep, or suffering from jitters, heartburn, belching, bloating, nausea, or palpitation.

Such a man may be well adjusted; he may be happy in his office and his home, and he may have no complexes or foolish thoughts, and still he may be nervously ill. He has one of those physiologic disturbances which are discussed in Chapter 9.

PERSONS WHOSE NERVES ARE PLAYING TRICKS ON THEM

As I point out in Chapters 9 and 15, there is a large group of persons whose troubles seem to be best explained as due to an erratic hypothalamus or to erratic and poorly controlled autonomic nerves which are frequently playing tricks with the several organs of the body, such as the lungs, the heart, blood vessels, kidneys, stomach, bladder, and skin. Most of these persons have greatly exaggerated reflexes. Some may have too great an outpouring of neuromimetic hormones, and some may be too sensitive to the actions of these substances.

Many of the persons with such a handicap make matters worse for themselves by overworking, worrying, fretting, losing their temper, or drinking too much. Such persons may fail to get any help from a psychiatrist because he cannot supply them with a stable type of nervous system; he may not be able to find in them many mental sins to correct. Their troubles originate in a disturbed physiology.

PERSONS WHO ARE TOO HIGHLY SUGGESTIBLE

Many a person is so suggestible that he or she can quickly feel an illness that someone else has. Such persons are like the medical student who daily suffers from symptoms of the disease that he has just learned about. Such people are constantly getting sick because of something they read or because a friend or relative dropped dead. I have seen men who got morning sickness when the wife was pregnant.

Other persons are too easily alarmed. Especially during World War II, many a woman with a son overseas became frightened and ill at the sight of a telegraph boy coming up the street. If the telegram proved to be for her, she became hysterical and telephoned for her husband to come and see what the message was. She would not open the envelope.

The physician must have sympathy and patience with such persons. He must remember that, given their poor nervous heredity and perhaps their poor up-bringing by excitable and uncontrolled parents, he would react just as they do.

PERSONS WHO ARE TOO SYMPATHETIC OR TOO PARTISAN

Some women get themselves into a state because they react so violently to their sympathies. I remember a woman who would weep all morning when she read of crowds starving in Europe or China. Another buxom merry woman wept for three weeks when her brother lost his money. Another belched for ten days when her brother died. Her "stomach was tied in knots" and she lost fifteen pounds. Another belched for two weeks after her mother died.

When upset in this way, an occasional woman of this type will go into an attack resembling a gallstone colic. I have known many such women who could become prostrated after seeing a dog or a squirrel run over in the street.

I remember a man who in his youth was manager of a baseball club. He confessed that his digestive and other troubles were due to the violence of his distress whenever his old team lost a game. He said he could be well if he could only keep from looking each day at the sports page of the paper.

THE PERSON WHO FEELS SORE AND ACHEY ALL OVER

The woman who feels sore and achey all over is likely to be suffering from a neurosis. Oftentimes she is fibrositic, but in some spells her trouble sounds like a psychic rheumatism. With a fibrositis she is likely to be helped by walking around, by taking a hot bath, or by getting physiotherapy. The person with only a neurosis is more likely to ache more or less all the time, and nothing then will help her. Some persons appear to have a combination of a fibrositis and a psychically produced pain.

PERSONS WHO FAINT EASILY

There are many nervous persons who faint easily, often after some emotion, or when they are very tired or hungry or under strain. Some young persons of both sexes will faint at the sight of blood, or when they get vaccinated, or when they see a hypodermic syringe. Some persons faint when they become nauseated or when they hyperventilate. The woman whose nerves play tricks on her often faints or feels as if she would (see Chapters 9 and 14). The migrainous woman sometimes faints easily, as does the person suffering from neurocirculatory asthenia. Older persons with cerebral arteriosclerosis may seem to faint, but I suspect it is often because of a small stroke. Rarely, what looks like a fainting spell is a variant of petit mal.

In rare cases fainting is due to hypoglycemia, but then one expects it to come in the early morning hours after the longest fast of the day, and one expects the patient to get quick relief from eating sugar. Often the history alone can practically rule out hyperinsulinism, as when the spells come soon after meals and are relieved by aspirin or black coffee.

Fainting may be due to a postural hypotension. In the cases of some frail persons the blood pressure falls badly when there is need for prolonged standing. In a common variant of this disease the person suffers a momentary dizziness when he or she straightens up after bending over, perhaps to look at a book on a bottom shelf. This failure of circulation in the brain comes because the mechanism which serves to maintain a normal blood pressure after a change in body position acts slowly or inefficiently.

A rare form of syncope is due to heartblock. Another one is due to an overactive carotid sinus reflex.

Treatment. There is no known treatment that can be counted on to keep persons from fainting. Probably a woman would be less likely to faint if she could keep herself always rested and in good physical condition.

I remember an unfortunate sailor who came to me during World War I, begging for some medicine that would keep him from fainting often, especially when he had to go near a doctor or see some blood. He said, "If something is not done for me I am going to become known as the number 1 coward of the Navy." Unfortunately, he had a neurocirculatory asthenia which I could not cure.

THE PATIENT WHO OFTEN HAS A BACKACHE

A common problem of the physician is to diagnose what is wrong with the person with an aching back. In many cases the trouble is due to arthritis of the spine or the sacroiliac joints, or there may be some fibrositis, with a number of hard nodules over the sacroiliac joints, or perhaps the muscles that hold up the body are just tired, or the person may have a psychic rheumatism. Or there may be a little slipping forward of the spine on the sacrum, or, rarely, little fatty tumors projecting through the fascia of the back. Or there may be poor curves in the back or a bad posture, or one leg shorter than the other, or the person may have become too heavy. Many persons with aching backs will be found to have congenital deformities such as an extra vertebra or a sacralized fifth lumbar vertebra, but commonly it is doubtful if these peculiarities have anything to do with the backache.

Often roentgenograms show arthritic spurs on the vertebrae, but, again, it is hard to know how much these changes mean at the time because so many persons have them without a backache. I remember patients with tremendous deformities of the vertebrae and no backache. I remember a man whose spine had slipped forward almost entirely off his sacrum, and yet he had no symptoms.

Often it helps to learn that the man has had bouts of lumbago, sciatica, sore neck, cricks, and neuritis of the intercostal nerves. This shows that in the past the arthritis of the spine has been producing symptoms. Marked curvatures of the spine are probably often due to an old unrecognized poliomyelitis which weakened the muscles on one side and allowed those on the other side to pull the spine into a bow. Sometimes nerves are then pinched on the concave side. I have seen cases in which such pain was treated on the supposition that it was due to a "colitis."

In many cases it is well to ask about overwork, fatigue, or psychic strain. I remember persons who suddenly found themselves almost unable to get up from a chair the day after a daughter eloped or the day after a loved husband died. I remember a woman who got a severe backache while waiting at the telephone to hear if her husband, in a distant city, was as seriously ill as she had heard he was.

A slipped disc. In the worst cases of low backache, often with sciatica, there is a slipped disc which is pressing on the nerves of the cauda equina. In such cases the story may be that the patient was seized suddenly with a pain which shot down one leg and perhaps weakened it. The patient may come in a wheel chair, or may be walking with a cane, with a list to one side. There may be a history of several such sudden spells, each severe enough to incapacitate the patient. In such cases the neurologist may find an absent or a weak Achilles jerk and changes in the spinal fluid, and the orthopedist will find marked spasm of the back muscles, limitation of leg-raising, and other signs of serious trouble.

In other cases the story is not so clear-cut: The patient will have signs of arthritis around the lumbar spine, and it will be hard to tell whether, in addition, there is a displaced disc. In all puzzling cases it is well to get consultations with an orthopedist, a neurologist, and a nerve surgeon who has had much experience in this field.

THE OVERCONSCIENTIOUS PERSON

Many women get themselves into a terrible state fretting over conscientious scruples and imagined sins of omission and commission. This is particularly true, perhaps, of overly religious women.

Many make themselves ill by overexercising some of their virtues. For instance, a woman may be so anxious to keep husband and children and parents well that she will fuss and fret at them all the time. She may be so anxious over aged parents that she will almost wear them out with her filial solicitude. Or she may be so anxious that her house be clean and neat that she will fret constantly at the children, fearing that they may track in some dirt. Or she will be so industrious that she will never get any rest, and, as a result, she will get tired and irritable and hard to live with. Or, she may be so devoted to good causes in her community that she will overdo, and drift into a nervous breakdown.

Occasionally, a woman working in industry will be so conscientious that she will keep doing her work over and over again to check it. Or, if she is a teacher, she may take the correction of papers too seriously, and wear herself down. If she is an economical, saving person she may overwork the virtue of thrift, and become penurious, or she may shop so long that she comes home exhausted.

A woman worried herself into a nervous breakdown because her mother had died during an operation. She blamed herself because she had insisted on having a certain surgeon whom the mother disliked.

Some good women worry themselves sick for fear that inadvertently they have broken some minor law or regulation. They wonder if they should give themselves up, confess, and take their punishment. The physician can usually get them to admit that they know this is silly; they know that if they were to confess, the authorities would be either amused or annoyed, and certainly they would be convinced that they were dealing with "a looney."

Occasionally, I see a priest who is ill because he fears that he may have said the wrong words while baptizing a child or administering the last rites to a dying man. The trouble is known to the "cloth" as scrupulosity. Or, rarely, a religiously inclined man will be worrying over Christ's saying that when a man looks after a woman with desire he has committed adultery with her in his heart. Other religious persons become ill, worrying for fear that they may have committed "the unpardonable sin," whatever that may be.

Treatment. Many of these persons can be helped by a kindly physician who will listen to their story and then tell them how a sensible person would react to the situation. Sometimes the patient is helped for a time, but later has to return for another boost. Many persons have to be shown repeatedly that they did not intend to do harm and hence cannot be blamed for what happened. Perhaps theirs was a disaster that no one could possibly have foreseen or avoided. It may be true that a woman's child got poliomyelitis after being taken to a picnic or being allowed to go swimming, but who knows that the infection was obtained in that place, or if it was, who could have foreseen the disaster?

Many persons who become fearful when they are happy need to be reminded that God is not "an old meany" who is always watching to trip them up with some little sin, or always trying to injure them simply because, for a while, they were happy or fortunate. Many persons actually believe that God took from them a loved one only because they had been successful or fortunate or had loved so deeply or were so happy in their love.

Many persons who keep thinking of confessing to the spouse some premarital escapade must be told in no uncertain terms to keep quiet. Their desire for confession is pure selfishness, and it may cause much unhappiness to the loved one, and endless trouble later to the confesser. Many religious persons with a constant fear of punishment for small sins or little mistakes are always trying to unburden their conscience onto someone else. A woman will want her husband to make many little decisions for her, or she gets him to assume the responsibility for many little acts. Or she arranges little subterfuges. Thus, if a woman's religion forbids her to employ contraception she may get her husband to assume the responsibility. Then he, and not she, will get the blame.

THE WOMAN WHO RULES HER FAMILY WITH THE HELP OF EMOTIONAL STORMS

There are some neurotic women who rule their families by threatening to have an emotional storm if things do not go just to suit them. Often nothing can be done to reform them, but the family can be advised that they need not fear that death will follow the tantrum. It may help to let them know that the disease is childishness and not heart trouble.

THE WOMAN WITH A MARTYR COMPLEX

The woman with the martyr complex is well known. While trying to appear as a most devoted mother or wife who has given up everything for the sake of her children or husband she may be constantly appealing for sympathy, and constantly making it mighty uncomfortable for the persons for whom, supposedly, she has sacrificed her life.

THE PERSON WHO PERSPIRES TO EXCESS

There are quite a few persons who complain mainly of perspiring too much. Some perspire all over, while others perspire to excess only in the armpits, or in the groins, or about the head and face or neck, or in the palms of the hands, or about the feet.

Some persons suffer from excessive perspiration most of their days, and in rare cases the symptom is most distressing. I know a stout man from whose face and head perspiration is always dripping onto his sodden coat collar. Many persons have such wet hands that they hate to greet anyone. Others have a similar wetness of their feet. In the office, as he examines a nervous woman, the physician will note that perspiration is running out of her armpits in little streams.

Usually in these cases one can instantly rule out hyperthyroidism just by reaching out and touching the patient's hand; the skin is cool. The pulse may be normal, and the patient may know from many tests that his basal metabolic rate is low. Furthermore, the sweating is not generalized, and the patient may know that it becomes excessive only when he is under strain, as when meeting someone, or when writing a business report, or when trying to make a sale, or when going out with a girl. As he works, the man who writes for a living may have perspiration pouring out of his right axilla.

Excessive perspiration under a little strain is often a salient symptom of a nervous breakdown. I have seen the symptom appear in older men and women when, perhaps with the coming of a little stroke, they began to fail in nervous strength. In these cases the sweating will come much as the "dumping syndrome" (see Chapter 18) comes, as soon as food or hot drink is taken. In the cases of usually healthy persons, such sweating after meals may follow an ordinary cold. It may come whenever the person feels weak, or it may be part of the syndrome of an over-reactive autonomic nervous system. It is one of the results of "nerves playing tricks" on the person. Sweating to excess is seen occasionally as a prominent symptom in the "relatives of the psychotic" (see Chapters 14 and 15). In many women about fifty, sudden short periods of sweating accompany the hot flushes of the menopause or they take their place.

Treatment. Unfortunately, there does not seem to be any good treatment for this syndrome. The only thing likely to do good in some cases is rest, which will tend to quiet the sympathetic nerves and the brain. A quiet brain will not send out so many storms to stimulate the glands in the skin.

Women suffering from the menopause should try using a drug such as stilbestrol, perhaps in a dose of 0.5 mg. once a day.

In rare cases of dripping hands the patient can be operated on. A skillful sympathectomy in the neck can make the hands dry. Perspiring feet can be corrected by a lumbar sympathectomy.

THE PERSON WHO CANNOT MAKE DECISIONS

One of the common causes of exhaustion in women is their tendency to lie awake half the night trying to make some decision. Usually they do only what I call squirrel-cage thinking; they keep going around and around without getting anywhere. They always come out by the same door through which they went in. It would help these women if they could avoid doing this sort of thinking at night. Many could quickly get out of the mess they are in by talking the problem out with some sensible person.

THE PERFECTIONIST

Many a person's health wears thin, and many a marriage is unhappy because of the great insistence on perfection on the part of one of the spouses. Every woman should see the play *Craig's Wife,* which is the story of a woman who was so fussy about having her house just so that eventually her fine husband and all her friends walked out and left her. All she had then was the house.

The migrainous woman is almost always a perfectionist about her house, and one of the causes of her fatigue and poor health is her tendency to clean too much and too long, and to spend too much time in putting everything exactly to rights. She may fret if things are not just so. I remember one such woman who so feared dust that she kept cellophane covers over most of the objects in her house. Similarly, at the office some perfectionists make much unnecessary work for themselves.

THE PERSON WHO THINKS HEALTH IS A PRECARIOUS THING TO BE WATCHED OVER EVERY DAY

Many persons have a strong feeling that health is a precarious thing that has to be struggled for and watched over every day. The least scratch must promptly be painted with some antiseptic. With the coming of a sore throat or a cold the person may go into a hospital and ask to be heavily dosed with antibiotics.

Every day the person must take vitamins, iron, calcium, and a tonic of some kind. Three times a week he or she may go to a physician to get a "shot" of something or other. Many such persons, when they have children, watch over them in the same way. Some well-to-do women with an only child would gladly have a pediatrician drop in twice a day to make sure that all is well with the youngster. Obviously, most such persons are a bit psychopathic, usually like some parent or grandparent before them. I have known prominent businessmen of this type who sampled every new form of quackery as it came out.

Treatment. Probably little, if anything, can be done in the way of reassuring these persons and getting them to change their ways. If, after examining such a person, the physician fails to find anything wrong, and does not care to treat strenuously, the patient is likely to be so dissatisfied that he will shop around until he finds some ardent therapist with whom he can be happy.

THE PERSON WHO FEELS NUMB HERE AND THERE

Many persons get alarmed over an occasional numbness in an arm or leg. Oftentimes it is there on waking, or it causes the person to wake. It causes some persons to fear that they have had a stroke or are going to have one, but in my experience this foreboding is rarely justified. A numbness that has been caused by a little stroke is not so likely to clear up in a few minutes as is the one which came from lying on the extremity.

It seems probable that older persons with their less elastic arteries can the more easily shut off the circulation from a limb by lying on it in some particular way. Some persons appear to have much more trouble with this distress than others do. Some try sleeping on the back and still they get the numbness, perhaps because they lie with the arms above the head. This puts tension on blood vessels. Another difficulty with some persons may be that they are not waking quickly enough when discomfort comes from the shutting off of the circulation in an arm or leg. In bad cases, and especially in the cases of younger persons, the physician should look for cervical ribs or a scalenus anticus syndrome. Fortunately, these troubles are rare.

Numbness and tingling in the legs, and more rarely in the arms and hands, should make one think of a primary anemia. Then the blood smears should be looked at and a gastric analysis should be made to see if there is any free hydrochloric acid in the stomach. The presence of such acid practically rules out a primary anemia.

A simple way of finding out if the arteries of the legs are patent is to ask the patient if he can walk at a good rate for several blocks without getting pain. If he can do this he must have pretty good arteries. The physician will also feel his feet to see if they are warm or if there is pulsation in the tibial arteries.

Occasionally there is trouble in a peroneal nerve because the person tends to sit too long with the legs crossed. Rarely, numbness and paresthesias in legs and feet will be due to a beginning tabes.

In older persons it is probable that many of the more lasting numbnesses and paresthesias complained of are due to arteriosclerotic changes in the brain or the spinal cord. Rarely are they due to a neuritis. In some cases the trouble may be related to arthritis or fibrositis, or narrowing of the smaller arteries of the affected part.

Treatment. Usually there is little logical treatment that one can carry out. One can try iodides such as lipoiodine, and one can try physiotherapy. Reassurance is often the most effective treatment.

THE PERSON WITH DISTURBING RELATIVES

As everyone knows, the mother-in-law in the home often wrecks the nerves of the daughter-in-law, and sometimes wrecks her marriage (see also Chapter 11). In the doctor's office many a woman breaks down and weeps when asked how she gets along with her husband's relatives. Perhaps the mother-in-law never liked her or approved of her, and perhaps she deliberately tried to wreck the marriage, or she demanded that her son keep her first in his affections and attentions. He, poor fellow, got caught in an impossible situation and did not know what to do. He could not bear to hurt his mother, but by not standing up to her he kept wrecking his marriage and his wife's health.

Naturally, the wife wanted to be first in his heart and in his consideration. She also wanted, above all things, some privacy with her husband. As one such wife once said to me, "I wish my husband would some day divorce his mother and really marry me!" Often the man reasons that since the mother is old and too rigid to change her ways, the wife should give in. Or he cannot afford a separate apartment for his mother, or if he tried to move her into one she would not go. Often the harassed man, with all his efforts to secure peace, finds that he is not pleasing or appeasing anyone.

Although it is a terrible thing for a son to hurt his mother, it is also a terrible thing for him always to give in to her and thereby wreck his wife's health and happiness. It is also a terrible thing for a man to wreck his marriage and thereby to injure the lives of his children. Often I think it would be better to insist that the mother live by herself. Even then there may be trouble if the mother insists that, on the son's way home from work, he always drop in for a visit with her. The wife is likely to resent this keenly.

Oftentimes in these cases there does not seem to be any comfortable way out of the tragic situation. This is the case when a young man's father has died, leaving the ownership of a business to the mother and the running of it to the son. If, as sometimes then happens, the mother keeps constantly dictating the boy's every move, or countermanding his orders, he is soon reduced to a nervous wreck. And the wife, seeing her husband harried and unhappy all the time, soon is so resentful at the mother-in-law and so angry at her spouse for not standing up for his rights that she is likely to steer the marriage onto the rocks.

Sometimes it is an old father in the home who is making things difficult by fighting with the husband or interfering with the boisterous life of the children. Or it may be the wife's own mother who still wants to run the kitchen or the house in her way, or who is constantly breaking into the hour or two of privacy which the young couple want to have at the end of the day. At any time of evening or morning she may walk into their bedroom without knocking, or she may fuss over *her* child while entirely ignoring the spouse. Brothers or sisters of the husband or wife, or their children, can also be disturbing agents when they all have to live in the same small house.

Treatment. Occasionally one can talk a couple into getting a separate little apartment for the disturbing parent. Or the physician may be able to help matters by tactfully talking to the person who is causing the trouble and selling him or her the idea that it would more comfortable to move out and live alone.

I remember a fine woman who, after enduring much distress from having her mother in the house, finally insisted that the old lady leave and have her own apartment some distance away. It turned out that even the mother was better pleased. She could then have her friends in whenever she liked, and, best of all, she and her grandchildren now enjoyed their visits together.

The woman whose life is wrecked by a psychopathic relative. Every so often I see a patient whose diagnosis is easy. It is that of a devoted woman who let her life be blighted by a psychopathic, alcoholic, or chronically ill or crippled relative. I have seen many such women who spent all they could earn helping a brother, sister, father, husband, or son who went on sprees, or cashed checks which had to be made good, or just kept the poor woman's nervous system in a miserable state. She never knew what the relative would do next.

I remember a fine woman who went into business with a weakling brother only to find that he could not leave the till alone; he was always taking out so much that there was little left for the payroll on Saturday night. In one case an able woman running a business left her useless husband one job to do and that was to sign the weekly checks for the employees. But either because of laziness or a desire to show who was boss around the place he would often refuse to prepare the payroll until he was good and ready! Then the wife would get a terrible sick headache.

Every so often one sees a man or woman whose troubles are all due to his or her having married a psychopath. For good measure, some have also begotten a psychopathic child or two. Often such a person needs expert advice as to what to do about a more or less intolerable situation.

THE PERSON WHO TAKES REFUGE IN ILLNESS OR USES ILLNESS FOR A PURPOSE

There are many persons who, perhaps in childhood, learned that illness could be useful. It enabled them to slide out of unpleasant situations, to avoid punishment, to gain an excuse for failure in some task, or for incompetence, or for flunking out of college. It enabled a weakling to avoid making decisions, or it helped him to escape from facing the world and its responsibilities, or it made it possible for him to keep his self-respect, or it enabled him to get his own way and to tyrannize first over his mother and later over his wife. I have seen children two years old who had already mastered the technic so well that when naughty they never were even scolded by their parents. All they had to do was to stiffen their muscles, or hold their breath, or imitate a stammer, and the parents gave in.

I have had migrainous women admit to me that they sometimes used their illness to get out of things they did not care to do. It was so easy. Sometimes, with the help of a headache, they could keep a husband in subjection or out of their bed. In other cases a painful pelvis was used to save a woman from the advances of an unloved husband, and in still other cases, illness of one kind or another enabled a woman to stay much of her time in hospitals or nursing-homes where the husband could not bother her sexually. In other cases illness got a woman out of a boring small town and into a more interesting large city. Several women confessed that their yearly trip to the Mayo Clinic was their way of getting a vacation from a boring husband.

Often I have suspected strongly that the patient before me had taken refuge in illness, but I hated to make the accusation or even hint at it. It would have been so awful if I had been wrong. I have heard physicians tell of having worked a cure by bawling out a woman and making her so angry that she pulled herself together and got well, but I cannot use this technic. I would so hate to use it, and later find that the patient had really had a multiple sclerosis or a brain tumor. Mistakes can be made; human beings are fallible, and I have seen many a man with an extremely painful posterior perforating ulcer who had been treated roughly by physicians and even locked up in a psychiatric ward. I prefer to work carefully and to feel my way.

At times I have seen that an illness was an asset to a person, but I wondered if he knew this, or if he could face the fact if it were to be pointed out to him. So often the person who takes refuge in illness has a poor nervous system to begin with, and a poor nervous heredity. If he had been stronger he could have faced life more bravely and worked out his problems.

Even a strong person can be knocked down into illness by disappointment or disaster. Then, if the man is not strong, or if his illness should turn out to be in some ways an asset, he may remain in bed. After flunking out, a college student may take to his bed or develop an illness which saves him from disgrace or blame, or the wrath of an indignant and hard-driving father.

Many a woman past middle age develops illness which serves to hold a husband or children in subjection so that they will remain in the home and will keep supporting her. Or a woman will fall ill to keep a son from marrying a girl not acceptable to her.

My impression is that most of the persons who flee into illness do not realize what they have done, because again and again they will allow themselves to be operated on.

A remarkable story of flight into illness was told by William Seabrook in his book, *No Hiding Place*. When he was a boy, suddenly and with no reason that he knew of, he told his mother he was ill, and went to bed and stayed there for months. So far as he could see, he gained no advantage from this illness. His feeling was that some force from outside had assumed control of him. In later years he became an alcoholic, and on several occasions he fled from life much as he had done when he was a boy. Eventually he fled from life by committing suicide.

Treatment. Sometimes one can tactfully get a person to see that he or she is using illness to get out of unpleasant situations, and then, perhaps, one can work a cure. Often, however, the person is too weak to do much in the way of self-rehabilitation. Occasionally, I help a young woman by getting her to see that it would be more fun to be well than ill.

THE TYPE OF PATIENT WHO LOVES TO BE EXAMINED REPEATEDLY

Physicians all know the type of person who loves to get examined, and who keeps going from clinic to clinic and physician to physician. I remember a man like that whose business took him all over the United States. Everywhere he went he dropped in either on an internist for an overhauling, or on a nose and throat man for an opinion as to whether his tonsils should be removed a second time. He was kept in a constant stew and state of indecision because while some men told him that all he had left in his throat were a few harmless tags, a few men were insistent that his "terrible tonsils" should come right out. A wealthy woman who spent her time going from one internist to another appeared to have had a little stroke which had left her with a mild agitated depression.

Some of these peripatetics are hypochondriacs, and others have a pathologic fear of death. Some curious persons travel about ostensibly looking for reassurance but becoming outraged whenever they get it! One of the surest ways of getting the undying hatred of a man of this type is to tell him that his supposed severe and soon-to-be-fatal "nephritis" is a harmless static albuminuria!

THE PERSON WHO THINKS HE HAS A FEVER

Each year a consultant sees a few patients who are supposed to have a fever. They bring reports of thorough examinations made by good physicians who tried hard to find brucellosis, tuberculosis, or some other chronic infection. In these cases I rarely find any sign of infection, and later the patients do not come to any bad end. I think it significant that the patient is usually a nervous, excitable woman who has an afternoon temperature ranging around 99.6° F. Perhaps when she is under great strain it will go up to 100° or higher. I call this a nervous hyperthermia.

One woman like this had a temperature between 102° and 103° F. for four days while her father was very ill. When he recovered, her "fever" disappeared. An anxious, very apprehensive Latin woman, when in my office getting examined, was found to have a temperature of 102° F. When told that nothing serious had been found, the temperature dropped to normal. She then said that she had done this sort of thing before. I remember several other tense migrainous or hysterically inclined women who ran a temperature of from 101° to 102° F. for weeks while all tests failed to show any sign of infection. One such woman ran a temperature around 101° F. for over a year after she discovered she had contracted an unhappy marriage. Interestingly, this "fever" was uninfluenced by months of rest in bed. Experts in the field of tuberculosis pointed out to me that this fact alone did much to rule out a smoldering tuberculosis.

Kleitman showed that after going to a movie in the evening, two girls usually had a rise of temperature of at least 1° F. Soldiers, while gambling, were found to push their temperature up a degree or two. I remember a very tired, tense young college woman who got married at the close of the last day of final examinations. She became hysterical and for a few hours ran a temperature of 106° F.

A choleric man of forty years had long been treated for brucellosis in spite of the absence of any sign of the disease. When I saw him I got the history that since boyhood, whenever he became extremely angry, his temperature would shoot up a few degrees, and he would feel ill and have to lie down. Five years later his doctor wrote me that he was still stout and healthy except for fever when he "blew his top." Dunbar (1946) summarized much literature on the nervous production of hyperthermia.

In recent years I have seen a number of elderly arteriosclerotics who for months ran a temperature around 101° F. They were studied extensively with every facility at my disposal and nothing wrong was found. A normal blood sedimentation rate and leucocyte count, plus a failure, with time, of a patient to go down hill, plus the fact that later he or she recovered, made me feel sure that the cause was not an infection or a cancer. I think it probable that the hyperthermia was due to arteriosclerotic changes in the hypothalamus which resulted in the changing of a setting in some little thermostat. A similar change would seem to cause the sudden losses of 30 or 40 pounds seen sometimes in these cases.

The physician, when dealing with patients with long-lasting hyperthermia, should remember, when he finds a slight leucocytosis, that it can be due to the same nervous tension that raised the temperature. This was shown by W. E. Garrey, years ago, and recently by Milhorat, Small, and Diethelm, and others.

It should be noted that Hobart Reimann, for years, has studied young persons who apparently were born to have a body temperature always a degree or two higher than the average. Thus far the persons studied have not come to any bad end.

The important thing in all these cases is not to diagnose brucellosis.

Treatment. The essential point in treating the patient who complains of a nervous hyperthermia is to explain (1) that a rise in body temperature can be effected by emotion, tension, and fatigue; and (2) that "normal" temperature, like all other bodily measurements, is not a dot on the scale: It is a band, within the range of which the figures vary in different persons and in the same person. Thus, normal temperature is not 98.6° F., but anything from perhaps 97° in the morning to 99.6° in the afternoon. In some persons the temperature tends regularly to be higher or lower than these limits.

THE PERSON WHO IS SUPPOSED TO HAVE BRUCELLOSIS

For awhile I used to see many nervous or constitutionally inadequate persons, nearly all women, who had been told that their troubles were all due to chronic brucellosis. In practically every case the almost life-long duration of the illness and the nature of it made me very doubtful if the woman had at the time, or ever had had, this disease. Also, she had never come in close contact with cattle or pigs. The so-called fever she had seemed more likely to be a nervous hyperthermia.

In these cases the bacteriologists of the Mayo Clinic reported that the concentration of agglutinins for Brucella in the blood was not high enough to be significant. Unfortunately, the skin test is not trustworthy; the sedimentation rate does not necessarily go up, and the spleen does not necessarily enlarge. Rarely can one find typical lesions in the spine, such as one finds in swine. In acute cases the best proof of the existence of brucellosis is the finding of the organism in blood cultures. Recently biopsies have shown that some persons can be carriers of Brucella, often without any symptoms.

Certainly, it does not seem wise to tell a frail sickly woman who has been ailing all her life that her troubles are due to brucellosis. Even if she did have the disease, the diagnosis would not help her much because no treatment has ever proved satisfactory for the chronic cases.

PERSONS WHO FEEL SET ASIDE, PASSED OVER, SUPERSEDED, AND NO LONGER NEEDED

A common source of neurosis and unhappiness, especially in older persons, is the feeling of being no longer needed or useful. One sees this so commonly in the case of the woman whose children have all gone to college or have married or moved away. When that time comes, unless she and her husband have remained congenial and in love, she will feel little responsibility to him; she will not feel needed by him, and she will feel that her work is done and her life largely over.

One sees this sort of thing in the case of many a man who has been retired by an employer or who has failed to get a coveted and long-awaited promotion. When he is superseded his enthusiasm and joy of work go; his devotion to his company and pride in it go, and with this he gives up: He just stagnates and lets his morale go down.

THE GRIEF-STRICKEN PERSON

Every year, because of illness or accident, hundreds of thousands of persons lose a loved one. Many then are so grief stricken that for a while they need psychiatric help. Some even go into a sort of agitated depression. This is especially true when, as often happens, there is some feeling of guilt, and the person keeps saying over and over again, "If only I had done this" or "If only I had not urged him to go out that day," or "If only I had called another doctor." So many persons of this type need to be told again and again that they are not responsible; they could not have avoided what happened; and no one could have expected them to see into the future. Some are the more upset because they had a quarrel with the loved one shortly before he or she died.

I remember a man who, shortly after a happy reconciliation with his estranged wife, was driving on the highway. Two cars racing each other around a curve forced him into the ditch where his car hit a pole. His wife was thrown out and killed. For months afterward he kept going back to see the highway police so that they might assure him again and again that he could not possibly have avoided what happened. For over a year he was not himself; he was so overwhelmed by grief.

After the terrible fire in the night-club in Boston, Lindemann (1944) wrote an interesting article about the persons who survived the loss of loved ones. He noted that the distress of great grief takes much the same form in different persons. They have a sensation of great bodily distress which comes over them in waves. They may feel a tightness in the throat, choking feelings, shortness of breath, a need for sighing, an empty feeling in the abdomen, a lack of strength, and great feelings of tension and misery and psychic pain. There is no appetite, and food has no taste. There is often a sense of unreality. There is a lack of contact with anyone, and love for the remaining relatives cannot be felt. Every bit of the day's work, instead of being largely automatic, has to be done as a special task. A sad feature of the trouble is that sometimes a worse attack of grief comes after the first numbing shock wears off, and the person sees even more clearly how empty and lonely and useless life is to be for long years ahead.

Many of the grief-stricken are so tortured every minute that they would welcome death. Some cannot find anywhere a moment's surcease, or forgetfulness, or peace. Work is about all that can help a little. These people feel that it is useless to go out with others, as to a movie, because nothing interests or diverts or pleases. Sleep is hard to get. There is a terrible restlessness. Some persons cannot sit still, and many smoke incessantly. So far as they can see, there is no longer any reason for living or carrying on.

Some persons feel terribly bereaved when a loved one deserts the home or gets a divorce, or when a child leaves in anger, or elopes with an unsuitable person, or gets disgraced in some way. Occasionally, then, the parent seems really to feel that if the child were dead the grief would be less. For such persons the term "heartbroken" is not inappropriate.

Treatment. These unfortunates are hard to help because there is little that anyone can say or do to relieve their suffering. The physician must be particularly careful not to make the patient angry by handing out platitudes. Sympathy should be implied rather than expressed. Some persons can be helped with sedatives to take at night so that they can get some sleep.

THE WOMAN WHO HUGS HER GRIEF

Occasionally, one sees a woman who, after the death of a husband or child or parent, dedicates her life to grief. With most persons, grief is eased by the passage of time, but the unusual woman seems to hug her sorrow and to become alarmed or ashamed at any sign that would indicate that she is getting over it.

After the death of a child a woman may pay little attention to her husband and at night may shut her door to him. She may greatly distress her remaining children by showing them no more attention or affection. As the child of one such woman said to his mother, "I know Johnnie is gone, but didn't you love us too?"

In Latin countries one can see such women clad in black, years after the death of a loved one. I doubt if such pathologically prolonged grief is ever seen in a normal person, free from some psychopathic tendency. A normal person realizes that there is no sense in remaining grief stricken for years. It can do the loved one no good.

Treatment. The physician must often beg these persons to resume their normal activities, or to find some useful job to do. I sometimes succeed in influencing a widow by saying, "If your husband, like some Greek hero, were to be released from heaven for ten minutes to see you, would he not spend most of that time begging you to stop this grieving, and to learn to be happy again?" Usually the woman says, "Yes, I think he would; he would not want me unhappy," and after that she behaves better.

If such a woman, by hugging her grief, is thereby hurting others and blighting their lives, often she must be shown how terribly selfish she is. Sometimes she can be made to see that so long as she cannot bring herself to suicide she must live—and if she is to live, she might as well begin to do a good job of it. The best thing she can do is to help others about her. That will help her.

NEUROSIS OR PSYCHOSIS FOLLOWING A BROKEN ENGAGEMENT

As everyone knows, many a neurosis in a young woman follows the break-up of a love affair. For instance, a girl much in love, but unable to marry because of her mother's strong objections to the man, for a few months lived a very active sexual life with him. Then they had a spat, and the man left town. With this, the girl promptly became badly nauseated. Later, she began to suffer from abdominal pain and vomiting. A surgeon explored the abdomen and, finding nothing, removed the appendix. A few days later the girl went raving mad and had to be committed.

When dealing with cases like this the physician should keep in mind the fact that a normal girl, with time, can usually recover her poise and get over her disappointment. When a girl cannot pull herself together it may be because she has a poor nervous heredity which makes it hard for her to live sanely.

NEUROSIS DUE TO A SCANDAL

Occasionally one sees a person who is in a miserable state of nervousness and sleeplessness due to involvement in some scandal. To illustrate: A college instructor came in a state of great nervousness and mental and physical distress. She had been accused of homosexual intimacies with some of her pupils. She denied the charges but resigned under fire. It was easy to see why she was so upset. Not only had she many humiliating memories to haunt her, but her career as a teacher was ended, and she did not know where next to find a job. There was little I could do to help except to sympathize and let her talk the thing out. Unfortunately she never regained her health.

A woman missionary in the Orient got herself so talked about because of her close friendship with a married man that it seemed best to her superiors that she be sent home to America. Naturally, she felt that her useful life was ended, and she wished for death. I suspected that this hopelessness and feeling of irreparable disgrace accounted for her abdominal pain and "fever." Later, when a surgeon explored her abdomen, she soon died without obvious cause, perhaps from a broken heart.

A tense migrainous woman of a lovely type came with a bad nervous breakdown. What happened was that one day her next-door neighbor had come upon her taking an injection of gynergen. Assuming that the drug was morphine, the neighbor maliciously spread the story all over town. What with brooding over the resulting scandal, and the difficulty of continuing to live next door to her enemy, she soon drifted into invalidism.

THE PERSON WITH RESTLESS LEGS

There are some persons, usually men past middle age, who complain of restless legs which distress them at night. They cannot sleep well because they wake with the discomfort in their legs. The trouble has been ascribed to many things, such as prostatic disease, and many treatments have been tried without success. The symptom appears at times in the cases of nervous women.

In some cases I suspected that the main cause was a poor nervous inheritance; in other cases it may have been arteriosclerotic changes in the nervous system.

Treatment. Among drugs that have been tried are sedatives, calcium, quinine, quinidine, hyoscyamus, the antihistaminics, artane, or tolserol (myanesin). In my experience, none of these drugs has been very helpful.

THE MAN DISTURBED BY CONFLICTS WITHIN HIS BUSINESS GROUP

There is many a businessman whose nervousness is due partly to the fact that in his business he is constantly being harassed or thwarted or given a feeling of insecurity because his fellow-executives are jockeying for power. Perhaps a new president or general manager has come in and he now wants to get rid of the men who were friends and protégés of his predecessor. He has his own friends whom he wants to put in, or he may fear disloyalty in the old crowd. Perhaps, unable or unwilling to come right out and dismiss the men he wants to get rid of, he will put his favorites over them and leave them with little or nothing to do. Then they will have to sit and wonder if they are going to be forced out or if they had better quit right off and go somewhere else to start over again.

Occasionally a new man will have been brought in to take charge of a department. He is happy about his rise in the world until he starts in the new job and finds every man's hand against him. No one is loyal; dirty tricks are played, and as a result the man cannot accomplish the things he was brought in to do. Worse yet, in a crisis, the executive who hired him fails to back him up; he balks at earning unpopularity by defending his new protégé.

In many companies there is a younger set of able college-trained executives who are struggling with the help of new scientific methods to build up the business and keep it in the forefront. They want to build research laboratories, to modernize plants, and to get along better with labor, but always they have to struggle with a few old stand-patters who would prefer to let things go on as in the past, just so long as they can skim profits. This conflict adds greatly to the nervous strain of the younger executives.

The man who hates his business. Many a man has a tendency to break a bit under business strain largely because he does not like what he is doing. Thus, a patient complained of one attack after another of supposed intestinal obstruction. He had had his abdomen opened four times but nothing wrong had ever been found. Then his wife spoke up and said she was sure that every one of the spells had been brought on by a tantrum over the mistake of some employee. Each time the man had blown up with extra violence because he so hated the work to which he was chained. At college he had planned a career of writing, but then his father had died, and with this he had to assume the management of the family business.

Occasionally a man's neurosis is due to his worry over the fact that his partners are doing dishonest things. He will want to get out of the business but, especially when it is a family affair, he will hate to lose his inheritance plus most of what he has worked for all his life.

THE MAN WHO IS RESENTFUL AND UPSET BECAUSE HE FEELS HE HAS FAILED

There is many a man who is bitter and resentful and upset nervously because he feels he has failed in life. He may have done well and lived well by the standards of most persons, but still he feels that with his talents he should either have done better or he should have been of more use in the world. He did not live up to the high hopes of his youth. Perhaps he set too high a goal for himself; perhaps all he did was to make money when he wanted to get a good education, and write, or be an artist. Or perhaps, like one of my patients, when he started working for a big company he expected soon to work up to be its president. Often, as Wendell Johnson has said, a man is in an unhappy quandary because he is not sure what he did want, or what he should have done, or even why he is so discontented, or what he could do to find happiness.

Johnson calls this the I.F.D. disease because it goes from a vague *Idealism* to *Frustration* to *Demoralization.* He says it is the commonest ailment of the university student who goes to a counselor for advice and guidance. Out of this unhappiness can develop a neurosis.

Dr. Coyne Campbell pointed out that all of these maladjusted unhappy persons have as their chief symptom an inability to say exactly what is making them unhappy. They will talk at length to a physician without leaving any clear idea in his mind. Campbell said that often, if one could only get such a person to state his difficulties clearly, one might perhaps make him well. Once the man saw clearly what was the matter, he either could see that it was not so bad after all, or he might do something to straighten himself out.

THE WOMAN WHO HATES THE TOWN IN WHICH SHE LIVES

Some women are mentally disturbed and ill, partly because the husband's business has compelled him to live in some unpleasant or lonely or boring place without interesting society or educational facilities. Perhaps the woman is terribly homesick, or she just hates the surroundings, or, after she moves in, she will not make the effort to begin a new life and find new friends. She frets and beats her head against the bars. She keeps constantly complaining to the husband and perhaps getting him much upset. Under these conditions, a woman can become mildly depressed.

Treatment. Treatment consists usually in asking the woman if she is going to ask her husband to give up his job and perhaps a fine opportunity, for her sake. If she is a good sensible woman she says, "Why, no, I would not do that to him and to us. Here is where we get our bread and butter, and hence here we must stay. " Then one can say to her, "Since you are not going to pull out and leave, you might as well settle down and get used to the town. You might as well start right now making new friends." In those rare cases in which the woman is desperate enough to want to go, no matter what happens to her husband's business, he may have to make the sacrifice and move. In that case she may spend her days regretting what she did and fussing about it.

THE TROUBLES OF A WOMAN WHO MARRIES A RECENTLY DIVORCED MAN

Occasionally I see a woman whose troubles began when she married a recently divorced man. Perhaps she had the great strain of having to go and live in the previous wife's house and to sleep in her old bed. Perhaps the husband saw no need for getting new things.

Then, perhaps, the former wife started calling up at all hours to revile the new one, and to call her unpleasant names. And when the new wife wanted a new dress or a new stove she had to run up against the unpleasant fact that she could not have anything because so much of her husband's salary was going out as alimony to the other woman. Perhaps, also, the second wife had to go without a wanted child of her own because she had to take care of the first wife's children, and the husband could not afford to have another baby added to the family.

Under such circumstances it is only a very sensible and self-controlled woman who will not get so resentful at these constant pin-pricks and big annoyances that she will start fighting with her husband and wrecking her nervous health.

THE YOUNG WOMAN WHO IS FRANTIC TO GET A "MRS." BEFORE HER NAME

There are many women who are so anxious to get a "Mrs." before their names that they are willing to marry almost any man who will have them. Some seem to be ashamed of their failure to find a mate. A few with an inferiority complex propose to marry far beneath them so that the man will be unlikely ever to leave. Others are frantic to marry so as to get out of the teaching profession, and others will marry almost anyone to get away from the tyranny of a mother or a stepfather.

Treatment. Many such women need to be advised that marriage to the type of man they have in mind will bring only sorrow, poverty, shame, more isolation, more lack of freedom, and more boredom. They may soon find themselves supporting the man or deserted by him and left to bring up a child or two.

Some lonely women need to change their occupation to one in which they can meet eligible men. Others, living in a small unprogressive town, need to move to a larger city. Many women might get married if they could spend their vacations in places where men go. Some women need to be advised to get more education and to dress more attractively. They must be reminded that when the fine man does come and does get interested, they must be attractive and educated enough to hold him. If they marry him they should know how to keep a nice home for him and to entertain nicely.

THE WOMAN WHO KEEPS HOUSE FOR HER FATHER UNTIL HE GETS MARRIED AGAIN

Several times I have seen a woman with a puzzling nervous breakdown who finally told how, when her mother had died, she had kept house for her father. Later, when he married and she had to leave the home or else stay on, not as the mistress but as a none-too-comfortable guest, she went to pieces nervously. Naturally, the same thing can happen to a daughter when she is living with a widowed mother who decides to marry again.

THE YOUNG WIDOW WHO HAS TO GO BACK TO LIVING WITH A DOMINEERING MOTHER

Many a young widow, living with her family again, is very unhappy, partly because of her mother's habit of treating her still as a girl who must be in by ten each evening. Naturally, this is not easily borne by a mature woman who has known the joy of having her own home and living independently like an adult. The strain of the new life builds up in the daughter a curious mixture of the old love for her mother and a new resentment against her.

Treatment. In all such cases the physician should see if it would be possible for the woman to get out and into a small apartment of her own. Often all that keeps her from doing this is a reluctance to hurt the mother or father. Then the doctor can tell the family that she must move.

THE WOMAN WHO ONCE SUFFERED FROM CHOREA OR FROM A TOXIC GOITER

Occasionally one sees a jittery, nervous, irritable woman who is having much poor health. She may have spells of excessive tension and irritability when she will shriek at her children and bawl out her husband. Her situation becomes more understandable when one learns that either as a girl she suffered from chorea, or later she suffered from a toxic goiter. She recovered, but for the rest of her days she was left abnormally nervous, jumpy, and trembly.

THE PERSON WHO BECOMES ILL BECAUSE HE IS BORED

A wide-awake pleasant businessman of sixty who had always been very active came up from South America to visit his daughter who had married in the United States. He stayed in her home for several months waiting for a grandchild to be born, and for the first time in his life, developed a distressing illness. Every evening he would get severe indigestion with nausea, bloating, and flatulence. He would sit up for hours rubbing his stomach; he would belch loudly; and in the middle of the night, to relieve his distress, he would get up and walk the streets. He would hope that on his return to bed he would be tired enough to fall asleep. He soon lost 20 pounds in weight.

Because of the man's age, the short history of indigestion, the previous record of perfect health, and the absence of any sign of nervousness,

I examined him twice in a couple of months, going over him very carefully, but each time finding nothing wrong. Later, he confessed that he was terribly bored by his unwonted inaction. He then flew home and went back to work. A year later he wrote that, before he reached the port of embarkation, he had lost all his symptoms. His case makes me wonder how many other similar ones I have seen in which I failed to make the correct diagnosis.

I remember an Army physician who, early in World War II, while taking a course of graduate training, missed the rush of his busy practice and began to suffer from severe migrainous headaches. Later he wrote that they must have been due to boredom because they disappeared the day he was assigned to a hospital where he had plenty of work to do.

THE PERSON WHO IS FULL OF RESENTMENTS

As psychiatrists are now constantly emphasizing, many persons are full of resentments against their parents or an older or more successful brother or sister, or against an employer or boss, or against society in general. Some of these persons can do themselves much nervous harm by their constant feelings of bitterness, and by their desire for getting revenge or for punishing or getting even. A law suit with a former wife will sometimes wreck a man's nerves.

THE SCHOOL TEACHER WHO IS WORKING FOR A MASTER'S DEGREE

Most physicians know the type of school teacher who, each summer, instead of getting a rest, goes to some college and picks up a few more credits toward a Master's degree. Naturally, because she never has a vacation, she gets worn down and full of aches and pains.

THE PERSON TROUBLED BY UNHAPPY MEMORIES AND ASSOCIATIONS

Some intense nervous persons have difficulties because of their fear of certain places and certain times with which they have unhappy associations. Thus, I remember a widow who still, after many years, cannot go into a certain store because in the old days she and her much-loved husband used to shop there so happily. Many a woman dreads a certain date on the calendar because it recalls some life tragedy. She is likely to spend that day brooding, or wondering how a certain disaster could have been averted, or the life of a loved one saved. If only she had not done this or that!

There are unforgiving persons who will not allow the name of someone to be even mentioned in their presence. Perhaps it is a former wife who was unfaithful, or who went away, or who was divorced with great bitterness and hatred, or a child who was disinherited. Persons so full of hate cannot hope to get any health unless they will forgive and try to forget.

THE WOMAN WHO CANNOT WEAR FALSE TEETH

There is a type of hypersensitive woman who should be urged to keep her teeth so long as she can because, when they are extracted, she will find it almost impossible to wear plates. She will keep going from dentist to dentist getting new plates, but she will keep them all in her handbag.

Before the proposed extraction her physician should have seen that with her fussiness, the oversensitiveness of her palate and fauces, and her inability to brush her back teeth without gagging, she would find it hard to wear plates. She may be unable, also, to wear bifocals because, with a glance at the dividing line, she will get nauseated. The wise physician advises such a woman to keep her teeth as long as she can.

THE PSYCHIC PROBLEMS OF THE PERSON WHO HAS JUST BEEN TOLD THAT HE HAS A CANCER

The person who has just been told that he has a cancer, and particularly an inoperable one, may profit from a little talk with his doctor. (See also Chapter 28.) I never like to slam the door of hope tight shut in the face of such a person. I usually say that there is some chance that the diagnosis was wrong, or I tell of those persons whom I have seen who fought the cancer to a draw, and lived with it until they died of something else, or I say that something may be done to slow the growth of the bad cells with the roentgen rays, or I say that some cure may come out of a laboratory in time. Such things have happened.

If there is some chance of getting the tumor out, the person may have to be encouraged to the point where he is willing to take the gamble. Usually he elects to take it. Often, as in the case of carcinomas in the esophagus or lung, he must be told that his chances of recovery are poor, but even then, he may prefer to take them. Sometimes, after a biopsy has been made or the growth has been removed, the patient can be cheered by the fact that the degree of malignancy was low. This gives a much better chance of a five-year cure.

In many cases the patient must be made to see that cancer is often curable if one can only get it out in time, and he must be told of the hundreds of thousands of persons who years ago had a cancer and are still going about well. Often the patient must be sent out to think things over and talk them over with his wife, and then to return for a decision. It must be remembered that for a while after being told that he has cancer, he is in such a state of mental shock that he cannot take in or remember much of what is told him. Oftentimes, also, the matter must be discussed with the family and friends who will influence the patient in his decision as to what to do and where to have it done. The family may have to be talked to and given hope before they will encourage the patient to be operated on. Often the wise physician will say, "This problem is a terrible one for you to face; you want to be sure before you accept operation, so why not go to a consultant for another opinion?"

Sometimes, as when there is a carcinoma blocking the pylorus or the cardia, the question arises, should there be a palliative operation? Would it really prolong life or give the person any joy or comfort? Here I think the physician and surgeon should be honest and frank. For instance, if I had a carcinoma of the cardia I would not accept a gastrostomy; I would not want to buy myself a few more months of pain, and hence I do not recommend the operation to my patients. A gastroenterostomy for pyloric cancer may prolong life and may be worth doing. Many persons ask for an operation because they hope they will die on the table.

When a growth is inoperable, or when the person returns with metastasis, he or she again needs psychiatric help. Often it is well to give some roentgenologic treatment, if only to maintain morale. If something is not done for these people they are likely to go to a cancer quack and be fleeced. Often the family will insist that something be done. They cannot bear to just sit by and wait.

Always the patient with great pain should be given enough sedative so that he can end his days in a fair degree of comfort. Families who perhaps, because of religious scruples, worry or fret about the giving of dilaudid or morphine or methadon should be assured that these drugs will not shorten life; rather they will decidedly lengthen it. Pain wears people down. Families who worry for fear that the loved one will get a habit should be reminded that even if he does get a habit in the four or five remaining months of life, it will not do harm. I have seen bedridden patients get up and work again for some months when given enough dilaudid to relieve pain. With rest and sleep some gained 20 pounds and looked and felt well.

THE PERSON WHO BECOMES NEUROTIC AFTER AN ACCIDENT

In this country hundred of thousands of persons are constantly getting hurt in accidents. Many of those who have a stable nervous system soon get well and go back to work. Farmers and persons who have skiing or hunting accidents usually recover quickly, partly perhaps, because there is no one to give them any compensation, and partly because they love their work and hate to be idle. Other persons after an accident get nervous and even somewhat psychopathic. Many strive hard to get compensation; some get into prolonged litigation, and some never work again.

Every storekeeper must have marveled at the difference between two women who stumble or slip and fall to the floor in his establishment. One picks herself up and goes on her way, while the other makes a terrible fuss, takes to her bed, gets scores of roentgenograms made, and sues for a large sum. Here, obviously, are two different varieties of the human species. As one would have expected, a study by Kozol (1946) showed that the psychoneurotic and the psychopathic are most likely to develop the traumatic neuroses.

Myerson (1938) once described the mental changes that take place in the injured. He noted first, the bad effects of our crazy laws which say that if a man is dying of a hopeless cancer, and a little accident somewhat shortens his life, the person who caused the accident is as responsible for the death as if the victim were an active young athlete. Similarly, if a psychopath who is highly predisposed to a neurosis or psychosis has a little accident which helps him over the edge into a state in which he never tries to work again, the insurance company has to shoulder all the blame for a complete disability.

As Myerson said, an accident with its resulting disability tends to disturb a patient's feeling of security as regards his health. If, also, it causes him to lose his job and the hope of getting another one, it makes him feel that he has lost his place in society. Then a sense of great resentment is likely to develop in him. He may become enraged at the law because it drags along so slowly. Any implication, also, by the insurance lawyers or adjusters that he is faking or "piling it on" will poison his mind, so that he may become somewhat paranoiac.

The law is supposed to be impartial, but a lawyer for an insurance company is naturally more valuable to his employers when, in many cases, he can beat down the amount of compensation to be awarded. Hence it is that legal battles take place, and the injured man may be made ever more bitter as he gets the idea that he, a poor person of little consequence, is being beaten down and treated shabbily by a great corporation.

Similarly, a veteran, asking for a big pension, may be the more upset because he feels he is a hero who is being let down. He may feel this way even when his nervous breakdown came the day he arrived in training camp. Such a man may become a professional ailing veteran, writing constantly to his congressman for special favors, and feeling that society owes him not only a good living but much sympathy and consideration as well.

Workers past middle age are likely to cling to any disability payments that they have obtained, if only because they realize that if on going back to the factory they should find themselves unable to do a full day's work, they would lose their job, and then not only be unable to get another but be unable to get back on compensation.

Today few men realize that the setting-up of pension schemes in many companies is making it very hard or impossible for an older man to get a job. To hire him would cost a company too much in the way of money that would have to be set aside for his retirement. These factors make it almost impossible to get older persons back to work after they have had a slight injury or have been placed on compensation of some kind.

After much experience with compensation cases, I came to feel that most insurance companies are foolish and stupid when they make it almost impossible for a man to even try to go back to work. Many men would try going back if only they were sure that if their health did not let them "make the grade" they could immediately and without the slightest difficulty get back on their old compensation. In many cases a wise and kindly insurance manager might help the man back onto half-day work or easier work. But, there again, one meets with customs in unions and businesses which make it imperative that on the first day of his return the man do a full day's work. This he may never be able to do.

PATIENTS WHO GET WELL SUDDENLY IN CURIOUS WAYS

Many a woman has tipped me off to the fact that her illness was psychic in nature by telling me of experiences she had had in which she was cured in a minute by some form of quackery. For instance, a stout woman who said that for years she had been having twenty bowel movements a day confirmed my hunch that she had a functional type of diarrhea by saying that once she had been cured instantly by a chiropractic adjustment. I then cured her for six months by giving her a hypodermic injection of typhoid vaccine. I suspected that this, too, was a vehicle for psychotherapy.

One of my bad bloaters was cured suddenly by a chiropodist who put a pad in her shoe "to raise the front end of her calcaneus." Another got cured suddenly by taking an Indian herb remedy.

Sometimes a patient who has been examined thoroughly and told that nothing organically wrong was found will leave angrily, refusing to accept the diagnosis. But later I hear that he or she was suddenly cured by some hocus-pocus, and then I suspect that that was the patient's way out. Probably he or she was ready to get well, but wanted to avoid having the appearance of being cured by psychotherapy.

CHAPTER 14

*Types of Mildly Psychotic
or Almost Psychotic
Persons*

A WISE OLD PHYSICIAN who sees sick persons every day should become skillful at classifying his patients and recognizing at a glance their peculiarities. The psychiatrist who probes deeply into the minds and souls of people and who sees queer persons every day should come to recognize quickly even more of the odd types than are known to laymen and general practitioners.

In this chapter I have gathered together brief descriptions of many types of troubled or handicapped persons whom most of us physicians know. Perhaps these descriptions will help young doctors to recognize the types, and to see that in them the pains or aches complained of are less important than is the abnormal personality.

The people here described are not those in asylums; rather they are those who often come to a doctor's office complaining of fatigue, "loss of pep," aches and pains, and feelings of weakness. Most of these people show signs of a tendency toward irrational behavior. For instance, as I write this, I am called to see a fine able lawyer, much respected in his large city, who apologizes for having been unable to keep on his face the mask of a machine for estimating basal metabolism. He became frantic and had to run from the room. And yet, as he said, he knew perfectly well that he was in no danger, and he knew he was making a fool of himself. He wonders if he is entirely sane and he is afraid he may be headed for trouble like his grandfather who wound up in the state asylum.

THE SCHIZOID OR SCHIZOPHRENIC PERSON

Schizophrenia is an exaggeration of a shyness, diffidence, unfriendliness, detachment, self-centeredness, touch-me-not-ness, or day-dreaminess that is found in many persons. It is the commonest form of psychosis, and there are all grades of it. Many of those persons who are only slightly affected are called schizoid. One can recognize them in a moment in any large institution where there are many secretaries. As they go through the halls and up and down the elevators the normal women will be looking about, observing their fellows, both men and women, recognizing all those whom they know, smiling and nodding at many, or saying a word of greeting. Some will go hand in hand, laughing, and talking of plans for the evening's fun. Not so with the schizoid girl. She keeps her eyes lowered; she does not seem to see that friends are near; she does not show any sign of recognition, and if spoken to, she may answer in a monosyllable with only a shy momentary glance. If someone takes her arm she may recoil as if touched by a hot iron. This is well described in a passage in *Wuthering Heights,* in which one reads that the psychopathic hero craved the love of a girl, but the minute she showed signs of responding, he drew away, almost angrily.

If a man tries to make friends with such a girl she will keep repulsing him again and again, often in a prudish way; she may appear distressed just because he is near. She has none of her well-sexed sisters' sureness of their ability to handle a man if he should become too affectionate.

Naturally, a girl of this type tends to be dull, lifeless, apathetic, uninteresting, mentally inaccessible, shut-in, and incapable of friendship. She may never go out with boys, and she may never have a beau. For reasons hard to understand, men do marry many of these girls, but they are not likely to have much happiness with them. Such girls are likely to be frigid, and many hate sexual intercourse. An occasional one remains a virgin throughout marriage, and some tolerate intercourse only a few times. Many suffer greatly from vaginismus or a sort of protective spasm of the thighs and the muscles around the vulva. The children of such women will say, "I cannot remember my mother's ever caressing or kissing me or saying that she loved me."

These are the persons of whom R. L. Stevenson was thinking when he said they were "tied for life in a bag which no one can undo. They are poorer than the Gypsy, for their heart can speak no language under heaven." Wrapped up much of the time in their own unhappy thoughts, they do not do well in industry; they are too likely to forget; they are often "wool-gathering" and so they make mistakes. Some live in a world of fantasy or symbolism. Some are likely to misinterpret what is told them.

In universities, according to Raphael and Himler 8.2 per cent of the students consult a psychiatric counselor, and many of these troubled youngsters are schizoid. The troubles of these students may begin with feelings of inferiority, rejection, shame, disappointment, and sadness, all of which feelings are easily understandable when one realizes that the victim is so cut off from human love and companionship and joy. There may be feelings of illness and fatigue, and there is likely to be trouble in concentrating and studying and keeping up with the class. Sometimes there will be a short episode of psychosis during or after an attack of influenza.

Later, if the person gets worse, there may be feelings of resentment and suspicion and ideas of persecution. There may be much day-dreaming, with a gradual withdrawal from life. Eventually the patient may be unable to distinguish between his fantasies and reality, and then he may depart in some way from orderly conduct. There will come delusions and hallucinations, and finally some mental deterioration.

Guthrie has commented on the great selfishness of schizophrenics. As he said, it isn't so much the schizophrenic who suffers, as his family.

Hoch (1910) wrote of the rigidity of these people; they cannot easily adapt themselves to situations; they are hard to influence and are stubborn in a passive way. They cannot see the other fellow's side of an argument. They show little interest in what goes on, and they do not care to participate in the pleasures and pursuits of those about them. Hoch found this type of personality in 68 per cent of the persons who later developed dementia praecox.

Weiss and English stated that in the early development of schizophrenia there may be a hypochondriacal phase, in which the patient complains of many discomforts. There may be anxiety, much as in cases of neurosis, but the schizophrenic is more vague about his symptoms than is the neurasthenic. He tends, also, to describe the symptoms in a peculiar way, saying, for instance, that it feels as if a snake or a tapeworm were moving about in his stomach. He may complain much of constipation, flatulence, belching, nausea, vomiting, or anorexia. (See the section in Chapter 15 on the relatives of the psychotic.)

The physical characteristics of the schizophrenic. It is interesting that the schizophrenic's body is often somewhat abnormal, much as is his brain. Many writers have commented on the poor physique and poor sexual development of these unhappy people. An expert could go through a crowd and pick many of them out just because of their pinched, ascetic, sad, apathetic, and lifeless faces. On examination, many of the women will be found to have small shotty breasts, and an infantile type of small uterus with a long conical cervix. Many have a dry or a greasy or evil-smelling skin, and a male distribution of body hair. Many have blue cyanotic legs, an irritable heart, and low blood pressure. Many are sickly, and some get operated on time after time.

Prognosis. Although some schizophrenics recover and have good years, psychiatrists say that their recovery can hardly ever be complete because they are so likely to go back only to their former schizoid state.

Treatment. The non-psychiatrist had better not attempt the treatment of a schizophrenic, but should turn him or her over to a psychiatrist. In the early stages something may be accomplished with shock treatments or institutional care.

The wise physician will be careful not to touch familiarly or "kid" patients who are reserved or schizoid. Patients of this type have told me how outraged they were at such behavior on the part of some physician whom they had consulted.

THE CYCLOTHYMIC, MANIC-DEPRESSIVE, OR MOODY PERSON

Some persons, while sane enough to live useful lives, tend to go through cycles in which they are either abnormally energetic, keyed-up, ambitious, social, and talkative, or else abnormally quiet, moody, uncommunicative, unhappy, discouraged, and tired. If such a person, on his swing back from depression crosses the line into hypomania, as a few do, he may for a time work too hard not only at his proper job but also at his hobbies. Going at top speed day and night without bothering to sleep much, he may accomplish more than two or three ordinary persons do: His brain may seethe with ingenious ideas, and because of his enthusiasm, the facile flow of his thoughts and words, and his certainty that some cause he has espoused is righteous and bound to succeed, he may be unusually successful in persuading his fellows to invest in something or to join him in some enterprise.

Salesmen and life insurance agents, during their spells of euphoria, may do wonderfully well. I remember a man of this type who, in a spell of hypomania, got an idea which was highly remunerative in his business. Later, during a spell of depression he became so neglectful of his work that his employers let him out. I doubt if they or the man's physicians ever thought of him as anything but unusually bright and a bit erratic, but as I drew from him his life-story, it was easy to see that for years he had been up and down as a mild manic-depressive. He saw it then clearly as he had never seen it before.

Another person of this type, when in a euphoric period, is a brilliant conversationalist and a delightful hostess; her brain then teems with ideas, she talks rapidly, she stays up half the night and, to work off energy, she writes books and plays and magazine articles. These contain brilliant passages and vivid imagery, but she can rarely bother to finish them and get them published. Perhaps partly because of this overdoing and lack of rest, she later slumps into a gloomy spell in which for months she hibernates and does little. If, when in a euphoric spell, she is warned not to do so much, she says that she must work fast and get things done while accomplishment is easy, because the time will soon come when it will be difficult for her to do anything.

To show how a person can slip into manic or depressive episodes, Kraines told of a stenographer, previously shy and retiring, who changed and became restless and talkative. Overnight she became a leader in civic work. She looked better than she had ever looked before; she had boundless energy; she never got tired; she stayed up late every night; she became the life of every party, and she became an unusually successful saleswoman. She talked rapidly; she was always vivacious, witty, laughing, and charming. However, after five months of this she began to get argumentative and cantankerous. Her speech became somewhat confused, and she would not finish sentences. She began to telephone people in the middle of the night; she ran up big taxi bills, and she gave big parties which she could not afford. Finally, she got so bad she had to be placed in an institution. Eight months later she was out of the hospital and her normal self again.

Hypomanics are likely to be the "live wires" of their community, but they tend to be erratic and easily diverted into some new line of activity. They love to write long letters to people whose names they have seen in the papers. Some travel and wander about making friends with strangers. A good description of such restless wandering can be found in the autobiography entitled, *Magpie, the Autobiography of a Nymph Errant,* the story of Lois Vidal.

In many cases of a mild manic-depressive insanity there are no definite spells of euphoria. In many cases of recurrent mild depressions one cannot get any story of spells of hypomania. Perhaps this is because on the upswing the patient's mood gets back only to the level that might be considered normal for most persons. In other cases the upswing does not carry the person quite back to normal, and then he or she tends always to be somewhat tired and moody. In other cases the mood of the hypomanic person never seems to drop down even as far as the line of normal for most people. Such persons may always be jittery and on the run.

Manic-depressives go through doctors' offices unrecognized. As Strecker and Palmer have pointed out, doctors' waiting rooms contain many manic-depressives whose real trouble is never even suspected. They do not tell their story well enough so that it is recognized. They talk only of fatigue, lack of pep, toxic feelings, aches and pains, or constipation, gas, and indigestion. Most get studied again and again for some focus of slumbering infection, and many get dosed with thyroid substance, sexual hormones, tonics, and vitamins.

If a psychiatrist were to tell the doctor that one of his patients was mildly psychotic and in need of shock treatments he would probably be incredulous. Every so often I have to tell a doctor that his wife, with all her gas and indigestion, is only a manic-depressive. It never occurred to him before what her basic trouble was, but when I tell him, a light may suddenly break over him.

The symptoms of manic-depressives may be a heavy feeling in the back of the head, a loss of appetite, an inability to concentrate or to work, physical inertia, tremendous fatigue, a tendency to cry, constipation, a loss of sexual interest, insomnia, precordial pain, a mental slowing-up, feelings of vague fear, a loss of interest in loved ones, and a loss of joy in life.

A typical case is that of a woman who, though decidedly manic-depressive, had lived sanely enough so that her banker husband was satisfied with her as a wife. At times he knew that he must not put any social strain on her, but when she was euphoric, she was a lovely hostess to his friends. The physicians who had taken care of her for twenty years had never noticed what was wrong with her, although at times she had been almost paralyzed by gloom, senseless worry, phobias, compulsions, terrible feelings of fatigue, and a desire to end it all with suicide. Interestingly, one of her brothers and her son are mildly manic-depressive.

Apparent causes. The typical depression comes out of what looks like a clear sky, but as one might expect, even hereditary depressions will often follow some strain, unhappiness, sorrow, disappointment, or financial loss.

Rosanoff, Handy, and Plesset examined the causes given for depressions in 1,410 cases and found listed: loss of employment or money, 370 cases; physical illness, 190; disappointment in love, 96; death in the family, 54; pregnancy or childbirth, 53; and alcoholism, 41 cases. Alcoholism is more likely to be the *result* of a depression than the cause. The alcoholic may be a manic-depressive who drinks to drown his suffering during his depressed stages. Strecker and Palmer stated that from 10 to 15 per cent of depressed persons take to the bottle.

Often the important point to note is that the trouble which sent a person into a depression was not such as would have tipped over a man or woman with a good nervous inheritance. He or she could have stood the disappointment or loss without much complaint. The fact, then, that a disappointment in love sent a man into a nervous breakdown lasting a year will suggest that he was by birth mildly manic-depressive. In mild cases, a slight illness such as hay fever may cause a cyclothymic person to feel depressed.

Mean spells. Sometimes a woman with a cyclic temperament, when in a euphoric spell, is so merry, communicative, and friendly that she makes an attractive wife, but, as she says, when she is in one of her "low spells," she is "a devil," and not fit to live with. Then the husband is lucky if he is only ignored; in many cases, no matter how warily he watches his step he soon "catches it." Many a woman of this type will say, "It is lucky for me that my husband is an angel; if he weren't he would have divorced me long ago. When I think how good and kind and patient he is it hurts me to remember how often, for no reason, I have lashed out at him and hurt him terribly." Sometimes one learns that this tendency to ugly spells appeared early in life.

How a depression may begin. It is interesting to read the descriptions some persons have given of their first symptoms when they were slipping into a depression. For instance, a Mr. A. C. Benson wrote in a magazine article that for six months he had been feeling vaguely unwell. He found himself disinclined to any exertion either mental or physical; he was easily depressed or elated; he was at times somnolent and at other times "irritably wakeful." Interestingly, at times the depression would leave him for a few hours and then, as he said, it would "leap upon me like an evil spirit in the middle of some social gathering . . . striking the word from my lips and the smile from my face."

One of the best descriptions of the lethargy that comes to persons as they start into a hereditary type of depression is that of Charles Lamb. He wrote, "Dear B. B.: Do you know what it is to succumb under an insurmountable day-mare—'A whoreson lethargy', Falstaff calls it—an indisposition to do anything, or to be anything; a total deadness and distaste; a suspension of vitality; an indifference to locality; a numb, soporifical good-for-nothingness; an ossification all over; an oyster-like insensibility to the passing events; a mind-stupor; a brawny defiance to the needles of a thrusting-in conscience? Did you ever have a very bad cold, with a total irresolution to submit to water-gruel processes? I have not volition enough left to dot my i's, much less to comb my eyebrows; my eyes are set in my head; my brains are gone out to see a poor relation in Moorfields, and they did not say when they'd come back again."

Spells of diarrhea due to feelings of panic. As I point out in Chapter 15 a high percentage of mildly psychotic persons complain of diarrhea which comes in occasional short attacks lasting perhaps a few hours. These episodes may be hard to explain until one gets the story that they come when the patient gets a bit depressed and perhaps panicky with fear that he is about to lose his mind. In some of these cases the panic brings on only an attack of noisy belching with air-swallowing. In other cases depression, with its slowing of peristalsis, brings constipation.

The diagnosis of a psychosis is easily missed. Henderson said so wisely that the average physician, faced by a mildly psychotic person "unconsciously acts as the patient's accomplice in disguising the real explanation." Even psychiatrists often seem unable to face the fact that a man is psychotic, or they fail to write this diagnosis down in the record. Commonly, all they put down is "anxiety neurosis," or "chronic nervous exhaustion." If they do this, what can they expect of us internists and general practitioners?

Because of everyone's faith in the need for medical overhaulings when one is ill, many a man or woman with mental disease easily recognizable by a psychiatrist is put today through one thorough examination after another and, worse yet, is turned out with a clean bill of health!

To illustrate: For a year a branch manager of a big company had been letting his office run down. On several occasions he had been sent by his superiors to prominent internists for a medical overhauling. Each time he had been "given the works," and each time he had returned with a report that he was in perfect shape. When I saw him I was impressed by a talkativeness, effusiveness, and camaraderie excessive even in the case of a crack salesman. Calling his wife out of the waiting room I asked her if he was always in so exalted a mood, and she said, "Oh, no, he is now in one of his excited spells; in a month or two he'll be depressed and then for weeks he will sit idly in his room, perhaps crying and thinking of suicide." Obviously, he had a short manic-depressive cycle, but always, when among strangers, he had been able to behave well enough so that no one outside of the family circle had suspected what was wrong. From the neck down he was fit enough to pass any laboratory test.

Another time I received a telegram from a physician asking me to look up an unmarried woman of thirty-two who had been operated on for a hernia. Every time I went to the hospital to see her she was out of her room and could not be found. The nurse then said, "You know, she is the most remarkable person; she is so sociable and friendly and talkative that she spends her time visiting all the other patients; I think she must know everyone in the place." When at last I caught up with the woman, I asked her if she was always that active. "No," she said, "soon I'll be in one of my blue spells, and then, for weeks, I won't talk to anyone, not even to Mother." Evidently she had a short manic-depressive cycle, but with never enough antisocial behavior to make a physician suspect what her real trouble was. To me it was interesting that my able young assistant who had worked up her case and the surgeons who had operated on her had not noticed anything wrong with her psychic status. When I questioned her, she admitted that she had always been a bit eccentric, too "screwy" in fact ever to hold a beau long enough to marry him.

Diagnosis. My impression is that in trying to make a diagnosis I can get most help from (1) a history of a cyclothymic personality; (2) a history of previous spells; (3) a family history of psychosis; (4) the history that some depressions came without cause; (5) a history that in a spell "the curtain came down," and (6) a history that the spell was not helped by rest or a vacation.

To show how suddenly the "curtain can come down": A pleasant healthy-looking woman was happy one morning with her children. About 10 A.M., her daughter called the father and said, "Daddy, come quick; Mommy is funny; she won't talk to us." The husband hurried home to find his wife deep in a depression which had come in a moment. Incidentally, when he took her to one of the leading internists in his big city, she was thoroughly examined from head to foot (as if that would do any good) and then she was given a diagnosis of amebiasis! The suddenness and causelessness of the deep depression should have been enough to make the diagnosis, but, in addition, there was the fact that the woman had had three similar spells before. The internist did not seem to even suspect what the disease was. He had never heard of it in college any more than I had.

THE UNHAPPY OR ANHEDONIC PERSON

As William James pointed out, there are persons who get spells of what has been called anhedonia or a distressing feeling of lack of all joy in life. Migrainous persons will sometimes have a joyless day when they feel little contact with the world. Often the person wakes feeling this way, or he will wake feeling all right, and later will suffer perhaps a couple of small annoyances that will hit him, one after the other, with a cumulative effect. Perhaps hours later he will come out of the unhappy state suddenly or slowly. Hamlet said, "How weary, stale, flat, and unprofitable seem to be all the uses of this world."

Some of these persons seem to be suffering from a mild depression, but Myerson thought that it is doubtful if the syndrome is related to a depressive psychosis. The victims usually have no delusions or feelings of guilt; they know that their feelings are illogical, and that their reaction to a little annoyance is excessive. They know, also, that they will come out of the state, and they have no tendency to commit suicide.

Myerson (1946) described a "constitutional anhedonic personality" with prolonged states of unhappiness. As he said, there are thousands of persons who go through life without any enthusiasm or sign of interest. They do not seem to get any joy out of living or working or even succeeding; they do not take joy in rest and sleep and vacationing; they may not find zest even in good eating and drinking, and they find little joy and no ecstasy in sexual intercourse. They may not care much for friends and sociability. They go through life, perfunctorily and stodgily, because it has to be done. I remember the disappointment of a friend when he took his neurotic bride West to see the Grand Canyon, the Bay of San Francisco, Yosemite, and the Sierra Nevada. She could hardly be bothered to look out of the train window. Beauty of scenery gave her no joy.

A fine-looking, husky young fellow recently back from his Army service had spells of two weeks or so when he wasn't particularly depressed; he just "didn't give a damn about anything." Until the mood was gone, even his attractive girl could not give him any pleasure with her body. I could get no history of manic-depressive troubles in the family, and after some months he straightened out.

THE OLD PERSON WHO BECOMES PECULIAR, PERHAPS BECAUSE OF SCLEROSIS IN THE ARTERIES OF THE BRAIN

As everyone knows, a considerable percentage of oldsters become queer, irritable, hard to get along with, childish, or actually psychotic. Many suffer mental deterioration because of cerebral arteriosclerosis, with many thromboses in the small arteries and arterioles of the brain. (See Chapter 12.) Others are suffering from other types of senile atrophy or sclerosis of the brain. Changes in character come, perhaps partly because of the escape of lower brain centers from the control of higher ones.

Fortunately, many physicians and some organizations are now interesting themselves in these mental problems of the aged. They are tremendously disturbing problems to many families, and many a man and woman has had his or her life ruined by the need for caring for a childish, psychotic, domineering, or demanding parent.

THE PERSON WITH A BAD INFERIORITY COMPLEX

As every physician knows, the world is full of persons with an inferiority complex, who suffer from shyness, fear of contact with others, feelings of inadequacy, and fears of not being able to make good. Often it is hard to see why a person feels this way because he or she is well built, has good features, a good presence, and a good brain and education. Perhaps the person has actually made good in the world.

Oftentimes the trouble is inherited from some odd or psychotic forebear, and sometimes it is exaggerated because throughout childhood, some sadistic relative kept hammering home the idea that the person was unattractive and bound to fail in life.

These people are ill at ease in the company of others. Some remain silent. If asked why they say so little, they may say that they cannot think of anything to say. One reason why some young people do not go out with members of the opposite sex is their fear of having to talk. They are so different from those other persons who can chatter by the hour without any effort.

Treatment. Some of these shy persons can be helped much by a physician's words of reassurance or of admiration and approval. Many can be helped by his interest and friendship. I fear, however, that most of them will always suffer somewhat from the feelings of inadequacy and insecurity.

Some few overcompensate in their efforts to free themselves, and then they become belligerent or overly aggressive. They try to beat the other fellow to the draw when usually the other fellow has no idea or intention of being unfriendly or unfair.

THE IRRESPONSIBLE AND THE DODGER OF UNPLEASANT DUTIES

The world is full of men whose main defect seems to be that they will not or cannot live up to any responsibility. They will not face unpleasant tasks, and they are inclined to walk out and disappear whenever the going gets tough. In boyhood they may get sick on graduation day so as to get out of taking part in the program. In the Army, thousands of such men were useless because they would not act like adults in the face of responsibility. If they did not like drill they walked off the parade ground and lay down under a tree; if they felt sleepy on watch they went back to the barracks and turned in. Officers at courts-martial often saw that these men were too childish to be punished severely, so they just sent them home. They shipped them home by the hundreds.

In civil life, also, these irresponsibles are of little use. They feel no concern over their job or of the property or interests of their employer. When they marry they are not much concerned with earning a living, and when the wife gets pregnant or has a baby they desert her and disappear. I remember well the young man whose wife I had to take care of forty-odd years ago. She was living in a mountain cabin where she was having her first baby and was going from one convulsion into another. I told the husband to go quickly into town and bring another doctor out to help me, but all he did was to go on a two-day drunk!

Many a woman has said to me when I suggested that she talk over a marital problem with her husband, "He won't talk; he never faces anything that is difficult; he just walks out and leaves me to do the best I can. His father and his brothers and sisters all have the same gift for dodging anything unpleasant."

I remember a man of this type whose wife died, leaving him with two small children. He married a school teacher who loved the children devotedly, and then he dropped out of sight. That was years ago, and today, unaided and often ill, the woman is still taking care of the children. The world is full of nice-looking, attractive slackers like that man.

Naturally, there are many women of the same type who do not do their housework, and who find a way out of responsibilities, often by getting sick.

THE UNDISCIPLINED MAN

The world is full of persons who are not only irresponsible, but undisciplined. They are constantly getting into trouble because they do as they please without regard for consequences or the hurt that may come to others or, for that matter, to themselves. They are irregular in their habits of eating and sleeping and working. When the family is sitting down to dinner the undisciplined son is likely to decide that he wants a bath or a hair-cut. When others want to go to bed he sits up. If at a bar he finds some interesting story-tellers of his own stripe, he will sit up with them all night, careless of the fact that at home his wife is frantic with anxiety, wondering what has happened to him.

Usually, such a person tends to be immoderate in the use of drugs. He or she is likely to become a chain smoker, or a chain coffee drinker, or a chronic alcoholic. If ever started on the use of any drug such as morphine, he or she will soon become addicted to it.

Much of this behavior is like that of a child who refuses to conform to the many disciplines of life at home or in school. Not only will a man refuse to conform but he may express contempt for the brother who settles down in one place and lives an orderly, disciplined, and respectable life, doing always as Cabell says, "that which is expected of him." The undisciplined person looks upon the disciplined one much as a timber wolf might look on a house dog: The wolf thinks he is the sensible fellow who is living a full life and having all the fun. The undisciplined fails to note that his sprees, his nervous breakdowns and other illnesses, and his aborted and deserted business ventures have cost his responsible and money-saving relatives thousands of dollars. He fails to note, also, that when sick, broke, or in debt he falls back on them for help and money, and perhaps the making-good of bad checks.

The black sheep is likely to forget, also, that often he is unhappy, frustrated, and bitter against society for what he feels are its injustices, its neglect of him, or perhaps its hostility to him. He will resent efforts of his family to guide him into a happier and more successful way of life, and will prefer to remain an Ishmaelite. Only occasionally, as in the case of a Richard Burton or a T. E. Lawrence, will an undisciplined man find a place in which his unusual talents can have great value and his eccentricities can be tolerated. Many such a man becomes successful only in some interesting or dangerous job, especially in a foreign, sparsely settled land, or among primitive peoples. There his courage and recklessness can be useful. Some of these men are decidedly gifted, especially in the arts. Many writers and newspaper men are of this type.

Naturally, when such an undisciplined person takes a wife he is likely soon to desert her because he cannot adjust well to marriage. He could not live happily even with an angel; there is too little consideration for others in his makeup, and too great a desire to live alone and in his own way.

Often I tell these undisciplined persons that, although they think they are free, they are not. Because they cannot or will not learn to get along well with society and make concessions to its mores, society will manage in one way or another to punish them and make them unhappy.

I have seen a number of these undisciplined men who drifted into a serious illness because of their unhygienic ways: their lack of regular hours of work and rest and sleep, and their tendency to yield to their appetite for drugs or food or alcohol until their bodies could no longer stand the strain.

Persons who crave drugs that will give relief from nervousness. There are many of these nervous or mildly psychopathic persons who so crave relief from their nervous tension that they must never be given repeated doses of any derivative of opium, except codeine and papaverine. They must not be given even dilaudid, demerol or methadone. It is too easy for them to get a habit, and once "hooked," as the addict says, they will never be safe again. With the least strain or disappointment or pain they will start trying to get some of the drug that used to keep them comfortable.

The problem of the poorly disciplined man shades over into that of the man with a psychopathic personality whose difficulties I will describe later.

THE POORLY DISCIPLINED WOMAN

There are women, also, who behave in undisciplined ways. Every so often I see a beautiful young woman who is married to her third or fourth husband before the age of twenty-five. She is unhappy and full of nervous troubles; she realizes that she is headed for disaster, but she cannot reform. She goes on smoking two or three packages of cigarettes a day, drinking one cup of coffee after another, and perhaps drinking too many cocktails each evening. She puts no curb on her temper, and she seldom goes to bed before two in the morning. One can imagine what a wreck she is likely to be before she is forty!

At night such a woman may get up and walk around the house, or she may sit up and smoke and listen to the radio. If one tries to get her to take sedatives so as to get better sleep she may either take a fraction of the dose advised, or she may take one pill after another until toward morning she falls asleep. Then she may say that she will no longer take barbiturates because she so dislikes that first uncomfortable stage of excitement through which she has to go before she can reach sleep. Because she is hypersensitive, nonstoical and afraid of many things, she may be loath to try out the medicines the physician wants her to take. Often she reports that the drug made her very uncomfortable, or she says it worked in a way just opposite to the one expected.

The physician may beg the woman to take a rest cure or to stay in bed mornings or to take a nap in the afternoon or to cut down on her activities or her smoking but she goes on as usual. Unfortunately, as she gets more and more tired from lack of sleep and rest, she becomes more sensitive and more subject to pains here and there: pains that may not be helped even by morphine. After months of this the woman may go into a semicomatose state, perhaps partly hysterical in nature, from which she can be rescued only after several days, perhaps after having been given large doses of paraldehyde or chloral by rectum, or sodium amytal intramuscularly. Sometimes rectal suppositories of nembutal (3 grains) will help. Her problem may be complicated by a severe migraine or some psychopathy. In a spell the woman may become a different person, sullen, abusive, or unamenable to reason. Finally, perhaps from sheer exhaustion, she may begin to drowse; she may get some rest, and in a day or two, she may come out of the spell.

Such women commonly have another difficulty and that is, they make little effort to keep up their nutrition. They may smoke so much that they have no appetite, and some drink too much alcohol. Most of them are so finicky as to what they will eat that they tend to live on coffee, a bit of meat, a little salad, and much sugar. Usually there are many foods the woman feels she must not touch, and it is hard to get her to make a study to see if they really are causing her symptoms. Because of semistarvation these women often go down pretty much to skin and bones, and then they stay that way for years.

Sometimes the woman is married to a man she does not love, and one may wonder why she, who was so attractive, married an older man whom she did not care for. Oftentimes one finds that she did it on the rebound from an unhappy affair, or after several men had dropped her because of her temper or her selfishness. Usually one learns that she fell in love with a "gay dog" who either jilted her or married her and soon left her. Whatever the reason, in many a case the woman is highly dissatisfied with her marriage, and this helps to make her even more reckless about her health.

When the physician tries to help such a woman she may say, "What's the use of trying to get better? Why should I make the effort?" He who wants to rehabilitate her has a hard road to go because she seldom does what he asks her to do.

Although most of these women have a charming side, they also have an unpleasant psychopathic side. Even when married to a fine man, they will at times abuse him like a fishwife. A few of the better characters of this sort do too much in the home, and thus wear themselves down. Some lack the ability to do things quickly and easily and without internal or external frictions. Others are too energetic, and in spite of their poor health they run businesses and do much for the community.

In my early days I used to expect these persons soon to go over the edge into a breakdown and a prolonged psychosis, but as years passed I noted that they rarely did this. They might have occasional ugly spells lasting days or perhaps a few weeks, but then they would get a little rested, and with this they would go back to work.

THE PERSON WITH A PSYCHOPATHIC PERSONALITY

The worst of these irresponsible and undisciplined persons have what is called a psychopathic personality. Every so often a physician will get a patient whom he will try hard to help but who will persist in going from one scrape to another. When on his good behavior the man may be attractive, ingratiating, likable, and highly entertaining, but often he is like a mischievous child, and when in a bad humor he may become a cursing, snarling, or drunken devil. Some of these persons are gifted, artistic, and musical, and often the first impression they make is an excellent one. But they take everything done for them as royalty would take gifts from a commoner, without any word or thought of thanks or appreciation.

Many are so debonair and charming that they are taken up and almost adopted by one well-to-do and kindly person after another. These persons take them into their homes and try to put them on their feet, but no real friendship is ever engendered in the protégé, and he shows no feeling of gratitude or devotion. For a while all goes well, but sooner or later there is an explosion of temper. Perhaps the protégé explains afterward, "I just got mad, and then I didn't give a damn what I did." Or, after taking offense at some little thing, he curses the benefactor and stalks out. If asked later why he did this, he will say that those people had it coming to them; they were not sufficiently kind and sympathetic and thoughtful for his comfort. I have seen a woman walk out in this way from the lovely home of her protectors when she hadn't a penny and did not know where her next meal would come from.

Many a man of this psychopathic type forges checks, drinks in sprees, or marries without waiting for a divorce from a previous wife. Hailed into court, he is likely to talk the judge into giving him a suspended sentence. The judge probably senses that the man hasn't the self-control of an adult, and hence cannot be held responsible for the silly things he has done. His crimes are not so much vicious as childish. For instance, when the fellow steals a car he does not try to erase its numbers and sell it; he just drives around town until the police pick him up; or when he forges a check, he does not make any effort to hide or keep out of the hands of the law—he just wanted some money so he reached out and got it.

Occasionally, such a man will do such a silly thing that he is taken to an insane asylum, but in a day or two the superintendent lets him out, perhaps saying, "I wish I had as clever a brain as you have" or "I wish I could play the piano as well as you do."

As Muncie wrote, there are many persons like this who keep their unfortunate families in hot water all of their days. For instance, a man of twenty-four had always been in trouble, stealing, lying, forging, and getting money under false pretenses. He was too unreliable for any work. He was overly critical of everyone, and always representing himself as important and powerful. When some of his skulduggery was exposed he would threaten suicide.

Even as a child he could always get his way by getting around someone. At the age of four he had a wild imagination and would talk for hours. He wet the bed until he was eight. At the age of twelve, he began to forge checks! As a youth he was fanatically religious and was trained for the clergy. But when the time came to take orders he blew up, became hysterical, and was let out. He was usually suave and sociable, but at times impulsive, irritable, secretive, talkative, imaginative, untrustworthy in his versions of things, and subject to short-lived swings in mood.

I think it highly significant that the man had a poor nervous heredity. His father was a spree drinker, seclusive, and hot tempered. The mother was a worrier; the maternal grandfather was aggressive, hot tempered, and a heavy drinker. One of the patient's brothers was alcoholic. This fellow may not have been "insane," but obviously, he was anything but sensible and sane.

The homes of this country are full of men and women of this kind, not psychotic enough to be locked up, and yet too abnormal ever to work consecutively at anything, and too childish and amoral ever to get along peacefully with society. When they break down nervously or physically one cannot put them into an ordinary hospital because they will not conform to the rules, and they are likely to clash with the superintendent and the nurses. One cannot put them in an insane asylum because they are not bad enough for that. And yet, when they keep going on awful sprees, forging checks, and running up big bills, the family can hardly leave them at large. Society much needs to devise some sane way of handling this terrible problem.

Years ago Goddard described these persons in a monograph entitled, very properly, *The Feebly Inhibited*. As he said, they always do what they please, never thinking of the cost of their escapades to them or anyone else. When asked why they did some foolish, lawless thing, their answer is always that of a child, "I wanted to," or "I felt like it."

Nielsen and Thompson have well described this type of person as he is met with commonly by the psychiatrists who, in certain states, are now advising police courts. As these writers said, it is useless to put the psychopath in jail because as soon as he is released he gets into silly mischief again. It is no use trying to rehabilitate him because he does not show the slightest appreciation of the efforts made in his behalf, and he does not stay rehabilitated. He will not do well in a job because of this unreliability and his conviction that he should be put immediately into a managerial position. He cannot settle down to any routine. He cannot stay married because of his complete selfishness, his many escapades, and his inability to earn a steady living. Apparently he seldom goes over into the ranks of the certifiable insane. He may be homosexual. In childhood he may have been difficult or incorrigible, and he may have spent his boyhood in reform schools.

Some of these people are kleptomaniacs, tramps, panhandlers, and narcotic peddlers. Some are eccentrics, cranks, and inventors of impractical gadgets. They usually are shameless braggarts and tellers of tall tales. Some love to pose as noblemen or army heroes. They are full of schemes, and if they lay their hands on any money they promptly blow it in.

Some women of this type may drift into high-class prostitution; a few, because of an exotic beauty, marry one wealthy man after another. Most of these women have bad tempers and are explosive, violent, occasionally alcoholic, and easily addicted to drugs. One minute such a woman will be entertaining and charming and the next she may be cursing like a fiend.

Most of these persons are overly touchy, and much inclined to look down on their fellows, and even on their battered relatives who pay their bills. I remember one gifted artist who "borrowed" several thousand dollars from a kindly friend who lent without any great expectation of getting his money back. He just wanted to get his gifted friend well established in a little business. But the artist kept coming back for more money, until finally the benefactor had to refuse to "lend" any more; as he said, he could not afford it. Whereupon the artist told me that his old friend was a heartless scoundrel who did not deserve to be repaid and hence would not be!

Some of these psychopaths have sense enough to see at times what a mess they have made of a life which, with their artistic gifts, could have been so successful. When this vision comes to them, they brood and perhaps get themselves sodden with drugs or drink. Usually they turn against society and curse the people whom they hold responsible for their troubles and their failures. They then are easily taken in by Communism or Fascism or some other scheme for changing the rules of life. Some are useful to a dictator because of their cleverness, their ability to write and talk, their love of power, their ruthlessness, and their complete lack of conscience.

A remarkable pen-picture of one of these likable scamps is in Wodehouse's series of stories about that master sponger, Stanley Featherstonehaugh Ukridge. Every physician and psychiatrist who wants to spend a few delightful and instructive hours should read these tales. The best clinical pictures of these people are to be found in Cleckley's *The Mask of Sanity*.

As I have said, these persons never express regret or sorrow over all the pain their indiscretions or thoughtless cruelties have caused others, especially those who love them. They are too self-centered, too full of self-justification, and too inclined to blame others for not being kind enough. Years ago, before I learned my lesson, I used to spend hours trying to save and rehabilitate some of these persons, and to get them straightened out and self-supporting and well. But they never stayed rehabilitated, and, in the end, all of them went away without a word of thanks.

Treatment. The wise physician will keep away from these persons because they can only cause him endless trouble. The experience of all psychiatrists with these people appears to have been bad. They do not care to change their ways; they do not think they are in the wrong; and if by some chance one of them should decide to reform he would forget all about it before the day was out. Typical is the story of one of these men who appeased a judge by promising him he would go straight and then paid his fine with a worthless check! That experience well sums up the situation as regards these people.

THE ALCOHOLIC

As everyone knows, much neurosis in American men and women is associated with the excessive use of alcohol. Obviously, any man or

woman who, every so often, gets drunk or goes on a spree cannot be
a satisfactory worker or spouse or parent, and if the habit is kept up,
he or she is likely to come to grief.

Often, if the physician is to make the correct diagnosis, he must
recognize the alcoholic facies because the person will fail to mention his
sins. Often one can recognize the reddish soft skin, the bleary eyes,
the trembling muscles, the appearance of dissipation, the loss of refinement, and either a certain coarse and bloated appearance or a gay-dog
look. Often the mouth is full of carious teeth. Perhaps the physician
will get a whiff of a tell-tale breath. I must confess I find it harder to
recognize the signs of alcoholism in women, and many a one has fooled
me.

Obviously, a tremendous amount of human wreckage in this country
is produced by alcohol. There are men and women who drink too much
every day, and there are others who drink only in sprees. They are the
dipsomaniacs. The heavy drinker or the dipsomaniac must probably be
born with the tendency. I have been impressed with the way in which
alcoholism runs through certain families (see Chapters 4 and 15). According to J. H. Wall and D. B. Allen, 30 per cent of the fathers of the
alcoholics they studied were alcoholic, and according to La Mare and
his associates, alcoholism appeared four times as often in the families
of alcoholics as it did in the families of normal men.

My studies of hundreds of families in which there is much psychopathy has convinced me, as others have been convinced, that chronic
alcoholism is an equivalent or a result of psychosis. Certainly, in my
experience, the descendants of alcoholics suffer from neuroses and
minor psychoses much as if the ancestor had been psychotic. I am not
inferring that the alcohol imbibed by the ancestor affected his germ
plasm; what I infer is that the ancestor drank because at times he felt
depressed and wanted relief from mental suffering.

The physician who would like to know why men drink themselves
out of everything that might make life happy and worth living should
read books like Maine's, *If a Man Be Mad;* Seabrook's, *No Hiding
Place,* or *Asylum;* or the volumes called *Behind the Door of Delusion,*
North 3-1: *Pick Up the Pieces,* or Charles Roman's *Man Remade.* Particularly in Maine's book one can see how psychopathic, inadequate,
insecure, and unhappy the alcoholic is, and how at times he drinks to
drown his sorrows, to make him forget what a failure he is, or to free
his inhibitions so that he can talk to his fellows in a barroom and can
become one of them.

Alcoholism must always be based on some serious defect in character
because no sane man would ever persist in ruining himself, his wife,
his children, and his business for a drug that makes him ill. As Maine

and Seabrook showed, even the love of a fine woman will not rest⌐ man in the slightest when he feels the call of the bottle.

The treatment of alcoholism will be discussed in Chapter 28.

THE HYPOCHONDRIAC

A hypochondriac has been defined as a psychopathic worrier who concentrates his attention for years on one organ which he is sure is terribly diseased. One cannot shake him in this view, no matter how much reassuring evidence one gathers. Talking to a man of this type, who for years had been sure he had a cancer of his stomach, I asked him if he would be reassured if I were to open his abdomen under local anesthesia and show him that the suspected viscus was normal. He said he wouldn't be reassured even with that! I told him then that I saw no sense in examining him further. He had given up a large business to spend all of his time getting his stomach roentgenographed. He had never married because he wanted to devote all his attention to saving his health.

Occasionally, after many years, a man like this will shift his fears from the stomach to the heart or to the colon. Many of those patients who fear intestinal autointoxication all their days are colonocentric hypochondriacs. My impression about these persons is that they are suffering from a mild psychosis. As Purves Stewart and others have pointed out, it is generally useless to try to cheer them; and it is useless to operate on them as some physicians do, and then to tell them that the supposed disease was found and removed. On waking from the anesthetic they still feel their old anxiety and discomfort. Ross agreed that these people are incurable. He thought that we physicians should give them some kindly attention if only so that they will not be so likely to fall into the hands of the quacks who stand ready to fleece them.

In respect to matters outside of health, these persons are often shrewd, intelligent, and sensible. A few of the wealthiest men I have known were unhappy hypochondriacs. Some, like the publishers of body-building magazines or manufacturers of "health foods" or patent medicines, have cashed in wonderfully on their intimate knowledge of the fears, beliefs, hopes, and desires of their fellow hypochondriacs. They knew how to write advertising copy that would appeal to them.

I must admit that I cannot stand wasting effort on many of these people. They take so much time, and it is almost certainly wasted.

THE PARANOID OR SUSPICIOUS PERSON

Paranoid persons are suspicious and inclined to believe that many things are being done by others just to annoy them. They think people have it in for them, or are talking about them, or would like to injure them. A paranoid man may say that when he sits down in a movie theater people around him get up and go out. "They do not like him." Because of his feeling that his neighbors are scheming against him or influencing his thoughts with the help of electric rays, he is likely to start lawsuits to protect himself or to strike back. Rarely, a physician will be consulted by a husband or a wife who wants help in avoiding the spouse's supposed attempts at administering poison.

The true paranoiac can be a dangerous man, and occasionally he gets so exasperated at his supposed "persecutors" that on the street he shoots and kills some innocent person. A good story is that of an able chemist in a big drug house who, one day, asked to see the head of the company. The president said, "Yes, send him in, I want to tell him I am promoting him to be head of a new section." But when the chemist came in he said to the president, "See here, I've had enough of your malicious mischief. You stop changing the labels on my bottles or I'll put a bullet between your eyes!"

A patient of mine, a sensible-looking man, once told me that he was constantly being hounded by the "Gehockers," a society of persons organized all over the United States to annoy him. These people followed him, and, standing behind him, would hawk phlegm noisily out of their throats! He said, "You know, the other day in New York one of them did it to me on a Fifth Avenue bus and I had all I could do to keep from turning around and shooting him through the head. If I had, he'd have had it coming to him!" Obviously, this sort of thing accounts for a number of strange murders.

THE SOLITARY PERSON WHO WANTS TO LIVE ALONE AND BE LEFT ALONE

I remember once reading in a brochure on Estes Park that in the early eighteen hundreds a man and his family lived there, but when someone moved in about forty miles east of him, the place "became too crowded" and he had to move west! I once asked an intelligent man why he lived alone on a desert ranch, without a wife or even a hired man. He said, "It is wonderful to be alone; there is no one then to bother me." Several of my patients with the same desire for peace each bought a little island in a lonely lake. When I was a boy in Hawaii there were on each island a number of Americans or Englishmen who lived alone in mountain shacks and seldom said a word to anyone. Even in a big city one can find any number of recluses who live alone in dingy rooms.

Naturally, such men are likely to be a bit odd and impatient with their fellows who, as they say, bother them. Some want to avoid the responsibilities, adjustments, conflicts, and restrictions of civilization, and the demands that society makes. Some hate women and want to get far away from them. Some probably have had an unhappy experience in life and want to run away and hide. I remember once meeting a big handsome man who was living alone in a shack in a dank gloomy forest in the West, miles from even a small settlement. One of my companions recognized him as a captain in the First World War who had gotten a beautiful, merry nurse into trouble. After a criminal abortion she died, and the man, perhaps by way of penance, buried himself alive.

THE RIGID PERSON

Every so often, when one talks to the relatives of a person who is having nervous and psychic difficulties, one finds that he is much too rigid for his own comfort or the comfort of those about him. Many a woman has told me of her difficulties with a husband who was fussier about the house and his belongings than any old maid could ever be. If the wife did not keep everything exactly as he wanted it he fussed and told her that if she really loved him she would grant him his desires and save him from annoyance. I knew a man who held a strict military inspection every evening when he came home! His wife and children lived in daily dread of these sessions. Another man, who in his early days had been a sea captain, ran his home and his children just as tyrannically as he had run his ship and his sailors.

Persons of this type are usually rigid in their religion. They force everyone in the family to go to church several times on Sunday. Many of these men are such tyrants in their homes that the children run away as soon as they can.

Women, of course, can also be very rigid, and many a matriarch is a tyrant in her home and perhaps in the homes of her children. I remember a woman who told me she traveled around from one to the other of the homes of her five married daughters, and in each house "soon put everything to rights." No one dared have a fight to a finish with her. To me the significant point is that among the forebears and descendants of a rigid person one is likely to find psychotics.

Treatment. The rigid person cannot easily be helped, if he can be helped at all. He prefers to stay as he is. He thinks his way of life is the best. The only argument that I have ever found helpful is that he ought to take note of what he is paying for his hobby in the way of loss of love of wife and children. He may be getting what he wants, but, Oh! at what a price!

THE ASCETIC AND THE OVERLY RELIGIOUS PERSON

Today one finds ascetic persons who, if they had lived in the middle ages, would have become hermits. Even today such persons sometimes withdraw from the world. The psychology of some of them is well presented by Thomas Merton, in his book, *The Seven Storey Mountain*. There he tells of the mental processes which led to his becoming a Trappist monk. (See also *I Leap Over the Wall* by Monica Baldwin.)

Many men and women who are overly religious live on the fringes of sanity. I remember a broken-down sad-looking, but fine young minister who thought that one night Christ had appeared before him. As he said, the vision might well have been a hallucination due to illness; he could not be sure. He rather doubted if the experience had been real because it had not lifted him up or made him a better preacher. In fact, he was so much worse after the vision that he could no longer compose a sermon. A psychiatrist who saw him feared that he was on the edges of schizophrenia.

Overly religious persons are usually rigid in their thinking; they may feel that they and God know what is best for everyone, and some are sorry that God is not as strict and severe as He should be with many people. Often such persons are pretty rough on their unfortunate children and think they should enjoy going to church several times each Sunday. Some torture their poor youngsters by insisting that they stand out as nonconformists in the community. The children must not attend even the school movies; they must not salute the flag; they must not drill, and the girls must not dress as the others do.

An excellent book to read in order to understand the behavior of these people is Hannah Smith's *For Heaven's Sake*. In this volume the author tells of her years of suffering and humiliation when, as a child, she had to be different from the other girls in school. Her father wanted her to be as a light before the other children. They only looked on her as a "nut."

Another remarkable and tragic picture of the sufferings a child has to go through, especially on Sundays, when born to an overly religious parent, is to be found in Edmund Gosse's book, *Father and Son* (1907). One sees there the picture of a man able enough to write charming books on natural history, but childish enough to spend hours on his knees, wrestling in prayer with God to get His advice as to whether his little motherless boy should go to a children's party in the neighborhood. The father thought that in some way such a party must be sinful. He wanted to bring up the lad to become another Messiah. Finally, the boy, unable any longer to stand the persecution, had to break with his father and leave him.

Another most enlightening book on the psychology of the deeply religious and the many saints of the church is William James' *Varieties of Religious Experience*. In this volume he quoted much from the writings of the saints to show that the main characteristic of most of them was their dislike of this life and their wish to escape from it. They got absolutely no pleasure from living, and hence they spent all of their time planning for the next world, in which they were so sure they would be perfectly happy, always praising God. As James said, it is obvious from their writings that these men and women were different from the rest of us.

THE PERSON WITH UNRECOGNIZED ENCEPHALITIS

Several times a year I see persons who are referred because of indigestion or a nervous breakdown or a supposed peptic ulcer, and soon I draw out a story of a previously unrecognized mild attack of encephalitis. My hunch is that with time we physicians will come to see that quite a few nervous breakdowns are due to a mild form of encephalitis which did not leave a typical Parkinsonian syndrome. It may be, also, that in some cases in which the nervous system was hereditarily subnormal an encephalitic virus was able to produce more incapacity than it could have produced in a strong healthy person.

A similar phenomenon is seen in cases of syphilitic infection. If syphilis is left untreated in, let us say, a nervously stable or insensitive man, it may injure only his aorta, but if spirochetes are left for years in the body of an eccentric intellectual, they are likely to produce in him a general paresis.

I am sure that today there is much encephalitis being missed, even by good consultants. One will surely miss it if one does not get a history, first, of a nervous breakdown and, second, of a fairly typical acute spell at the start of the trouble.

THE MENTAL DISTURBANCES OF THE PERSON WITH A TUMOR OF THE BRAIN

A tumor of the brain may show itself first through alterations in personality. The patient may do strange things that puzzle his family. He may keep his hat on in the house or urinate on the floor. At times the patient may clown and may keep wise-cracking, and later he may become apathetic, depressed, mentally deteriorated, or disorientated in space, with some failure of vision, or with headache, loss of memory, aphasia, ataxia, or sudden vomiting.

As soon as curious alterations in personality show up the patient should be put in the hands of a neurologist. I tell elsewhere in this book of a minister who was brought in by his head deacon simply because he had been coming late to church and making mistakes in his ritual. Once he started to marry a couple with the baptismal service! The deacon was right; something was seriously wrong, and on examination a brain tumor was found.

An interesting story written by a newspaperman who suffered from a brain tumor is that of Frigyes Karinthy; it is called *A Journey Round My Skull* (1939).

THE PERSON WITH A DUAL PERSONALITY

Some of the men and women cursed with moody spells may complain of a somewhat dual personality. They may have a fine, lovely, and idealistic half which has to keep struggling to hold in subjection an unpleasant, mean, hard, and evil-tempered half. More than one such person has said to me, "How I hate and despise this other person who lives in my body with me!" One beautiful woman, about to divorce her fourth husband by the age of twenty-five, said feelingly that she would give anything to be either saint or devil; she didn't care which, just so long as she could get rid of the eternal conflict between the two persons within her. That was what was wearing her out. Half the time she was good and religious, like her aristocratic, church-loving English father, and the rest of the time harum-scarum, violent, and stormy-tempered like her Irish mother. She had never been able to fuse these two discordant components of her character.

He is a fortunate man whose parents are enough alike in their temperaments so that he does not have two warring factions within him.

THE PSYCHIC PROBLEMS OF THE STUTTERER

Stuttering is found commonly in persons who have a poor nervous inheritance. Berry stated that the trouble is hereditary in at least 65 per cent of the cases. He might have added that in many of the near relatives the nervous defect shows up not as a stuttering but as a mild psychosis, alcoholism, a bad tic, or a great nervousness.

Speech is dependent on such a highly complex mechanism that it can easily be disturbed by nervous tension and self-consciousness. One finds defects in speech, also, in persons who are clumsy, whose muscles are all under poor control. Berry found, on studying 500 stuttering children and comparing them with 500 normal children, that the stutterers were retarded in acquiring motor skills. They were slow to learn to walk. James S. Greene and S. M. Small (1944), who have had an enormous experience in the field of speech defects, also noted that the stutterer is usually an awkward person whose motor integrations are not good. They speak of a stutter-type of person. Such a child often suffers from nightmares; he wets the bed late, bites his nails, and shows other symptoms of inborn nervousness. He is often asocial, shy, and seclusive. While trying to talk, his palms may become cold and wet. He may have difficulty in meeting people, and when he has to shake hands his heart may pound, he may feel tight around his neck, and he may have a sinking or empty feeling in his stomach.

Some 25 per cent of stutterers were found to have an abnormal electroencephalogram. One would expect from this that some of them are relatives of the epileptic. Some are emotionally immature. Some remember that when their trouble started in childhood they had been frightened or made to feel insecure and apprehensive.

According to Wendell Johnson, stuttering children have an average mental development, and are not retarded in the development of speech, walking, or teething. Johnson doubts if right- or left-handedness has anything to do with the trouble. From the time of Aristotle onward, the defect was thought to be due to some abnormality in the frenum of the tongue, but today we know this is not true.

The stutterer is too much concerned with what others are thinking of him. His real problem is not the ability to talk—he can do that; his trouble is that he is afraid he will not speak fluently, and that he will not measure up properly to what the world expects of him.

Stutterers usually are able to talk without difficulty when alone, with sibs, other stutterers, or a dog. They can sing without difficulty. They are more likely to stutter when talking to a stranger and on a subject that disturbs or distresses them. Greene believed that stuttering usually points to some defect in personality and some difficulty in adjustment.

Wendell Johnson believes that much stuttering starts as an effort of the child to hold the center of the stage when he has nothing to say. Certainly all of us have seen spoiled or only children doing this, especially when company was present. Johnson thinks that this practice would not go on to stuttering if the parents would not become alarmed over it, but would just say quietly, "Junior, wait until you know what you want to say, and then we will listen to you."

Johnson thinks, also, that the beginning of some stuttering is only the hesitation and repetition commonly seen in the speech of normal children. Everyone knows that young children love to repeat syllables and to say things like "pinky panky poo," or "hickory dickory dock," or "by the hair on his chinny chin chin." From 15 to 25 per cent of their words figure in some such repetition. Similarly, primitive peoples commonly use double words like "hana-hana" or "wiki-wiki." Such doubling of syllables comes naturally, then, to children, and from this the transition to stuttering is possible. Because children have trouble learning to form sentences their speech is not fluent. They stop to "er" and "uh," and they do this more whenever they are in a hurry or when they feel embarrassed or when they are being scolded or disapproved of.

It is said that such children might not become stutterers if they were not labeled as such—if they were told repeatedly that it is normal to speak nonfluently; that most persons repeat words, fail to finish many sentences, and hem and haw. Even public speakers do this sort of thing, and often a man's mind and his speech mechanism seem to get separated and out of phase. One trouble with the stutterer is that he thinks he should be as fluent as a radio announcer on a give-away program. When he finds he is not, he gets panicky, and starts trying to force out his words. He should be encouraged to speak nonfluently and to accept this as natural and commonplace.

Johnson says one should never praise a stutterer for not stuttering, but only *for speaking nonfluently without concern*. The more worried the parents become over the child's speech the worse he will stutter. Johnson suspects that often the stuttering child's worst trouble is that his parents are perfectionists who complain about many things he does. Sometimes one or both parents are a bit violent or unpredictable or choleric or hard to live with. Nothing, then, can be done for the child until his people can be helped by a good psychiatrist. The child cannot get self-control until his parents do, and until they learn to maintain a happy home in which there always is peace without tension. As Berry said, especially at the start of treatment, the psychiatrist must treat the parents more than he does the child. Discipline for the child should be firm but not harsh. Evenings should be quiet so that sleep will be good.

Treatment. There are several theories of treatment and with any one of them most experts can help or cure many of their patients. Greene stated that it is important to get the stutterer into expert hands quickly before the habit is well established.

According to Berry, the child should be encouraged to talk both at home and at school, but never forced to do so. He should never be ridiculed or embarrassed or punished for stuttering. He should never be made to feel different from other children or an object of pity. He should be told often of the love his parents feel for him, and he should be made to feel that his place in the home is secure.

It often helps the stutterer to dress him well so as to bolster his ego. It improves his self-esteem and confidence. The stutterer must try to relax his tension. He should talk slowly and, so far as possible, without effort. Some of the patients take a deep breath every so often, with the hope of relaxing.

In speech clinics the patient is made to study his own voice as it comes back to him out of a recorder. He is also made to practice talking before a mirror, and he is urged to talk freely to others about his difficulty. So long as he tries to run a bluff that he never stutters he cannot get well. He should practice talking with a number of other stutterers who will try to help him just as he will try to help them. One of the most thrilling experiences of my life came one evening as I sat with Dr. Greene in a hall in his college in New York, listening to the speeches made by ex-stutterers at a meeting of their club. There, one ex-stutterer after another got up and made a remarkably good short talk.

Interestingly, at the Speech Clinic of the University of Minnesota, the major problem is not stuttering. Where most of their patients need help is in overcoming the tendency to make a "th" sound for an "s," or a "w" sound for an "i." Help has to be given, also, to the foreign-born who often have great difficulty with some of the sounds used in English. Thus, it is a good Swede who eventually learns to say "just" and not "yust."

THE SORROWS OF THE HOMOSEXUAL MAN

According to Kinsey and his associates, among the young unmarried males he questioned, 27.3 per cent had had homesexual activity to the point of orgasm. This certainly is an astounding figure. Among married males from the ages of twenty to forty-five years, less than 1 per cent of the total "outlet" was homosexual in character.

The homosexual is likely to be neurotic and unhappy, if only because Nature has played him a miserable trick; it has deprived him of so much that can give happiness and purpose to life. To him marriage and a home are often out of the question. He may not be able to stand even just living in the same house with a wife, with no physical intimacy. Every physician should read the autobiography called *Monsieur Montcairn,* or Norman Hall's poignant story, *Death on an Atoll* (Atlantic Monthly, March, 1931), in order to realize what an awful shock it can be for a young man one day to discover that he is not made as other men are, and that love for a woman will probably never be possible for him.

Every physician and psychiatrist should read the fine study of male and female homosexuals by George W. Henry and others (1941). This book shows that the defect is found usually in persons of more than average intelligence and artistic ability, who have had a number of odd forebears and sibs.

A good example of the sort of heredity some bisexual males have is given on page 42, of Volume I of Henry's work, where it will be seen that a certain man's several uncles and aunts and sibs had to be classified as "bisexual, epileptic, impotent, frigid, musical, neurotic, drug addicts, psychotic, psychopathic, alcoholic, and promiscuous." Another enlightening pedigree is to be found on page 844 of Volume II. There one learns that a homosexual woman described her paternal grandfather as a tyrant. One of his sons was avaricious, and another son and a daughter were overly religious. The maternal grandmother was so strict that her children could not stand her. Late in life she had delusions. This woman had one son who was a mean drunkard. A daughter was a selfish, narcissistic person who lived only to be admired.

Another daughter was headstrong and a nagger. The daughter who bore the homosexual girl whose case was being studied was obviously schizoid. In spite of homosexual leanings she married and bore nine children, *none of whom married!* One of these, a boy, had a vile temper and was sadistic and childish. Another boy was epileptic and eccentric and choleric, another was a cold-blooded miser, and another was overly religious and trained to be a monk. One of the girls was also overly religious and wanted to be a nun.

It seems obvious from these family histories that there is much psychopathy in the forebears of homosexuals. With so much poor nervous heredity, one would expect the variation in the person's character to be far more inborn than developed. Actually the abnormality often is recognizable early in life, when a little girl wants to play only as a boy and to dress as a boy, and when a boy wants to sew and play like a girl, or wants to dress as a girl.

A sympathetic write-up of the problems of the homosexual male is to be found in the book entitled *The Invert and His Social Adjustment, by Anomaly*. It tells of the unhappy problems of the invert and what he had best do about them. Interesting is homosexualism as it is discussed and classified in the language of the underworld. An analysis of this subject was made by Dr. Samuel Kahn, psychiatrist to several New York prisons. He published a number of ardent love letters which passed between homosexual prisoners. He also noted that most homosexuals come of families in which there is much psychopathy. He told (p. 126) of a homosexual woman who said, "When you are young you do not care, but when you are older, you want to be normal but you can't."

Louis H. Loeser (1945) described 270 homosexuals found in the armed forces. They were all highly intelligent. Some 40 per cent came of families in which there was psychosis, alcoholism, and neurosis. About a third were neurotic, and about a third drank to excess. Only some 40 per cent had a feminine appearance and temperament. Some homosexual men are big, strong, and finely built.

Rosenzweig and Hoskins (1941) described a homosexual Negro whom they treated for a while. He was an effeminate person who loved to design women's clothes. He was a short, stocky man who except for his large masculine genitalia was in every respect a woman. He showed an exaggerated female gait and speech and had all the mannerisms of the clinging-vine type of woman. With men he was coy, silly, and affected, but with women he talked like one woman to another. Because of some peculiarities of behavior he was placed for a while in the Worcester State Hospital for the mentally deranged.

No one should hazard an opinion on homosexualism until he has read a number of the studies made of these people and has read some of the autobiographies they have written. No physician who hopes to be worthy of the name of scientist should approach the study of this subject with prejudice, preconceptions, disgust, or a desire to blame or punish. The physician who thinks that these persons are debauchees and criminals who should be put in jail should go into kindergartens and grade schools and there study the boys who want to be girls and the girls who want to be boys. As I said, the pattern of what a person's life-behavior is to be is often obvious in the nursery, *when no possible blame can be attached to the individual.* I often think of the situation as one in which a wicked elf went into the infant's room of a hospital and, while no one was looking, switched the genitalia from boys to girls and vice versa. As a result, here is a boy with a vulva and vagina, and there a girl with a penis and testicles.

Naturally, it is not all so simple as this because sex is a quantitative thing ranging through several grades, from that of the man or woman who must have intercourse three times a day to that of the man or woman who never wants it. There are also all grades of homosexualism in men and women, with different grades of abnormality of body.

As G. Legman showed in his chapter in Henry's second volume, the underworld has names for homosexuals of the several types, with the several tendencies and idiosyncrasies. In the cases of both men and women, some individuals tend to be aggressive while some like to be submissive. Some, who are called "white-livers," are completely indifferent to persons of the opposite sex, while others called "queer birds," are at times heterosexual. There are "papas" or "daddys" and "mamas" or "wives," and there are "one-way" or "two-way" or "double life" men. A "bull-dike" or a "horse-woman" is a very mannish Lesbian; a "girl" is a very effeminate man, and a "person-on-the-fence" hasn't yet "discovered his gender." There are "triangles" in which a male homosexual and a Lesbian live with a Lesbian whom the two love.

Treatment. Because of the poor heredity, and sometimes the decidedly feminine appearance and behavior and walk of homosexual men, and the decidedly masculine appearance and dress and walk of homosexual women, one would never expect any amount of psychotherapy or anything else to change these people. *One might as well try to talk a normal heterosexual person into being a homosexual.* Doubtless in many cases the pattern of a homosexual's brain is just as abnormal as is the pattern of his body. We physicians cannot change the pattern of the body, so why should we think that we can change the pattern of the brain?

As one would expect, the giving of male hormone in huge amounts to a homosexual man does not change his behavior in the slightest

(Rosenzweig and Hoskins, 1941). The trouble is apparently in the brain and not in the glands.

It is a disgrace to society and civilization that these unfortunate and much-to-be-pitied men are often blackmailed, and hounded by the police. Curiously, their homosexual sisters, many of whom live together for years like man and wife, are not bothered.

The man who wrote *The Invert* said (p. 99), "Having witnessed numerous attempts on the part of well-intentioned inverts to find happiness in an attachment, the sacred permanence of which was to be assured by a setting of approximate domesticity, I am forced, regretfully, to the conclusion that the idea is impracticable. The prospect of success is remote." Kahn and others have also testified to the folly of advising these persons to try marriage. I have talked to a number of them who had tried it and soon had had to give it up. Some could not stand it for more than a day or two even when they liked the spouse a good deal. Some, however, were able to stick it out for several years.

THE SORROWS OF THE HOMOSEXUAL WOMAN

A considerable percentage of women are more or less homosexual. Many, when young, have marked "crushes" on older women, but gradually they escape from this minor form of homosexualism. Many become sufficiently ambivalent to marry and to be happy or reasonably happy with a husband. The physician will see many married women who are obviously somewhat homosexual in their makeup. Many a one marries a small mild man who perhaps likes to be mothered. A decidedly eunuchoid minister who had never shaved told me that he had had many proposals of marriage from such women, some of whom apparently wanted marriage and a home but no "annoyance" from the husband. They evidently thought he would make the sort of husband who would not trouble them.

Homosexual women appear to be less promiscuous in their amours than are men. They share with their heterosexual sisters a desire for deep love and affection in a lasting union. The male homosexual, like many male heterosexuals, often prefers a great variety of experience, and hence he resorts regularly to male prostitutes. The male is more interested in physical sex while the woman is more desirous of tenderness and friendship.

The best way in which to get an understanding of the psychology and sufferings of these persons is to read some of the fine autobiographies they have written. The two best that I have found are *The Stone Wall,* by Mary Casals, and *Diana,* by Diana Frederics. Another is called *The Scorpion.* In these books one gets a vivid picture of the feelings of frustration, unhappiness, great jealousy, and despair when one union after another breaks up. The homosexual woman is more handicapped in "marriage" than is her heterosexual sister, because she is likely at any time to lose her "wife" not only to another woman but perhaps to a moderately homosexual man. The "wife" may prefer marriage with a man, granting that she can stand the intimacy.

The physician is usually afraid to discuss with a homosexual person his or her difficulties and strains, and perhaps this is just as well, because if he cannot talk about the subject with sympathy and understanding and freedom from any tendency to recoil or blame, he had better leave it alone. I doubt very much if a psychiatrist can ever cure a born homosexual; about all he can do is to supply an outlet for mental catharsis. He can bolster self-respect and, if he knows enough about the subject, he can give the victim a better understanding of it than he or she may ever have been able to get before. No one should ever think of reviling anyone for being homosexual, any more than one should think of reviling a person for being psychotic or impotent or castrated. No one should attempt to treat homosexualism until he has read at least the few books I have mentioned here.

Every physician ought to be able to recognize at a glance a considerable percentage of homosexuals. Curiously, many women love to flaunt their peculiarity by affecting mannish ways and dress. They get a man's hair-cut, they wear mannish clothes, and they have a man's strong stride. Probably many a doctor fails to recognize the borderline cases because the subject of homosexualism was never even mentioned to him in medical school. It is curious that we physicians can be so prudish and prissy as to refuse to study or even mention sex in men and women. I have even had a medical editor refuse to let me mention homosexualism in an article on neuroses! He said he was proud that the word had never been mentioned in any publication of his house! I remember a fine homosexual woman of fifty who told me of her life-long loneliness and suffering because of her defect. One day she tried to talk of her problem to one of America's leading internists, but all she got was a tongue-lashing!

Treatment.   Sometimes the worst thing a physician can do to a strongly homosexual woman is to tell her to marry and try to adjust to heterosexual intercourse. She may be just as unable to stand sexual intercourse with a man as the doctor would be. In Henry's book there are statements from women who, in a desperate attempt to become normally heterosexual, forced themselves to attempt intercourse with men. The result was only disgust and nausea. I remember a number of such women who told me that after marrying, they soon had to leave the husband. They were fond of the mild little man, but they could not stand even living in the same house with him.

THE PERSON WHO THINKS HE SMELLS BAD

There is a type of elderly woman, usually single, who goes to a gastro-enterologist complaining that she smells so bad that people in a movie theater get up and go out when she comes in. She goes to a stomach specialist because she thinks her feces are smelling so terribly that the odor is going through her body and into her clothes.

I have seen a number of these persons, all of whom were almost certainly psychotic, but who were so well behaved in my office that I could not prove anything against them. Unfortunately, all of them came in alone, and so I could not learn anything from relatives or friends. I could not learn of any other hallucinations. In one case I suspected that the patient was smelling her own crusted nose which had a considerable odor to it, but she was probably psychotic in addition. In no case could I or my assistants or nurses ever smell anything wrong.

One woman, a bookkeeper, was so convinced that the books she had worked on for years had picked up her bad odor that she took her savings and hired someone to copy all the old records onto clean paper. I put her in a hospital room for a few days and nurses, interns, and all who came in were instructed to watch for an unpleasant odor. No one ever smelled anything unusual. As I feared, this did not reassure the woman in the least; she thought we were all lying to please her.

Rogerson (1939) wrote of a farmer with this syndrome who appeared at first to be mentally normal, but who later was found to be psychotic. Davidson (1938) thought that olfactory hallucinations come from a lesion of the uncus or hippocampal gyrus. This may be arteriosclerotic in origin.

Patients with tumors of the temporal lobes have been known to complain of a bad odor as also have patients suffering from epilepsy and syphilis of the brain. The schizophrenic is sometimes subject to hallucinations of smell. Davidson studied eighteen such cases in which there was either a psychosis, hysteria, epilepsy, or arteriosclerosis of the brain.

One woman thought that foul fumes were coming up from the radiator into her room. A man thought that he smelled so bad that people were objecting to having him around. He thought, also, that fumes were coming through the window of his room. Another man smelled fumes, and another smelled a strong odor, like that of a medicine. About 4 per cent of a group of 500 unselected psychotics confessed to these hallucinations of smell. In most cases the symptom appeared late in life.

THE TROUBLES OF THE PERSON WITH A LOW INTELLIGENCE

Physicians would have less trouble handling some patients if they realized more quickly that they were dealing with an individual with so low an intelligence that he could not understand what was being said to him. Especially in free clinics, a great deal of medical effort is wasted because the persons on whom it is spent cannot profit from it: Their I.Q. is too low. They have no insight into their situation, and none can be put into them. The physician can talk to them by the hour without changing them or influencing their behavior. All these people know is that they feel sick, and they want a bottle of medicine or an operation. They can be dismissed happy with some medicine, but they cannot see that they should be doing something to ameliorate the situation at home that is producing the illness and prolonging it.

To illustrate the troubles one can have with some persons, a while ago I saw the wife of a wealthy man who had traveled several thousand miles to the Clinic because her physician, alarmed over a slight harmless variation from normal in her sella turcica, had told her that she had a pituitary tumor, and that, to avoid blindness, she must immediately be operated on. She promptly developed a hysterical type of tubular vision and a hysterical patch of painful anesthesia on her face.

When told by able roentgenologists, neurologists, internists, and neurosurgeons that her sella was normal, that her slight blindness and the painful spot on her face were of no importance, and that she didn't need any operation, she was incredulous, angry, and outraged. I tried to explain to her how it came about that her physician had made a mistake, and why the oculists and neurologists knew that her symptoms must be functional in nature and due to her anxiety, but soon I saw that her I.Q. was so low that she could never understand the mental processes of the specialists who had seen her. We were wasting our time talking to her. An electrician might just as well have been trying to explain to her what had gone wrong with her television set.

She left us in anger to go to another medical center where she said she would be operated on, no matter who opposed her. With this woman the only way to a cure would have been through the use of some spectacular hocus-pocus. I am sorry that I do not know what happened to her later. She was the sort of person to whom the opinion of a chiropractor was just as good as that of a distinguished consultant. It was not to be discarded simply because several nationally known specialists did not think much of it! When I find myself dealing with a person who behaves this way I feel inclined to bow myself out because other patients are waiting whom I *might* be able to help.

ANOREXIA NERVOSA

The gastroenterologist sees each year a number of young women who are eating very little, and who are perhaps regurgitating a good part of that. Many of them go down to skin and bones, but, curiously, they tend to keep up and about. Usually by the time they have become very thin, menstruation has stopped, and their basal metabolic rate has dropped. These changes do not appear to be due to any disease of the glands of internal secretion. The giving of thyroid substance may help the woman a bit but it does not work any miracle. For some years an attempt was made to explain this syndrome on the basis of a supposed Simmonds' disease of the pituitary gland, but this idea has now been given up. In the cases of most of these young women the essential trouble appears to be an inherited psychopathy, plus strain in an unhappy home.

Commonly, the home is run by a domineering sex-hating mother who has little use for a weak or futile or alcoholic father. The patient seldom has much sexual interest, and if she gets married her adjustment is often poor; in some cases she is soon back with her mother.

In a series of these cases studied by psychiatrists, some of the girls were found to be schizoid, and all had psychic problems. Several of them had a low intelligence. In some cases the girl's troubles followed an attempt to reduce weight. Because people teased her about being overweight she went on a restricted diet. When she reached normal weight she couldn't seem to stop and kept going on down.

Another story is that the girl started regurgitating, and soon, not content with this, she cut down on the intake of food. I remember a nun who regurgitated her food as fast as she swallowed it. For a time she had to be fed by tube so that she could get a start on the way back to health. Occasionally one will see a fairly normal girl who started losing weight when trapped at home and deprived of a chance to marry by a selfish and tyrannical mother. Such a girl may get well rapidly if helped to escape. In one such case the girl trapped herself by entering a convent and staying on after she had found that she was not suited to the life. She got well as soon as the Mother Superior told her to go out into the world again.

Many of these girls, if taken away from their family and urged to eat and to keep the food down, will behave fairly well and will gain back their weight. I have helped a few to start eating by giving some insulin each day, or by giving amino acids by mouth, or by giving food by stomach tube. It has been suggested that with extreme emaciation the body's supply of protein gets so low that digestive ferments cannot be formed in the intestine. Be this as it may, I have seen a few of these girls who started eating only when "the pump was primed" with amino acids. In some cases the secret of success is to get the girl to stop regurgitating her food because it gives her much epigastric pain. She is too willing to relieve her distress by letting the food come up. It takes courage and determination to hold it down, but this is essential to success.

Unfortunately, although one can often fatten these girls and can get them back to a fair degree of health, one cannot keep them from slumping again, especially when they have to go back into an unhappy and perhaps broken home, either with a psychopathic mother or an unloved or unloving husband.

Occasionally, one sees the syndrome of extreme anorexia in older women who have run into psychic problems bigger than they can solve. I remember one such woman who faded away to a walking skeleton after she suspected her husband of unfaithfulness; another little constitutionally inadequate woman got a severa anorexia when her husband died and left her with responsibilities too big for her, and another had anorexia for years in spite of the fact that she was a merry, delightful person without serious life problems that I could learn about. The significant point in her case appeared to be that she came of a family in which there was much insanity.

Rarely I have seen what looked like this syndrome in men. In one case the cause was a tuberculous abscess arising in a thoracic vertebra, and in another, at necropsy, there was found a large cyst in the cerebellum. I cannot remember having seen in men the type of disease that is common in girls. I have seen a few cases of severe anorexia in men and women due to their conviction that their food was poisoned or that Christ had told them not to eat.

Usually anorexia nervosa is a disease that might well be handled by a psychiatrist and a gastroenterologist working together.

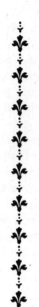

CHAPTER 15

Mild Equivalents of
Psychosis and Epilepsy

RELATIVES OF THE PSYCHOTIC

MANY YEARS AGO I became interested in syndromes which it seemed to me must be due either to the autonomic nerves playing tricks on the person, or to an erratic hypothalamus, or to sudden outpourings of neuromimetic hormones. I described some of these syndromes in Chapter 9.

I soon learned that most of the persons with illness of this type had psychotic or highly neurotic or alcoholic or epileptic relatives. As years passed and I studied more and more of these jittery or overly worrisome or neurotic patients I found it ever more easy to recognize the ones who had a bad nervous inheritance. Often a glance at the person and a quick look over the history, and I could guess correctly that back of him was a poor nervous ancestry. I would sense that that man had more trouble than could be accounted for by ordinary nervousness or fatigue.

Naturally, there were a few cases in which I could not get the expected history, even when the person was so peculiar that I felt sure that some ancestors must have been odd. A common reason for this failure to get a history of psychosis was that the patient did not know much about his older relatives. Perhaps they were left behind in Europe, or one or both parents died early, or the sibs scattered and dropped out of sight. In other cases the patient concealed what he hated to face; in others the psychoses, if there were such, appeared long ago, perhaps in unknown great uncles and aunts, and in other cases there was much oddness and eccentricity in the family, but no insanity. In these cases, the psychotic tendencies, instead of being concentrated in one or two persons, were so diluted and scattered through the whole family that they could be detected only by someone who had lived alongside of the people.

Muncie reported a case of this type in which a young man with a psychopathic personality had a violent-tempered, unreasonable mother, a queer maternal grandmother, a queer maternal aunt, a maternal aunt hospitalized twice for a depression, a nervous, irritable father, and a maternal grandfather who, in his later years, withdrew from society and eventually committed suicide. To me, an interesting point about this history is that if the maternal aunt had never been depressed enough to be committed, or if her illness had been unknown to the patient, many a psychiatrist might have said, "Here is a good example of a psychosis due purely to sexual traumas in infancy."

Lessons to be learned from a large family made up of mildly depressed persons. Many years ago, in California, I knew a large family whose members taught me much about the inheritance of small doses of a tendency to depression. It is significant that, with all their great reticence, I would never have learned what I came to know about them if I had not become well acquainted with a number of them and their spouses. Only gradually over several years did I get enough information to piece together the story.

The first member whom I saw was a nice-looking, intelligent, well-educated and likable woman of forty who complained first of backaches and headaches but later told of spells of nervousness in which she felt strange and not herself. Ordinarily she was a lovely person, idealistic, and devoted to her husband and children. At times she was too active, ambitious, and restless and inclined to get up at daybreak so as to get done all the things she wanted to do. In other words, she was then hypomanic. Later, she would quiet down and go into a spell in which she felt slowed-up and tired. She then realized she was a bit unreasonable, and her temper was hard to control. Interestingly, as a girl she already had these wide swings of mood, and when in a depressed spell she would tie a handkerchief around a post on the front porch to tell her beau that she was in no mood to see him, and he had better keep away! Evidently, she had been somewhat manic-depressive all her life.

When I asked her where she got this tendency she said it came from her father who was stern, domineering, selfish, evil-tempered, and often moody and mentally inaccessible. He wet the bed until he was fifteen.

At times he would disappear for months, leaving his wife to keep the ranch going as best she could. The wife of the odd father, the mother of my patient, was an able, hard-working and determined woman.

A son was a silent moody man who, after an unhappy love affair, scarcely spoke to anyone for a year. A daughter seemed to be a fine, well-balanced, pleasant woman. Another son was odd and eventually became miserly. Another son had spells in which he was too depressed to talk to anyone or to go to work. Another son was able, but he had spells of mild depression, and one "nervous breakdown" following a love affair. Another son was a fine, gifted, highly successful, well-adjusted and kindly man, but even he admitted that at times he was cursed with the family tendency to slip into silent and moody spells. A daughter was able and idealistic but often dreamy and "up in the clouds." Another daughter for a time was insane, and so depressed that she would not recognize anyone. Another daughter was once depressed over a love affair. She was irritable, odd, and at times "difficult," so that the family feared her.

Most of the sibs tended, like the father, to escape anything difficult or unpleasant by refusing to face it or discuss it; they just "went into the silence." I haven't much information as to the next generation, but already one descendant has suffered from late bed wetting, one probably has suffered a spell of major hysteria, and another has been depressed and silent. One man, at the age of thirty-four, sat down and never worked again.

To me a most interesting point about this family is that only one of the ten sibs can be classified as having been insane, but nearly all of them have a manic-depressive temperament. Interestingly, also, is the fact that although in any psychiatric survey made by an investigator the father would probably have been classified as "sane," he wasn't quite that. As sometimes happens in these families, there is much good mixed with the bad, and several of the father's brothers were distinguished university professors.

It seems obvious to me that unless students of mental disease and general ill health learn to pay particular attention to men like this father, and to recognize the great significance of his traits, they will never get anywhere with their statistics and their genetic interpretations. When one follows up the trail of a psychopathic inheritance, the minor manifestations may be just as important as the major ones.

How often can one get a family history of psychosis? Some readers will doubtless feel inclined to question my ideas; I can hear them say, "Oh, you can get a history of insanity in any family if you will only dig back a bit." To see if they were right my assistants and I questioned with care 479 intelligent patients, one after the other. All of them were seen by me. In 77.4 per cent we were unable to get a history of any psychosis in the family. In all cases in which the person was suffering from nervousness or a "functional" disease, I was particularly careful and pertinacious in going over the family history already taken by an assistant. In some cases of non-nervous disease I trusted to the history taken by the assistant.

Actually, I could obtain a history of psychosis in near relatives in only 13.2 per cent of the 479 cases. I found a family history of alcoholism or dipsomania in another 5.9 per cent of the families; of psychopathic behavior in 0.8 per cent, of epilepsy in 2.5 per cent, and of feeble-mindedness in 0.2 per cent. This gives a total incidence of poor nervous heredity in 22.6 per cent of the cases.

Doubtless this incidence of 22.6 per cent is higher than in the general population because so many of the patients I see are referred to me because the home physician thinks I will be interested in some bizarre neurosis or equivalent of a psychosis. Accordingly, I next questioned 100 patients, seen consecutively, who did not have signs of a neurosis, and from them I obtained a family history of psychosis in only three cases, of alcoholism in five more, and of psychopathic behavior in one. That gives a total incidence of 9 per cent.

Patients lie about their family history. As I said in the chapter on the art of getting from patients a family history of insanity, it is unfortunate that many persons will lie like troupers when they get onto this topic. Thus, one day I was called to see a physician's wife who demanded that I find some focus of organic disease to explain all of her many neurotic and hysterical symptoms. Again and again I tried to get a history of bad nerves in the family but each time she swore there was none. Then I got her husband off by himself and learned from him, first, something that she had not admitted, and this was that she had been drinking heavily. Second, the doctor told me that one of the woman's uncles drank himself to death, a brother is a psychopathic simpleton, one aunt went into a depression and committed suicide, and two other aunts have been in and out of asylums! Whenever, after having been lied to by a patient, I get a story like this from relatives, I realize how valueless many routinely taken family histories are.

Particularly interesting is the story of a sullen young woman whom I saw one afternoon. Her appearance and her story of spells of "smothering," tachycardia, and abdominal pain all made me suspect an equivalent of epilepsy. Appealing to the red-faced, surly-looking father, I tried repeatedly and as tactfully as I could to get a family history of "fainting spells" or short dreamy spells, but always I ran up against a wall of denial. Perhaps there was ironic justice in what happened next; anyway, driving home that afternoon, the father had a convulsion, ran off the road, and smashed his car up against a tree. If I hadn't seen the report of the accident in the paper next day, I would have been short one case record in my file of the "relatives of the epileptic!"

Minor neuroses that run down through a family. Many an old country physician could tell of families in which mild neuroses of one or more types keep cropping up in every generation. In the family of this type which I will now describe it will be noted that except in the case of one person the troubles which keep occurring are different from those met with in the California family.

About 100 years ago a family came from Germany. The father was a genial, very social, and friendly vineyardist. Nothing is known of his wife, but he had half a dozen children all of whom appeared to have had more than average intelligence and success in life. Two were hotel keepers. A daughter was nervous, irritable, and hampered by a quick temper. Her children by three husbands were frail and sickly and almost all died young. The best of the lot grew up to be a big, handsome, highly intelligent woman. But for all her appearance of health she suffered almost constantly from nervousness, an atypical migraine, an over-irritability, a most uncomfortable colon, insomnia, and a quick temper. She could not even contemplate a journey without getting diarrhea, and after starting, she would get feverish and have to stop and spend a day resting somewhere. With all her distresses she was never seriously ill, and in later life she tended to gain weight. Many medical and surgical examinations failed to show any organic disease.

She married a man who came of a sturdy, rather stolid tribe, without any nervous symptoms. The one of their children who inherited the largest dose of the mother's nerves tended from infancy to be odd, solitary, and sad. He became a chain-smoker and constant coffee-drinker. He was a poor sleeper and often would walk the streets much of the night hoping to get tired enough to fall asleep. For months he would overwork and then he would get a mild nervous breakdown in which he would have to take an easy outdoor job. When in a spell in which he couldn't work his trouble was fatigue more than depression. He did not care to marry because he realized no woman would want to share his erratic ways of living; besides, he preferred living entirely alone. Under psychic strain he had tremendous mucous colics like his mother's. He was an artist, a linguist, a raconteur, and a traveler on the face of the earth.

A brother inherited a mild migraine, a highly sensitive and troublesome colon, some of his mother's distress when traveling, some insomnia, and much sensitiveness and nervous tension. He had a fatigue state after years of overwork but there was no element of depression. Another brother inherited a mild migraine with some nervousness and much insomnia due to nervous tension. A sister inherited the mother's tendency to become ill on going out into crowds and was so oversensitive that all her life she suffered from nervousness. She was able, however, to work every day.

In the next generation a daughter during girlhood was frail, nervous, and highly sensitive. When on a journey, she tended to become ill and feverish for a day. As a child she became nauseated and afraid she would vomit whenever she started a new term in school. A son had mild migraine and a number of nervous tics; another son and daughter, from infancy onward, were very poor sleepers. The daughter had hay fever and her grandmother's habit of becoming ill after starting on a journey.

In the next generation there are again some signs of the family nerves. One child had enuresis and a prolonged regurgitation of food, but, of course, these troubles may have come down from the other side of the family. One child had temper tantrums, another was for the first few years excessively shy, and one appears already to have the family migraine.

It is interesting that in this family, with all the nervousness and oversensitiveness and tendency to discomfort, there has never been any tendency to hypochondriasis or worry over illness. That apparently was not in the genes. All of the adults have kept at their work; they all have achieved success, and they rarely go to a physician. Even the highly nervous man, after trying several occupations, finally found one in which he could be happy and successful.

SYMPTOMS AND SYNDROMES OBSERVED IN THE CASES OF 410 PATIENTS
WHO HAD PSYCHOTIC OR ALCOHOLIC ANCESTRY

To see what the syndromes are that afflict the relatives of the psychotic and the alcoholic I first abstracted and then analyzed in detail the records of some 410 patients from whom I had obtained a family history of psychosis or alcoholism. All these patients were so well studied at the Mayo Clinic that I could fairly well rule out or recognize any organic disease that might be present in thorax or abdomen.

The relatives of *alcoholics* were studied along with the relatives of *psychotics* because in a preliminary survey I could not see that there was any difference in the syndromes presented by the persons in the two groups. I gained the impression that the troubles of the relatives of epileptics are somewhat different, and hence their syndromes are described separately.

The essential story is often missed. Internists have sometimes remarked to me that they do not see the borderline-psychotic type of patient whom I keep talking about. My answer is that they must be seeing him, but they are not taking the sort of history that will reveal his essential trouble. One can easily let a psychotic person go through the office without suspecting the nature of his illness.

For instance, as I was writing this I was called to see a prominent industrialist who was dissatisfied because, after a thorough examination, he was being dismissed with the diagnosis of "digestive neurosis." I asked him what he really was worried about, and he said, "You're right; I am not worried about that little indigestion; what frightens me is a feeling of mental depression, together with a recent failure of my mental powers. I am not thinking clearly as I used to, and at times I am so jittery I can hardly sign important papers." It was these things, which he had not even mentioned to my younger colleagues, that had frightened him into making the long journey to Rochester.

When I could not get from him any history of either overwork or a little stroke, I asked about his family history, and at first was assured that his stock was excellent. Later, when I kept after him, he admitted that several of his father's brothers had been drunkards, and finally he broke down and told me that his father, on four occasions, had become so maniacal he had had to be locked up! The patient feared he was going the same way. What I wonder is: How many men like this are going through our offices each month, with their real disease not even suspected or mentioned?

Psychotic tendencies. On looking over the lists of distresses of the relatives of the psychotic I was surprised to find how large was the number with symptoms which suggest to me more a psychosis than a neurosis. For instance, there were 105 persons out of the 410 who mentioned or complained of spells of mild or fairly severe depression. Some thirty-one, as they chatted with me, came to see that for most of their lives they had had a manic-depressive temperament, which caused them to swing from moods of elation and overactivity to moods of lethargy, depression, and great fatigue. Some fifty-six of the women said they had "jags of senseless crying."

Nineteen were so hypomanic at times that they were much too talkative and social. One such woman, a physician's wife, remarked that once for six weeks she was so keyed-up that she had to have company for dinner every night; then she collapsed and went into a mild depression. Eight persons suffered from an agitated type of depression in which they walked the floor in an agony of restlessness. Eight more felt that life was not worth living since there was no sense to it or joy in it. At least ten women became depressed or psychopathic before each menstrual period, and seven others, who probably were mildly depressed, said they spent their days brooding over ill health. Some of the nineteen alcoholics apparently drank because they were depressed;

most of the seventeen who suddenly and unexplainedly lost weight were depressed, and some of the twenty-two who often thought of suicide were depressed.

At least forty-three persons were schizoid in temperament: They were shy, retiring, silent, undemonstrative, unfriendly, timid, dreamy, or uninterested in sex. Twenty-two women were frigid; at least five were sexually immature, and some of the twelve who complained much of painful intercourse were schizoid. One was a virgin after many years of marriage. Most of the twenty-one persons suffering from anorexia nervosa were schizoid.

There were thirty-seven who, from time to time, suffered from hysteria, and many of the bloaters were almost certainly hysterical. There were twenty-three persons who had compulsions, obsessions, and occasional delusions or hallucinations. There were sixty-six with some disorder of personality, and I learned later that five wound up in an asylum. Others had to have shock treatments.

Epileptic tendencies. There were sixteen who had epilepsy or suffered on rare occasions from a convulsive disorder, and four more who appeared to have an equivalent of epilepsy. Thirty-six admitted having an explosive temper, such as goes often with an epileptic inheritance. Twenty of those whom I suspected of having a tendency to epilepsy showed some dysrhythmia in the electroencephalogram, which somewhat reinforced my clinical suspicions.

Nervous troubles. Under "nervous" symptoms the commonest complaint was great fatigue. This was mentioned in eighty-five of the records. There were eight persons who felt almost too tired to get out of bed in the morning, five who dragged around, forty-one who felt exhausted, and thirty-four who were too tired to do any work. At least twenty-one could not read much, and twenty said they could not concentrate or think.

Seventy-three persons said they were nervous, and sixty-three more were "very nervous," a total of 136. Forty-two said they had had a "nervous breakdown," or they were in one when they came. Seventy-two were constant and often unreasonable worriers. Twenty-seven suffered because of hypersensitiveness; twenty-nine were very irritable; sixteen were highly emotional; eleven high-strung, and sixteen excitable. Ten said that everything bothered them. Probably more than a half of the 410 complained of symptoms due to their nerves playing tricks on them. Eighteen fainted easily; twenty-six complained of numbness here and there; at least twenty had been operated on again and again to little purpose. One woman had been operated on each time she had gone into a depression! Thirty-six complained of burnings, quiverings, and sorenesses in the abdomen. Sixty-three complained of aches and pains either all over, or else here and there, and seventy-three complained particularly of pains, aches, and distresses in the abdomen.

At least seventeen could not stand crowds, and nine could not even go to a movie; they got so tense and frightened that they had to leave and go home.

Persons who felt queer. I was much impressed with the number of persons who *felt queer* in various ways. Sixty-three had a poor sense of balance; fifty-two were terribly tense; forty were jittery or shaky; thirty-nine felt dopey or dazed or slowed-up; twenty-six were numb here and there; eighteen felt miserable or odd or queer and not themselves; sixteen felt terribly restless; another sixteen felt burnings here and there; fifteen felt strange things in and about the head; thirteen felt chilly; twelve felt weak, and eleven felt insecure. Others complained of all sorts of strange sensations, many of them suggesting a schizophrenic type of distress or a hallucination. For instance, they felt as if there were a snake crawling under the skin, or as if their whole body was acid, or as if a hand were clutching the bowels.

Fears. Interesting was the number of persons who were full of fears, phobias, and abnormal worries. Thirty were constantly afraid of going insane; twenty-two feared they would commit suicide; nineteen said they feared everything; twelve feared being alone; seven feared close places and a low ceiling; nine greatly feared heart disease; six were in a constant dither over cancer; five were acutely afraid of death; and five feared fainting. In addition there were fifty who each feared one or more of some thirty types of disaster.

Digestive troubles. As one would expect, many complained of symptoms suggesting something wrong with the stomach or bowel. To me a big surprise was the high incidence of diarrhea. At least eighty-eight mentioned it, and in some cases it was the outstanding complaint. In none of them was there any sign of organic disease in the bowel. The spells of diarrhea commonly followed panics of fear or they came with excitement or tension or fatigue, or with even such a mild worry as anticipation of a journey. It is easily understandable why some persons should get diarrhea when seized with the idea that they were "going crazy," perhaps "like Aunt Lizzie." One man who happened to live in Louisiana had his stools studied with the utmost care by several eminent bacteriologists. No one had noted that his trouble was due to the fact that he was having panics of fear, sensing that he was going insane like his uncle before him.

Sixty-eight persons bloated, most of them with gas, and forty-nine complained of flatulence. Curiously, only twenty-eight complained much of the irritable bowel syndrome with mucous colics; some of those who did had an extreme form of the syndrome, and had lived for years on only a few foods. Some seventy-six complained of constipation, but it is hard to know if this incidence was excessive. Fifty-seven suffered from functional forms of indigestion, and thirty-two, who had a normal-appearing stomach and duodenum, complained of hunger pain. This is an interesting finding, which suggests that pseudo-ulcer is at times an equivalent of psychosis. Seventy-five, and doubtless more of the patients, were often belching and swallowing air. Many of them were accomplished air-gulpers. As I said before, twenty-one suffered from anorexia nervosa.

Fifty-three had a tendency to vomit and this is worth noting. At least fifty complained of nausea. This finding was one of the important ones because so often the internist cannot guess why a person is often nauseated. Forty-one persons suffered from regurgitation, which shows, again, what I have long felt, that regurgitation is always functional in nature, and often based on an inborn tendency. Seventeen suffered from heartburn. Curiously, four persons told of spells of bulimia in which they felt compelled to eat large quantities of food. Bulimia has long been known as a symptom of psychosis.

Miscellaneous distresses. Eighty-one persons complained of various types of headache, and as will be noted later, eighty-one suffered from migraine. There probably is some overlapping of the two groups of "the headachey" and "the migrainous." Forty suffered from palpitation, ten from tachycardia, and eight more from paroxysmal tachycardia. Twenty-three were troubled with air hunger, and thirty more with a cardiac neurosis. Interesting is the fact that fourteen sometimes had difficulty in swallowing. Ten complained of a severe type of globus; eight had ear noises and seven had a failure of vision of a functional type. Twenty-three of the women complained of severe dysmenorrhea, and I have long suspected that women in psychotic families have more than their share of menstrual troubles. The schizoid women often had poor pelvic organs.

As was to be expected, eighty-one persons complained of insomnia or restless sleep. Fifty-seven complained of feeling dizzy or giddy, or of having lost to some extent their sense of balance. This is an observation that should be remembered by all internists, neurologists, and otologists. Thirty-five complained much of backache, and twenty-nine women complained of urinary distresses and frequency of urination for which the urologists could find no sufficient local cause. Twenty-seven persons perspired to excess in spite of a normal basal metabolic rate, and this is worth noting. As was to be expected, twenty-four had cold, wet, clammy hands. At least seventeen felt sore and pounded all over; twelve itched, and what is very interesting, fourteen complained of a so-called fever. Most of these had been told on inadequate evidence that they had brucellosis. Ten complained of nervous chills, and seventeen, of sudden unexplained losses of weight. The fever, the chills, and the loss of weight seem all to be due to a change in the setting of regulating mechanisms in the hypothalamus.

The meaning of the study. Some readers by now may be protesting, "But, surely you are not asking us to believe that every person who feels blue or shy, or fears to go into a phone booth is related to the psychotic." No, of course not; all I am doing is analyzing the medical records of 410 persons who had one or more psychotic or alcoholic near-relatives. On looking over the lists of their symptoms, I am struck by the frequency with which certain distresses occurred. I think all internists who read these findings should be impressed by them as I am. These figures should make us think and observe further.

Unfortunately, I haven't yet prepared a control study of the symptoms of 410 men and women who went to the Mayo Clinic for the treatment of, let us say, a boil or a fracture. I can only say that I am almost certain that in such a group I would not find more than a few depressed or schizoid persons, or more than a few complaining of great fatigue, queer feelings, extreme nervousness, pathologic fears, great worry, nerves playing tricks, pains and aches all over, regurgitation, dysphagia, vomiting, nausea, bloating, anorexia, hunger pain, diarrhea, headache, migraine, palpitation, dizziness, dysmenorrhea, or sweating.

Intercurrent diseases or abnormalities discovered during this study. Some readers may be wondering why I have not gone into details as to the physical and laboratory studies made in these cases. I haven't done this because in almost all cases the physical and other examinations failed to show much. Aside from some signs of constitutional inadequacy there was rarely anything physically wrong with these persons. Some thirty-eight complained of arthritis or fibrositis but this probably does not mean much. Twenty had a definite hypertension, and eighteen more had a slight or beginning hypertension. This sort of thing is so common that I doubt if the finding has any significance. There were ten persons who appeared to have suffered from encephalitis and this incidence is so large that I suspect it means that persons with a poor nervous heredity are a little more subject to inflammation of the brain. I think this incidence is higher than normal. Eleven persons had had trouble with a goiter. Sixteen had had a duodenal ulcer; and six had had asthma. Curiously, seven had had for years an anemia for which no cause could be found. Four had diabetes, and five had had tuberculosis. The schizophrenic is said to be rather subject to tuberculosis. Thirty-four persons complained of decided food sensitiveness.

To me one of the most striking findings was the great incidence of migraine in these patients. Eighty-one, or 20 per cent, had had the typical headaches, and twelve others suffered from syndromes which may well have been migrainous. I do not know what the normal incidence of migraine is. It is hard to estimate it, because it varies so markedly with the percentage of intelligent and upper class persons in the group studied. However, I believe the incidence in this group is excessive. My impression is that one of the factors which tends to make migraine severe and prostrating is a psychotic inheritance. One can easily see how the nervous suffering due to manifestations of a poor nervous heredity might easily convert a "carrier" of migraine into a bad sufferer from the disease.

Weird Nervous Syndromes of the Relatives of the Psychotic

Some of the relatives of the psychotic suffer from weird syndromes in which their autonomic nerves play tricks with them (see Chapter 9). Usually the trouble comes in spells, sometimes induced by emotion, fatigue, eating, or defecating, but sometimes coming at any time, even at night.

For instance, a person will suddenly get jittery and numb all over, perhaps with feelings of chilliness and pins and needles; or ants crawling on the skin; sudden perspiration; palpitation and pounding of the heart; missing beats; air-hunger; a feeling of choking, or globus; a feeling of faintness, impending death, and great weakness, together with much belching, blurring of vision, fear of going insane, and a fear of impending diarrhea or vomiting. There may be a feeling of tightness in the head, with salivation, trembling, reddening of the face, a feeling that the head is getting bigger and bigger, a desire to hyperventilate, a feeling of going into a trance, butterflies, or cramps in the abdomen, numbness of the tongue, bursting feelings here and there, feelings of great exhaustion, sometimes fever, causeless crying, inability to think, semiconsciousness, or feelings of great burning or tightness somewhere.

After one has seen a few of these attacks one can be fairly certain as to their nature and etiology. They seem to be due to storms coming out of the brain and running out along autonomic nerves.

These persons should not be operated on as they now often are. In making a diagnosis the physician is faced by a choice of such diagnoses as an equivalent of psychosis or epilepsy or migraine, hysteria, or a tantrum of temper, or a curious allergic reaction.

It helps in many cases to get an electroencephalogram and to either find or else rule out a dysrhythmia.

The treatment must consist usually of reassurance plus sedatives and sometimes anticonvulsants.

MILD EQUIVALENTS OF EPILEPSY

As Cobb has said, many epileptics live out a long life without ever having a fit. Innumerable persons with a dysrhythmic electroencephalogram never have a fit, but many have queer nervous storms which seldom are recognized for what they are; that is, mild equivalents of epilepsy. Cobb has spoken of "sensory fits" with curious visceral distresses, and sometimes temporary disturbances in vision, hearing, smell, and touch. These people will feel a bit "woozy," or their eyes will not see well, or they may suddenly get a vile taste in the mouth, or a pain or a distress in the abdomen. Lennox has mentioned attacks of palpitation, difficult breathing, choking sensations, hot flushes, sweating, shivering, trembling, nausea, feelings of impending death, the passage of much urine, sudden rises in blood pressure, lacrimation, salivation, or spells of hyperventilation.

As I grow older I find myself recognizing more and more patients with equivalents of epilepsy, sometimes from their rather surly appearance, or often from their irritability and irascibility, or from the nature of their story; and then I draw out a history of epilepsy in the family. Some of these persons have sulky spells, many are hard to get along with, and a few are dipsomaniacs. I have seen a number who had spells of hunger pain, due apparently to a great irritability of the stomach, because no ulcer could ever be demonstrated. Others suffered from spells of abdominal pain resembling a migrainous equivalent, and a few had painful attacks closely resembling a gastric crisis of tabes.

Many of these persons have tremendously exaggerated knee jerks, and probably because of this over-reactivity, some suffer from a distressingly premature seminal ejaculation. A few are so irritable they cannot eat when anyone is present at the table. These persons will admit, if asked, that they never dare spank a child because they fear they might not be able to stop. Actually, such a man once, when left as a baby-sitter, beat the child to death because it cried. Once he started slapping the child, he could not stop. Some of these men avoid getting into an argument, because they are fearful they might attack and kill the opponent.

Some have touch-me-not moods when they growl at anyone who comes near, or they have spells of ill humor lasting hours or days, or they have spells in which they feel like being cruel. In other spells, the man will wander away from home. I have seen a number of these men who were sleep-walkers, and some of these, when half awake, would attack a roommate or wreck the bed or the room.

Some have panicky spells in which they tremble all over or perspire heavily. Some feel giddy and dizzy, the heart may race and pound and the victim will feel weak and very tired. He may feel numb here and there; he may ache all over, he may get abdominal pain and indigestion, he may bloat, and he may pass large quantities of flatus. With the panicky spells he may get diarrhea. He may belch loudly and repeatedly, he may regurgitate his food, and in spells he may be severely constipated.

Strecker, Ebaugh, and Ewald, under the heading of epileptic psychoses, mentioned twilight states, perhaps with mental confusion; and states of delirium in which the patient is somewhat conscious.

Lennox, Gibbs, and Gibbs found that only 10 per cent of persons with an apparently good heredity have a dysrhythmic electroencephalogram, while 60 per cent of 183 relatives of the epileptic showed dysrhythmia. Lennox and his associates concluded that the persons with only a submerged predisposition to epilepsy outnumber the epileptics with seizures 25 to 1. This would mean that in this country about 12 per cent of the population carry this tendency.

Some day, we physicians must get much more interested in recognizing these persons with their curious nervous storms, and their tendency to get embroiled with other people or with the law. Some day the handicap of more of these persons must be recognized in infancy and childhood. In later life, when they contemplate marriage, they should compare their electroencephalogram with that of the loved one so as to avoid a union with another dysrhythmic. Some day in all states the highway police will want to have an electroencephalographic report before issuing a driver's license. One hears of many tragedies due to lack of this precaution. The papers are constantly reporting serious accidents due to a man's "falling asleep at the wheel."

Some syndromes. I remember a jolly woman of fifty who complained of "choking spells." They came at any time and anywhere, often while she was playing cards happily with friends. Often she would be so ill she had to lie on the floor. Her friends, much alarmed, would fear she was dying. Some attacks woke her out of sleep. In these spells she would get air hunger and would hyperventilate. She would feel a band of iron around her chest, contracting down. Sometimes her legs would become numb. In mild spells there was only the numbness. Sometimes she felt so faint she feared she was going to fall down. She had had most of these spells in the year before I saw her, but it was significant that in girlhood she had had them when she began giggling or laughing. Like other persons suffering from cataplexy, she had had to train herself not to laugh heartily.

One of her troubles was that she had a curious difficulty about getting up in the morning. She would feel so weak she would fall back onto the pillow and would have to wait a while until more strength came. Ten years before I saw her she had a spell in which, for a time, she lost her sense of balance. She also had a spell of burning in the mouth. At times she would drop things because of lack of control of her hands.

Good physicians had diagnosed a neurosis but against this was the fact that she was merry and stout and easy-going. So far as I could find, she had no sorrows or worries, and she was happily in love with a fine husband. I thought it significant that her mother and a brother were choleric, morose hypochondriacs, difficult to live with. As I expected, her electroencephalogram showed a decided dysrhythmia, and the taking of dilantin put an end to the spells.

Another fine woman for years suffered from violent attacks of what looked like gastric crises of tabes. Even large doses of morphine would not stop the pain and vomiting. Then I learned that on rare occasions she had fallen heavily, and when an electroencephalogram was obtained it showed a dysrhythmia. Dilantin relieved her.

According to Liveing, Dr. Erasmus Darwin, the grandfather of the great evolutionist, called attention to the fact that, in children, bad nightmares, somnambulism, and trances are sometimes equivalents of epilepsy.

M. T. Moore reported a series of cases of periodic attacks of severe abdominal pain, sometimes with vomiting or diarrhea, or headache, nausea, or rumbling sensations in the abdomen, perhaps with subsequent headache and feelings of aching all over, or a peculiar feeling of being dazed, or a feeling of imminent collapse. In most of these cases the electroencephalogram showed typical changes, and the starting of anticonvulsive therapy stopped the spells, perhaps after 10 or 15 years of suffering.

The common symptoms. On studying the records of a group of 56 persons who had one or more epileptic relatives, I found that most of them had curious nervous symptoms and syndromes. The following table lists the symptoms most commonly mentioned. Besides these, there were dozens more complained of by only a few patients. Most of the symptoms suggested a nervous origin.

SYMPTOMS OF PERSONS WITH EPILEPTIC RELATIVES

Irascible and overly irritable 22	Spells of depression 8
Tired and tires easily 20	Very tense 8
Very nervous 17	Bloating 8
Fainting or dizzy spells 16	Premature ejaculation .... : 8
Curious spells 15	Lack of sex interest and early loss
Strange feelings 14	of it 8
Many fears 14	Heartburn 7
Headache 12	Aches and sorenesses all over 7
Much belching 11	Spells of vomiting 7
Abdominal pain 11	Petit mal 7
Much constipation 10	Nausea 6
Migraine 10	Terribly restless 6
Distresses in the head 10	Abdominal soreness 6
Tachycardia 10	Nervous breakdowns 6
Diarrhea 10	Regurgitation 5
Worry, anxious and frightened states. 10	Pseudo-ulcer 5
Burning here and there 9	Cries easily 4
Spells with much flatus 8	Weight goes up and down markedly .. 4

CHAPTER 16

Hysteria

E VERY PHYSICIAN SHOULD know hysteria in all of its bizarre manifestations. The disease is so common and so important that every
week teachers of medicine should be showing examples of it in the college amphitheater. Because they are not doing this the students graduate without the ability to recognize much hysteria at a glance, and as
a result, later in their practices they tend only to examine these patients
at great length, confirming them in their conviction that they must be
very ill.

Every specialist should know those particular manifestations of hysteria that he is likely to see often in his type of practice, and every
surgeon should know the disease well. The orthopedist and the physician who does industrial accident work must know it well. Often it
embroiders the picture of organic disease, and then it takes all the
knowledge and skill the physician has to unscramble the two conditions.
As Ross said, a girl coming down with multiple sclerosis can easily
get so frightened she will show some manifestations of hysteria. I remember a woman with gastric crises of tabes who sometimes got so
frightened that she had a pseudocrisis that was hysterical in nature.

As some have said, hysteria is the great mimic of disease. The only
fortunate feature is that usually it fails to mimic perfectly enough to
deceive an expert. It tends to follow the pattern of what a laywoman

thinks the symptoms should be. One great difficulty is that although a physician may strongly suspect hysteria, he may not be sure enough about it so that he can convincingly insist that the patient come out of the attack. Even a good neurologist will sometimes have this difficulty. All his clinical sense will tell him that certain symptoms are hysterical, but perhaps there is a suspicious Babinski test on one side, or signs that may or may not represent the residue of a small cerebral accident or an old polio-encephalitis.

What is hysteria? No one knows exactly what hysteria is or how much the patient is deceiving herself while deceiving others. Probably most Army psychiatrists would say that there is a decided difference between the malingerer and the hysteric, even when both are attaining the same end, which is to get out of combat duty. The hysterical person is gifted with a great ability to fool himself into illness. He may lose confidence in his ability to move his limbs. The anesthesias are evidently referred out from the brain. Just as a hysterical soldier can suggest himself into illness, so his physician can sometimes talk him out of it. Some writers have called hysteria "unconscious malingering," which is not a bad definition. As Mapother once said, "The infinite capacity of the human race for self-deception makes the additional gift of malingering almost unnecessary."

Ross said that the physician should not waste his time spying on a hysterical man with a paralysis because the fellow really believes that he cannot move his leg or arm, and hence he will remain paralyzed even when no one is around. Ross thought that, to the patient, the paralyzed arm or leg hardly exists in consciousness. Hence, to bring back function in it the man must make a big effort to think of the member and to think of it as in a new position. For instance, if his hand is contracted into a fist he must try to think of it as open.

Ross' impression was that there is no one whom the hysteric is more anxious to deceive than himself. He thought that if a person suffering from organic disease plus hysteria were to lose the organic disease he would not know it and would stay on in the hospital indefinitely. Many a time I have seen this happen. I have also seen persons suffering from hysteria who became much disturbed and worried when a symptom cleared up. I think they were afraid this would put ideas in my head.

The patient's suggestiveness. Bernheim pointed out that the symptoms of hysteria are such as might easily be produced by hypnotic suggestion. Furthermore, they can sometimes be removed or moved about on the body by hypnosis and suggestion. For instance, a woman was in a house which was struck by lightning. A few minutes later, when I saw her, she said that a ball of light (St. Elmo's fire) had come into the room and had struck her foot; whereupon the limb had become paralyzed. I said I would drive the electricity out by the way it came in, and, taking a faradic battery, I stroked the limb from the groin to the foot. This seemed to her and the family so logical a treatment that in a few minutes she was up and walking around again.

Similarly, with a little hocus-pocus, such as by applying a magnet, an area of anesthesia or analgesia can sometimes be transferred from one side of the body to the other. Some writers have claimed that many hysterical anesthesias are produced when the physician gets out his pin and his bit of cotton. Always in questioning a hysterical person the physician should try to avoid producing the symptoms. This is particularly needful when handling patients with traumatic and compensation hysteria.

On self-deception and deception of others. It is true that a hysterical girl will sometimes fake things to keep up the interest of her doctors in her case. For instance, the impression I have gained from much literature on the subject is that a girl who has regurgitated lumps of feces will later secrete some fecal matter in her bed and will say that she vomited it. Another girl, after perhaps running a hysterical hyperthermia, will start putting her thermometer on a hot water bottle. I remember a nurse who, after four futile abdominal operations in a year or so, suffered a week-long attack of hiccups. When these spasms, due to a virus (?), stopped, she went on for a day with a voluntary poor imitation of hiccup.

After seeing in Mexico an enormous amount of hysteria, my impression is that although, to a large extent, the girl is deceiving herself, she has something decidedly wrong with her brain. Often she gets into the grip of strong forces which are arising in a brain made abnormal by heredity and also influenced by environment. We must all remember that a hysterical woman will often remain ill for years, wrecking her life, when it would seem as if, with a little sense, she would pull herself together and choose health. Evidently her brain is not normal enough to realize the folly of what she is doing. Occasionally I have cured a hysterical girl by getting her to see that it would be more fun and more profitable to be well. She apparently had not thought of that.

Ross used to tell of an able superintendent of nurses who should have had good sense, but after a slight injury, she drifted into a state of complete disability with a compensation neurosis. She was so fooled by herself that in her efforts to get well she sacrificed a mouthful of good teeth. Finally, Ross cured her by making her see what she was doing, and by persuading her to give up the small compensation payments she was receiving. It was hard to get her to see that full pay for all-day work would be better than her partial pay for disability, and that it would be *much to her advantage to get well!* Like all these patients, she wanted that compensation for the principle of the thing, and she had great difficulty in facing facts and doing what was sensible.

The hysterical person knows what is going on and has some control. The hysterical woman in a trance knows what is going on and she can be influenced by commands. Scores of times in Mexico I would quiet a girl who was having hysterical convulsions simply by taking out my stethoscope and asking her how she expected me to listen to her heart while she was thrashing around. Although women in such spells would not obey an order to quiet down, they always obeyed my request for quiet so that I could listen to the heart. They did this because in their folk medicine the "attacks" are supposed to be due to disease of the heart. Similarly, if I would put a cup of soup to the lips of a girl in a pseudocoma, she would be likely to drink. A woman walking in her sleep knows what she is doing and may even talk to a person she meets. Many a woman, after "playing possum" a while, has confessed to me that she knew all the time what was going on but did not feel like answering questions or talking.

That hysterical persons can often control themselves was shown by Ross in his Army experience. For instance, when every night in a ward several men were having fits which disturbed their mates, the offenders were told that since they couldn't safely be out on the streets, their leaves would be cancelled until they got well. With this, in that ward fits immediately became unfashionable. In the county hospital where I was an intern, I often stopped patients from having nightly hysterical attacks by telling them that for their own safety, I was going to take them from the ward and put them off by themselves in a lonely room in the attic. In an hour they called me to say that they thought they were getting better and would not be having any more spells.

As I have said, a hysterical girl will sometimes get worried when she sees that a physician is suspecting what is wrong with her. Then she may make extra efforts to put on a good show. One day such a girl, alarmed at the coming of a resident to make a lumbar puncture, suddenly lost the contracture of her abdominal muscles. She was as apologetic about this as would have been an athlete after falling off his trapeze.

One day a woman in my office with a hysterical contracture of an arm became so alarmed when she sensed that I was onto her, that her breath became so horribly foul and fecal that I had to open the window and door. After she left I had to air the room for a while before I could use it again! Next day her breath was all right.

But there is more to hysteria than faking. In my intern days in a big city hospital we used to see women with such complete anesthesia of their tissues that my old professor would pass a long hat pin from one side of a thigh to the other. I could not imagine a normal woman with enough self-control to permit this without flinching. There must have been a marked degree of anesthesia. Similarly, I cannot imagine a woman's being able to keep from gagging when someone tickled her fauces. And yet a woman with an apparently anesthetic hand may button her clothes or pick up a pin, which shows that she can feel well enough.

Some hysterical persons, like an Indian holy man, will hold an arm in a certain position until the joints almost ankylose. I knew a woman who did this simply to injure the reputation of a physician whom she had come to dislike. Another did it to avoid marrying a man ten years her junior, but she kept it up after he departed.

It is hard to see how any amount of conscious and deliberate will power could throw a woman into one of those pseudo-encephalitic states in which she lies stuporous for weeks, perhaps with a fever, until she has to learn to talk and walk all over again. I cannot imagine, also, how a hysterical girl of fifteen years whom I found once in a shack in the mountains of Mexico could have known that in the cases of children the world over the common manifestations of major hysteria are mutism and paralysis from the neck down. She had never read Charcot or Bernheim, and yet she knew exactly what to do! How, also, could a person consciously maintain marked mydriasis in one or both eyes for a few months? Or how could women, apparently hysterical, maintain for months a pulse rate of 120 beats a minute?

That hysteria is associated with changes in the involuntary nervous system is shown when the skin of unused limbs quickly becomes blue, cold, shiny, or somewhat boggy. The fingernails in an unused hand may soon atrophy, and the muscles may waste more rapidly than they should from disuse alone.

The great difficulty in many cases seems to be that the patient has lost confidence in his muscles and nerves. In other cases he may be so upset that he contracts flexors and extensors at the same time. I remember a fine intelligent man of sixty who was well until he fell and broke his leg. After recovery he developed a sort of astasia-abasia with an inability to take a step without help. His explanation was that he had become terror-stricken for fear if he walked he would trip and fall and break his leg again. With explanations and much encouragement he soon was walking fairly well with a cane.

Another fact about hysteria which shows that it is due to something wrong with the brain is that the disease appears usually in a certain type of odd, self-centered person, often a person with a poor nervous heredity or a tendency to psychosis. I found this when studying the relatives of the psychotic (see Chapter 15).

Hysteria is a syndrome which can be superimposed on almost any form of neurosis or psychosis. It is seen most commonly in lowly and ignorant persons, but it is met with occasionally in persons from the higher walks of life. In the British Army, Slater (1943) found its incidence positively correlated with a low intelligence. Cobb thought that hysteria is usually seen in women with an infantile body and mind. Some of them show a boyish build, an infantile uterus, and a baby face.

Types of persons subject to hysteria. My impression is that hysteria of a stormy type is most likely to appear in women of certain ethnic groups who, from childhood onward, have been taught by example to explode violently whenever they are either angry or grief-stricken or frightened. If some Latin American women did not get hysterical, in the lay sense, on the death of a mother, husband, or child, they would lay themselves open to the criticism of the onlookers who might assume that they had not loved the deceased.

Hysteria has been observed commonly in certain racial groups such as the Latins, the Jews, and the Celts. During my years in Mexico, not a week passed that I didn't see examples of major hysteria with convulsions, opisthotonus, hemi-anesthesias, paralyses, pseudocomas, blindness, and what-not. In this country, with a large clientele, I seldom see such cases. In Mexico, I noted also that a tendency to hysteria ran in certain families. With such people medicines usually worked wrongly, and even a minor operation was dangerous because it was most likely to be followed by a long spell of some bizarre syndrome. I remember once, preparatory to ophthalmoscopy, putting a weak mydriatic into the eyes of a husky-looking brother of a hysterical girl. One of his pupils remained widely dilated for the next six weeks. After I had seen a few things like this happen, I learned to leave largely untouched the relatives of the hysterical. A colleague of mine who, against advice, performed a diagnostic spinal puncture on one of these persons, had her on his hands for two months afterward, screaming with headache.

According to some psychiatrists, hysteria appears in persons who live in a zone somewhere between sanity and insanity. Some few of these patients eventually drift into a psychotic state. One thinks of hysterical women as being emotionally unstable, and overly desirous of attention and sympathy. They tend to react too dramatically, emotionally, or stormily to annoyance or sorrow or boredom. Slater found hysteria but rarely in schizophrenics.

Most lay persons think of a hysterical person as one who laughs and cries with the same breath but this is not hysteria as the psychiatrist understands and uses the term. The average physician thinks of the hysterical woman as thin and scrawny but she may be stout, well proportioned, beautiful, calm, or "perfectly sensible." One of the best hysterical shows I ever saw was put on by a young woman weighing 250 pounds.

Hysteria is thought of as largely a disease of girls and women, but any amount of the disability can be found in men. I once saw manifestations of it in a man who, in his youth, was one of the country's most powerful and scrappy hockey players! As Dr. Brosin once said, during World War II he saw in a month more hysteria than he now sees in a year in his office. One does not expect to see hysteria in the aged. When one suspects that certain symptoms in a middle-aged person are hysterical it is helpful to inquire and learn of episodes, probably hysterical, that came in the earlier years of the person's life.

Women are said to get hysteria from boredom and lack of proper emotional outlets. Tremendous epidemics of violent hysteria are said from time to time to attack the East Indian women who live out their lives shut up in a Rajah's harem. Many persons use hysteria to escape from an unpleasant situation or to punish someone; hence whenever one sees hysteria it is well to look around to see who is being punished or hurt. It may be a mother to whom the girl seems devoted but who once outraged her in some way.

Hysterical indifference. One sign of a psychopathic personality in many hysterical patients is their apparent indifference to the disease that is wrecking life for them. They may go on contentedly with it even after they have been assured that if they were to make an effort they could get well. I remember a young woman who, apparently to punish her mother for having borne her illegitimately, remained a chronic invalid for most of her life, from the time she discovered the facts about her conception until the mother died. Then she got well. During those twenty years the girl had chances to marry. She seemed to be somewhat in love with a few men and very anxious to have a sexual life, but she would not give up what almost certainly was a severe form of hysteria.

What was happening when the first attack came? Usually it is helpful to find out what the circumstances were when the symptoms first appeared. Thus, one may learn that there was a death in the family or a family row or a broken engagement or an impending divorce. Although at the moment when an attack of hysteria comes a woman may seem to be happy and at peace and without any disturbing thoughts, investigation will often show that for some time she had been under great strain. When told that her trouble is of nervous origin a woman may say, "But it can't be, because when I took sick I was at a party having a grand time." I used to be puzzled over this type of happening until I saw enough cases to realize that if the trigger gets set fine by some strain it does not take much to set it off. It will often then seem to go off by itself. For instance, suddenly one afternoon a nervous bloater went into an attack of vomiting and bloating such as she had been experiencing for twenty-five years. Her basic strain was life with a dipsomanic husband. She protested that on this occasion when I saw her she had been happily shopping with her mother, not thinking about the husband, 500 miles away, who had been on the wagon for some time. The instructive point about this case was that after all her years of almost constant ill health, she quickly recovered when the husband died and freed her from anxiety. She then went into business and was successful at it. She could never have run a shop before that.

On the importance of diagnosing hysteria from the history and the appearance of the patient. It is unfortunate that today even in the offices of some neurologists, there is a tendency to diagnose hysteria by exclusion. Actually, in many cases, the best evidence available to rule out a supposed physical injury is to be found in the history. For instance, a young man, while scuffling with a friend, felt a pain in his neck. If he had been an ordinary college student he would have done nothing about it, but since he came of a family of wealthy and patho- logic worriers, he went to his doctor. The fact that he walked to the doctor's office is good evidence that he did not have a broken neck. Unfortunately, on the basis of a roentgenologist's misinterpretation of a congenital anomaly, namely, two fused cervical vertebrae, a broken neck was diagnosed and the boy was put into casts and collars and braces and kept for many months in bed. Then came World War II, and he decided to do his bit. Accordingly he got up out of bed, joined the Marines, and served with them throughout the Pacific campaign! At no time was he ill. Certainly that does not sound like the doings of a man with a broken neck!

On his return home he again felt some pain in his neck, and, again, he fell into the hands of his pessimistic family physician who promptly put him back to bed and for months kept him there in a collar and a cast! A few years later, when he came to see me, he was weak, apathetic, and in a wheel chair. He had an expressionless face and a monotonous voice, and he held his neck stiffly. It seemed to me then that *from the history alone* I could rule out a broken neck and could diagnose hys- teria. I probably was right because after half an hour of exhortation I had him out of the wheel chair and his braces, and walking about. For a few days he clung to a cane but then I got this away from him. In this case one could think of a slipped cervical disc, but I think my col- leagues, the neurologists and orthopedists and nerve surgeons who saw him, were wise in not wanting to operate and look for one. The sad thing about this man was that he seemed to prefer his doctor's pessimism to *my* optimism. His wife also kept saying, "But if he hasn't a broken neck, why did good consultants say he had?" She acted as if she did not like my diagnosis and efforts to cure. I suspect that by now his old doctor has him back in a cast.

In many cases it is very helpful to learn that the accident that was supposed to cause a serious syndrome was a minor one which *caused no immediate disability*. For instance, rising up in the kitchen one day, a young woman bumped her head on a cupboard door, as all of us have done more than once. *A few weeks later* she broke down nervously and for weeks was in a hospital being studied by able neurologists who kept searching for signs of a blood clot. They could have saved themselves the trouble if they had only insisted that the accident was a minor one and the symptoms had come too late. Also, if they had only talked to the girl's friends they could have learned that her trouble came when her mother had broken up her engagement to a young man and had sent him packing. This the girl would never admit to anyone, but she got well when she found a new beau.

As I said, often it is diagnostic enough that the symptoms came *some time after the accident* and especially when some lawyer suggested that compensation might be obtained. Good examples of this were found often in the Army where the soldier did not get his hysterical symptoms at the front; he got them later at the base hospital, where he was examined too thoroughly, and where he got ideas from the man in the next bed.

A typical case of compensation neurosis with hysteria. A beautiful example of all the disasters that can follow when the first physician consulted does not have the knowledge or the courage to diagnose hysteria and then refuse to examine further is to be found in the following case report. The patient was a rather beautiful but impassive unmarried woman of thirty-two. She walked into my office one day bent way over and looking back up in a typically hysterical way. Her story was that she had gone on an auto trip as the guest of friends. On a wet, slippery curve the automobile went off the road and turned slowly over on its side. The passengers got out unhurt, turned the machine back on its wheels, and drove on.

Two weeks later, after a good vacation, playing tennis and swimming, she returned home, and a friend, an attorney, said to her, "We might as well get some compensation for you out of the insurance company. It could pay for your vacation." The lawyer sent her to a roentgenologist to see if he could find any change in her bones that would support the claim. When the roentgenologist reported what he thought was a crack in a cervical vertebra, the girl became alarmed, and with this her neck and back became twisted. Several orthopedists then saw her, some on her side and some on the insurance company's side. She was hospitalized and examined from head to foot. Neurologists and internists were called in, and after long and expensive examinations she was put into a collar and later into a back brace. While in a hospital for weeks of physiotherapy she developed a limp due to pains and contractures in the muscles around one hip joint. All this time she was unable to work and barely able to dress herself.

As soon as I saw her and got her story I started explaining to her that she couldn't possibly have sustained a broken neck in the accident because the symptoms all came weeks later. I showed her the close relation between the development of the symptoms and the roentgenologic diagnosis of a cracked vertebra, and I told her that I knew that her contraction was a typically nervous one because I had seen it many times before. I eased the blow for her by saying that the situation was not all her fault, and that the whole thing had followed suggestions by others.

With this she straightened right up; she lost all of the remarkable contracture of the muscles of the neck and back, and she walked well again except for a slight limp. I tried hard to get her to give this up too but she would not let it go—she needed it. She explained that at home she had run up hospital bills, doctor bills, x-ray bills, and lawyer bills totaling about $2,500. She was only a secretary, and unless the insurance company paid these bills she would be on a spot. She just had to win her suit. I tried to get her to see that she would be better off back at work and well again, without the money, but I had no success. I do not know what happened to her when she got home.

Certainly this case shows beautifully the need for an immediate diagnosis of a neurosis before a huge debt has been run up. As the girl said, once the debt had been built up she had felt forced to sue. If the first orthopedist consulted had only taken a good history, or had recognized a hysterical contraction, and had then refused to go any further, or if then he had talked to her like a kindly father, all the mess might have been avoided. She or the insurance company might then have been willing to pay a hundred dollars or so for her examination and that would have been the end of it.

Hysteria often should be recognized at a glance. In many cases the physician should know in a moment that he is dealing with hysteria as when he finds an anesthesia that is not limited to any nerve distribution, or one which is dissociated from motor weakness, or which is not associated with any changes in the deep reflexes. The gag reflex is sometimes absent, but the abdominal reflexes are likely to be present, and there should be no Babinski reaction. The pupillary reflex to light should be present, and the sphincters of bladder and rectum should be behaving normally. There is no reaction of degeneration in the paralyzed muscles of the hysterical person. Typical are glove or sock or arm or leg anesthesias which do not follow nerve distributions.

An expert can often recognize a hysterical paralysis as the person tries to sit up or get off the bed. At times there is something a bit wrong with a hysterical hemiplegia in that a few muscles on the normal side of the body may be involved. This would not be the case with a hemiplegia of organic origin. Furthermore, in cases of hysteria all the muscles on the affected side are likely to be paralyzed while in organic disease some may escape.

It is said that one can tell a hysterical weakness of a leg by asking the patient to walk backward. A person with a true weakness will keep favoring the bad leg. The hysterical girl may get confused and use the bad leg well. Usually a supposedly paralyzed arm or hand or leg can be moved a bit and this will give the thing away.

A trick that Ross used was to take a flaccidly paralyzed arm and raise it up in the air. Then he would say, "Keep me from pulling it down," and the man would resist. Then Ross would let go and there the man would be, holding his arm up in the air. Even the man could see then that the muscles were not paralyzed. Of course, Ross had then to go on quickly and say that this did not mean that the man had been shamming, but that he was deceived by his feelings into thinking that his arm would not work. Now he could see that it could work.

The importance of a bad family history and past history. Oftentimes one can get a helpful history of psychopathy in the family, or, as I have said, a history of previous attacks of illness that probably were hysterical in nature. Perhaps the diagnosis of encephalitis was made at one time, but this will seem highly improbable because of the severity of the symptoms during the comatose state and the lack of any residue afterward. These patients tell of having to learn to walk and talk again, but later they show no sign of any injury to the nervous system. Some of them will tell of being "unconscious" for a day or two after a dental extraction or a minor accident or after giving birth to a child. Questioning will show that although the woman would not talk, she was conscious of what was going on about her.

An unhappy homosexual woman whose symptoms appeared to be hysterical in nature made me the surer of this when she told me that once on a journey she got to feeling lonely and something seemed to snap in her mind. She suddenly went dumb and could not answer people's questions. She walked around the corridors of her hotel with her eyes closed. She felt she was dying, and she began crying and laughing. Soon she recovered and was all right again.

TYPES OF HYSTERIA

Of late, psychiatrists have taken to speaking of *conversion hysteria* which, as the term implies, is a hysteria which comes when the person has some strain from which he can escape by going into a hysterical syndrome. Other patients are supposed to have an *anxiety hysteria*. It is doubtful if these terms are of much value. It would seem more important to note that in many cases hysteria comes in occasional episodes at intervals of months or years, while in other cases a hysterical syndrome will last for years, or until the person dies.

The fit or convulsion. In Latin countries one of the common manifestations of hysteria is a big convulsive attack. Summoned in haste, the physician will come into a room full of people, and there, on the bed or the floor, will be a young woman throwing herself about much as if she were trying to make it difficult for the several men who are holding her down. Once one has seen a number of these attacks one can recognize them at a glance, and there is no possibility of confusing them with an epileptic fit. With epilepsy the convulsive movements are more like big purposeless twitches and the patient looks very different, with a livid convulsed face. The hysterical fit usually lasts much longer than an epileptic one, and it may quiet down and flare up again. Rarely the girl will get up on her heels and her head with her back arched, and she may move her pelvis as if sexually excited. She may make noises in her throat but they are not like the epileptic's cry which comes at the beginning of the seizure. She will also maintain a good color and her face will probably not be convulsed. Her breathing will not be stertorous, her eyes will probably not be rolled up, and her pupils will be normal. It may be hard to see them because she will probably hold her eyes tightly shut. The epileptic in a fit is completely unconscious and cannot be waked, while the hysterical woman may respond to a sharp command or she may wake when the physician digs his thumbnail into her supra-orbital notch. Often after a moment she will go back to playing dead again. The hysterical person can come right out of a spell while the epileptic is likely to remain dull for a while after he wakes. Of course, some epileptics have curious halfway spells, but even these are different from hysterical attacks. The epileptic more often is a man, and he is likely to be surly and anxious to be left alone.

As I said before, in Mexico I could always stop a hysterical convulsion by listening to the heart. As I did this, I would get the family to clear the room of spectators. If, after quieting down, the girl tried to start up again I would say, "No, you've had enough," and she would subside without giving more trouble. These women never bit the tongue nor voided urine, and they rarely hurt themselves. As the fit passed, the woman might clown a bit or cry for a while.

The only type of hysterical spell that is hard to tell from an epileptic seizure is the one in which a girl, perhaps on entering the doctor's office, drops to the floor and twitches a bit and bats her eyelids. Rarely will she fall hard enough to hurt herself. She may grind her teeth but not as an epileptic does. In a few seconds she may come to and get up. She will not then show any sign of dullness, and she will not have a headache.

Usually the hysterical spell is precipitated by some annoyance or excitement and it is said that it never occurs in the absence of an audience. It rarely, if ever, wakes the woman out of sleep. I have seen much hysteria in men but I cannot remember ever having seen a man in a hysterical fit.

The pseudotrance or unconscious spell. Another type of hysterical spell is the one in which the patient "plays possum" or acts dead. Commonly a Latin woman will do this, perhaps to frighten a husband after they have had a quarrel or after they have been drinking. In such a spell the woman can be aroused either by a painful stimulus or by tickling of the soles of the feet. The only difficulty with these spells, from the point of view of the physician, is that the family is insistent on his bringing the woman to before he leaves the house. If it weren't for this he could just leave her alone and let her sleep off the spell.

The anesthesias. As every physician knows, the hysterical person sometimes complains of areas of anesthesia. These can usually be recognized in a minute because they do not correspond to any nervous or segmental distribution. There is the typical glove type of anesthesia of a hand, or a sock anesthesia of a foot, or anesthesia of an arm or leg or half the body. There may be a pantslike anesthesia from the waist down. Interesting is the anesthesia of only the front of the thigh, the patient apparently having forgotten the back!

As I have said, this anesthesia may be so marked that a long hat pin can be passed through the thigh. Worth remembering is the inability of many of the anesthetic and apparently paralyzed persons to stand tickling of the soles of the feet. Many a time I have tickled an apparently paralyzed girl until, in desperation, she suddenly pulled her foot out of my hand. With this, of course, she gave herself away.

In most cases of hemianesthesia there is likely to be some diminution of smell, vision, taste, and hearing on the bad side.

Sometimes the limits of an anesthetic area will not be sharp everywhere at the midline as they should be in organic disease. This happens especially around the crotch. According to Nielsen and Thompson the external genitalia may escape, perhaps because the patient cannot decide to which half of the body they belong! A hemianesthesia is said at times to involve, also, the mucous membranes of mouth, nose, and pharynx, but usually not the conjunctiva. Hysterical cutaneous anesthesia may include all types of sensation or it may be limited to the pain sensation.

According to Janet (1925), one can confuse a hysteric patient by telling her to say "yes" when she feels a touch or a prick and "no" when she does not. The hysterical person does not accidentally burn or cut the anesthetic hand.

Hyperesthetic areas. There may be hyperesthesias and hyperalgesias and so-called hysterogenic zones. Pressure in such an area in the left groin may start or stop a hysterical spell. Scratching of an area on the middle back near the spine may cause violent belching. I have seen this in the cases of several women.

The paralyses and contractures. The hysterical person can have all sorts of paralyses and contractures which may come on gradually or suddenly. Often the experienced physician can see in a moment that the trouble is hysterical, just from the way in which a paralyzed arm is held. The contracture is not of the type which results from the overcoming of weakened extensors by stronger flexors.

The commonest form of hysterical paralysis is a left-sided hemiplegia. It does not involve the face but it may take in some of the muscles of the neck. A marked twisting of the neck is seen occasionally. Spasticity from the start suggests hysteria. The "organic" paralyses are likely to go first through a flaccid stage. Very suggestive is the ability of the patient to move the paralyzed extremity a little. A curious trick of an occasional hysterical person is to contract a segment of one rectus abdominis muscle so as to produce a phantom tumor.

Astasia abasia. One of the most striking and amazing forms of hysteria is that in which a man with strong and well-coordinated leg muscles cannot stand or walk. Sometimes he can walk if he is helped by a man on each side. His difficulty is fear and lack of confidence in his legs and his balance. He is like a man who can walk a plank lying on the ground but could not walk it if it were a hundred feet up in the air.

Gaits. There are a number of strange gaits which hysterical persons assume. There are limps, shuffles, near-fallings, walks with the body twisted and bent, and a walk with one apparently paralyzed leg being dragged behind.

Pain. Pain is a common complaint of hysterical women. It can be in the back, the abdomen, the head, the cecum, or the ovaries. One must always suspect a pain which, after an operation or an injection of the part with procaine, moves over to the other side of the body. Today many pains are being recognized as probably psychic in origin, but it is hard to say if they can be called *hysterical*.

Difficulties in swallowing. There are types of hysterical dysphagia in which a person is afraid to attempt the swallowing of anything solid. Usually the patient is a woman who puts the food in her mouth and chews it but then has trouble starting it down her throat.

Disturbances of digestion and abdominal distresses. There is no doubt that many digestive disturbances and abdominal discomforts are psychic in origin but, again, as with the pains, it is hard to say if they can be called hysterical. Sometimes a distress may be hysterical and at other times not. For instance, anorexia nervosa with regurgitation might at times be called a hysterical syndrome, but sometimes it seems to be due to fatigue or a situational neurosis, or constitutional inadequacy, or a psychosis with the delusion that the food is poisoned or that Christ forbade the eating of it. The same things can be said of the regurgitation of food. Hysterical women have the faculty at times of passing material from the rectum up to the mouth. There appears to be a remarkable tendency to reverse peristalsis. See Alvarez: *Introduction to Gastroenterology,* and McLester, J. S.: J.A.M.A. *89:* 1019, 1927.

Hysterical bloating. In Chapter 18 there is a description of a hysterical type of bloating, sometimes associated with pain and vomiting. I have described another almost certainly hysterical and very rare syndrome (Alvarez, 1945), closely related to the bloating one, in which, in spells, the abdomen is boardlike and there are rhythmic labor-like pains.

Hysterical troubles of the eye. Many hysterical persons complain of either loss of vision or great photophobia. Usually the blindness is unilateral, on the side of a hemianesthesia, and it is not complete. Even when both eyes are "blind" the patient can usually see enough to get about, and he does not bump into things. One must always be suspicious of a sudden loss of vision in both eyes. I have seen it in women for a while postpartum. Often one can suspect a hysterical disturbance of vision when the patient is wearing heavy black glasses in the house where he does not need them. The pupillary reaction to light is normal, and examination of the retinas shows nothing wrong.

Common is the so-called tubular vision, with narrow fields. Usually the oculist who handles the perimeter becomes suspicious because the results of repeated tests are discordant, or the line as marked on the card tends to take a spiral shape. The person with tubular vision must see better than he thinks he does because he walks about comfortably. I once found bilateral tubular vision in a businessman who seemed to have no consciousness of it and no other sign of hysteria. He came to see me about some gallstones.

The ear. Hysterical deafness is seen often in soldiers, sometimes associated with blindness or mutism. It may be total or partial or unilateral. If unilateral, it may be on the side of a hemiplegia or hemianesthesia. It may be associated with anesthesia of the external auditory canal and the drum.

In recognizing hysterical deafness it helps to find normal responses of the labyrinth to heat and to whirling. That would tend to rule out an organic lesion. It may help to see if there is the normal psychogalvanic response to a loud sound. The patient may be deceived by the use of a stethoscope with the tube to the "good ear" blocked. Another method is to use an instrument which makes a terrible racket in the supposedly bad ear. If it is not deaf, the person will be likely to raise his voice in answering the physician's questions.

According to Rodenberger and Moore it is fairly easy to cure hysterically deaf soldiers with the help of a sodium amytal seance in which they tell about the terrifying experience which preceded the loss of hearing.

Aphonia. Hysterical whispering or loss of the voice is fairly common. It is said to be due at times to feelings of guilt. The patient may accept it and go on whispering for years. There may be a weakening of the adductors of the vocal cords with pharyngeal and laryngeal anesthesia. Many a hysterical whisperer has been cured, at least temporarily, with a little faradism applied to the outside of the larynx.

There is another hysterical type of speech defect in which the patient stops to take a breath between syllables.

Mutism. There may be a hysterical mutism, perhaps particularly in children and in soldiers. It is said that these persons can write, which shows that they are not aphasic.

Loss of smell. There is a rare type of anosmia in which the patient is unable to smell even an irritating substance, such as ammonia.

Loss of taste. The sense of smell and taste can be lost together. The loss of taste may be associated with analgesia and anesthesia of the tongue. I have seen loss of taste as the first symptom of a true depression. According to Hughlings Jackson, bilateral loss of taste is practically always hysterical.

Respiratory disturbances. The respiratory organs can be affected by hysteria with the production of a dry hacking cough, perhaps asthma, uneven breathing, or hiccup. One can sometimes tell that the hiccup is forced. Someone has suggested that an excellent way of diagnosing neuroses would be to get a spirogram from all suspected persons. The neurotic person's spirogram would probably be uneven.

Hysterical joints. Painful and lame joints are often seen in hysterical persons, especially after a slight injury. The most commonly affected joints are the hip, the elbow, and the knee. These joints may in time become stiff, and the nearby muscles may become sore. The joint and muscle senses may be lost. There may eventually be swelling of the joint.

Fever. There has been some argument as to whether there is a hysterical type of fever. I think there is. I remember a highly nervous bride who had a temperature of 106° F. on her wedding night. When she calmed down next day the temperature became normal. A woman's temperature went up to 102° F. when her father was operated on, and I have seen a Latin woman run a "fever" of 102° F. while being examined in the office. She admitted she had performed the stunt before. Certainly, a nervously produced hyperthermia is common; the question is, how often can one call it "hysterical?"

Pseudo-encephalitis. A number of women whom I have seen suffering from hysteria have told a story of a long-lasting attack of coma and fever, thought to be an attack of encephalitis. This seemed to me very doubtful because these women all recovered without any residue.

Fugues and amnesias. Some authorities have described hysterical fugues and amnesias.

Miscellaneous symptoms. Hysterical persons have many symptoms and, as I have said, it is hard to say how many of them should be called hysterical. Neurologists have listed a number of troubles such as unexplainable bleeding from the mouth or rectum. (I have seen a number of cases of this, all in women who were mentally odd.) There have been described also regurgitation or a nervous vomiting of food, gagging, the hyperventilation syndrome, the pseudo heart attacks such as I have described elsewhere in this book, marked aerophagia, globus, a sort of tetany, some types of palpitation, perhaps some types of headache, some tics, marked dermographia, a great desire to be operated on, some diarrheas, perhaps occupational cramps, some forms of lack of balance, or pseudo Ménière's disease, many forms of fainting, some types of flatulence, crisis-like attacks of abdominal pain, and some disturbances of the functions of the bladder and the sexual organs. Ross listed, also, somnambulism, double personality, certain types of delirium, and certain hallucinations.

Helpful points in a diagnosis. Hysteria is hard to recognize when it is added to the clinical picture of some organic disease. Sometimes one attack will be organic in origin and a subsequent one will be hysterical and due to fear.

Often one can suspect hysteria from the nervous makeup of the patient and perhaps of the family. One will suspect it because of certain events which just preceded an attack, and one will suspect it, or be sure of it, because of the nature of the syndrome. As I said before, in many cases the physician need hardly make any neurologic examination; a glance is enough. It is suggestive, I think, when the family notes that a contracture disappears during sleep, but some neurologists say this is not a sure sign. It will add to the physician's suspicions to find that the syndrome is getting the patient out of some unpleasant situation, or is causing inconvenience to some disliked person.

The cases which have puzzled me most have been those in which I quickly removed most of a contracture with a calm talk, but then was unable to get rid of a little residue. The question then was: Was this residue organic in nature or was it a bit of hysteria hung onto for the benefit of the industrial accident commission or the family, or for some saving of face? Often in such cases the expert neurologists whom I called in to help me also felt puzzled even after they had made all their tests.

There are a few tricks of diagnosis which may be useful. If one raises a hysterically paralyzed leg and then lets it go there may be an appreciable interval before it falls. There may also be a slight sense of resistance or of assistance as one handles the supposedly paralyzed limb.

Malingering. Occasionally the question arises, as in cases of war or compensation neurosis, is the patient malingering, or is he eking out hysteria with some faking? Fortunately, out-and-out malingering seems to be fairly rare, and the persons who do it are not quite right in the head. The malingerer can be suspected from his uneasiness and watchfulness during the examination. He is anxious and on the alert because he fears that his imposture will be detected. He is likely to overact and thus to give himself away. In compensation cases one suspects the patient when one finds him misrepresenting known facts about his accident. If he lies about these things, he will probably lie about his symptoms. He is not likely to be cooperative with the physician, but his distrust can be understood, especially when the physician is employed by an insurance company and is going to testify against him in court. Many persons may seem to be malingering when they are just following the common human custom of believing what they want to believe.

As can easily be imagined, it is a terrible thing to accuse a hysterical person of malingering, because it can greatly injure his ego and his attitude toward the medical profession.

THE HANDLING AND TREATMENT OF THE HYSTERICAL PERSON

The successful handling of the hysterical patient is an art some of which can be learned but much of which must be God-given. To have much skill in the game a man must be born with certain gifts. Certain men with a subtle power of command over their fellows can convince a paralytic woman she is no longer crippled and she will be cured. Others try the same method and are cursed for their pains. As Osler said, "The successful treatment of hysteria demands qualities possesed by few physicians." Ross used to say that if a man does not possess the skill he should not try to treat these people because when he has failed he has made it much harder for the next man to succeed.

Often a quack cures hysteria because he was born with the gift, or he has a great sureness in himself, or he comes along at the right time when the patient is tired of the illness and ready to get well, or he cures by some hocus-pocus, such as adjusting a vertebra, which does not bring any humiliation to the patient. It is wonderful what a "holy man," or a "layer on of hands" can do in the way of relieving hysterical symptoms.

One of my old teachers of medicine was an artist at curing hysterical persons. Thus, one day when a man was brought into the City Hospital with astasia abasia, unable to walk a step, Dr. J. O. Hirschfelder started telling him that three days later, on Saturday morning at 9 o'clock, he would walk again. Each day the professor kept promising the man this, and telling him that doctors and students were coming from all over the country to see the miracle. In the meantime the man was told repeatedly that his legs were all right and that he had only lost confidence in them. The situation at home that had led up to the "paralysis" was also talked over and suggestions made to ameliorate it. On Saturday morning, with much ceremony and suppressed excitement, a hundred students were gathered about the man's bed in the big ward. A little faradism was given to the legs, and then two interns picked the man up by his arms and walked him up and down while everyone applauded. Feeling very important, the man went home, walking as well as anyone.

One can see how, in this case, the so-called "atmosphere of cure" helped much. Mesmer had this idea when he had his apartment fixed up with luxurious hangings and subdued lights.

Often the doctor must present a cure in such a way that it can be accepted without humiliation. One must not do the work in such a way that the family will think the trouble was always psychic in origin. Then they will be angry and vituperative and the patient will be on a spot. While assuring the woman that the trouble must be a functional one, I keep telling her that what happened was that she lost confidence in the arm or leg and for a while lost the knack of using it. Now she will learn to use it again. If a woman has difficulty in walking I tell her the story of the man who can walk a plank when it is on the floor but could not walk it if it were stretched across a chasm.

Ross used to say, "Keep bolstering the patient's self-respect. Never leave the impression that you thought he or she was shamming." Ross would never remove a paralysis until he had found out why the patient had slipped into it, and what could be done about his psychic problem. If he did not help the patient with his psychic problem, the man would slip back again, or become depressed. For instance, a fine military aviator, when he at last broke down and developed a hysterical syndrome, had to be cured in such a way as not to be left with the devastating thought that he had been a quitter and a coward. It had to be made clear to him that his sensitive nervous system, unable to take the strain any more, had begun to play tricks on him.

As William James pointed out years ago, the reactions of the body to fear are very disturbing to the victim and can produce more fear. The type of soldier who, in battle, has no reactions in his body due to the outpouring of nervous hormones can easily be a brave man, while the other type of soldier who, under fire, gets palpitation, a dry mouth, nausea, retching, diarrhea, sweating, or a great impulse to urinate will be a sick man. Under such conditions it will be very hard for him to be brave.

After convincing a hysteric soldier that his brain and nerves were undamaged, Ross seldom had difficulty in getting the man to move a paralyzed limb. Ross would explain that no man could have undergone such awful experiences as the soldier had without feeling fear. Fear is a normal human reaction, and no discredit attaches to a man when he gets scared. All men get scared, and then their limbs are likely to shake. The important point is that, in this situation, some person's limbs shake until they give way. This giving way is likely to leave the man with the idea that he has become paralyzed. If, later, he were to discover that he was not paralyzed, then he could get up and walk again. Ross felt that the physician must keep on saying this sort of thing until the patient is using his legs normally. It is bad to stop in the middle of such a session of treatment and say, "Come back tomorrow," because the patient may then remain for a long time at the stage in which he was left.

In trying to restore the self-esteem of intelligent soldiers and aviators who had broken down under great strain, Ross used to say that a nation which consisted only of the physically tough might, like the ideal dictator state, become largely a nation of savages. The physically and nervously frail are often the most highly intelligent, sensitive, imaginative, and inventive people in a country. They are so badly needed in the world that they should not be allowed to go to war. Even in World War II some inconceivably stupid brass hats wanted to send gifted physicists and instrument makers and inventors into the fox holes. One such man, put to work inventing or improving radar equipment or bombsights was worth 100,000 men in the infantry! The very fact that a man is a splendid architect or musician commonly disqualifies him as a shock-trooper. In war there are many places back of the lines in which a delicately built and overly sensitive man can serve his country well.

A soldier may force himself to be brave but his autonomic nerves may make him too ill to go out on another mission. Thus, Fetterman described the case of a gunner on a bombing plane who lost his nerve after having been wounded several times. He insisted on going back over Germany with his buddies but each time, before starting, he would become so ill with nausea, abdominal pain, and diarrhea that he would have to be left behind.

Most of the bravest men I have known were without fear, evidently because they were stolid persons without much capacity for any emotion. Their internal organs did not react to fear. Many, also, did not have the ordinary instincts of self-preservation. Thus, I know mountain climbers who, in the depth of winter, love to go alone into the Sierras, where, in case of an accident, they would perish miserably.

Ross disapproved of curing hysteria with faradic electricity because he so wanted the patient to know that, through an understanding of his illness, he had cured himself. Then, if, as might easily happen, he were to slump again some day, he would not have to go back to the doctor for more electricity: He could again cure himself.

Ross used to treat soldiers suffering from mutism by teaching them, first, to whisper the sounds of P and T. Then he got them to whisper "pack," "packed," and "put"; then the patient was told to put more sound into these whispers, and soon he'd be talking.

Naturally, in puzzling cases the physician should not attempt psychotherapy until a competent neurologist has studied the patient carefully, and has decided that he can rule out a brain tumor, multiple sclerosis, and other "organic" causes of the symptoms. It would be most embarrassing to a physician to start psychotherapy and then to have to admit that the disease was grossly organic. One of the most important things a neurologist can sometimes do for a clinician is to answer his question, "How much of this syndrome is hysterical and how much is organic?"

An interesting point about the hysterical person is that some day he is likely to get well either by himself or after the laying on of hands or the taking of some herb tea. A "blind man" will suddenly announce that he can see, perhaps after a chiropractic "adjustment." I suspect that this cure comes when the person no longer needs his hysteria or perhaps has tired of it.

More on hysteria will be found in the several sections on the neuroses as they are met with in the specialties.

CHAPTER 17

The Headaches

H EADACHE IS ONE OF THE commonest of the afflictions of nervous persons. It should be differentiated from pains in the head or face such as come with an acutely inflamed paranasal sinus, an ulcerated tooth, tic douloureux, or, perhaps, a small stroke. Headaches may be mild or severe, dull or splitting, or steady or throbbing. There may be feelings of constriction around the skull, or of internal pressure, or of boring or burning, or of a spike being driven into the head.

It should be noted that some persons are much inclined to headache, while others never have any, no matter what happens to them. In the first group the ache may often be an equivalent or manifestation of fatigue, nervousness, tension, annoyance, hunger, lack of coffee, worry, or boredom. Headachey persons probably inherit their tendency from some headachey ancestor. Women are more likely to be headachey than men, or they are more likely to be prostrated and invalided by their distress. The man takes some aspirin and keeps at his work.

For details as to headache the student should turn to Harold Wolff's great book on the subject or to my articles in Oxford Medicine.

Types of headache. The commonest types of headache are those due to nervousness and nervous tension, fatigue, being in a closed room, going without breakfast and coffee, getting constipated or having indigestion, taking too much alcohol the night before, or using the eyes too much. Headaches can come, also, at the beginning of an infectious disease, with fever, or at the beginning of menstruation. There is a constant type of headache due apparently to nervous tension. There is the morning headache of high blood pressure, the throbbing headache of migraine, and the dull headache of food allergy. There are severe headaches due to brain tumor and syphilitic periostitis. The headache of a sinusitis is often more a pain in the face. Trigeminal neuralgia, the neuralgia due to a putrescent tooth pulp, and the atypical neuralgias of the aged are more pains than aches.

A common type of headache is the one which arises, apparently, in the muscles at the back of the neck. Researches by Harold Wolff indicate that a high percentage of headaches are produced by tension in the muscles *outside the skull.*

With the ordinary types of headache that afflict millions of persons, the physician does not expect to find any cause besides the inborn predisposition and the strain of life.

The nervous tension headache. Many headaches are doubtless due to marked nervous tension which causes contraction of the muscles either in the forehead or around the back of the neck. This is a headache that is often relieved when the person goes on a vacation. The man in the street doubtless senses that headaches are due to nervous tension when he speaks of an obnoxious person as "a pain in the neck." Many a headache of this type disappears when the patient takes a journey to consult a specialist. The fact that such relief came can be very helpful diagnostically.

Constipation headache. Most persons think that a constipation headache is due to the absorption of toxins from feces in the colon, but this can hardly be the case because in all but a very few cases the ache disappears within a minute after the rectum is emptied. This fact means that the ache must be produced in a mechanical way; the feces pressing on nerves in the rectum which affect the brain. Occasionally the pressure in the rectum serves as a trigger to set off a migrainous type of headache.

Allergic headaches. Some headaches in allergic persons are due to the eating of some food to which the person is sensitive. With this headache may go considerable lethargy and mental dullness, and in serious cases, even symptoms of slight meningeal irritation such as a jab of pain on coughing.

Hypertension headache. According to Wolff, the hypertension headache is probably due to the distention of blood vessels just as is the migrainous headache. Injections of ergotamine can help in some cases. In other cases it helps to sleep with the head of the bed much raised. The severity of the headache is not correlated with the height of the blood pressure, and the distress may be entirely absent in cases of rapidly increasing pressure such as is noted in cases of malignant hypertension.

Nuchal headache. A nuchal headache can sometimes be helped by physiotherapy. It is often made much worse by nervous tension. Migrainous headaches can start in the back of the neck. Some writers think that this type of pain is related to fibrositis, but others deny it. Certainly, as Hench says, innumerable persons have much cervical arthritis without ever having a headache. Even when they are suffering much from a wryneck and sore cervical muscles they will not have any headache.

Long-lasting, constant headache. A most refractory type of headache is the constant one which persists day and night for years without let-up. Sometimes such a headache will begin intermittently and later become constant. Usually the patient is young, but occasionally one sees this type of headache in older persons.

When a patient comes with a constant headache I never expect to find any physical cause or any effective treatment. Some of the patients are definitely neurotic but others do not seem to be abnormal in any way. Perhaps a constant headache is like a constant ache in the abdominal wall or loin; we know that that is almost always of psychic origin. The cause may be a poor nervous inheritance.

Histaminic headache or facial pain. Horton has described and studied for years a type of facial pain which is an entity. This pain almost always comes in one cheek and with it there is watering and congestion of the eye on that side together with stuffiness of the nose on that side, and an extra amount of secretion in it. The pain may be severe. It often comes around 4 o'clock in the morning, and then it may last from one to three hours. Often the disease is demoralizing because of the severity of the distress. There are no gastro-intestinal symptoms. An attack can be brought on in a few minutes by a subcutaneous injection of 0.1 to 0.2 mg. of histamine. The patients can usually be relieved by a desensitization to histamine.

There are cases in which an injection of histamine will bring on an attack of migraine, and there are some cases in which a headache has some characteristics of a histaminic headache and some of a migrainous headache. In addition, there may be allergic factors.

Headaches due to infection and fever. As everyone knows, many persons have a headache when they are coming down with some respiratory or other infection. It appears to be due to a stretching of intracranial arteries.

Trifacial neuralgia, or tic douloureux. This is a severe affliction in which there are sharp and flashing pains which come in paroxysms lasting half a minute or so. The pain is limited to the distribution of the fifth cranial nerve or one of its branches *on one side*. It is often precipitated by talking, chewing, or touching the face. There may be trigger zones where a touch will start the pain. The patient converses with his lips as immobile as possible so as to avoid starting a pain. The disease appears usually in persons past middle age. Unfortunately these patients usually get all their teeth removed on the affected side. Relief can be obtained either from an alcohol injection of the nerve or by the operative removal of the sensory root of the ganglion.

Atypical facial pains. There are a number of atypical neuralgias or pains in the face, usually seen in old arteriosclerotics or in psycho-neurotic or psychotic patients. It seems probable that in some cases the lesion is an arteriosclerotic one in the brain, and then no amount of local treatment can do any good. Occasionally a violent neuralgia comes when a dental pulp has died under a filling. The application of heat to the tooth will cause gas to expand and this will bring jabs of unbearable pain; the application of cold may bring some relief. These facial pains have been studied by Fay and by Glaser.

Headache due to trouble with the eyes. Enthusiasts used to claim that most headaches were due to eyestrain, but this is not generally believed today. Perhaps one reason is that nowadays most persons who need glasses get them and wear them. Errors of refraction or mus-cle imbalance may occasionally be the cause of headache. One would then expect the headache to come at the end of the day or after a day in which much close eye work was done. One would not expect to find such headache due to errors of refraction in the short-sighted because they cannot strain their muscles of accommodation. It is significant that many persons with tremendous refractive errors and marked muscular imbalance never have a headache. Evidently in those cases in which headache comes there must be an added factor of hypersensitiveness or a tendency to headache.

Headache may come, of course, with glaucoma, iritis, or uveitis.

Facial pain due to disease in the sinuses. With all puzzling facial pains a good nose specialist should examine the sinuses. If sinusitis is present, pain is likely to come only with an acute exacerbation of the inflammation. A person who has suffered from sinusitis can quickly tell whether a hurt in his head is due to a sinusitis or an ordinary head-ache. There is a decided difference in the feeling.

The let-down headache. There is a type of headache which comes when a strain lets up. A nurse may get it on her day off, a minister may get it Monday morning, many persons get it Saturday noon, and some get it if they sleep late on Sunday. Some of the headaches come in migrainous persons, and apparently are equivalents of migraine.

Some can be relieved by an injection of gynergen. I have known migrainous physicians who, during World War II, had much headache when they were stationed in a hospital where there wasn't much to do. They got well as soon as a big batch of patients came in.

Headache due to a brain tumor. The headache of brain tumor does not seem necessarily to be due to an increase in intracranial pressure. According to Wolff it is steady and dull. It is seldom throbbing. It is usually intermittent but it can be constant. Sometimes it is severe, but rarely is it as intense as that of a bad migraine. It can usually be relieved by the taking of aspirin or the putting on of a cold compress. It rarely interferes with sleep. It is aggravated by coughing or sneezing or straining at stool, and sometimes it is worse if the patient stands. It may be made much worse by a bad cold. It may wake the patient in the morning. When not severe, it is not likely to be accompanied by nausea.

Unusual and rare headaches. The headache of the cerebral form of malaria can be very severe. Some forms of heart disease are associated with headache. Polycythemia vera sometimes causes a headache which may be due to too great a fullness of the arteries of the brain. Periarteritis nodosa may cause a pain felt in a small area in a temple. The examiner may then be able to palpate the tender nodular vessels. There is a rare form of patchy inflammation of the temporal artery, associated with fever and prostration.

Epileptics often have a headache after an attack. Headache can be produced by alkalosis during an old-fashioned Sippy treatment for ulcer. Severe headache can be due to infection of some ganglion with the virus of herpes. Headache can follow anesthesia, and it can be produced by vasodilators. Diabetics sometimes suffer from headache.

Some points in the diagnosis of headache. A headache that is relieved by a tablet of aspirin is mild. It is mild, also, if it permits the person to sleep. The clinician should know if the person has two or three types of headache. One due to fatigue can be relieved by aspirin; a migrainous headache may be untouched by aspirin but relieved by gynergen; a menstrual headache may come with the period, and a histaminic headache may come at 4 in the morning. An allergic headache will come after eating some food.

The fact that one can relieve a headache with an injection of gynergen or DHE 45 is generally a sign that it is of migrainous origin. In trying to diagnose migraine it is always helpful to find that the person, usually a woman, has a distinctive migrainous personality and build. It is helpful, also, to find that in childhood the patient suffered from attacks of bilious or cyclic vomiting. A scintillating scotoma, with bright zig-zag "fortification figures," coming just before a headache, is typical of migraine. It is helpful, also, to get a family history of migraine. Often most helpful of all is to see the patient in an attack of migraine, utterly miserable, and fishy-eyed. A migrainous headache is often throbbing.

An acute sinusitis can be identified in a moment by looking at the patient's handkerchief full of pus. There may also be tenderness of the cheek.

In some cases it helps to find that some relatives suffer from a convulsive disorder, and then it may be very helpful to find that the person has decided dysrhythmia in the electroencephalogram. In all puzzling cases of headache stereoscopic roentgenograms of the skull should be obtained. The hyperostoses of the frontal bones which are seen in many roentgenograms are usually harmless. Similarly, no significance need usually be attached to calcification of the falx or of the pineal body, or of the choroid plexuses. Sometimes the roentgenogram shows calcification of the internal carotid arteries, and this is significant. Small changes in the sella turcica in older persons can usually be ignored. Increased density of the shadows of the nasal sinuses can be ignored if there is no pus in the nose.

It is always well to look into the backgrounds of the eyes where rarely one can find a choked disc or the changes that go with severe hypertension, nephritis, or diabetes. The ocular tension must be estimated in order to rule out glaucoma.

Sometimes the otolaryngologist will cocainize the sphenopalatine ganglion, or he may shrink a nasal spur, or wash out a sinus to see if that helps.

Treatment. The treatment of headache naturally depends on the cause. Migraine is discussed later in the chapter. The histaminic headache can be much helped by a slow daily desensitization of the patient to histamine. I know of no treatment that does any good in cases of constant headache.

For the ordinary headache aspirin appears to be as good a drug as any. Measurements of the threshhold for pain have shown that aspirin is about as effective as phenacetin, acetanilid, antipyrine, amidopyrin, sodium salicylate, or alcohol. It does not seem to help to combine two or more of these drugs, and it does not help to increase the dose. It may help to add ½ grain of codeine to aspirin or one of the other drugs of its type. Fortunately, codeine very rarely produces a habit. If one wants more relief one has to go to the group of morphine, dilaudid, demerol, and methadon, but this is to invite disaster.

There are several proprietary headache remedies on the market, but an analysis usually reveals a combination of aspirin and phenacetin. Cibalgine is a useful combination of pyramidon and dial. It must be remembered that in rare cases pyramidon will produce a fatal agranulocytosis.

In cases of puzzling headache it is well for the physician to show the patient how to look for an allergic cause. I have described the technic in Chapter 18 in the section on food allergy.

Constipation may have to be combated. An oculist should check the eyes. Many a patient could be helped most by a rest. The teeth should be roentgenographed, and badly abscessed ones should be removed. A dead pulp may be hard to recognize. It can produce unbearable facial pain made worse by eating.

In cases of severe morning headache due to hypertension it may help to sleep with the head of the bed raised a foot and a half or more.

In some cases of muscular headache, results have been obtained by injecting into the tense tissues a solution of procaine or some similar anesthetizing drug. Nuchal headache may be relieved by massage of the back of the neck and by diathermy.

In cases of post-traumatic headache an able neurologist and a brain surgeon should get together and decide if there is any use in operating. In some cases of headache with dysrhythmia in the electroencephalogram, dilantin should be tried. The dosage can be 1½ grains three times a day. Some neurologists combine this with ½ grain of mebaral.

I know of no treatment which will help an arteriosclerotic type of facial pain. An occasional headache is relieved by shrinking or removing a septal spur that was impinging on the nasal wall.

MIGRAINE AS A CAUSE OF NEUROSES

Migraine is such a common complaint of educated persons, and a tendency to it explains so much of the illness that is seen in them that every physician should know the disease well. He must constantly be on the watch for it because so many of the sufferers, when in a doctor's office, fail to mention their sick headaches. They talk only about indigestion, fatigue, or frequent illnesses. Then if, as usually happens, no organic disease is found, the physician will not know what the trouble is.

The need for recognizing the migrainous person at a glance. Every good internist ought to be able to recognize the migrainous woman the minute she walks quickly into his office. Perhaps she starts blinking at the light coming from the window, and he must pull down the shade for her. Usually she is short in stature; she is well and trimly built, and well dressed. She is obviously intelligent, wide awake, alert, quick in her thought and her movements, with bright eyes and social attractiveness. As she grows into her sixties, she often maintains this attractiveness, and she rarely puts on weight.

On noting this type of person the physician should ask if she ever had unilateral or sick headaches. Sometimes she will say, "I had them when I was in my twenties, but now they seldom come, and they are not my trouble." I have talked to many a woman who could remember having had in her lifetime only two or three sick headaches, but she was so typically migrainous that I could understand why she had been ailing all her days. Such persons sometimes have migrainous equivalents such as dizzy spells or attacks of vomiting or abdominal pain.

It helps much to ask and to learn that in childhood the person used to be sent home from school because of "bilious vomiting spells." Perhaps a doctor diagnosed cyclic vomiting, which I feel sure is an early manifestation of the migrainous constitution. It helps to know that others in the family have migraine. The knowledge that a woman is migrainous is very helpful in understanding her lifetime of illness. It explains why she has always been rather frail and subject to sudden and devastating attacks of fatigue. It explains a tendency to ill health with perhaps "dizziness," a sore bowel, and backache. It explains why a woman who has had so much illness has no demonstrable organic disease, and it explains why, perhaps, she is either childless or has only one or two children. On asking, one will usually learn that the bearing and rearing of her first child were so hard on her that she and her husband decided she had better not have any more.

The characteristics of the headaches. If a physician depends for his diagnosis of migraine only on the description of the attacks, he will often be confused; in many cases the migrainous headache is atypical. It may be on both sides of the head or it may start in the back of the neck. Often there is no scotoma and no vomiting. Confusing, also, may be the fact that the woman has other headaches due to fatigue or to getting her breakfast and coffee late, or to menstruating. It helps to unscramble the story so as to identify these several types of distress in the head. It helps much to learn that the worst type of headache comes in a typically migrainous way, after fatigue, excitement, or some disturbing experience.

Often the patient will say that when a headache starts she hopes it will be a mild one that will be relieved by breakfast or a cup of coffee or a dose of aspirin, but after a while the head begins to throb, and then she knows she is in for serious trouble. Sometimes she can tell that a true migraine is coming by sitting and bending over so as to get her head low between her knees. Then, if it throbs, she knows she has "the real thing."

The physician cannot depend for his diagnosis on the history of a scotoma because only one patient in three or four has one. The typical scotoma *comes before the headache,* and is associated with blurring of vision and a bright zig-zag line that shimmers. Many migrainous women say they see bright spots during the headache but I am not sure that these manifestations are diagnostic.

There are some persons, usually men, who have a typical scintillating scotoma without any subsequent headache. This fact, when established, is important because it shows that the person has the migrainous constitution. The doctor should know well that headache is only one manifestation of migraine; in many cases it is a minor one, and what bothers the patient most is her lack of stamina and her great tendency to get tired.

The migrainous personality. It is remarkable that migrainous women have not only a certain type of body but also a certain type of temperament. Commonly, the woman suffers from great sensitiveness to sounds, light, smells, pains, and discomforts. She cannot stand much gabble of conversation about her, and she cannot stand a crowd. She is usually a poor traveler and often a poor sleeper. She cannot shop long or look around long in a museum. Next to this great sensitiveness as a source of distress is the great tendency to fatigue. The woman tires suddenly, and then she may be "flattened" and have to go to bed. To keep going well every day she usually needs a midday nap.

Migrainous people are perfectionists who like to work fast and accurately and perhaps to plan for several things at a time. They get tense figuring what they will do next. Everything out of the ordinary routine is likely to upset them and bring on a headache. The migrainous woman often overworks because she wants her house to be spotlessly clean and run just so. Because her relatives have learned greatly to respect her ability and judgment and skill in getting things done, they all go to her with their problems and sorrows, and these burdens often help to wear her down. If she is to give a dinner party, she has her table set by noon, and perhaps by the time the guests arrive she is too sick to see them. She can never promise to be anywhere at a certain time, because a headache may suddenly strike her down. Often she hides the fact that she has her spells because she is so ashamed of them. She hates to be so unreliable with appointments and dinner engagements.

If the physician knows from the start that a certain woman is migrainous, then when the results of her tests are negative he will not be puzzled. He can say, "I expected that because few of you people with sick headaches ever have any organic disease." Furthermore, he will know why the woman has been sickly and ailing, and he will be prepared to draw out quickly all the essential details about her life and its tensions and problems. Knowing well the common faults and strains of the migrainous person, he can quickly find out the particular strains of the woman before him. Perhaps there is tension at home, or some marital dissatisfaction, or an effort to do too much for the community.

Highly important, also, is the physician's acquaintance with the woman's basic migraine, because, with this, if the examination should reveal gallstones or a myomatous uterus, he will not be enthusiastic about operating; he will know that removal of the gallbladder or the uterus will not make the patient over into a strong, well person. It would leave her with the same old fatigue, dizziness, and headaches. Such knowledge, if it were widely disseminated throughout the medical profession, could save thousands of these women from needless operations.

A highly important point, not yet recognized sufficiently by most internists, is that there is no sense in looking below the neck for the cause of migraine. I once made a study of 1,000 patients with migraine, and in only a very few cases did I find even a trigger mechanism in the form of disease in the abdomen. I can remember perhaps three women whose headaches were for a time helped by the removal of gallstones, and one who was relieved for a while by the removal of the appendix. Actually, migrainous persons seem to be largely immune to serious organic disease, and their blood pressure is usually normal.

Migraine in men. The man with migraine is usually over his headaches by the time he is thirty. Occasionally they will return in later years, but then it is due to the coming of much strain in life, or possibly to a thrombosis of a small blood vessel in the brain. In some cases I suspect migraine is particularly severe because of the cropping out of some hereditary psychopathy.

Warnings of an attack. Some persons can tell the evening before that they are going to get an attack. They may be unusually wide awake or talkative, or they may have a bad breath or a big appetite. Sometimes the spouse knows the signs, and can prophesy that an attack is on its way.

The nervous storm. The sick headache appears to be due to a storm which starts perhaps in the visual center at the back of the brain and then, in bad cases, spreads to the vagus center and on down into the abdomen. In the worst cases, it reverses peristalsis in the duodenum and stomach and causes bilious vomiting. The storm may spread also to the cervical sympathetic ganglions, and this causes some of the arteries supplying the surface of the brain to dilate. With this dilation the blood goes pounding through to produce a throbbing headache. Often the person suffers from chilly sensations and a fear of impending disaster.

The headache. A typically migrainous headache is usually so severe that it is not helped by the taking of aspirin or any other drug of similar analgesic power. It can often be relieved by morphine or dilaudid but such drugs should never be taken. During this type of headache the scalp often gets sensitive and an eye may hurt. All sensations are heightened. There is often photophobia, and noises pound in on the brain. The patient usually does not want to be touched or talked to. There may be repeated vomiting spells in which all that is brought up is some bile-stained fluid. The events that take place during the headache are not well remembered later. In a bad headache a woman may be unable to work for a day or two. Usually, she does not want to eat, or she is unable to eat. If food is put into the stomach it is likely to stay there or in the duodenum for hours. The finding of this stagnation during a roentgenologic examination sometimes leads to a wrong diagnosis, and in years past it led sometimes to the performance of a futile gastro-enterostomy. There may be frequent urination. There is usually a feeling of detachment from the world and from loved ones. There may be weakness of some muscles with poor control over them. In the worst cases the patient may be a bit disoriented and unable to speak clearly. A letter written during a headache may be full of mistakes.

In many cases, especially in men, there is a headache without nausea or vomiting or abdominal pain. Especially in later life, these headaches may disappear, leaving spells with only vomiting or nausea or abdominal distress: the so-called equivalents of migraine.

The diagnosis. The diagnosis of migraine can usually be made with certainty when a typically migrainous person describes spells which come typically, after fatigue or strain or annoyance. If before the spells there is a scintillating scotoma, I think there can be no doubt. A physician who knows migraine can make the diagnosis in a moment by just seeing the person in a spell, with dull eyes, utterly miserable and detached from the world. There is no other disease, except sea-sickness, which produces such a picture of dejection.

It is helpful to find that there is migraine in the family, and that in childhood the patient suffered from "cyclic vomiting," or that, as a girl, she used to come home from school because of vomiting. A woman with this story may say that she never was able to go to a school picnic or graduation because the anticipation and excitement kept her at home vomiting.

As I have said, it is important to find out if the migrainous woman has two or three types of headache. Often she has. It helps to know that aspirin will not touch the severe headache; it helps to know that this is throbbing, prostrating, and nauseating, and I think there can be no question as to its nature when gynergen or DHE 45 gives relief. There are atypical cases in which the diagnosis is difficult. The nature of a headache may be hard to determine when, as rarely happens, there is some extra disease present, such as gallstones. Then the physician should try to unscramble the two stories, one of migraine and the other of the abdominal disease.

Twilight spells. The migrainous woman sometimes has dark days in which she is a bit depressed, apathetic, dazed or confused, uncommunicative, and disconnected from the world. She may be utterly miserable during these times. The impression is that she is having a migrainous attack without the headache or nausea. She may go on with her work but she will pay little attention to the people around her.

Equivalents or atypical syndromes. Migrainous persons nearly always have peculiar symptoms of a functional type which are not necessarily equivalents of migraine, but are due to the nervousness and oversensitiveness. Especially in later life the migrainous woman or man is likely to have equivalents which can be deceiving. In the worst cases the patient gets operated on because she vomits for two or three days. The surgeon should have been warned by such facts as: (1) that the patient had many similar attacks before which cleared up quickly and left no sequelae; (2) that he or she was migrainous in temperament; (3) that there was no fever; (4) that there was no great pain; (5) that there was no rigidity of the abdominal wall; and (6) that there was no great leucocytosis. A count of 12,000 or 14,000 cells can be due purely to nervousness and pain. It could have helped, also, to find out that the attack followed an emotional storm. Perhaps, also, careful questioning would have shown that there was a little unilateral headache before the spell.

In the case of a bad vomiting spell a surgeon usually fears intestinal obstruction, but the patient's bowels keep moving, there is no typical bloating, and a scout film of the abdomen will show no segment of bowel filled with gas. In these cases the coming of abdominal pain has no relation to meals or anything else, except perhaps an emotional storm. Digestion often is good enough between the spells, and this tends to rule out a slight obstruction in the bowel.

It would appear that the feeling of giddiness or light-headedness or top-heaviness is more common in persons with migraine than in others. Some physicians believe that Ménière's disease, paroxysmal tachycardia, and some other nervous troubles are equivalents of migraine, but this has not been demonstrated conclusively. Such syndromes can easily afflict a migrainous person because of his or her great sensitiveness.

Some physicians think that migraine is just a form of allergy, but I am sure it is not. Many migrainous persons are allergic to one or more foods but this is what one would expect, because of their great sensitiveness. Allergy is just one of the triggers that can start a migrainous headache. The eating of chocolate often causes trouble. Another trigger in some cases is constipation, another is menstruation, and a rare one is eye strain. The oculist should look for muscular imbalance, and if there is a tendency to a squint he should try the effect of grinding in a prism or two.

A number of writers have claimed that migraine and epilepsy are related, but in 1,000 cases of migraine studied in recent years, I have found little evidence for this view. Several other students of the problem feel as I do. Certainly migraine and epilepsy attack two very different types of persons. The migrainous patients are bright and pleasant, while the epileptics are more likely to be dull and sullen. Furthermore, drugs such as phenobarbital, bromides, and dilantin, which usually help the epileptic, have no effect in lessening the number of the attacks of the migrainous. These drugs often have no effect on the frequency of the headaches, even when the patient has a dysrhythmic electroencephalogram.

Complicating factors. Some migrainous persons have a psychopathic inheritance, but this seems to be a coincidence. Psychopathy and migraine are both so common that often they should meet in the same person. When a migrainous person inherits a tendency to psychopathy, hypertension, or epilepsy, one would expect her to have a more severe type of migraine, and sometimes she does. Some women with migraine are constitutionally inadequate, and this extra defect adds greatly to their misery.

My feeling is strong that whenever a woman, especially past middle age, is having two or three migrainous headaches a week she has some extra factor that is making things worse. Usually she is just fretting and stewing and worrying too much, but she may have a psychopathic inheritance, or a severe hypertension, or she may be under great strain, or she may be using her brain foolishly and unwisely, or she may have had a little stroke.

Factors that can bring an attack. Several biochemists have tried to find something wrong with the body chemistry of migrainous persons, and especially of persons while they are suffering from a headache, but nothing definite has ever been found. There is some evidence to indicate that an excess of prolan from the pituitary gland will produce headaches. Certainly, the giving of pituitary extracts to migrainous women can start a headache. Occasionally, an injection of histamine will start a headache.

That the glands of internal secretion have something to do with bringing the attacks is suggested by the fact that most migrainous women are free from their headaches during pregnancy. A few are relieved at the menopause, and perhaps one in seven is better after ovariectomy. A curious finding is that the migrainous person who develops cirrhosis of the liver or hepatitis, especially with jaundice, will usually be freed of headaches for some months. Many physicians and laymen think that migraine is produced by disease of the liver but, actually, the coming of disease of the liver tends, for months, to stop the headaches.

Unfortunately, practically nothing is known about the microscopic pathology of migraine. Persons do not die of it and hence their brains are not studied at necropsy. I know of no adequate research done in this field of pathology.

Migraine represents a life-long tendency that is so built into the body and the personality of the patient that no one can ever hope to eradicate it completely with any treatment.

TREATMENT

There are two parts to the treatment of migraine: one, that of trying to keep the spells from coming so often, or at all; the other, that of aborting or shortening or making milder the attacks when they come.

Efforts to prevent attacks. I know of no drug that will lengthen the interval between spells even by one day. Many drugs have been advocated and I have listed most of them in an article in Gastroenterology for December, 1947. The fact that one sees an article or two about a drug and then never hears of it again suggests that the first favorable results were not duplicated later.

A few persons are helped by desensitization to histamine but it is hard to say whether the relief is due to the drug or to the rest secured while the person is at a medical center getting the treatment. Every so often one hears of a new "cure," but if one tries it on a half-dozen women it does not work.

I have tried dilantin in cases in which there was an epileptic inheritance and a dysrhythmia in the electroencephalogram, but so far I have not had much success. Still in severe cases I always have an electroencephalogram made.

Occasionally a person is made much better by being taught to leave alone some food to which she was sensitive. Chocolate is a common offender. Cutting down on the amount of water consumed may help, because dehydration can make attacks less severe.

A woman should for a while keep a record of happenings and strains and of foods eaten before spells so as to see if she can learn of any exciting causes or triggers. She should learn that if she gets tired and irritable a trigger may get set so fine that it can go off by itself. The plan should be to so live as to get the trigger set coarsely.

I often tell patients of the woman running a big office who had three migraines a week in spite of everything several able physicians could prescribe. Then she lay on a beach every day for two months and got well. Usually only rest seems to be able to set the trigger in the brain coarsely. I remember the prelate who had frequent headaches while he worked his way through college and divinity school and then up the ladder to success in a fine big church. About this time he got a pastor's assistant, and thenceforth until he was sixty he never had a headache. Then he was made a bishop, and moved to a big city where he had to work hard all day at tasks, many of which were uncongenial to him. With this he began again to have several migraines a month. As he said, he knew the one thing that would cure him, and that would be an easier job.

Every migrainous woman should try for better mental hygiene, with an earlier bedtime; good sleep, obtained with sedatives if necessary; shorter hours of work; less tension in it; the avoidance of conflicts and annoyance; less fussing and fretting and trying to have everything perfect; more acquiescence to things that cannot be changed; less responsibility outside the home and, very important, a nap in the afternoon. All these things can help greatly.

Oftentimes the husband can work a cure by avoiding doing something that distresses his wife, or by getting his mother out of the house and into a separate little apartment. When out somewhere, the husband should watch his wife for signs of fatigue, and when they come he should quickly get her home. He should not try to take her into crowds or noisy restaurants or night clubs, or to football games or New Year's Eve parties.

Some women may be the better for the expert fitting of glasses; others are better when they take an enema every day to control constipation.

One in seven can be relieved of headache by a hysterectomy or application of radium in the uterus, but since one in three is made worse by this castration it should never be done just with the idea of curing migraine. Many women do not lose their migraines with the menopause.

Treatment of the attack. There are two main things to be remembered in treating a migrainous headache: One is that anything, if it is to help, should be given quickly; later it may not work because the artery walls will be edematous and will not contract. The other is that after nausea has set in, it is of no use to take medicine by mouth;

it will not be absorbed. One must then give it either per rectum or sub-cutaneously or intramuscularly.

Some fortunate women can abort a headache by immediately taking a tablet or two of aspirin, and then lying down for a while. Others get relief by taking black coffee or a saline laxative or an enema. Some now take a couple of tablets of cafergot which is ergotamine plus caffeine. A few get relief by taking from 2 to 4 tablets, each containing 1 mg. of gynergen. Occasionally one hears of a woman who gets immediate relief by putting her head under a cold shower.

The surest relief comes from taking quickly a hypodermic injection of 1 cc. of a solution of gynergen. If this should cause much nausea or tingling or numbness in arms or legs, the patient should try either 0.5 cc. of the gynergen solution or 1 cc. of a solution of DHE 45, which is dihydroergotamine. This is much less toxic, but, also, not so effective. Some persons are delighted with it, and use it regularly. If an injection relieves for an hour, and then the headache starts to come back, another injection can be taken. Gynergen or cafergot should not be taken every day as a preventive measure; that might cause injury to the arteries.

Many physicians fear gynergen immoderately and will not let their patients use it, but I am sure they are mistaken. Incidentally many of these men now prescribe cafergot freely, which is not logical. There have been a very few cases of cancer of the liver in which many injections of gynergen a day, given to relieve itching, caused injury to arteries. But I know of hundreds of persons who have taken gynergen frequently for years and I know some who have taken it every day or every other day for many years without coming to grief. I have been prescribing the drug for twenty-five years without disaster, and hence I have no fear of it when used with any sense at all. I am afraid of cafergot because I fear some persons will take it three times a day, and that might cause trouble.

If a migrainous spell gets out of control, or if gynergen does not work and there is much vomiting, a good way of quieting the vomiting center in the brain is to insert in the rectum a suppository containing 3 grains of nembutal. Then the person should lie down in a quiet, darkened room to sleep off the spell. More such suppositories may be taken later if necessary. In very bad spells an intramuscular injection of 0.25 or 0.5 gm. of sodium amytal may help, or paraldehyde or chloral can be given per rectum. Only rarely should morphine, dilaudid, or demerol be given because thereby a habit can easily be started.

Dramamine in 50 mg. doses may stop nausea if it is given quickly enough. The drug can be a great boon to migrainous persons when they have to go on a journey.

In a few cases the breathing of pure oxygen for an hour or two will stop an attack. The patient can get it out of a doctor's basal metabolism machine, or a hospital anesthetist can give it. I know a few persons who get such perfect relief from oxygen that they have it piped from a tank in the basement to an aviator's mask at the side of their bed. Unfortunately, it is inconvenient to get the oxygen and the mask; the gas does not work for many persons, and in the case of some of those who are helped, the effect later wears off.

I have seen a few persons whose spells were relieved by the slow intravenous injection of from 20 to 50 mg. of nicotinic acid. They would stop the injection when the flush came. The intramuscular injection of the drug did not work so well.

THE PATIENT WHO HAS HAD A HEAD INJURY

As Woltman and others have pointed out, after a person has sustained a blow on the head it is often impossible to say how much of the disability or headache is due to the accident, how much to a constitutional tendency to neurosis or psychosis, and how much to a desire for compensation.

The wise neurologist will want particularly to know if the patient was normal nervously and a steady worker before the accident, and he will want to watch his attitude and his behavior as he goes through his examination. The more normal he was psychically before the accident the more probable it is that his symptoms are due to a hematoma or to the late results of concussion. One must remember that in the Army, hundreds of healthy men who got shot through the head, and who later recovered, did not complain afterward of headache or disability. It is said that among these men the incidence of a convulsive disorder was no higher than in the country at large. As I write this I am seeing a man who is working hard every day in spite of the fact that his skull contains slugs shot into him during a hold-up a few years ago. His only remaining difficulty is a remnant of a hemiplegia that followed the shooting.

A. E. Bennett (1946), in a good article on the psychiatry of head injuries, emphasized the need for combating neurosis *from the start*. If the syndrome, together with the temperament and behavior of the patient, suggests a neurosis, the physician should avoid running up a big bill for hospitalization and repeated examinations. These examinations alarm the patient; they tend to confirm him in the idea that he is seriously ill, and if he acquires a lot of big bills he may feel compelled to demand that some insurance company pay them.

An electroencephalogram may help if it shows signs of a localized injury to the surface of the brain. According to Bennett, shortly after the accident there may be random delta waves with disorganization of the alpha rhythm and epileptiform discharges.

Part V

*The Psychosomatic
Features of the
Several Specialties*

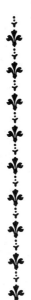

CHAPTER 18

*Neuroses and Functional
Diseases of the
Digestive Tract*

As everyone knows, there is a tremendous amount of indigestion
and abdominal discomfort which is functional in nature. Much is
due to emotion and fatigue, and much appears to be due to the inheritance of a sensitive nervous system or a peculiar digestive tract. A
stout, strong, insensitive man or woman is likely to be endowed with
a digestive tract which can handle without complaint any kind of
food and large amounts of it. Furthermore, in the cases of such persons the tract may be practically unaffected by emotion. It is of the
type seen in the murderer who can enjoy and digest his last breakfast,
when he knows that in three hours he will be hanged! An entirely different type of tract is that of the sensitive Irishman, a great admirer
of Lincoln, who one day found himself in Lincoln's old house in Springfield, Illinois, with the privilege of having lunch served on his hero's
old table. He was so overwhelmed with emotion that he could not
swallow a bite!

The wise clinician will remember that even when a patient has organic disease such as peptic ulcer or chronic ulcerative colitis, his main
difficulty may be a psychic one. In 1938, Rivers and Mendes Ferreira
concluded that one patient in four who complains of indigestion has a
functional trouble.

347

CASES IN WHICH THE PRESENCE OF A CARDIAC NEUROSIS HELPS THE GASTROENTEROLOGIST

The fact that a patient has a typical cardiac neurosis can often greatly help the gastroenterologist when he is puzzling over the nature of an abdominal discomfort. Since the autonomic nerves are playing tricks with the heart they are likely to be playing tricks, also, with the stomach and bowel. When one suspects the presence of a digestive neurosis it is helpful to learn that there are neurotic symptoms elsewhere in the body, as in the urinary bladder. The patient may be running to the toilet every fifteen minutes and passing perfectly clear urine. It helps, also, to learn that in the past the patient has had episodes that suggested an attack of hysteria or depression.

THE SYNDROME OF REVERSE PERISTALSIS

There are many persons, some highly nervous, who complain of symptoms, all suggesting a tendency to a reversal of the waves in the upper part of the digestive tract. These symptoms are regurgitation of food, repeated belchings, heartburn, water brash, occasional hiccups, sometimes nausea and vomiting, and a feeling as if waves were running back from the stomach to the pharynx. See the chapters on reverse peristalsis in Alvarez: *An Introduction to Gastroenterology.*

In many families there is a hereditary tendency to this sort of reversal of waves in the digestive tract, and in several generations there will be individuals who regurgitate, ruminate, suffer from heartburn, or vomit with ease.

A large meal which overdistends the stomach commonly causes waves to run off from it in both directions. Hence, after a banquet one will often note that a number of the men sitting nearby are burping and suffering from waves coming up. Strong emotion may start some regurgitators to vomiting. As one would expect from the gradient theory (Alvarez: *An Introduction to Gastroenterology*) reversal of peristalsis is more likely to appear when the person is constipated, or when a woman is pregnant, or menstruating, or when there is acute inflammation around the lower end of the ileum, as in cases of acute appendicitis. In cases of constipation one suspects that the reverse ripples are arising in the distended colon, because often the minute the plug of feces is removed by an enema, the nausea, distress in the esophagus, regurgitation, heartburn, or vomiting stops. In children, constipation can take away appetite, and the minute the fecal plug is removed, the child will want to eat.

The reversal of the gastric and intestinal currents can be exaggerated, also, by the giving of certain somewhat emetic drugs, such as digitalis, or by the eating of slightly emetic foods, such as cucumbers or cantaloupes. Reversal of waves can be produced by stimuli coming down the vagus nerves as from a brain tumor, or from the brain of a woman suffering a bad attack of migraine, or from the brain of a man having an epileptic equivalent.

The syndrome of reverse peristalsis can be marked in cases of hysteria, or it can be produced by a lesion of the bowel which serves as an ectopic focus for waves which run orad. If a physician fears the presence of intestinal obstruction it is a hopeful and reassuring sign if there are no symptoms of reverse peristalsis.

If one accepts, as the simplest and most helpful working theory, the idea of a polarized digestive tube with a gradient of forces down the stomach and another down the small bowel, then one must suspect that some persons were born with steep gradients and others with flattish or easily reversed ones. The ones with steep gradients are likely to have a perfect digestion, while those with flattish or easily reversed gradients should often suffer from the symptoms of reverse peristalsis. They will have most trouble when the gradients are flattened by fatigue or infection or emotion. Some persons can vomit very easily, while others vomit with the greatest difficulty.

Treatment. Persons with a tendency to reverse peristalsis should avoid constipation and the eating of foods such as fats and melons. Sometimes, when waves are coming up, the person can drive them down again by sipping water, as one does to cure hiccups; or he can eat some food, or in bad cases, he can take a laxative. In some cases fatigue, anger, overexertion, or work done bending over must be avoided.

BELCHING

I have noted in this book that air-gulping with belching of the explosive and long-repeated type is often an equivalent of a psychosis rather than a manifestation of indigestion. The person's digestion may be perfect.

Obviously, then, any treatment should be directed only toward helping the neurosis or mild psychosis. Perhaps fear must be combated and a bad habit must be fought against.

HEARTBURN AND ACID STOMACH

Heartburn is a burning or rending distress which is felt usually along the course of the esophagus, sometimes as far up as the pharynx. The easiest way in which to diagnose it is to ask the patient to take his hand and show where the distress is. Practically always he points to the epigastrium and then runs his hand up the sternum. If his hand remains over the epigastrium he has a different type of burning. That is a paresthesia in the skin. Much information as to the probable mechanism of heartburn can be found in my book, *An Introduction to Gastro-enterology,* and in my article on the subject (1944).

The distress appears to be due largely to the regurgitation of gastric juice into an esophagus which, for some reason, has become irritated and sore. Perhaps acid has come up into it and stayed there long enough to somewhat burn the mucosa. In most persons, just as in normal cats, acid gastric juice appears to be regurgitating often into the esophagus and then running down again, and usually this cannot be felt. But occasionally the regurgitation becomes painful, and with this the person may be in distress for days or weeks or months. Later the trouble will disappear, perhaps as suddenly as it came.

My impression is that the syndrome is practically always functional in nature, even when it is found associated with a peptic ulcer. Curiously, in these cases, when the ulcer symptoms are present there is no heartburn, and when the ulcer becomes quiescent the heartburn may return. It is interesting, also, that the heartburn is seldom relieved by the taking of food as hunger pain is. This would indicate that the mechanisms producing the two distresses are different. The treatment most likely to relieve the distress of heartburn is the washing out of the esophagus with a solution of sodium bicarbonate. As one would expect, a tablet is not so helpful. It is a puzzle why some persons suffer from heartburn even in the absence of free hydrochloric acid in the stomach.

There is a decided family tendency to heartburn. It is particularly common in the case of the Jewish people. An attack can be brought on by excitement, emotion, getting angry, having an "aggravation," or by the eating of certain foods, the drinking of certain liquors, or the smoking of too much tobacco. Many persons with heartburn have told me that when they got good and angry they were "on fire" for four or five days. But many an attack comes when the patient cannot see wherein he has sinned.

Treatment. The patient must keep a record to find what habits of living, thinking, eating, drinking, or smoking bring his attacks, and then he must reform.

REGURGITATION

Regurgitation is very different from vomiting in that usually there is neither nausea nor retching, and the stomach is not emptied. The food or fluid runs back into the mouth with ease, and without effort on the part of the patient. It comes up in mouthfuls or small amounts just as it does in the case of a baby who has taken too much milk. The process may go on for hours. Apparently it is due to reverse peristalsis in the stomach and esophagus, and the vomiting center in the brain has nothing to do with it. In vomiting, the stomach will be more or less emptied usually some time after a meal. Regurgitation commonly starts during a meal or right after it, and then mouthfuls keep coming up.

The syndrome is seen usually in women, but it appears also in quite a few nervous men. The tendency to it runs in families, and it is more than usually common in persons who have a psychopathic inheritance. (See Chapters 14 and 15 concerning the relatives of the psychotic and types of mildly psychotic persons.)

The symptom is often severe in the cases of girls who go on into an attack of anorexia nervosa. There are some persons who have a life-long predisposition to regurgitation. In some cases it starts up whenever the person gets tired, or when he or she gets angry or excited or comes under strain. In some cases the symptoms may be a part of hysteria.

Some persons who regurgitate say they do it because it is so distressing to keep the food down. As soon as they eat they begin to have a discomfort in the epigastrium. Some of these people are able to hold the food down, especially when they are dining out, but some seem unable to control the situation, no matter how much they wish to do so. No matter where they are, the food comes up. Some of these persons regurgitate more after eating fats or certain foods to which they may be allergically sensitive. Usually the bad regurgitator is a bit immature or even psychopathic. Sometimes regurgitation begins when a girl feels caught in a trap (see Chapter 8).

I can remember having seen only two women whose regurgitation was complicated by the presence of organic disease in the digestive tract. One had a duodenal ulcer and the other had gallstones. In these two cases some of the symptoms were removed by operation but the regurgitation went on. Regurgitation appears, then, to be practically 100 per cent functional in origin, and the surgeon should never operate with any hope of curing the disease.

The essential point in the diagnosis is that the patient is not vomiting, she is only regurgitating. To show how different the two symptoms are, a physician once told me that all his life he had *regurgitated* with the utmost ease. But occasionally, when sick from drinking too much whiskey, he had a terrible time trying to *vomit;* he could not retch.

Treatment. I am sorry to say I know of no good treatment for this condition. Some women learn to control it by will power, and some lose it when they become rested or happier, or when they get out of a miserable trap. I remember a nurse who eventually learned that the coming of regurgitation was always a sign that she had been too long on a hard case. It may help some regurgitators to keep free from constipation, and it helps a few to avoid certain foods like fats or spinach. I know of no drug that helps.

FUNCTIONAL TYPES OF VOMITING

True vomiting, with nausea and retching, can be produced, of course, by psychic stimuli. It may be caused by emotions both agreeable and distressing; it may be due to pain, and it can be produced reflexly from disease in almost any organ of the body. Some persons vomit under slight provocation and with great ease while others vomit rarely and with great difficulty.

According to Cabot, in the fine study he made of the subject, vomiting was seen commonly in cases of (1) toxemia of pregnancy; (2) acute dyspepsia—whatever that was; (3) alcoholism; (4) sea-sickness; (5) the onset of some infectious disease, and (6) postoperative "shock." *In the hospital,* during the period of the study, Cabot noted 2,126 cases of vomiting due to "gastric neurosis"; 1,819 cases due to acute appendicitis; 1,512 to heart disease; 309 to peptic ulcer; 209 to so-called gastritis; 167 to intestinal obstruction; 113 to gastric cancer; 45 to uremia, and 42 to tabes dorsalis. I found a history of vomiting common in the relatives of the psychotic (see Chapter 15).

In a given case, one can learn most about the cause of vomiting by taking a good history. For instance, one can often say right off that there is no pyloric obstruction, simply because the patient never vomits food; he vomits only bile-stained fluid. Incidentally, the vomiting of bile does not mean that there is anything wrong with the liver, as most persons assume; it means only that there has been reverse peristalsis in the upper part of the small bowel which has pushed intestinal contents back into the stomach. When a woman is vomiting bile-stained fluid one must always ask if she ever suffers from migrainous headaches. That is a common cause of the trouble.

Whenever a patient has definite pyloric obstruction he is likely to vomit large amounts of rancid food; he is likely to sleep poorly at night because of constant gastric peristalsis, and usually he loses much weight because there is so little absorption of food from the gastric mucosa. It helps to learn that some of the food noticed in the vomitus had been eaten from twelve to twenty-four hours previously. This does not always mean serious pyloric obstruction, but it suggests its presence.

Hysterical women often vomit violently and for long periods of time. Hysterical bloaters (see a section in this chapter) sometimes vomit for half a night. The patient with anorexia nervosa may vomit much but she is more likely to regurgitate. Some women vomit on the first day of menstruation.

As Woltman has pointed out, the so-called projectile vomiting of brain tumors is perhaps better described as sudden or unexpected vomiting, not preceded by nausea. In older persons the sudden coming of nausea, vomiting, and perhaps dizziness or loss of balance, especially if it is not associated with any sign of disease in the ear, is likely to be due to the thrombosis of a small intracranial artery.

In children, spells of so-called bilious or cyclic vomiting are usually equivalents of migraine. Often when one is puzzled as to the nature of a headache it helps greatly to find that when the patient was a child he or she sometimes came home from school because of vomiting, and then lay for hours in a sort of stupor or an apathetic or mentally inaccessible state. Children of this migrainous type may start vomiting if they are to go to graduation exercises or to a picnic, or if they are to start on a journey.

In some cases of vomiting it is helpful to know that the patient always produces it by sticking the finger down the throat. Then it may be found that he or she is doing this to get relief from a little gastric discomfort. In such cases there may not be much reverse peristalsis in the digestive tract.

Vomiting can occur with disease of the heart, kidneys, gallbladder, spleen, thyroid gland, ovaries, uterus, and suprarenal glands. As everyone knows, vomiting can be severe during pregnancy. As one would expect, the nervous or hysterical or constitutionally inadequate type of woman is more likely to have a hard time during pregnancy than is her strongly built, unemotional sister. Some nervous persons are likely to get to vomiting on the second day of a journey. Some are easily made sick by travel by car or ship or plane.

In the cases of sensitive persons, vomiting can be produced by eating when the individual is upset or tired or disgusted with the food. It is said that even a certain baseball hero will vomit if he eats when depressed over losing a close game. Some persons can vomit easily when startled or even overjoyed.

Vomiting can be brought on by much coughing as in cases of whooping cough or tuberculosis. When a person complains of morning vomiting one must ask about chronic alcoholism and must look for tuberculosis.

Persons highly allergic may vomit after eating some food to which they are sensitive.

Treatment. The treatment must depend on the cause. If there is marked pyloric obstruction the only sensible thing to do is to operate. If the cause is migraine, an intramuscular injection of a solution of gynergen or DHE 45, given at the very start, should give relief. Sometimes a rectal suppository of 3 grains of nembutal or an intramuscular injection of 0.25 or 0.5 gm. of sodium amytal will quiet the vomiting center and bring relief. Morphine is usually a poor drug to use because it tends to increase the irritability of the vomiting center.

Some nervous women and girls will stop vomiting only if they are liberated from some form of trap in which they are caught (see Chapter 8). They must, for a time, be gotten out of the home and into a hospital.

Some women can best help themselves by refusing to bring their food up the minute it distresses them. They must put up with some discomfort. They must not be like the woman who runs to urinate the moment she becomes conscious of urine in her bladder. They must break themselves of the habit of vomiting on slight provocation.

It might be well to try injections of DHE 45 or gynergen in cases of cyclic vomiting in which the child becomes apathetic and uncommunicative. It should be tried in cases in which a girl is often sent home from school because of vomiting.

Many very tired and nervous women will stop vomiting only if given a rest cure with plenty of sleep and freedom from strain and annoyance.

Dramamine (50 mg.) appears at present to be the best drug to use for the avoidance of motion sickness.

NAUSEA

Nausea is a most distressing symptom for which until recently we physicians had no good remedy. Studies in man and animals indicate that the symptom is often associated with changes in the activity of the duodenum or the upper jejunum. It is practically never complained of by patients with peptic ulcer. It is common when there is obstruction in the small bowel, and I have seen it as the first symptom of tumors of the small and large bowel.

Sometimes nausea comes in waves and this may mean that the patient is feeling actual waves of reverse peristalsis running up the bowel. The fact that in many cases a person who is suffering from nausea can suddenly get complete relief after a big burp, or one retch, suggests that with the running out of a big reverse wave, peristalsis in the stomach or bowel quiets down or starts running normally caudad again.

In many frail women nausea comes with fatigue or disgust. That nausea is due to disgust is indicated by the phrase, "you make me sick." Nausea can easily be produced by a bad smell. That the sensation can originate in the brain is indicated by many facts, such as that it can come in an attack of migraine, Ménière's disease, or motion sickness, or after a small stroke, or an attack of encephalitis, or when a woman mistakenly thinks she is pregnant, or when she gets the idea she has eaten dirty food. It can come with the stormy emotions resulting from the sudden break-up of a love affair. I have seen it come in sensitive men when the wife was pregnant! Nausea is a common complaint of the relatives of the psychotic, and this fact should often be remembered (see Chapter 15).

Persons who are overworking and very tense may wake at night and suffer with nausea for an hour or two. Nausea can be produced by emetics which act mainly on the vomiting center in the brain. I have seen persons suffering from chronic nausea which proved to be due to the taking of digitalis, or aminophylline, or to the chewing of too much tobacco. It can be produced by the intravenous injection of certain amino acids. At operations on man, it has been found that stimulation of the vagus nerves can cause nausea.

Nausea and even vomiting can be produced by pain, or especially by pain due to distention of a hollow organ. Nausea can also be a very distressing symptom of a failing heart. It can be severe after a large hemorrhage which has produced anemia of the brain. It can come suddenly in severe spells in cases of mountain sickness, even when the climber has been resting and is not cyanotic or dyspneic.

During the World Wars, soldiers became nauseated from fear or disgust. Some highly sensitive persons can be nauseated by unpleasant smells, or by disgust at the unattractive appearance of some food, or at the thought that they may have eaten spoiled food. A woman, once badly poisoned by the paste in a cream puff, always thereafter avoided going into a pastry shop because if she saw a cream puff she became ill. I have known women who suffered nausea following sexual intercourse with an unloved husband.

Curiously, the symptom can be helped or made much worse by lying on one side or the other of the body. It may be lessened if a person is kept busy, as is a sailor on a ship. Nausea, of course, is severe during some pregnancies, or it may be troublesome at the beginning of a menstrual period. Severe nausea is observed in some cases of food allergy. I know a man who lost his every-morning nausea and vomiting when he had his teeth extracted to cure a bad pyorrhea.

When a person comes complaining of nausea and abdominal discomfort one should think of an obstructing lesion low in the bowel, and should get a scout film of the abdomen to see if a segment of small bowel is full of gas. In an interesting case, a previously healthy ranch woman began to suffer much from nausea right after a herniotomy. A scout film showed a distended loop of ileum, and operation showed the bowel kinked where the surgeon had inadvertently run a suture through the wall of the bowel and fastened it to the abdominal wall. The minute this kinked segment was freed the woman was well.

I have seen nausea as the earliest and, for a time, only symptom of cancer of the colon.

Treatment. The first thing to do in cases of nausea is to look for the cause and to treat that if it can be found.

Dramamine, which comes in tablets of 50 mg., has been a very helpful drug in many cases, especially of motion and travel sickness. Some persons feel unsteady if they take more than one-half a tablet. Another prescription that may help will consist of some barbiturate, or bromural, plus some hyoscine. This type of prescription was used for motion sickness during World War II. Benadryl also helps.

The taking of food or the sipping of milk or the cleaning-out of the lower end of the bowel with an enema or a laxative may help in some cases.

Nightly nausea can be helped most by a vacation, by having a restful evening, or by going without supper. Often the patient should use the technic described in this chapter to see if some food is responsible for the nausea. A heavy user of tobacco should cut down on his allowance to see what happens.

SALIVATION

Salivation is commonly associated with nausea and can probably be produced by some of the conditions which produce nausea. I have seen it come from the eating of some food, such as chocolate, to which a person was allergically sensitive. It was associated with the canker sores that were produced by the chocolate. It is conceivable that salivation might be due to a little stroke, to disease of the salivary glands, to lesions about the teeth, or to encephalitis. Unfortunately, little is known about the symptom.

WATER BRASH

The term *water brash* has been applied to the type of morning regurgitation of fluid which shades into vomiting. One sees it in some cases of chronic alcoholism. In my intern days we used to call it the old bartenders' disease. Sometimes the fluid was acid or burning and sometimes it seemed to be just water.

Treatment. In attempting treatment, the physician might ask that a foul mouth be cleaned up, and the excessive use of alcohol and tobacco be stopped.

BILIOUSNESS

It is not always easy to learn what a person means when he says he is bilious or liverish. There is certainly little evidence to suggest that the syndrome has anything to do with bile or the liver. Often all it means is that the person is constipated and uncomfortable because of this. Or it may mean that he is suffering from an attack of migraine without much, if any, headache. In some cases there may simply be a tendency to reverse peristalsis. In other cases there may be a reaction to the eating of some food to which the person is allergically sensitive.

Treatment. Many persons say they can relieve their biliousness by taking a laxative or a little calomel or an enema.

DIZZINESS OR UNCERTAINTY ABOUT THE BODY BALANCE

Because, so far as I know, dizziness is not a symptom of disease of any abdominal organ, a discussion of the subject hardly belongs in this chapter, but I feel I must include here some discussion of the syndrome because so many patients and physicians look to the liver or colon whenever a patient gets an attack of giddiness or vertigo, especially with nausea and vomiting. They cling to an old-fashioned idea. Often the patient says he is bilious. I feel sure the liver has nothing to do with vertigo because I see so many patients suffering from cirrhosis or hepatitis who never complain of any feelings of imbalance.

Most of the people I see who complain of dizziness or vertigo do not mean that they see things spinning around. Their trouble is more a feeling of uncertainty as to balance. Some say they are so top-heavy, light-headed, or woozy that they fear to go around a corner fast. Sometimes the desk or the table-top before them seems to move a bit, or things will seem to swim before them. In bad cases the sense of position in space will suddenly be gone. Many times the person fears he will fall, but he rarely does.

It would seem that the source of the trouble should be either in the semicircular canals of the inner ear, or in those parts of the brain, such as the cerebellum, that have to do with maintaining the sense of balance. The lesion can be either a thrombosis of a little artery, or, less likely, some spasm in it. The otolaryngologists say that in necropsies on a few of these persons they have found a hydrops of the inner ear.

It helps much to learn if the trouble came suddenly because this suggests a thrombosis of a vessel. The presence of a cold will suggest that the disease is in the ear. Often the diagnosis of a little stroke is easily made when, with the dizziness, there came some mental changes, some loss of memory, or a patch of anesthesia or numbness somewhere, or a weakness in some muscle, or a clumsiness of a hand. One wants to know about nausea and vomiting such as would go with a Ménière syndrome. This can be produced by injury to either the brain or the ear. One wants to know if the ear was already the seat of disease, or if noises or some deafness came with the spell.

Often sudden deafness and tinnitus, together with positive results of tests of the labyrinth, show that the point of injury was in the inner ear. In other cases the lack of any abnormality in the ear will force the physician to diagnose a lesion in the brain. Often the physician dodges the issue by making a diagnosis of "toxic vertigo," whatever that means. Today there is too great a reluctance among doctors and laymen to face the fact that many of the bad dizzy spells in older persons are due to tiny strokes.

Usually the diagnosis must be made largely from the history and from an expert examination of the ears. Much depends on the age of the patient. The older ones who have always been well before are likely to have had a little stroke (see Chapter 12), but a momentary loss of balance occurring in the case of a young hypersensitive migrainous woman, or a young person with neurocirculatory asthenia, or a hysterical girl is not likely to mean much. A woman may even drop to the floor but all she will have is an ordinary fainting spell. Rarely, a person who gets faint on long standing will be found to have some static hypotension. In such a case the blood pressure, standing, will be found to be decidedly lower than that measured when the person is lying down. Such persons usually get dizzy for a moment on standing up suddenly after stooping over. In them the nervous mechanism which pushes blood up into the brain works too slowly or inefficiently. This tendency can run in a family.

Dizziness often means nothing in the cases of women suffering from a difficult menopause. In a few cases dizzy spells are equivalents of petit mal, or they are due to a mild encephalitis or perhaps to too much smoking. In other rare cases the trouble is a brain tumor, or a metastasis to the brain from a bronchial cancer.

Treatment. For those momentary losses of balance due to migraine, asthenia, or static hypotension, little can be done. Neither can much be done for the person who has had a little stroke. For trouble due to edema in the inner ear the patient can take nicamin, or a diet poor in sodium chloride, or frequent injections of histamine to effect desensitization. Time often works a cure. The woman whose dizzy spells are due to the menopause can be given some estrogen. The migrainous woman must learn to put up with her slight dizzy or faint spells. Dilantin may relieve the dizzy spells which are equivalents of epilepsy.

DISTURBANCES OF DIGESTION DUE TO EMOTION

Emotion can cause the rapid formation and even perforation of peptic ulcers. It can produce severe abdominal pain, perhaps with spasm of the stomach and bowel, and it can cause blanching or flushing of the gastro-intestinal mucosa. It can produce a gastric mucosa that is more friable or subject to injury. It can produce the clinical picture of a mucous colic, and it can produce a reversal of peristalsis which shows itself in burping, nausea, regurgitation, and even vomiting. Sometimes strong emotion, pain, or great fatigue will paralyze the stomach so that food will stay in it overnight. Pain or other emotion can cause the bowel to fill suddenly with gas. Emotion can also affect profoundly a diseased digestive tract, so that it will speed the development of a peptic ulcer, a gastric cancer, a chronic ulcerative colitis, or a sprue.

Obviously, if emotion is this powerful in affecting digestion and nutrition, physicians should more often inquire to find out if there is any unhappiness or worry at work, and if there is, they should make great efforts to straighten things out.

Indigestion due to eating under unpleasant circumstances. Many irritable and overly sensitive persons who complain of attacks of abdominal pain and indigestion are perfectly comfortable and can eat almost anything with impunity when they go on a vacation or when they go to some distant medical center where they stay ten days or so for an examination. During this time they are free from strain, tension, and annoyance. A hundred times I have had a patient remark that the day he left home to go to the Mayo Clinic his pain or diarrhea stopped; and this one fact showed how dependent his trouble was on emotion. Usually, then, I found that he got into trouble whenever he was tense, or whenever he ate when nervously upset, or very tired, or annoyed.

Emotional jaundice. I have seen several patients from Latin America, with and without cholecystitis, who got brief attacks of jaundice whenever they got angry enough. Evidently the ancients had observed this phenomenon because in Greek the word *choler* means both bile and anger. In Spanish, the word *cholera* is used both for a rage and for an attack of jaundice. We say, in English, that a man with a bad temper is choleric, or full of bile. To me it is an astounding fact that the Aymara Indians of Peru have the same trick of speech in which bile and anger are synonymous. They are so independent in their ways that it does not seem likely that they took the idea from the Spaniards. The word that they use probably came down from time immemorial.

No one knows what the mechanism is through which emotion produces the jaundice.

PSYCHIC ASPECTS OF FLATULENCE

In the cases of sensitive persons, gas in large quantities can accumulate in the bowel a few seconds after a fright or a hurt. This is well demonstrated every day by the urologists. The roentgenogram taken just before catheterization of the ureters may show only the usual small amount of gas in the colon and none in the small bowel; but the next one, made after the catheters have been pushed up, commonly shows not only the colon but the small bowel full of gas. This does not appear to be swallowed air, and hence it must have been poured out of the blood vessels into the lumen of the gut.

A nervous young man out with a girl may suffer from this type of rapid accumulation of gas in his bowel. As the colon fights to move this gas onward, more is excreted into the bowel. I think this phenomenon is most often seen in the cases of persons with a highly sensitive and mucus-forming colon.

Some nervous persons will fill with gas a few minutes after drinking a glass of cold pop on an empty stomach. They may also wake bloated after a nap. Many persons pass much flatus when they get constipated. In them the gas seems to keep pouring into the rectum so long as it contains feces. It stops coming out as soon as the bowel is emptied.

I have seen manic-depressive persons who were full of gas during their depressed phase and free from it during their euphoric one.

To me it is interesting that the two ends of the digestive tract, the esophagus and the colon, seem to be most under the influence of the emotions. This perhaps is to be expected because of the proximity of these segments to branches of the central division of the nervous system.

Treatment. Many sensitive persons who, when out to dinner, tend to fill with gas can be helped by taking from ¼ to ½ grain of codeine before they leave home.

DISTRESS DUE TO GAS IN THE SPLENIC FLEXURE

Occasionally, persons complaining of a feeling of pressure under the left leaf of the diaphragm will be found to have a large accumulation of gas in the splenic flexure. I have a hunch that quite a few of these persons have a rectal ring irritated by hemorrhoids. They may also be constipated.

Treatment. Persons with this trouble can get relief by getting into the knee-shoulder position; then the gas is likely to rise into the rectum, whence it can easily be ejected. Often the pain due to gas locked in some part of the bowel is relieved instantly by the assumption of the knee-shoulder position.

THE SORE COLON, OR THE SYNDROME OF "MUCOUS" OR "SPASTIC COLITIS"

One of the commonest causes of distress in the abdomen of many nervous persons is the overly sensitive· and mucus-forming colon. We physicians should try hard to avoid the terms mucous or spastic *colitis* because in the syndrome here described there is no colitis: There is no inflammation, and the only trouble is that the person's nerves or some neuromimetic hormones in his blood are playing tricks with his bowel. Since the genitive ending "itis" has come to mean inflammation, it would seem best not to use it for the naming of a disease in which there is no inflammation. It can be confusing and even alarming to designate a harmless neurosis with the term usually reserved for a serious and often fatal disease.

It is unfortunate when a physician shows an alarmist type of woman the roentgenograms of her colon and points to the haustrations as signs of spasm and colitis. Actually, such haustrations are normal and are found in the colon of every normal person. It is bad, also, to say that the colon is ptosed or too big or too long or poorly rotated. To give a nervous woman the idea that she has a diseased colon can only do harm. I am sure that ptosis does not produce symptoms. It is found in almost all women.

In most cases when a woman comes with the diagnosis of "mucous colitis" the physician who would like to really help her must spend time assuring her that her bowel is normal. He should tell her that if she were to have her abdomen opened the colon would look perfectly normal, just like that of any healthy person. The doctor should have the colon studied roentgenologically if it has not already been done, and he should look into her rectum with a sigmoidoscope. Usually then he can assure her that he saw a perfectly normal mucosa.

To a large extent the term *mucous colitis* has been a placebo, helpful in getting fussy women quickly out of the office. In his *Story of San Michele* Axel Munthe told how pleased the fashionable women of Paris were when "this new disease was devised for them."

The underlying causes of the syndrome. I think the sensitive colon or the tendency to get attacks of colic is usually inherited, and the bowel tends to remain sensitive throughout all of the affected person's days. Perhaps the essential point is that it is a colon which responds easily to emotion and to nervous tension.

In many cases the syndrome is so mild that no complaint is ever made of it; in others, it is severe, and in them the attacks may come frequently and cause much discomfort.

Common causes of attacks are going out to dinner with others, or having guests come into the home. Especially in the cases of young persons, going out with a member of the opposite sex can bring on an attack. Some persons get a flare-up when they eat some food to which they are allergic, and some get distress as the first sign of an approaching cold. Some upset their bowel by taking laxatives, or by letting themselves get constipated. Many nervous women suffer from a sore colon most of the time. Usually the descending portion is contracted so that it feels like a solid rod, very tender to pressure. Sometimes the cecum, also, is tender to pressure. Some persons are comfortable for weeks at a time, and then they get an acute spell that lasts for hours or a few days.

Curious features of the disease. Often a woman will say that her trouble is a diarrhea, but careful history-taking will show that this is not true. At times she may have an urgent desire to go to the toilet every half-hour or so, but no feces will come; what comes is only some gas with brown slime or foam and perhaps an ounce of fluid. In many cases the woman's misery arises from the fact that, in spells, she cannot pass gas except in the toilet, because of the presence in the rectum of a small amount of fluid. And when the colon keeps struggling to force out the gas, it is stimulated to produce more and more. The minute the rectum is emptied a great peace falls upon the bowel, and for a while no gas is formed.

Interestingly, a teaspoonful of paregoric or ½ grain of codeine will usually, for some hours, stop the formation of the gas and fluid and mucus, and this will permit the person to go out to dinner without suffering tortures. Going to bed and falling asleep is also likely to put an end to the formation of gas and mucus, but sometimes there will be a residue of the trouble present the next morning.

A curious feature of the disease is that often a big psychic strain will not bring on a spell, while just going out to dinner with old friends may bring much distress. The spell may start an hour or so before the person is to go out, apparently because of a subconscious tension. I remember a public official who was always late to banquets because, at the last minute, his highly nervous wife would have to rush back to the bathroom and take another enema. The cleaning out of the distal colon gave her a little respite from her distress. As some of these persons say, "My colon is constantly yelling at me." Many a physician who feels only contempt for the victims of this disease would certainly change and become very sympathetic with them if only for a few days he were to suffer as they do from a constant misery in the colon and rectum and anus. He would never again sneer at the woman who, in order to get some surcease from suffering, takes three enemas in a row.

Interestingly, if during a bad spell the person takes a couple of large enemas, one after the other, he is likely to discover that the distal three-fourths of the colon contains no feces. Spasm in the muscle of this region is apparently holding all the material back in the cecum.

In bad cases, and especially after a severe psychic strain, the patient may pass a sort of mucous cast of the inside of the bowel. Most physicians, at some time, have had a patient bring in a Mason jar full of this material to ask what it was. The largest such cast I ever saw was passed by a temperamental young Latin, who, at a house party, on a Wednesday met a very affectionate and passionate young lady. By Friday they were engaged. But on Saturday a great revulsion came over the man and suspecting that he had got himself into a mess, he went home. Naturally, he was all in from excitement and worry and loss of sleep. Next morning he passed a big cast of the whole colon. It appeared to be made of mucus which had become coagulated.

A woman in a bad spell may get a rectum so sensitive that she will be distressingly aware of the presence near the anus of even a small lump of feces. The misery will be so great that she will be unable to do any work until she gets this lump out. Also, in a person like this, during a mucous colic, the colonic waves can cause much distress by running right down to the anal ring, where the victim becomes acutely conscious of them. During health the descending waves apparently fade out in the upper part of the rectum where they are not felt.

Diagnosis. The person with mucous colics can easily be recognized, especially if the attacks are typical. But always the colon should be studied with the roentgen rays as a barium enema is being run in. Sometimes air must be injected after the enema is let out and stereoscopic films must be made. Then the roentgenologist can recognize polyps. I remember two persons with typical mucous colics due to business tragedies, in whom I missed a carcinoma of the colon because I did not think I needed to look for it. I remember, also, a woman with severe mucous colics who lost her life because when she suffered volvulus of a segment of jejunum, the physicians who saw her thought she was having only one more colic.

Treatment. Obviously, if the tendency to the disease is inherited, one cannot expect to cure it; one can only explain the situation and then help the patient so to live that he or she will not have so many spells. One can also give sedatives to help during a bad spell.

Usually the physician must first explain the nature of the disease. Here he must be tactful and persuasive and patient because often a woman will resent his analysis of the problem. She may answer angrily that if the physician would only quiet the distress in her bowel her nerves would be all right. To some extent she is right, but the nervousness seems usually to come first, and certainly little can be done to help the colon so long as its possessor is fretting and fussing and getting tense. Often the only way to break into the vicious circle is to give the woman a rest and some peace. Sometimes her only hope for a cure is to get out of some difficult and unhappy situation, such as that created by an unfortunate marriage.

Often the physician must combat disturbing ideas that the patient has picked up along the way, such as that the colon is inflamed, or ptosed, or possibly cancerous. It is not diseased, and in my experience there is no more danger of cancer developing in a mucus-forming colon than in a normally functioning one. I have never seen any of my patients come to any bad end because of mucous colics. Some patients have to be reassured about the passage of the mucus. They can be told that the body will not miss it or be the worse for its loss.

In the cases of sensible persons, reassurance and explanation of the syndrome are most of what is needed. Then the person must be taught to keep a record of foods eaten before spells and events preceding them so as to learn what causes them. In a section in this chapter I tell how to watch for offending foods, and in the section on constipation I give suggestions for controlling that. In the cases of persons with a highly sensitive bowel, treatment with rough diets and bulk-producing diets may work badly. Enemas of physiologic saline solution are likely to work better. A smooth diet, low in roughage, makes many of the patients more comfortable.

I don't think much of belladonna as a treatment for the sore colon, because I have seen so many hundreds of these patients who had been thoroughly dosed with the drug without getting much, if any, benefit. A few, however, said they could get temporary help from belladonna. I have seen no permanent benefit from the use of any of the newer relaxants, and so I do not prescribe them. I doubt the wisdom of giving bromides or phenobarbital every day, the way many physicians now do. Bromides can accumulate in the blood and produce a mild psychosis. I give some bromural only at those times when the person is unusually jittery or under heavy strain. Often what seems to be needed is a drug which will start peristaltic waves running smoothly and normally caudad again. Unfortunately, as yet, no such drug appears to be known. Occasionally a dose of castor oil will terminate a bad spell.

In acute spells and especially when the patient has to go out to dinner or to some public function, it usually helps greatly to give ¼ or ½ grain of codeine sulfate, perhaps with ½ grain of papaverine. This usually quiets peristalsis in the colon, and stops the formation of gas and mucus. By the occasional use of these sedatives I have rescued many women from a solitary life, and have made it possible for them to be social beings again. I have never seen any tendency to habituation from such a use of codeine. So far I have not seen anyone to whom it gave any feelings of euphoria such as would make her want to take the drug "just for fun" or for a "pick-up."

As I have grown older I have had much less tendency to prescribe a smooth diet and much more tendency to study the patient with an elimination diet or a food diary to see if any of the spells are due to eating some particular food. It can so easily be milk, eggs, chocolate, or some other supposedly highly digestible and "smooth" food.

CONSTIPATION AND THE DISCOMFORTS IT CAN CAUSE

There are some persons who, for days, can tolerate the failure of the colon to empty. Some can go a week or two without a bowel movement, without getting abdominal discomfort, indigestion, or headache.

But other more sensitive persons must have a movement every day, because if they do not they promptly become distressed in one way or another. Sometimes the bowel will move several times but because much fecal matter remains in the rectum or the descending colon, the person still feels full and distressed. Some persons will promptly get a headache which is relieved the minute the bowel is emptied; others will keep passing gas until the rectum is emptied; others will get hunger pain, while others will bloat, and a few will feel toxic. Some will suffer from constant awareness of the fact that the rectum is full. An occasional person, when constipated, will get a mucous colic.

Many delicate women should be constipated, as they are, because they eat so little food and so little roughage that it must take days for the colon to fill up. If not distressed by constipation such women might do well to let the bowel alone until it is full and ready to move by itself, unaided. Others can start a movement by taking an enema of warm water with a tablespoonful of salt to 2 quarts of water.

The physician need get excited about constipation only when it appears for the first time in a person past middle age. That will suggest the coming of a carcinoma. Perhaps, then, there will be pain shortly after eating, due, perhaps, to food driving down against the obstructed place. There may be borborygmus and perhaps the rising up at intervals of a loop of bowel, which then goes down again with a gurgle. This alone is enough to make the diagnosis of organic obstruction.

Always, in cases of recently acquired constipation, the stomach and colon should be examined by a roentgenologist, and the rectum should be examined with the finger and the sigmoidoscope. In older persons constipation can come suddenly with pyloric obstruction, or sometimes after a stroke, or the extraction of all teeth, or the coming of a mental depression, or of hypothyroidism or a diverticulitis.

Treatment. When faced by a man who insists that his constipation be "cured" I explain that so long as he lives the tense life he leads he will have to fight constipation. I explain that his colon is perfectly normal; the trouble is that his nerves are producing spasm or disorganized action. I may get him to admit that when he is on a vacation his bowels move well.

Then I reassure him by telling him that in constipation the stasis is always in the lower end of the colon and never in the small bowel. I also reassure by saying that today authorities do not put any stock in the old idea of intestinal autointoxication.

Finally, I take a piece of rubber tubing and remind the patient that there are only three ways of getting a plug out of it. In the case of the intestinal tube, one can either force it out from above with a laxative or a bulky diet or plenty of water, or one can wash it out from below with an enema. One should choose the method found most convenient or most uniformly successful. But one cannot expect a "cure." By talking in this way to a worried patient one can give him a great deal of comfort and often send him away happy.

Today it is the fashion to try to cure constipation in only one way, with a rough diet or with bulk-producing gummy substances. In many cases this works well for a while, but in others it does not work, or after working well for a while it no longer has any effect; the colon adjusts in some way. The most tasty of the bulk-producers is the canned Kadota fig. Perhaps three or four of these, eaten every morning for four or five days, will work beautifully. Then the patient can alternate with canned plums so that the bowel will not get so accustomed to one type of bulk that it will stop functioning. A few persons can get results from prunes or prune juice, but most cannot. A few get help from a glass of sauerkraut juice taken with two glasses of water. This should be taken before breakfast. Many take mixtures of several gums with cascara or they take preparations of cellulose.

There are some persons who get along beautifully with a daily dose of hydrocarbon oil, but after a time the colon may get accustomed to it and then it may begin to come through unmixed with feces. It is probably best taken in an emulsified form.

Some persons with a rather insensitive makeup correct their constipation satisfactorily with a laxative. Others cannot use laxatives because on some days they work too violently or not at all. A mild and useful saline is calcined magnesia.

Occasionally, a person with bad hemorrhoids will lose his constipation and flatulence after a good hemorrhoidectomy.

For persons with a very sensitive colon the best treatment is likely to be a daily enema of 2 quarts or a quart and a half of warm physiologic solution of sodium chloride. A tablespoonful of table salt should be added to the bag full of water. This enema should be run in all at one time and let right out again. An ordinary short tip should be used, and the patient should be seated on the toilet. There is no need of lying down or assuming the knee-chest position. If one runs in enough water it has to go over to the cecum; there is no other place into which it can go. When the patient suffers distress he can clamp the tube for a few seconds until the colonic muscle relaxes. There is much less difficulty getting physiologic saline solution in and out than is experienced with ordinary water or soapy water.

Before the physician can get many patients to use this simple and very useful measure he must combat the exhortations of several physicians who have told the person under no circumstances ever to take an enema. I do not know why physicians are so hostile to enemas. For thirty years I have been looking for a person whose colon was injured by them and I have not yet found one. I have heard of a few cases in which a stupid person managed to force a long enema tip through the rectum into the abdomen, but I do not see why we should give up the use of enemas simply because of these rare accidents. As I said, I have yet to see a colon stretched out of shape by enemas or in any way injured by them, and I have seen many women who had taken at least one enema a day for fifteen years or more. Physiologic saline solution cannot injure the colonic mucosa.

There are some persons who maintain that they cannot take enemas, or that, for them, an enema will not work. Since the taking of an enema is often a painful process due to the intermittent or constant spasm of the colonic muscle, I think we can assume that many nonstoical or hypersensitive persons haven't the courage and determination to run in more than 8 ounces of fluid at a time. This, of course, can empty only the rectum or the sigmoid colon. Since in many cases the distal two-thirds of the colon is contracted down so firmly as to hold all the fecal material back in the cecum, such a small enema will not bring any results.

FOOD SENSITIVITY AND ALLERGY

Many physicians have been unwilling to take much stock in the idea of food sensitivity or food allergy because they say the patients are all hypersensitive neurotics. To some extent this is true; probably no one can be highly sensitive to allergens without being highly sensitive to other stimuli. But this does not mean that there is no such thing as food sensitivity. All it means is that fatigue and nervousness can increase a man's sensitiveness to foods and other allergens. For instance, a friend of mine, a surgeon, after a bad night spent in patching up a lot of people injured in auto wrecks, will have trouble next morning scrubbing up. The skin of his hands and arms will not stand the soap. But if he has had a restful night in his bed, next morning he can scrub all he likes and there will be no rash. Another man I know gets asthma from inhaling certain dusts, but only when he is upset nervously by the presence in his house of his mother-in-law!

Most persons are unable to eat one or more foods, and some bizarre syndromes, commonly diagnosed as neuroses, are really due to food allergy. I have seen a few cases in which the patient, after eating some particular food, went into shock, and looked for a while as if he or she were going to die. In one case this was due to eating Roquefort cheese hidden away in salad dressings, in another, it was due to the eating of a bit of oyster in the dressing for a duck, and in another case it was due to a taste of clams.

I have seen persons who had terrible headaches due to the taking of very small amounts of milk or chicken or egg. On finding what the foods were, and eliminating them from the diet, these patients became well; they fattened up, and went back to work.

I will never forget the stupid-looking boy who for years had not been of any use, even on a farm. He came of an able family in which all the sons had distinguished themselves. This boy did well at college until his sophomore year. Then he broke down and was no longer able to study; he had constant headache, mental dullness, and abdominal pain. An exploratory laparotomy in his home city showed nothing wrong. The astounding fact was that when he was put on an elimination diet he not only promptly lost his stomach-ache but also his mental dullness; he became bright and able again. He proved to be highly sensitive to eggs, and what he had been doing was eating, each morning on the farm, a half-dozen of them!

I knew a famous surgeon who retched and purged if he ingested a milligram or two of cottonseed oil, and I remember two women who could show the perfect picture of a gallstone colic, one after taking a cup of coffee and the other after eating eggs.

A certain physician, if he were to take a large plate of chicken soup would be acutely ill for forty-eight hours or more with a dull headache, signs of meningism, perhaps weird hallucinations, an inability to read, and a marked indigestion. There is no question that a food allergen can depress the functions of the brain and can make the person feel dull. Whenever I put an allergic person on an elimination diet and the next day he remarks that his head is clear, I know that I am going to cure him.

The physician should always think of food allergy when there is a flatulent indigestion, with perhaps a sore bowel, and some diarrhea. In severe cases there may be headache, abdominal pain, urticaria, nausea, canker sores in the mouth, and migraine. Rarely there may be a stuffy nose, an irritable bladder, pains in the joints, and a sore liver.

Methods to be used in searching for the foods that are causing distress. Most patients who try to find the offending foods never identify them because (1) they leave out of the diet first one food and then another, usually leaving in something that can cause trouble; (2) they do not keep a record of their experiments; (3) if they keep a food diary, they put down everything they ate every day and soon get a record so bulky they cannot make anything out of it. They would do better to put down only the unusual foods eaten. (4) When they try an elimination diet to begin on they often choose one containing foods like milk and eggs which are very likely to be offenders. As I show a little farther on, they should have started eating a few foods which rarely cause trouble.

There are several ways of finding out what the offending foods are, and what can be used in one case may be out of the question for another.

The diary method. When the indigestion or pain or headache comes in attacks at intervals of weeks or months the person should make, each time, a written record of all the unusual foods—foods not eaten every day—consumed in the twenty-four hours before the upset. Most suspicion should fall on the foods eaten at the preceding meal because they are the ones most likely to be at fault.

After three or four attacks, the record should be searched to see if any one food was eaten before each upset. If one is found, it should be omitted from the diet for a while to see if this brings a cure. If it does, the food should be taken a couple of times again to see if each time it produces the distress. If so, it should be banished from the diet. If the patient is comfortable for three or four weeks between spells he may do well to list the common foods eaten during that time, because they are likely to be safe ones for him.

Often the physician can be fairly certain that painful upsets that come once a month are not allergic in origin, because if they were, they would have to be due to the eating of some unusual food such as shell fish, and then the person would quickly have noticed the association between cause and effect. There is the possibility, however, that the patient can eat a food such as milk or cantaloupe twice a week but not every day. Some foods cause trouble only after they have been eaten for three or four days running.

The elimination diet. When a distress is present almost every day the problem of finding an offending food must be simplified by reducing the number of unknowns. The best method would be to have the patient eat nothing for forty-eight hours to see if he then gets comfortable, but people hate to fast, and hence I usually give them *for forty-eight hours* a diet consisting of nothing but oatmeal, lamb, beef, rice, carrots, butter, sugar, water, and canned pears. These foods have been chosen because experience has shown that they rarely give trouble allergically. The oatmeal is eaten at breakfast with butter and sugar on it, and the canned pears are used for dessert. The rice is cooked in water and eaten with butter and sugar. During the two days no other substance must be put in the mouth: no drinks or laxatives or candy or gum.

If, after the two days, the patient still has his distress, the assumption must be either that his troubles are not allergic or else that one of the foods in the elimination diet is causing trouble. Often one can tell which is which by having the person fast for twenty-four hours. I see no sense in keeping people on an elimination diet for weeks because allergens produce their symptoms usually in a few hours. If, during the two days, the person is comfortable, he should start right in trying out foods, *one at a time,* keeping a record of how he reacted to each. Any food that seems to cause trouble should be tried at least three times before it is given up. Good ones to start with are potato, gelatin, asparagus, turnips, string beans, arrowroot cookies, rye krisps, thin toast, and cream. Milk, chocolate, eggs, and coffee should be tried out later because they are common offenders.

The overeating method. Oftentimes when a patient keeps wondering if a certain food is really hurtful he should eat a large amount of it at one meal. Then, if he experiences no discomfort he can stop worrying about it and can eat all he wants of it.

The rare person who is highly allergic to many foods can find help in the booklet on Food Allergy in the Harper Series, obtainable from Harper and Brothers, 49 East 33rd St., New York City. It costs $1.00. It contains a list of unusual or exotic foods which can be tried, and which, because they have never been eaten before, are not likely to give trouble in an allergic way.

PSEUDO-ULCER

There are quite a few persons, usually men, who complain of hunger pain much like that of peptic ulcer. It will usually be relieved by eating or taking milk or antacids. The trouble may come in attacks lasting days or weeks or months, or it may be fairly constant for years. The gastric acidity may be normal or there may be hyperacidity or hypoacidity.

In these cases good roentgenologists examine the patient again and again without seeing any sign of ulcer, and in an occasional case a surgeon will explore the abdomen without finding anything to explain the pain. It is significant that with the passage of years these persons do not develop any of the symptoms of a complicated ulcer: They never suffer from hemorrhage, perforation, or pyloric obstruction. Rarely are their symptoms severe, and rarely are they awakened at night. They almost never have to vomit.

The causes. There are several ways in which a susceptible person can get an attack of hunger pain. Probably first he must be born with a sensitive digestive tract which can easily become crampy. Then, perhaps, he must eat for several days some food to which he is allergically sensitive. He may not get hunger distress if he eats the food once, but if he eats it for several days running he may get into trouble. In two of the most troublesome cases reported, the patients, both physicians, were highly allergic to the milk they were taking every hour to relieve their pain. When, accidentally, they discovered this sensitiveness and stopped drinking milk, they were well. In another case, a physician would get severe hunger pain at 11 A.M. whenever he had eaten two eggs for breakfast. Then, because he was so distressed, at luncheon he would decide to go easy, and he might eat two poached eggs! When he did this, by 4 P.M. he would be in such pain he could not stand up straight. This went on for many years, until by keeping a record of foods eaten before spells he discovered his sensitiveness and stopped eating eggs. Later, when he noted that he would get a particularly long and severe spell of hunger pain in August, it occurred to him that he might be sensitive to the cantaloupe which, at this time of year, he liked to eat every day. On giving up the cantaloupe, except for an occasional taste, he never again had a bad spell lasting more than a day or two.

Another common cause of hunger pain has proved to be constipation. Some men cannot go without a bowel movement for forty-eight hours without getting hunger pain, relieved for a while by the taking of food and more permanently by the taking of an enema. This pain feels as if it were due to gas trapped in a segment of jejunum. This gas can be forced onward by the peristaltic waves that start running after the taking of food.

Finally, when persons with this type of illness get rid of their allergies and their constipation, they can still get short spells of hunger pain whenever they are coming down with a cold. It would seem that the toxins of the infection make the bowel overirritable or they interfere with the evenness of peristalsis. They may also upset the mechanism which normally takes gas out of the gut. It is possible that in some persons the presence of a diseased gallbladder will make the duodenum oversensitive and subject to painful spasm.

Some persons get the pain in a few minutes if they sit or squat bent over so that perhaps a fold of the abdominal wall keeps pressing on the stomach or duodenum. Because of such pain, a man may be unable to bend over to weed his lawn, or he may have to be careful to sit up straight when driving his car. A patient of mine who had suffered for years from hunger pain lost it when he changed the height of his chair at the office so as to avoid bending over. He had noticed that his pain followed any bending forward.

I have seen a number of relatives of the epileptic who suffered from pseudo-ulcer. Most of them had a dysrhythmia in the electroencephalogram. Their trouble appeared to be due to their greatly exaggerated reactivity and irritability. The nervous system in the bowel was probably as over-reactive as it was in the rest of the body.

Treatment. The treatment will be obvious from what is written here. It must be based on a study of the causes of the pain in the individual case. All allergens to which the person is sensitive must be sought out and removed from the diet, and constipation must be avoided or relieved by a daily enema. Some persons should carry a bottle of malted milk tablets. A half dozen of these, chewed up and swallowed with a little water as soon as the pain starts, will usually give relief. Patients with pseudo-ulcer should quickly learn the unwisdom of ever leaving the pain unrelieved for long. To leave the pain unhelped by food for an hour or more may enable the gastric acid to so irritate the duodenal mucosa that, for a week or two, the pain will keep returning two or three times a day. But if food is taken within a few minutes of the appearance of the pain, and if the rectum is kept clean, the pain, once relieved, is not likely to return.

PSEUDO-APPENDICITIS

There are many persons who complain for years, or much of their life, about an ache or pain or discomfort or misery, or a "sense of something there," in the right lower quadrant of the abdomen. Usually, at some time during the early days of the illness, the appendix is removed, but without results. Sometimes the surgeon will open the abdomen again and explore without finding any cause for the distress. What, then, causes the trouble? Often I cannot guess what it is. It may be significant that most of the patients are nervous, tense, complaining, hypersensitive persons. Some have a poor nervous heredity, and I think this often is important. In a certain type of case the cecum is decidedly tender and this is probably part of the syndrome of the sore colon. In one case like this a surgeon removed the right half of the colon without lessening the distress. The woman's real trouble was a depression. In some cases the soreness is definitely in the abdominal wall and is due to a fibrositis or to an irritation of the nerves coming out of an arthritic spine. In rare cases the trouble may be a myositis or fibrositis involving the iliopsoas muscle. One would think that in such cases this muscle should be sore on straining or on lifting the thigh.

When the ache is constant it may well be of psychic origin and referred out from the brain. I know of a few cases in which in the end it became clear that the patient had always been slightly psychotic. Oftentimes the story shows that the distress has nothing to do with the digestive tract; it is no worse for eating and no better for emptying the colon. In a few cases there is much distress and gurgling as the small bowel empties into the colon. Then it is conceivable that there is a disturbance of function in the bowel about the ileocecal sphincter. In many cases the distress is made worse by standing and getting tired, and then it is relieved by lying down and getting rested.

Occasionally, if the distress is low in the groin it may be due to a large internal inguinal ring into which a loop of bowel is trying to bore.

In such a case the distress comes if the person stands much in the evening when he is tired and his muscles are relaxed. Such pain is immediately relieved by the patient's getting off his feet. In some cases the pain seems to be related to sacroiliac disease.

There is a group of cases in which the distress is so great that one has the feeling that there should be some local cause, but I do not know what it is.

The important point about all these cases is that practically never does one do any good by operating and exploring the abdomen. The only cases in which one can hope to do anything with appendectomy are those few in which the patient, nearly always less than thirty years of age, has recently suffered from one or more attacks of pain which suggested acute appendicitis.

A pain that is not worse with menstruation is not likely to come from the pelvic organs. A pain that is worse with menstruation will suggest a lesion in the ovary or perhaps an endometriosis.

For me, the most puzzling cases are those in which some of the symptoms point to a fibrositis of the abdominal wall or an arthritis of the spine, while others point to some malfunction in the terminal ileum with a loud gurgling of liquids through the ileocolic sphincter. When, in addition, the patient has symptoms of a bad neurosis or minor psychosis, I feel stumped.

PSEUDOCHOLECYSTITIS

There are quite a few persons, nearly all of them women, who complain of pain and soreness in the right upper quadrant of the abdomen. Occasionally one will be found who has attacks which resemble colics.

In a few of these cases in which the gallbladder functions well with the dye the organ doubtless contains small stones or some sand which is not visible in the roentgenograms. Hence it is that occasionally, when the gallbladder functions normally, the clinician will have to recommend a surgical exploration of the abdomen simply because the symptoms are so definitely those of gallstones. At the Mayo Clinic, a new and often very helpful technic is now used for showing stones. The dye-filled gallbladder is roentgenographed as the patient lies on his right side. Then any stones present are likely to become visible, lying against the lower or right wall of the organ.

In other cases, because of the constancy of the ache, the clinician will decide that the cause of the distress is more likely some psychic strain, or a fibrositis of the thoracic and abdominal walls or a hepatitis or a lesion in the right kidney.

I have seen cases in which the drinking of coffee or the eating of eggs produced the typical picture of a gallstone colic, even after the gallbladder had been removed. I remember cases in which the pains kept up even when there was a T-tube in the common duct, or when the common duct had been destroyed. In some of these cases, the cause of the pain could never be learned. In a few cases, with a T-tube in place, I was much interested to note that whenever the patient had a colic, the material coming out of the common duct changed from the normal yellow bile to a blackish, stringy, sticky material. In the case of one woman this change could be produced by the giving of chicken soup or chicken fat. It suggested that there was a marked change in hepatic chemistry coincident with the pain.

In some of these cases the liver edge was tender. Always in such cases the physician should check the liver function because there can be pain with subacute hepatitis.

POSTCHOLECYSTECTOMY SYNDROMES

Many persons who have recently submitted to cholecystectomy come back to complain that they are still suffering from abdominal discomfort, flatulence, and even attacks of severe pain in the upper part of the abdomen. Then the questions are, was a stone left in the common duct, is there a hepatitis, is the trouble nervous in origin, is there a tendency to spasm in the common duct or the duodenum or stomach, or is there a dyskinesia or abnormality of muscular action in the duct? Will the patient have to be operated on again or should he wait a while longer?

In such cases most information can usually be obtained from a good history. The first thing to do is to find out why the gallbladder was removed, and to get some idea as to whether or not it was diseased. If, before operation, the patient's symptoms were those of a neurosis, if there never were any colics, if the diagnosis of cholecystitis was based on the roentgenologist's report of a "poorly emptying" gallbladder, and if at operation no stones were found, the chances are that the diagnosis was all wrong and the gallbladder was normal. In that case it is highly improbable that there is a stone or any inflammation in the common duct. The chances are that the syndrome is functional or nervous in origin *just as it was before the operation.*

Occasionally there is trouble after a needless cholecystectomy, but then it may be because the patient gets diarrhea (due perhaps to the steady draining of bile into the bowel), or there is pain and perhaps jaundice due to some injury to the common duct. Then a very expert surgeon may have to reconstruct the duct or make an anastomosis between a hepatic duct and the duodenum.

If the story indicates that there never was any cholecystitis, the physician may be able to draw out a history of some psychic strain or of a food allergy or a fibrositis or migraine. I like always to check the liver function to make sure that I am not dealing with a painful hepatitis or cirrhosis. In rare cases the trouble may be a pancreatitis.

When there were colics before the operation and stones were found, there is a good chance that one or more concretions were left in the common duct. The physician will want to know if the surgeon explored this duct, and if so, if he found stones. If he did not explore the common duct, or even if he did, there is one chance in seven that stones either were left or else came down from the hepatic duct after operation.

If the common duct was opened and a T-tube was put in, one should find out how long the bile kept draining. If it kept running for more than six weeks it is probable that there was a stone partially blocking the sphincter of Oddi.

Often it is well for the person to wait a while even when he or she goes on having colics after cholecystectomy, because in many cases, after some months, the trouble quiets down. Perhaps the common duct gets used to stones, or small ones pass into the duodenum, or perhaps the colics were due to spasm somewhere in the duodenum. After years of inflammation in the biliary tract, it or the duodenum or stomach may perhaps become so irritable that its muscle occasionally goes into a painful spasm. With time this tendency may go, and peace may descend on the digestive tract.

In deciding whether or not an attack of pain originated in the common duct it helps to know if, the day after a spell, the titer of serum bilirubin rose. Suggestive, also, is a chill, a sharp spike of fever, and a slight leucocytosis, with soreness in the right upper quadrant. If the patient had colics before the operation it is helpful to know if those that are now coming are the same as the old ones. Do they produce a catch in the breath as a gallstone colic often does? Sometimes the patient will say, "These spells are different from those I had before, and the pain is in a different place." That is against the diagnosis of a common duct stone.

It can be very helpful if an observant and experienced physician can see the patient in a spell. I remember a woman who had had colics until a stone was removed from her common duct. When she went on having severe attacks of pain in the upper part of the abdomen I feared she would have to be operated on again. But, fortunately, about that time, I was able to see her in a spell, and in a few minutes recognized a gastric crisis.

Treatment. Occasionally one can relieve postcholecystectomy pain with inhalations of amyl nitrite or tablets of nitroglycerin. In the worst cases morphine or dilaudid will have to be used. It sometimes helps if, for a time, the patient will get a rest cure so as to quiet his reflexes. It may help, also, to live for a time on a smooth, low-roughage diet.

In the cases of excitable persons it may help to have the patient keep a record to see if the colics always follow an emotional upset, a quarrel, or the eating of some food to which the person is highly allergic. I have seen several cases in which the "colics" were due to violent quarrels, or to drinking-bouts, or to drinking coffee or eating eggs or some food to which the person was sensitive.

THE DYSPEPTIC

Although today we physicians know that few persons lack pepsin and few owe their indigestion to a lack of this ferment, some of us think of a certain type of thin finicky man as a dyspeptic: a person who, with but little appetite or capacity for food, looks on his meals with little interest, and is practically certain that whatever he eats will disagree with him. He insists that his food be simply prepared and cooked, without fancy seasoning. He will prefer foods such as steak, which have not lost their identity, and he will eschew ragouts, stews, hashes, meat balls, and mixtures in casseroles. These dyspeptics, at necropsy, are usually found to be without gross disease in the digestive tract.

INDIGESTION DUE TO A SMALL GASTRO-INTESTINAL LABORATORY

There are many dyspeptics who suffer from indigestion whenever they eat a large meal of any kind. The secret of comfort for them is to eat little at any one time. Then they get along fairly well. I suspect that their gastro-intestinal laboratory is small and poorly equipped. Some of them probably have a short small bowel or, more important, a bowel with few folds or few or defective villi so that the surface area is much less than normal and the absorbing surface is small. Others may have a somewhat achylous bowel, much as they often have an achylous stomach.

Treatment. Obviously, there is only one thing such persons can do and that is to go on living frugally. They must eat simple foods, simply cooked, and they must get up from the table the minute they feel they have had enough.

THE SYNDROME OF THE HYPERSENSITIVE DIGESTIVE TRACT

There are some hypersensitive persons, often with greatly exaggerated knee jerks, who have what I call a hypersensitive digestive tract. In them the eating of any food or the drinking of a glass of ice water may bring a sort of dumping syndrome, with feelings of warmth, faintness, nausea, fullness in the abdomen, bloating, or impending diarrhea. The fact that these persons can get the syndrome with pure ice water shows that when it follows the eating of food it is not due to indigestion or allergy, but to the physical impact of the food.

In some cases the main symptom complained of is a sudden filling of the bowel with gas, especially when cold water or pop is drunk on an empty stomach. Gas must pour out of the blood vessels into the bowel.

Treatment. Persons with this syndrome will do well to avoid drinking anything on an empty stomach. They will avoid iced drinks and drinks with much sugar in them. Ice cream may cause trouble.

It may help to eat slowly and to begin the meal with some solid food such as toast. In bad cases it may help to give a tablet of bromural twenty minutes before the person eats so as to quiet the reflexes. It helps to take food and drink at body temperature.

FUNCTIONAL DIARRHEA

One must always find out what a patient means when he says he has diarrhea. He may mean one soft, watery stool a day, or two or three soft stools in the morning and, after that, no more trouble; or he may mean the passage of a little watery mucus with gas when he is highly nervous (a mucous colic), or he may be going to the toilet frequently to pass a few small hard lumps of feces (perhaps due to hyperthroidism), or he may have a true diarrhea, with many soft or watery movements a day.

It is very helpful to find out if the diarrhea wakes the patient at night because, if it does, it is much more likely to be due to some organic disease. The presence of blood in the feces always suggests ulceration of the bowel. Great urgency with tenesmus indicates a lesion of the rectum.

Perhaps nine out of ten persons with diarrhea must have a functional trouble of some sort because no ulceration of the bowel can be found; their gastric juice will be full of acid; the roentgenologist will report a normal-looking digestive tract; the sigmoidoscopic examination will reveal a normal mucosa; the stool will contain no pus or parasites, and the blood sedimentation rate will be low. It is significant when in these cases, in spite of many movements a day, the person remains well nourished or stout for years and years. It is important, also, to note that in functional types of diarrhea it does not make much, if any, difference what the patient eats. Treatment with drugs, also, may have but little effect.

One must always think of the nervous type of diarrhea because it is so common, and one must think of it especially when the story is that the patient occasionally has one or two large movements and then is normal for days or weeks. Often, on questioning, it will be found that the large soft movements appeared when the patient became alarmed or panicky over something. The more I see of the relatives of the psychotic the more I am impressed with the fact that many of them suffer at times with a functional type of diarrhea due to panic and alarm. It might conceivably be due, also, to some abnormality in the brain center for the bowel or for the autonomic nerves. This abnormality can be a small share of the disease which in some relatives affected the brain so as to produce a psychosis. It is possible that diarrhea can sometimes be a symptom of hysteria. It certainly can be a troublesome symptom in the cases of some hysterical women.

It helps much in the diagnosis of functional types of diarrhea to find that the patient always had a tendency to loose stools, especially when he was excited or anxious or tense or about to start on a journey. It helps, also, to find that other members of the family have had a similar tendency.

I have found very helpful as an index of organic disease in the bowel a high blood sedimentation rate, often around 60 mm. in an hour Westergren. Such a rate usually means that the patient has an extensive stenosing enteritis or chronic ulcerative colitis. A normal rate goes far to rule out any long-lasting or extensive disease of the bowel.

There are some diarrheas due to the drinking of milk or to the eating of some food to which the person is sensitive. This food should be discovered by the technics described in the section on food sensitiveness. Milk is probably the worst offender. If the person is sensitive to the eating of fresh fruit he will be worse in the summer than in the winter.

It is well to inquire and make sure that the person is not drinking too much water or beer. One can test the gastric secretion for hydrochloric acid, but in my experience, achlorhydria rarely produces diarrhea.

Efforts to learn something by studying the bacterial flora of the bowel are nearly always disappointing. A patient's story may show that his diarrhea started acutely and probably with an infection with some dysentery-producing organism, but apparently this germ soon died out because the bacteriologist cannot find any of the common pathogens in the stools or in swabbings from the rectal mucosa.

In all cases, of course, amebas should be looked for by someone expert enough to recognize them or their cysts. *Giardia lamblia* will sometimes be found, and at times it produces malaise and ill health. Occasionally one must think of pellagra, sprue, or a primary anemia as causes of a puzzling diarrhea.

Treatment. It is very difficult to help many of the persons with the common types of functional diarrhea because they fail to respond to diet or to drugs like bismuth. But always one can try. One must be sure that the person is not eating or drinking some food to which he is highly sensitive. A smooth diet without much fresh fruit or many rough vegetables may help. Always, for a few days, milk and milk products should be avoided to see if this will help. A low-residue diet should be tried. It should consist largely of meat with pure starches, such as rice, white flour, sago, and tapioca, with some butter and fruit juice. In some cases a few days of almost starvation will cure a diarrhea. It allows the intestinal mucosa to recover. A dose of castor oil may also bring a cure.

It may help to talk over the person's life problems and to see if panics and fears can be relieved. Better mental hygiene with more rest and sleep may help. Some persons can be cured just by putting them to bed for a week. Cabot showed this many years ago. It may help much to lower the liquid intake. An enema of warm physiologic salt solution, taken morning and evening, may save the patient many trips to the bathroom.

If the person has no hydrochloric acid in the gastric juice one can try giving *with meals* and well diluted, a teaspoonful of a mixture of equal parts of dilute hydrochloric acid, U.S.P., and water. Many physicians give too little acid, and they keep giving it for months when it does no good. In my experience if the acid is ever to work it does so immediately. I have little faith in the drugs that are designed to turn into acid in the stomach. They have been shown to have very little effect in lowering the pH of the gastric juice.

One can try giving heaping teaspoonful doses of bismuth subgallate or kaolin with the idea of drying the feces. Some of the gummy laxatives will, at times, relieve diarrhea, apparently by taking water away from the intestinal contents.

One can try giving sulfasuxidine or sulfathalidine or aureomycin or chloromycetin to see if almost sterilizing the colon will do any good. This might also show if the diarrhea is due to a dysentery-producing organism.

In all difficult cases, even if no amebas can be found in the stools, it is well to try an intramuscular injection of 1 grain of emetine. If the diarrhea is due to amebiasis it should immediately subside a bit. I have seen an occasional miracle worked in this way. One can also give in one day 6 capsules, each containing 0.25 gm. of carbarsone. These will constitute one course of the drug, which should not immediately be repeated because of the contained arsenic. Such a course usually causes amebas to disappear. If *Giardia lamblia* are present one should give atabrine for a day or two. It is said that if it is going to work it will do so the first day, and this has been my experience.

In many cases, when I cannot help in any other way, I give the patient capsules containing ½ grain of codeine sulfate, perhaps with ½ grain of papaverine. One of these capsules, taken before the person goes out in public, may insure comfort and relief from embarrassment. In some cases, one or two capsules a day will work a cure. In a few bad cases I have given a woman back her health and morale and a normal social life with three or four such doses a day. So far, I have not heard of any of these persons showing any tendency to habituation, or any desire to increase the dose of the codeine.

A few persons do not feel comfortable when the diarrhea is stopped. This stoppage gives them so much gas that they prefer to keep the diarrhea.

If a patient has no free acid in the stomach, and if he has numbness or tingling in the legs and some blood changes, the administration of liver, folic acid, and B_{12} should be tried out.

DISTURBANCES IN SWALLOWING

It is curious that many patients who have difficulty in swallowing fail to mention it when they go to a doctor. Why they do this I do not know, but this quirk of human nature leads to the making of many wrong diagnoses. Oftentimes the patient complains only of a distress or pain around the lower end of the sternum, and then the physician may direct all his efforts toward finding a lesion in the stomach, gallbladder or duodenum.

When a person says he is not swallowing comfortably, the several troubles that must be thought of are a hysterical reluctance to swallow, or a fear of swallowing solids, or an esophagospasm, a cardiospasm, a short esophagus, a diaphragmatic hernia, a diverticulum of the esophagus, a cancer somewhere along the way from the pharynx to the fundus of the stomach, a tumor of some kind pressing on the esophagus, or perhaps a little stroke that has affected the glossopharyngeal or vagus nerves. Always there must be a careful examination with a barium meal, and if necessary, with an esophagoscope.

Especially in the cases of older persons, the physician will want to be sure that the patient has not suffered a bulbar injury. In that case the story is that perhaps after a bad dizzy spell, food started entering the larynx and causing violent coughing spells. Always when the physician suspects there has been a little stroke, he should ask about difficulties in getting the food down the right way, because a history of strangling and coughing, when obtained, may settle the diagnosis. Sometimes a laryngologist will report that there is loss of normal function of the vocal cords or epiglottis, or he may note a lack of normal sensation in the pharynx. Roentgenologists will often diagnose a little stroke when they note that some of the barium meal given an elderly person went into the lungs. Also, after a stroke, the roentgenologist may note a curious diffuse spasm along the esophagus.

Typical of an arteriosclerotic bulbar injury is the complaint that one day the mucus in the pharynx became ropey or gluey and hard to cough out. This can be loosened perhaps with the help of ipecac or lipoiodine. I have seen it clear up beautifully for a while after an injection of emetine.

I suspect that in rare cases esophagospasm is a residue from an injury to nerves caused by a mild unrecognized attack of encephalitis or perhaps polio-encephalitis or diphtheria. I know men who sometimes, when tense and nervous, can be thrown into an attack of painful esophagospasm by exposure to a cold draft. Other persons suffer from diffuse esophagospasm when placed under nervous strain.

All persons with dysphagia must be examined carefully for carcinoma of the esophagus, the cardia, or the fundus. In some cases the lesion is small and hard to find. Occasionally, dysphagia will be due to the pinching of the esophagus in a diaphragmatic hernia. Then an esophageal ulcer may form at the point of constriction in the diaphragmatic hiatus.

In rare cases, peptic ulcer of the esophagus has been found. Rare, also, is the esophageal diverticulum which, when full of food, presses on the esophagus and causes obstruction.

CARDIOSPASM

A number of writers have claimed that cardiospasm is a neurosis, but it must be more than that. I have seen some stout jolly persons who suffered from cardiospasm in spite of the fact that they had no reason to be under psychic strain; and then, again, I have seen some who did have serious nervous troubles. I have seen several persons who, with cancer of the cardia, got their symptoms only when under psychic strain.

In most of the cases of cardiospasm in which a necropsy was obtained, the ganglion cells in the nerve plexus at the cardia were found to be absent or diseased. As I have shown (Alvarez: 1949), this fact can easily explain the spasm and the lack of function at the cardia. Against the idea of a purely psychic cause for cardiospasm is the fact that most of the patients cannot be cured until the cardia is dilated forcibly with the Russell-Plummer bag. From this it would seem that some fibrous tissue must have formed, or muscles must have become stiffened. Actually, histologic studies of cardias removed at necropsy from the bodies of persons who had suffered from cardiospasm failed to show any thickening of the muscle or any formation of connective tissue.

Porter Vinson, who has seen many hundreds of persons with cardiospasm, does not believe that the disease is a neurosis.

Occasionally, a person who is having trouble with gallstones will show mild transient spasm at the cardia.

Treatment. At the Mayo Clinic most patients with cardiospasm are quickly relieved by dilation with the Russell-Plummer bag. Some have to return for one or more dilations. First the esophagus and cardia are examined with the roentgenoscope, and if there is any suspicion of carcinoma, the esophagoscope is used. A silk thread is swallowed, and when this has become anchored in the bowel, the tip of the dilator is threaded over it, and with it as a guide, the instrument is passed through the narrow place.

In the hands of an expert, this dilating method is safe, and the results usually are very satisfactory. Immediately the person starts eating again. Only rarely does he or she have to return for an operation. Details as to the technic of the dilating procedure can be found in Vinson's book.

HYSTERICAL DYSPHAGIA OF THE PLUMMER-VINSON TYPE

In 1912, H. S. Plummer wrote about spasm at the upper end of the esophagus, and in 1922 Vinson reported a group of cases in which this difficulty was present. Practically all of the patients were Scandanavian women past middle age who had a great fear of choking on solid food or on small boluses or pills. Because they soon were living on a narrow diet, they tended to become anemic. They did not attempt to swallow any but liquid food. Eventually they got a sore tongue, and sometimes pain back of the larynx and in the abdomen.

Treatment. These persons can usually be relieved by the passage of a thick rubber sound through the fauces, especially if the physician keeps assuring them that this will work a cure. A third of the patients will have to come back occasionally for another dilation.

A GREAT RELUCTANCE TO SWALLOW

There is a syndrome in which the patient chews her food but cannot bring herself to swallow it. She may keep it in the front of the mouth for minutes at a time, and as a result she may take an hour or two to eat a small meal. Naturally, with so much chewing, the muscles of mastication may get to feeling sore and weak, and the physician may fear a beginning myasthenia gravis. The presence of strangers at the table often adds to the patient's distress.

Treatment. According to Vinson these persons must be trained and encouraged to swallow normally again. The physician must sit with the patient and encourage her to attempt the swallowing of a piece of bread. Usually the trick can be taught the woman in a couple of lessons.

LOSS OF APPETITE

It is not clear why some persons have spells in which they have no interest in food, or why some seldom have any appetite. Some women go on living well enough for many years in spite of the fact that they do not seem to eat much more than their coffee and a little salad. Usually, one can examine them from head to foot without finding any serious disease.

A youth, who after an acute abdominal upset loses appetite, may have had either a bad cold or a smoldering appendicitis, a beginning tuberculosis, a beginning mild psychosis, or an unhappy love affair. Rarely one must think of Addison's disease. Most of what is known about the physiology of appetite and hunger is summarized in a chapter of my book, *An Introduction to Gastroenterology*.

It is curious how some persons with a normal desire for food will lose it after taking a few mouthfuls. Some of these persons have symptoms suggesting a poor intestinal gradient of forces, or even some reversal of it.

Now that hepatitis is so common, the physician must think of this disease when a person begins to lose appetite and to suffer from a puzzling indigestion and feeling of illness. Jaundice may later appear. Tests for liver function should be made, and the amount of serum bilirubin should be estimated. I have seen a number of cases in which a loss of appetite, together with a feeling of ill health, was puzzling until jaundice appeared.

Treatment. The physicians of fifty years ago treated loss of appetite with "tonics" and bitters, but modern doctors have lost faith in them, and many do not ever prescribe them. Today almost everyone gives vitamin B, which may or may not help.

PUZZLING TYPES OF BLEEDING FROM THE DIGESTIVE TRACT

There are puzzling types of bleeding from the digestive tract for which no cause can be found. Even in some of the rare cases in which the person bled to death, no source of bleeding was found by the pathologist.

PSYCHIC PROBLEMS OF THE PERSON WITH A PEPTIC ULCER

Almost everyone with a peptic ulcer has some psychic problems which at times will appear to be the cause of a flare-up in symptoms. Sometimes the man is a hard-driving fellow who needs to let up on strain and to mend some of his ways. Perhaps the ulcer started when he was meeting heavy competition or taking big losses, and later, recurrences came with unhappiness or worry or resentment. The first patient who taught me this was seen in 1912. He had several hemorrhages about six months apart, every one of which came when an important invention of his gave trouble, so that the machinery had to be quickly redesigned.

Many persons with ulcer lose their symptoms the day they shut up the desk at the office and start off for a vacation or a trip to some medical center for a diagnosis. Others lose their pain the minute they enter a hospital. Often I have said to such a patient with a bad ulcer, "Why submit to an operation with all its hazards when you know you can get well simply by cutting down on the strain of work and life? Why have the ulcer cut out or sidetracked when you are going to go right back into the sort of life that caused this ulcer and may easily give you a new one?"

The big difficulty usually is that a man cannot go easy on his job. He must either drive hard or quit entirely. Often he gets his ulcer just about the time he has learned a business or acquired a certain skill, and then it is hard to give up and adjust to a smaller income.

Today physicians talk of calling in a psychiatrist to help the patient remake his personality, but my impression is that what he needs usually is to get away from too tough a job or too severe a boss or too strenuous a life. Many a man could be cured if only a wealthy uncle would die and leave him a good annuity so that he could take life easy.

A helpful hint. To my way of thinking the most important thing many a man with ulcer can be taught to do is to start taking food every hour as soon as he runs into some great psychic strain or sorrow. It is then that he will be in great danger of an acute flare-up of symptoms with, perhaps, a perforation or a hemorrhage. Then is when his gastric acidity will greatly increase. The worst danger comes after 10 P.M. when the stomach is empty of food but still full of a highly acid juice. Then is when the man should be taking milk and antacids every hour. I say to these patients, "Why wait until you get a bad flare-up of the ulcer? When a life crisis comes, start treatment immediately to combat the gastric conditions that you know will soon be present, and which can easily bring a new ulcer or can greatly deepen an old one." Much of the time a man with an ulcer hardly needs any treatment; he is comfortable, and it may be that his ulcer is healed.

What patients should do when they run into such a crisis is to take milk and antacids at 10 P.M. and then keep setting an alarm clock to wake them every hour until perhaps 3 A.M. This can give much the same effect as a continuous drip treatment with a tube through the nose.

Many persons with an ulcer are much more in need of good advice than they are of a Sippy cure. I have seen many a man with a severe type of ulcer lose his pain when he calmed down and stopped "blowing his top."

DISTRESSES AND BURNINGS AND BAD TASTES IN THE MOUTH

There are quite a few women and a few men, usually around fifty years of age, who complain bitterly of a sore mouth or tongue, or a burning in the mouth, perhaps a feeling as if it had been burnt with hot food, or perhaps an acid or a metallic or a foul taste. Practically never can one see any local changes to account for this, and the fact that occasionally the distress is on only one side of the tongue or the mouth suggests strongly that the trouble is due to injury to a cranial nerve or some tract in the brain. My impression is that many of these persons have suffered thrombosis in some small artery in the bulb. I believe this because (1) in some cases it is clear that the distress in the mouth came with a small stroke, (2) the symptom comes usually at a time of life when little strokes are common, and (3) the misery seems always to remain unchanged through the years, in spite of every form of treatment physicians can think of.

Treatment. Because the lesion is up in the brain local treatment of the mucosa of the mouth does not do any good.

A loss of taste. A sudden loss of taste, especially on one side of the mouth, should make one think of thrombosis of some small intracranial artery. One might think, also, of hysteria. I remember a man who lost his sense of taste whenever he was going into one of his mild depressions. Sometimes the loss of taste is associated with a loss of smell, due either to a central lesion or to a bad sinusitis.

CANKER SORES IN THE MOUTH

Some persons suffer from little white, painful patches in the mouth. Physicians often call these "aphthous ulcers," but this is not a logical term because in many cases they are allergic ulcers. All the person has to do to avoid getting them is to keep a record of foods eaten the day before they appear. Then he may find that they are due to chocolate, tomatoes, pineapple, banana, pork, peanuts, or some other food. With the exclusion of the hurtful food from the diet the patient is well.

Often the lesions start with a little bleb, the top of which becomes necrotic. In this way the little ulcer forms. In many persons such an ulcer always lasts five days and then heals. I have known a few women who had these ulcers, not only in the mouth, but also in the vulva and vagina.

In a few of the cases I have seen, great anxiety proved to be the cause. In other cases mild canker sores seemed to be associated with colds.

Treatment. No local treatment seems to do any good. The best way to a cure is to find the offending food and to leave it out of the diet. If this does no good one must look for psychic strains. I doubt if vitamins or antibiotics do any good.

THE COATED TONGUE

Many persons worry about a coated tongue. Usually we physicians cannot do much about it. Some persons seem to have a life-long tenddency to a furred tongue. Perhaps the coating is formed by material which, during the night, has run back from the stomach into the mouth.

About the only thing one can do then is to take a wash rag and rub off some of the fur. This may help to sweeten the breath. To scratch off the "fur" the Japanese use little hoes or bamboo loops.

HALITOSIS

Some persons always have a sweet breath while others suffer often from a bad breath. In the worst cases, I think this must be due to some abnormality in metabolism or in the function of the liver. It may be like the changes in metabolism which occur shortly before death and result in a foul breath. The bad breath of many persons past sixty years of age may be due to changes in metabolism caused by aging.

Strong emotion, great anxiety, great grief, or the excitement of making a speech can quickly produce a foul, fecal type of breath, and this can clear away in a few minutes when the person is at peace again. Many women are distressed and handicapped because their breath becomes somewhat fecal in odor during sexual excitement. It is hard to say what the mechanism is, but a marked drying of the mouth may be the important factor.

Any change in the liver which would allow the passage to the lungs of foul intestinal gases should produce halitosis, and some persons suffering from hepatitis and cirrhosis have a bad breath.

Interesting was B. B. Crohn's observation that the eating of much pork can produce a bad breath. Many Europeans have a very bad breath which may be due in part at least to their fondness for large quantities of garlic, onions, and other spicy seasonings. The smoking of Turkish tobacco can also permeate a man's body and breath with a strong odor. Paraldehyde injected into the rectum may be smelled on the breath. The drinking of much alcohol can, of course, produce an unpleasant sourish breath next day. As is well known, a very foul breath can be due to ozena, a crusting destructive disease of the nasal mucosa. Fortunately, this disease is now rarely seen.

Other forms of bad breath can be due to pyorrhea, large cavities in teeth, or subacute sinusitis. Such odors can usually be recognized and differentiated by anyone who has often smelled them. The person dying of nephritis may have a urinous odor on the breath, and the diabetic often has a bad breath. Sometimes a woman's breath is bad during menstruation. Hypodermic injections of sodium cacodylate cause the breath to smell of garlic.

A useful trick to see if one's breath is bad is to lick the back of the hand and then smell it.

Treatment. Unfortunately, not much can be done for persons with the worst forms of halitosis: the ones that seem to be due to some metabolic defect. But all persons can keep the mouth clean and in good condition with the teeth and gums well attended to. Persons with severe pyorrhea should have the teeth removed and plates made. Bad tonsils full of plugs can be removed, and persons with antra full of pus can have windows made into the nose. Persons with a badly coated tongue can try scrubbing it every morning with a wash rag.

Many a man with a bad breath could help matters much by stopping heavy smoking and the drinking of alcoholic drinks. He should avoid pork, garlic, and onions and should not eat highly seasoned ragouts. He should, for a time, keep a record of unusual foods eaten to see if any of them produces the halitosis. If constipation is a problem, this should be corrected by a daily enema to see if this helps. A liver function test should be made to see if there is any deficiency in function there. A low fat diet can be tried. Any measure that improves health or gives mental peace may help the situation. Recently the claim has been made that one can sweeten the breath by taking pills of chlorophyll. Eating spinach should be just as good.

THE PERSON WHO SUFFERS A MARKED LOSS OF WEIGHT

In an older person a fairly rapid loss of weight without other symptoms or findings to suggest the presence of a carcinoma should always make one think of something wrong with the brain. I remember a woman who rapidly lost 100 pounds when she discovered her husband's infidelity. I have seen other women lose from 50 to 75 pounds because of a small, unrecognized stroke. Apparently the setting of some little "thermostat" in the hypothalamus becomes changed.

More than once I have seen a slightly psychotic girl in boarding school lose from 30 to 50 pounds because of homesickness or the discovery that her parents were thinking of divorce. I remember a priest who, on two occasions, suddenly lost 40 pounds, when he became doubtful of his fitness for the ministry, and much disturbed over this thought. As I show in Chapter 15 quite a few relatives of the psychotic will suddenly lose weight; and a decided loss of weight is sometimes one of the first signs of a serious mental depression. Often the rapidity with which the weight goes off suggests a psychic cause, or a stroke.

Obviously, whenever a person suddenly loses much weight, the physician should order an estimate made of the basal metabolic rate. Usually one can tell it is up from the appearance of the patient, the rapidity of the pulse, and the warmth of the hands, but in rare cases one can be deceived by lack of these signs. In puzzling cases the physician can try the effect of giving a little iodine or thiouracil.

ABDOMINAL DISTRESS DUE TO A LITTLE
UNRECOGNIZED STROKE

Every year I see several old men or women complaining of an abdominal distress and perhaps loss of weight for which several gastroenterologists have tried in vain to find a local cause. Then a carefully
taken history shows that at the beginning of the illness, a pain, or wave
of heat, or rending feeling came *suddenly* one day with other signs of
a little stroke. Several of the symptoms, such as a change in character,
will point to an injury to the brain (see Chapter 12). Sometimes the
abdominal distress soon fades, but in other cases it remains for years.
Sometimes with it there are signs of cramping in the stomach the minute
food is swallowed. In such cases the muscle of the stomach seems to be
spastic, much like the muscle of a hemiplegic arm.

DISTRESSES DUE TO GASTRITIS

In recent years, with the widespread use of the gastroscope, there has
been a flare-up of interest in gastritis, and for a while there was a tendency
to explain much illness on the basis of a little atrophy of the gastric
mucosa. In many a case the mucosa is a bit abnormal: There is no doubt
about that, but what it means is a question, and it is doubtful if it is producing symptoms. I much doubt if we ought to dignify these atrophic
changes with the name *gastritis* because that implies the presence of an
inflammatory process.

No one has been able to define the symptoms of mild forms of "gastritis," and it is now well established that commonly the mucosal changes
are present in the absence of any symptoms. It has been shown, also,
by Walter Palmer and his associates that over the course of years, in the
case of any one patient, "gastritis" can come and go *independently of
any symptoms* that may also be coming and going.

Under these circumstances, the wise physician will rarely tell a patient
that his symptoms are due to gastritis. To make this diagnosis may only
do harm by adding to the man's anxiety. Hypertrophic gastritis with
some acute inflammation of the gastric mucosa can produce the clinical
picture of ulcer, and in rare cases I have seen it followed later by extensive cancer of the stomach. Watching individual patients for years, I
have seen polyps come and go in the stomach without changing into
cancer. Accordingly, I haven't the fear of them that I used to have.

Treatment. As yet, physicians do not know what the treatment of
gastritis is, granting that in a given case it should be treated. In some
cases, a bad pyorrhea might be cleared up; certainly it would seem that
much pus coming down from the mouth should do harm to the stomach.

In cases of hypertrophic gastritis, if the acidity of the stomach is high,
and there is hunger pain, frequent feedings and antacids should be pre-

scribed. In cases in which there is an atrophic mucosa with achlorhydria one might try giving liver extract or riboflavin or folic acid with vitamin B_{12}. In my experience the giving of hydrochloric acid seldom does any good.

DISTURBING RESULTS OF DRINKING UNNECESSARY WATER

For years many self-appointed health advisers have been preaching that everyone should force himself to drink several unwanted glasses of water or even 2 or 3 extra quarts a day. So far as I know, there is no scientific basis for this advice. Walter B. Cannon used to say that a person's thirst tells him exactly how much water his body needs to maintain his fluids at the right level. To drink more water than is needed is only to put a burden on the heart and kidneys.

One reason why I object to the fad of indiscriminately loading persons down with unneeded water is that occasionally it does harm. Every so often I see a person whose insomnia is due to his having to get up several times at night to get rid of his extra quart of water. I remember, also, a woman who came half across the continent because of a diarrhea which no one in her state could cure. It stopped the minute I took away from her the extra 2 quarts of water she was taking each day *on instruction from her doctor's office nurse!* Occasionally I see a man whose diarrhea proves to be due to drinking more beer than his bowel or kidneys can handle comfortably. I have seen tubercular patients whose diarrhea was due to the drinking of too much milk. They had reasoned that if a quart was good, several quarts would be better and would cure more quickly!

ABDOMINAL DISTRESS DUE TO A SEVERE SINUSITIS

There are a few cases in which sudden and complete relief from a chronic abdominal distress follows the making of a window between the nose and a badly infected antrum. It would appear, then, that at times infection in the nose can upset the behavior of the digestive tract, just as it is upset when a cold is coming on.

THE MAN WHO HAS TO RISE NEAR DAYBREAK TO PASS GAS OR MOVE HIS BOWELS

There is a syndrome which is very disturbing to some people, because it causes them to get up around daylight to pass gas or to move the bowels. I do not know what the cause is. It was once thought to be due to achlorhydria, but we know now that this is rarely the case. My impression from studying many persons with this syndrome is that some are hypersensitive and cursed with too active reflexes. Others, with their overly sensitive and reactive rectum, also have an overly irritable bladder. I think most of the patients I have seen with the syndrome were men between the ages of forty and fifty.

The physician should always ask the patient to go to bed supperless for a night or two to see if the trouble is due to the eating of any particular food. I remember a case in which the waking was due to drinking coffee. Especially if a man with this trouble is overworking, one should find out if the symptom disappears when he takes a vacation. In that case, one knows that it is due to the hypersensitiveness and overactivity of the brain that come with overwork.

One of my patients with this syndrome recovered quickly when he got rid of a lot of bad teeth and thereby cured a severe pyorrhea.

The syndrome here described must be differentiated from that in which the patient has to get up at daylight because of the distresses that go with a fibrositis. In this disease rest in bed brings stiffness and pain, and relief comes when the victim gets up and walks around.

In all cases in which the early rising is due to gas or a loose bowel movement, the common causes for diarrhea should be thought of and looked for. One should examine the gastric juice to see if there is any acid; one should examine the colon with the roentgen ray, and one should examine the rectum and sigmoid colon with the sigmoidoscope. The stools should be examined, and in older men the prostate gland should be examined and the amount of residual urine measured.

Treatment. One can try giving the patient bromural when he wakes at three to urinate. This will help him to sleep until seven. He may try eating a light supper, and he may try taking an enema before retiring, so as to have the colon cleaner. In bad cases in which the person's rest is much disturbed, ½ grain of codeine can be taken at bedtime or when he wakes to urinate.

GREAT DISTRESS AFTER DEFECATION

A few highly sensitive, nervous, or somewhat psychotic patients complain bitterly of a pelvic or abdominal distress or of a jittery spell which closely follows defecation. This syndrome is not due to any gross disease that can be found in the rectum or pelvis, but appears to represent an exaggeration of that feeling of weakness and distress which affects some sensitive persons when, perhaps during an attack of diarrhea, they have a large loose bowel movement. Jittery persons with markedly exaggerated reflexes can get this same distress after a *normal* bowel movement.

I once reported sixty-three cases of this disease (Alvarez: 1944). All of the patients were more than usually nervous, tense, sensitive, and reactive to stimuli. Thirteen had psychotic relatives, and several were psychopathic. Some had episodes of nervous diarrhea, and some had a typically sore colon.

Treatment. It may help the patient to take a tablet or two of bromural 30 minutes before trying to move the bowels. This may quiet the reflexes. Some persons may have to take the sedative also before eating. Some should live on a concentrated, roughage-free diet without milk, fruit, and vegetables, so as to cut down on the frequency of their bowel movements. In this way they will have fewer ordeals to face. In some cases, and especially those in which there is dysrhythmia in the electroencephalogram, one should try the effect of dilantin.

ANOREXIA NERVOSA

This subject is discussed under the heading of the mild psychoses.

MARKED ABDOMINAL BLOATING NOT DUE TO GAS BUT TO A HYSTERICAL CONTRACTION OF THE MUSCLES OF THE ABDOMINAL WALL

In 1949 I reported ninety-six cases of a remarkable syndrome in which the patient, usually an unhappy woman of poor nervous heredity, bloats markedly because of the contraction of muscles at the back and top of the abdominal wall (Alvarez: 1949). Often the patient assumes a lordotic posture which helps to throw the abdominal contents forward and downward toward the pelvis. In most cases it is easy to recognize the syndrome from the history. The patient either bloats suddenly, or her abdomen gets larger and larger during the day. At night the swelling usually goes down, either partly or completely. The diagnostic point is that the deflation is not accompanied by the passage of any flatus. Diagnostic, also, is the fact that when the patient is bloated a roentgenogram of the abdomen shows no excess of gas in the stomach or bowel.

Sometimes, in these cases, under the influence of great emotion, the bloating takes place suddenly, and occasionally it will disappear just as suddenly. The fact that, under the influence of vomiting or of a general or spinal anesthesia or the injection of a dose of morphine, the abdomen goes flat suddenly without the passage of flatus shows that the bloating is not due to any increase in the volume of the abdominal contents. It is due purely to a shifting forward of these contents.

Pseudocyesis, or false pregnancy, is probably produced in much the same way, but it is a different disease in that in it the woman imagines herself pregnant, and she maintains the swelling for months. The nervous bloater seldom remains distended for more than two or three days, and she never has any idea that she is pregnant.

One way of making the diagnosis is to have the woman lie on her side and then quickly to pull her knees up to her chin. With this, the bloating may disappear. When a bloated woman lies on her back, especially with her thighs flexed on the abdomen, the distention either disappears or is much less prominent. Much depends on getting rid of any lordosis that may be present. As soon as the woman stands up and slumps into her old lordotic posture the distention returns.

In some of these cases the bloating is associated with abdominal pain, and because of this a few of the women get into the habit of taking morphine. In some women even the bloated abdomen is soft and easily palpated; in others it is tense and tender to the touch. In quite a number of them, segments of the rectus abdominis muscle on one or both sides will contract into a phantom tumor. A few of these women can bloat on one side of the abdomen or in only one quadrant of the abdomen. In a rare case the woman will have labor-like pains when she is bloated.

Many of the women are most likely to get their spells when they are tired or angry or upset. Between attacks they usually have a normal digestion. A number suffer at times from other signs of hysteria. A few have had spells of hypomania and some have been depressed. A third of the women seen by me had suffered or were suffering from migraine, and all were hypersensitive and overly reactive. Many were decidedly allergic and sensitive to many foods, but this allergy appeared to be only a complicating factor.

Many of these patients had been operated on, some many times, without any lesion having been found. None was helped by surgery. A few recovered later when they achieved a better adjustment to life or got out of some unhappy situation.

Treatment. I never found any good treatment, and some of the women remained ill for years. A few got well when a marital situation got better. A few got by by eating little. Some, when they wanted to go out in the evening, ate nothing all day. Some could wear a corset but others could not stand one when they became distended.

THE MAN WHO CANNOT EAT AT THE SAME TABLE WITH OTHERS

I have seen men, most of them with an epileptic inheritance and all the irritability that can go with that, who could not eat at table with anyone else. At home, the wife and children had to eat by themselves, and if at a restaurant someone came to sit at the man's table, he would have to get up and go out, leaving his food uneaten. Such men act in this way because they say that the near presence of someone bothers them beyond all enduring. If such a man were to force himself to stay and eat, he would get indigestion. I remember a man who resigned from the Rotary Club because he was so distressed over eating with others.

FIBROSITIC AND ARTHRITIC ACHES IN THE THORACIC AND ABDOMINAL WALLS

It is unfortunate that today one of the commonest causes for aches and pains around the thorax and abdomen is not thought of, and as a result, many patients are needlessly frightened with a diagnosis of angina or gallstones or ulcer, and many get a futile operation. I refer to that arthritis about the spine or fibrositis in the thoracic and abdominal walls which cause aching and neuralgic jabs of pain.

Oftentimes, if a patient were to be asked if his ache was inside the body or out in the wall he would say, "It is in the wall; when I am in pain some of my ribs are sore, or my abdominal wall is sore." In such cases if the doctor were to press on the ribs, or if he were to lift up a fold of abdominal wall and pinch it, he would see that the tenderness was superficial or mainly superficial. Often, also, he could learn that the patient had long been arthritic or fibrositic, and that he had suffered occasionally from backache, lumbago, wryneck, cricks, sacro-iliac pain, sciatica, so-called neuritis, or arthritis in the several joints of the arms and legs.

Very helpful is the story that the patient's ache becomes worse when he has been sitting a while, or lying in bed. Sometimes when in pain he has to get up to walk around a while to get "warmed up." This story is pathognomonic. Helpful diagnostically, also, is the fact that getting into a tub of hot water, or having some massage, brings relief. Helpful, also, is the story that the patient often gets along all right until he has an acute cold, and then he has a flare-up of his aches. Some persons of this type will note that the aches get worse as a storm is approaching, and this reveals the fibrositic or arthritic nature of the process. The aches may get worse, also, whenever the patient gets very tired.

A physician can usually tell in a minute that an ache is not anginal in nature because it lasts so long and has no relation to exercise; in fact it gets better if the person gets up and walks about. However, if he overexercises, as by digging in his garden, and thereby gets his muscles sore, he is likely to suffer next day, and this, again, is diagnostic. Persons with an ache in the lower ribs on the right side will sometimes be advised to have the gallbladder out, but usually it can be shown that the gallbladder functions well with the dye and the pain has no relation to eating. In other cases the xiphoid appendix of the sternum is sore and tender to the touch, due to a perichondritis. This soreness is sometimes mistaken for that of peptic ulcer. Sometimes there is some arthritis in the joints at the end of the tenth rib, and between its movable tip and the rib above. Arthritis in these little joints causes the side-ache of runners.

Often it helps in ruling out disease in the thorax to show that the ache in the chest wall occasionally moves on down into the abdominal wall. Sometimes the ache on one side can be made worse by having the patient bend to that side so as to put pressure on the nerves emerging from the spine. There is a type of pseudo-appendicitis which is probably due to a myositis or fibrositis of the iliopsoas muscle.

In some cases the diagnosis is a bit difficult because, associated with a fairly acute arthritis around the spine, there will be some distressing flatulence, possibly reflex in origin and due to irritation of spinal nerves.

There is a rare acute disabling form of this fibrositic disease which sometimes produces a puzzling picture. The syndrome has been called infectious pleurodynia, or the devil's grip. In this disease the patient may start with what looks like a severe lumbago on one side. Because of the pain on movement, for a few nights the victim may have to sleep in a chair with a board behind him. The pain may spread up to involve the diaphragm and the muscles of the thoracic wall. With the splinting of the diaphragm and the thoracic wall and perhaps some involvement of the pericardium, the patient may get decidedly dyspneic on exertion. For a time he will be unable to lie down or to lie on the affected side. In some cases the pain may run into the epigastrium and be mistaken for that of peptic ulcer. Usually, after a few days or weeks, the disease quiets down. The cause would seem to be a virus, but it has not been identified. The disease is self-limited and usually does not leave sequelae.

Treatment. Obviously the treatment for pains of fibrositic or arthritic origin must consist largely of physiotherapy—heat and massage. A hot tub bath will often help much. Many persons use a lamp or a baker for the application of heat. Aspirin will help. Unfortunately there is as yet no specific drug.

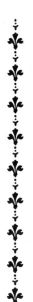

CHAPTER 19

The Psychic Problems
of the Patient with
Heart Trouble

THE IDEA OF DISEASE in the heart is particularly frightening. Because of the widespread idea that heart disease is commonly fatal many men and women are thrown into a panic the minute they suspect they have it, and a cardiac neurosis, when once established, is one of the hardest of all neuroses to get rid of.

As Willius once pointed out, there is much in our mother speech and folklore to make all of us heart conscious. We often say a person dies of a broken heart or of a heart attack. Hence, just let a man get a pain in what he thinks is his heart, let him feel a missed beat, let his heart race for a minute, or let him feel a little harmless air-hunger, and he may instantly become a badly frightened man. As a man once wrote to his physician, an extrasystole always affected him as if it were a cannon ball shot at his brain!

Let a man be turned down for life insurance or for Army service because of a little murmur or some slight change in his electrocardiogram, and he may become so disturbed that he will start going from physician to physician, getting opinions.

Every month the internist sees patients who have been badly frightened by a questionable diagnosis of coronary disease, usually based on an inadequate history and an inexpert interpretation of an electrocardiogram. In the worst cases of cardiac neurosis the patient appears to be mildly psychotic.

The common symptoms of a cardiac neurosis. Probably the commonest symptom complained of by heart-conscious patients is palpitation, with a fast, pounding beat. Perhaps an attack starts without obvious cause, or it follows excitement, a fright, a cold, or some fatiguing experience.

When a woman with a tendency to palpitation comes into a physician's office her pulse may be running as high as 130 beats a minute. Usually, after a while it will be found to have slowed down to perhaps 80 beats a minute, and early in the morning, if the husband will count it while she is still in bed, he will find it running only 60 beats a minute. Vagal stimulation, effected by asking the patient to take a deep breath and hold it, may slow the pulse to normal. These facts all make the diagnosis of a nervously overactive heart, and they rule out hyperthyroidism. Especially if the patient's hands are cold, as they are likely to be, there is little need for having the basal metabolic rate estimated.

Some worrisome persons with a fast heartbeat will be fearful that, with the excess beats, the heart will wear out. They can be assured that it will not. Others who have a slow pulse are afraid that it will slow still more and stop. It will not. Nervous persons sometimes suffer from paroxysmal tachycardia. In this disease the pulse suddenly starts going so fast it can hardly be counted. Later, it as suddenly resumes its normal rate. Especially when the electrocardiogram is normal, this syndrome rarely gives any serious trouble.

Another common symptom of persons with a nervous heart is the extrasystole. As most physicians know, these extra beats commonly go with an essentially normal heart. Obviously, one should never make a diagnosis of heart disease on the mere presence of the premature contractions. Furthermore, in such cases it is unwise to spend a lot of time examining the patient's heart and perhaps hospitalizing him. This is likely only to increase his fear. In the case of nervous persons a fast pulse or a missing beat may appear for the first time after some trying psychic experience or during convalescence from some illness such as influenza, or it may come as the result of smoking too much or drinking too much coffee. It is worth noting that many rather insensitive persons remain unconscious of extrasystoles while others, probably more sensitive, are much upset by them.

The treatment of this condition consists of education and reassurance. For years I kept in my consulting room a copy of Sir James Mackenzie's great book on heart disease with a mark at the page on which, in one sentence, he gave the treatment of extrasystoles. He said that the patient must learn to get used to them and disregard them! I have cured many a person by just showing him that statement. I have helped many, also, by telling of my father who had them from the age of forty-eight to the age of eighty-four. They never did him any harm. I have found it helpful, also, to draw for patients a diagram showing how a nervous impulse throws in a little extra beat which blocks out the next regular beat. The beat after that, because of the longer rest, is a powerful one, which gives the patient the impression that the heart has turned over or thumped.

When the patient becomes convinced that his heart is essentially sound, and that it is only his nerves that are playing tricks with it, he is likely to be much reassured, and he may go away happy.

Another common symptom, usually seen in a woman who fears heart disease, is *air-hunger,* or a feeling that air is not getting down deep enough into her lungs, or is not supplying enough oxygen. This is not dyspnea and it should never be called dyspnea. It has nothing to do with the heart but is nervous in origin. Some women will say that they are smothering, and they will then fan themselves. Waking at night with the distress, they may jump out of bed and run to a window with the idea of there getting more air, or air with more oxygen in it. Occasionally a person whose nose has been stuffed up may wake out of sleep with an air-hunger which can be relieved by taking a few big deep breaths. In such cases it is possible that with shallow breathing there came some oxygen deficiency in the lung.

The important point is that the symptom comes at any time and is not brought on by exertion or anger. It may be brought on by the psychic impression of being in a closed room. Many sensitive and migrainous women cannot stand a closed, air-conditioned room. They feel the need for an open window and a bit of draft. In an air-conditioned room the air may be moving very well but the woman still wants an open window.

A woman suffering from air-hunger will sometimes, in her fright, start hyperventilating, or panting rapidly, and with this there will soon come an alarming wooziness, giddiness, or faintness, together perhaps with numbness and tingling in the hands and around the mouth.

Many nervous women who often *feel faint,* or tend to *faint easily,* think they are subject to heart disease or liable to get it. Actually, faintness in a person who is up and about is seldom due to heart disease. It is much more likely to be due to overemotionality, poor nervous stability, or the migrainous constitution. Still another symptom sometimes ascribed to a supposed heart disease is a *pathologic sense of fatigue.* This is usually due to a poor nervous inheritance, and often to constitutional frailness or neurocirculatory asthenia.

Some persons get upset and frightened because of a feeling of *gas under the heart.* Perhaps they do have an excess of gas either in the stomach or in the splenic flexure, but this, of course, need not have anything to do with the heart. Other highly neurotic persons are frightened by what they call *choking spells,* probably a form of globus hystericus.

Some young women, too young ever to have a real angina pectoris, complain of an ache over the heart and down the left arm. It may cause them to drop things out of the left hand. It comes, not with exercise, but with fatigue, and it may come off and on during a lifetime. Obviously, it is not an angina. In some such women it may perhaps be a forerunner of hypertension.

Pseudo heart attacks. A neurotic woman sometimes wakes at night, perhaps with a big thumping extrasystole, and gets panicky with the idea that she is about to die with a heart attack. What with air-hunger, hyperventilation, and some hysteria, she is soon putting on a good show. Perhaps several physicians are called. When the first one arrives much depends on his good sense and ability to handle excited persons. If he recognizes a nervous storm, reassures everyone, tells them that nothing has happened to the heart, gives the woman a sedative, and sends the whole family back to bed, all may be well. But if he gets excited, rushes the woman to a hospital, puts her in an oxygen tent, has a series of electrocardiograms made, and announces that a coronary artery has become thrombosed, the woman may get launched on a career of neurosis that no one can ever stop. Anyone who later tries to take her "heart disease" away from her may get no thanks for his pains.

Sometimes it will be noted that the woman has her attacks of panicky "heart disease" when she is out in the country where it would be hard to get a physician quickly. When she is in town, or when she has a nurse with her, there may be no trouble. This story makes the diagnosis. I remember a woman like this who, one night, shortly after her husband's death, got a panicky spell while alone in her big house out in a suburb. When a physician finally got there, he thought she had had a heart attack. She went on having such attacks almost nightly until she came to Rochester. With many doctors just across the street from her hotel, she had no spells. Following this hint, I had her move out of her lonely home to take an apartment next to the one occupied by her trusted family physician. After this she was well.

A common cause of a cardiac neurosis is the sudden death of a relative or friend or business associate. This takes away the person's sense of security, and the more he concentrates his thoughts on his heart the more symptoms he can feel in his chest. A vicious circle is set up because the more he feels in his "heart," the more frightened he gets.

Many persons are the more concerned about heart disease because they know it runs in the family. Perhaps it has caused several relatives to drop dead before they were fifty. Unfortunately, a man with such a family tendency has good reason to be fearful, especially when the titers of his blood cholesterol and fats are high. The unfortunate feature is that a man with such anxiety is likely to interpret any little fibrositic ache in his thoracic wall as due to heart disease.

The effort syndrome or "soldier's heart." During World War I, one of the commonest diagnoses made was "effort syndrome," "soldier's heart," "disordered action of the heart," "irritable heart" or "over-consciousness of the heart." The syndrome had been observed in the Civil War and many wars before that. DaCosta had spoken of the rapid heartbeat, palpitation, shortness of breath on the slightest exertion, vague pains in the chest, disturbed sleep, giddiness, flatulent indigestion, and sweating. He also noted the cold, blue, mottled legs that go with a neurocirculatory asthenia.

Later, Kilgore noted in these patients signs of constitutional inadequacy, such as flabby muscles, a tendency to low or high blood pressure, often poor nutrition, cold dripping hands, dripping axillas, and dermatographia. He noted the tendency these persons have to faint easily, and he noted the consciousness of the heart action, and the somewhat irregular pulse.

Gradually, as World War I came to a close, more and more physicians came to see that these men did not have heart disease. Their trouble was in the brain and, to a large extent, scattered all over a poorly built body. These men were born frail, with poor materials in them. In most cases they developed their symptoms in the induction stations *before they had a chance to fight.* Then it was found that if they were put to bed and coddled they got worse. They did much better when sent out to play baseball or to raise vegetables for the hospital. Most of them got better when the Armistice was signed.

Later, it was discovered by Oppenheimer and Rothschild (1918) that over two thirds of these men had psychotic relatives, and this was the essential point. They belonged in the group that I describe elsewhere in this book as "relatives of the psychotic," and "their nerves were playing tricks on them." Most of their troubles were due to anxiety and fear and an inability to "stand the gaff" of Army life, or, for that matter, of any life.

In the years that followed, other men such as Wolfsohn, Campbell, Douglas-Wilson, and Wood confirmed the findings of Oppenheimer and Rothschild. Dunn and many others confirmed the fact that these patients were primarily psychoneurotic.

Interestingly, in World War II the knowledge of psychiatry had advanced so much that little was ever said about the effort syndrome or "shell shock." The patients were recognized quickly for what they were and were mustered out or turned over to the psychiatrists. Recently

Meyer Friedman has studied a group of these men and has emphasized a few points such as their tendency to tremor and to hyperthermia after a little excitement, such as that attendant on gambling. They have cold wet hands, their faces flush easily, and they have a labile pulse and but little ability to hold the breath.

After careful study, Friedman concluded that the pseudo-angina of these men can arise in the chest wall. It appears to be due to an insufficient use of the diaphragm and to too great a use of the intercostal musculature in breathing. There are reasons for believing that the respiratory spasms of these men come out of the hypothalamus.

On recognizing the person with a nervous heart. The person who is likely to have a nervous heart usually appears nervous and behaves in a nervous manner, as is described in Chapter 3. Rarely the man arrives in a wheel chair which he does not need. At a glance the physician can see that he has neither dyspnea nor cyanosis nor edema.

Often the wise physician will suspect a *cardiac* neurosis as soon as he notes that the patient has one or more typical *abdominal* neuroses such as air-swallowing, regurgitation, or burning in the epigastrium. The doctor can then tell the patient that the same nerves that are playing tricks with his good stomach are playing tricks with his good heart.

As shown in Chapter 4 it helps to note how the history is given. The person with a functional trouble is more likely to be vague and rambling and to emphasize his fears. It helps greatly to know that spells of distress follow psychic upsets and not exertion. It helps to learn of poor nervous heredity, and it helps to get the story of nervous breakdowns, perhaps episodes of hysteria, or symptoms like unreasoning fear which suggest more a psychosis than a neurosis.

In Yaskin's (1936) group of 100 cases of bad cardiac neurosis, most of the patients were neurotic and had several neuropathic or psychopathic relatives. Six of the patients later developed psychoses, which shows that a supposed "neurosis" is sometimes really a mild or a beginning psychosis. There were thirteen patients who suffered from compulsions.

The first attack. Sometimes it helps to learn the details of the first attack which frightened the patient. What had he been doing? Had he been under great psychic strain? For instance, a woman got her first spell after wrangling for several hours with a sister-in-law. A man got his first spell after the distressing experience of having to discharge an old employee, and another became heart conscious the night his brother dropped dead and his mother promptly followed suit.

Anginal pain. If there is a question about coronary disease the physician must question the patient in great detail as to whether the pain comes always with exercise. Real angina is especially likely to come after breakfast or when the person is walking into a cold wind or carrying suitcases. One wants to know if the patient's pain compels him to stop, and how soon it is before he can walk on again. How far can he go without being stopped? Does he take nitroglycerin, and does this help?

I remember a man who gave me what I thought was a perfect story of angina. Then Dr. Willius drew from him the admission that he got the pain only when he was on his way to solicit an advertising contract. If he got it, he could blithely walk back to his office, and run upstairs without distress. Dr. Willius decided that his trouble must be psychic in nature. Often a patient will say that he stops when he feels pain in his chest, but a question will show that he does this not because he has to, but because his doctor told him to do it. One may then have reason to doubt if the man really has angina. Sometimes true angina comes with sexual intercourse.

Often, careful questioning will bring out the fact that the "pain" in the "heart" is a typical fibrositic ache in the thoracic wall which lasts for hours and has no relation to exertion. It is actually cleared away by walking. Perhaps, with an arthritis of the spine, there will be short sharp neuralgic jabs of knifelike pain. Usually in such cases one can get a story of arthritis along the spine, with a wryneck, lumbago, cricks, and sciatica.

Often a little questioning will show that a patient has several types of chest pain: One may come with exertion and will suggest angina; another may be an ache in the chest wall; another, a sudden jab; another, a peculiar rending, expanding, or burning feeling, originating probably in abnormal peristalsis in the esophagus; another may be originating in a gallbladder full of stones; or another may be originating in a diaphragmatic hernia. I have seen a few persons who had not only coronary disease, but also gallstones, and even a diaphragmatic hernia. Sometimes a patient has a constant ache on one side of the thorax and perhaps part of the abdomen: an ache which is typically psychic in origin and made worse by depression, fatigue, or annoyance.

In rare cases angina is brought on by attacks of paroxysmal tachycardia. They bring out a latent tendency to the disease. Other causes for a distress in the chest may be heartburn, or globus, or a bit of lumbago involving the diaphragm and the thoracic wall. I have seen short spells of severe thoracic pain due, apparently, to spasm in the esophagus brought on by emotion, or a draft of cold air, or eating certain foods.

The little stroke. In older persons what at first was looked on as a heart attack may prove later to have been a little stroke with a paresthesia shooting down into the thorax. Electrocardiograms will then be normal, and the subsequent course of the patient's illness will show that the injury was to the brain and not to the heart.

Why a person so fears heart disease. In many cases it is very important to find out why the patient fears heart disease and why he fears it so terribly. Usually the answer is that heart disease runs in the family, and the patient saw one or more near relatives die of it.

The person who has recovered from coronary heart disease and now suffers only from fear. There are innumerable persons who have ridden out the storm of a coronary thrombosis and have been left with only a small almost symptomless scar. They have a good cardiac reserve and can walk around comfortably. If such a man has only a normal concern about his health, and a lack of paralyzing fear, he can go back to his office and work hard, perhaps for another fifteen years, or until he is ready to die of old age. But just let him be a worrisome type of man, easily frightened and predisposed to hang onto his fears, and then there is trouble. He may continue, for the remainder of a long life, to go from physician to physician, getting endless electrocardiograms made.

Interesting is Dry's story of a man who, in his late thirties, had a coronary occlusion so bad that he nearly died. When he was well, Dry commented on his lack of fear which helped to save his life. The man answered, "Oh, I wasn't scared because in the last thirty years I have watched Dad weather successfully three bad attacks of coronary thrombosis, so I knew it could be done!"

The man who gets angry when told he hasn't organic heart disease. A man with a normal mind and a normal reaction to disease will rejoice when a cardiologist tells him that his local physician was mistaken as to the interpretation of an electrocardiogram, and that he can now go back to his work, his hunting, and his golf. He will not argue with the cardiologist and will not try to trap him in inconsistencies of statement. He will go back to work and will not bother to get more electrocardiograms. Another type of man will cling to some home doctor's diagnosis of heart disease, and will seem to be angry with the specialist who tries to take it away from him.

The significance of electrocardiograms. As Dry has well said, more diagnostic errors result today from the incorrect interpretation of an electrocardiogram than from the failure to have one made.

Today, many physicians, and even many who call themselves cardiologists, seem to interpret any deviation from the textbook electrocardiogram as indicative of myocardial damage. It is most unfortunate when they fail to note that the deviation is due to the fact that the patient is old, or that abdominal fat has pushed the heart up into a horizontal position, or that the man has hypertension, or is taking digi-

talis. It is sad, also, that often the physician fails to ask what the heart
can do, and thus fails to learn that the patient is still playing good
tennis or still hunting in the mountains. According to my cardiologic
colleagues at the Mayo Clinic, such facts are far more significant than
the one that he has a few slurrings and notchings in his electrocardiogram. I often marvel at the amount of deviation from the normal
textbook electrocardiogram which these colleagues of mine commonly
ignore as within normal limits, considering the person's age or shape
of thorax. They are always more interested in what the man's heart
can do in the way of handling strains on his circulation.

I was much impressed once, hearing how impatient Sir James Mackenzie used to get with physicians who, at a consultation, kept talking
about the patient's electrocardiograms. Sir James, who had popularized
the use of electrocardiograms, would say, "Throw those things away,
and tell me how long is the man's rope." In other words, how far he
could walk without being compelled to stop because of pain in his
chest. If this distance was short the man's condition was serious, but
if it was long the prognosis was good.

As Dry has said, he who would diagnose heart disease correctly
must be capable of recognizing in a moment in the electrocardiograms
the disturbing influences of digitalis. Many a man has been told
that he had coronary disease simply because the physician failed to
recognize a digitalis effect, and did not think to ask if the drug was
being taken.

The influence of emotion on the electrocardiogram. Dry listed
among the electrocardiographic findings noted at times, in cases of a
purely irritable heart, a prolonged P-R interval, a prolonged QRS complex, which is usually preceded by an unusually short P-R interval or a
sino-auricular block, also changes in the T-wave in the second and third
leads. These changes appear to be dependent on the vagus because they
can often be abolished by the giving of atropine.

A number of men have studied the changes in the electrocardiograms
which can come while the patient is under the influence of strong emotion (see Am. J. Psychiat. *101:*697, 1945).

These studies should cause physicians to remember how anxious some
persons are when the first electrocardiogram is taken. When they feel
that their life depends on that little record, how can they approach the
ordeal without emotion? Perhaps the technician should always make
note if the person seems overly worried while his electrocardiogram is
being taken. Many persons, of course, will not be upset, but some will
be. I tell elsewhere of the anxious physician who went into a state
of noisy hyperventilation when I got out his electrocardiograms to
look at them.

I remember a company official who went to be examined for a $250,000 life insurance policy. He arrived late and all upset because, while hurrying through sleety streets, he twice had skidded into a snow bank. Probably, as a result of the mental state he was in, his electrocardiogram was so abnormal that the insurance company turned him down. That they were wrong was shown by the fact that for years afterward he remained well and strong, and during these years dozens of electrocardiograms were normal.

Deaths due to fright. Mainzer and Krause spoke of the fact, which is well known to surgeons, that some persons die on the operating table just before the starting of the anesthetic. Some of the deaths apparently due to anesthesia appear to have been due to fright because they came as the patient took the first few whiffs of the gas. I have seen several such cases in which death came while the abdominal wall was being painted; in others it came with the start of the anesthesia or with the introduction of a hypodermic needle. On several occasions I have seen patients die or almost die after they said they would go out on the table. Such cases have taught me never to force an operation on a patient who fears greatly that he will die, or on one who, for some reason, wants to die. One should not force an operation on a badly frightened patient who, on several mornings, has had to be sent back from the operating room because of a sharp rise in temperature. I remember a woman who had such emotionally produced rises who died with the first whiff of the anesthetic.

Puzzling cases. There is a type of case in which the cardiologist may have to withhold a positive opinion, and that is the case of a person who tells a story of angina on exertion or after anger: a story so good that it cannot be disregarded, and yet, one with decidedly inconsistent features. Perhaps the man gets attacks of pain while lying quietly in bed, and then at times he walks rapidly without discomfort. He may show no signs of heart failure and he may not get angina when made to breathe air deficient in oxygen. The puzzle about this is that one would think that a man who gets so much angina while at rest should be in such bad shape and with so little cardiac reserve that he would be almost unable to walk. Often in such cases the electrocardiogram does not help much. Then, about all the cardiologist may be able to say is, "Carry on as you are doing, stopping when pain comes, and taking nitroglycerin when you need it." These people often cannot be given a diagnosis when they first come in; only a period of observation will show what the situation is. The fact that nitroglycerin helps does not prove the presence of coronary heart disease; it may be relieving pain due to spasm in the esophagus or in the common bile duct.

The psychic disturbances that occur during the course of serious heart disease. The cardiologist has to be a bit of a psychiatrist not only to care for the neurotic persons who have only a fear of heart disease but he has to be ready to handle wisely those many persons who have become mentally disturbed over some serious organic heart disease. Occasionally, also, the cardiologist will have to take care of a person who becomes psychopathic or a bit maniacal during an attack of endocarditis.

As Yaskin (1936) has pointed out, especially if a patient has a poor nervous heredity, during decompensation of the heart he may become confused, disoriented, and hard to handle. He may get hallucinations and ideas of persecution, and he may go into a mild delirium. Milder mental disturbances may come simply as the result of hospitalization with its restricted activity, discouragement, and worry. Other causes of mental symptoms may be renal failure, acidosis, cerebral anemia, and the toxic effects of drugs being administered, such as digitalis.

Lewis A. Connor wrote once of the peculiar mental makeup of persons who have had mitral stenosis from childhood. Just as they often have a small head and face, they may have somewhat peculiar mental processes. The person with aortic regurgitation may suffer from bad nightmares.

The handling of the patient with a cardiac neurosis. No cardiologist can be a good therapist until he has learned how to handle his worrisome patients. He must learn what to do and not do and what to say and not to say. As I pointed out in Chapter 8 if he is not wise and well schooled and watchful always of his tongue, he will often be upsetting patients and making worried wrecks of them. Often the best thing he can do is to start reassuring the minute he hears the story of such things as extrasystoles, air-hunger, or a fibrositic ache in the chest wall. In many such cases, if the patient accepts the doctor's opinion and trusts him, it may be best not to go on and give a thorough examination. Just taking a history and listening to the heart may be enough. It may do harm to send the patient to a hospital for an extensive study. It may intensify fear, and it may fasten on a neurosis.

So often a physician can send a patient home reassured and happy within a few minutes after he comes in. For instance, a fine businessman came a long distance, much frightened over some extrasystoles that followed a very trying experience. Worse yet, he had received an alarming diagnosis based on a cardiologist's pessimistic interpretation of slight changes in an electrocardiogram. Immediately on hearing his story, I said, "Do you mean to say all you have are missed beats? Why, one of my relatives began to have them when she was twenty-two and still has them at the age of sixty-five." With that statement alone the man began to breathe easier, and that night he slept again. My cardiologic colleagues at the Mayo Clinic could not see anything alarming about his electrocardiograms, and two days later, looking like a different man, he went back to work.

In many such cases, of course, a good examination, with the making of electrocardiograms and roentgenograms, is necessary if the patient is to be dealt with fairly and properly reassured, but it helps much if the patient sees that the physician knew right off what was wrong and was not alarmed. It is a physician's evident alarm that is bad. It may be essential to get from the home doctor the electrocardiograms on which the serious diagnosis was made, and then to say that the changes in them are within normal limits or explainable on the basis of some such thing as hypertension, a high diaphragm, or digitalis. If the consultant were to say only that the electrocardiograms *he made* were normal the patient might say, "You missed the abnormality but it showed up in the electrocardiograms that I had made at home."

A good and careful examination is sometimes the best part of psychotherapy. As Paul White has said, there is no reason why a psychopath cannot have a coronary thrombosis. A well-taken history commonly cures a patient if it helps him to see that the pain is in his chest wall, or if it shows him the connection between his syndrome and an unpleasant experience. Many a time I have had a patient go home satisfied, reassured, and happy just because the points brought out in the history convinced him that his heart was all right and strong. Obviously, one has to spend time with the patient, and often one must cross-examine him to see exactly what he meant by a certain statement. If an intelligent man feels that the doctor's explanation fits the facts of his illness and is logical and reasonable, he will go away happy.

The need for showing the patient what an electrocardiogram means. Sometimes one has to get a patient to understand a little of what an electrocardiogram is. He may think it is like the slip of paper that comes out of a scale when one sticks in a penny and gets weighed. He may think it will tell whether he is ill, and how long he will live, and that it will do this with certainty. He may have to be shown that this is not the way an electrocardiograph works. The records it makes have to be interpreted by an expert, and in poor hands they can be very misleading.

Often it helps to show the victim of a coronary thrombosis a roentgenogram of an injected heart, with one coronary artery closed off and the collateral circulation carrying the burden. Then he can see that he has a scar in his heart muscle; he can see why he did not die with the plugging of an artery, and why he can now live on for many years in good health. I often tell these patients of the many friends I have in the medical profession who are still doing good work fifteen years and more after a bad coronary attack.

In many cases the physician must answer an intelligent patient's question as to the limits of what an electrocardiogram can do in the way of ruling out serious disease. The patient will say: "You say my electrocardiogram is normal, but I know of a man who was told one morning that his electrocardiogram was perfect, and that night he dropped dead." Surely, of course, this can happen. A man with a narrowed coronary artery can suffer from angina on exertion because not enough blood is getting through to his heart muscle. But so long as there is no thrombosis, the electrocardiogram can be all right because there is no dead or scarred heart muscle to deflect the course of the impulse as it travels over the heart. An electrocardiogram is only a record of the changes in voltage that take place as the contraction wave moves through the heart muscle.

The man who has had a coronary attack, or who has a narrow coronary artery that gives him angina when he walks fast, must be told the truth so that he can guard against disaster. It helps to tell him that his anginal distress is useful and valuable in that it will always tell him to stop when he should. It is his constant mentor and guide, taking the place of a personal physician. With this he does not have to be asking his doctor all the time what he can do: His angina will tell him.

Probably a letter of findings should usually be given because otherwise the patient is bound to get things all mixed up. As in the case of the person being told for the first time that he has tuberculosis, the patient told that he has heart disease is likely to black out. Hence, it is often advisable either to write a report or to see the patient again after he has had time to come out of the shock of hearing the bad news.

On mentioning harmless findings. Often, also, the physician has to explain why he is not concerned over an old cardiac murmur which evidently has not greatly increased the work of the heart muscle. As I showed in Chapter 8, a big question that frequently arises is whether the physician should tell of such a harmless murmur. This is particularly important in consultant practice where the patient often goes from one physician to another getting opinions. If Dr. A does not mention a functional or congenital murmur or a left ventricular preponderance or an inversion of the T wave in lead III, what will happen in the patient's mind if Dr. B or Dr. C tells him about these things and marvels that Dr. A missed them? If one either tells or does not tell, a worrisome type of patient may get into a bad state of mind. Dr. Dry thinks it better to tell about the changes found even if they are of no significance. Then, if they are found later, they will not cause so much alarm.

The doctor should be positive. In treating persons with heart disease the unpardonable sin is indecision and a wish to straddle the fence or to hedge and keep a way open for retreat. The doctor who does this will never cure an anxious patient; he will only make him worse. In order to cure persons, the physician must be definite. If he decides there is no disease in a heart he must say so flat-footedly. He must not say, "Your heart *seems* all right," but rather, "It *is* all right." He must not say, "I think your heart is all right"; he had better say, "I can find absolutely no sign of heart disease." Furthermore, he must not say, "But you had better go easy," or "You might take a little digitalis."

The doctor cannot just say, "There is nothing the matter with you"; because if the patient feels ill or has a pain there must be some cause. The important point is that the distress is not arising in the heart. It is nothing to occasion concern. Then the doctor must go on to explain in simple speech how he thinks the distress came, and what it means. He may have to find out exactly in what part of the thorax the pain comes. Often, for a time, he will have to keep seeing and reassuring the patient because, and this is an important point, *each day the man's pain or ache will be suggesting to him that the doctors are wrong and he really is ill*. Or he may keep saying to himself, "If I am all right why do I not get well immediately?" He will forget that it took him a long time to get tired and ill, or he will forget that annoyances in home or office are still going on, or that a great burden of strain is still on his shoulders.

As Willius has said, the physician must try not to leave the patient with the idea that perhaps the seat of his trouble has not yet been found, and that a more thorough examination would reveal it. This is such a common attitude of patients today, and we physicians foster it by our expressions of uncertainty.

Sometimes I think it is wise when a worried patient comes back to beg for another electrocardiogram to tell him, "No, the one you had was normal and that is enough. You can't get well if you keep trying to prove that one wrong." If the physician gives in and orders another electrocardiogram the patient may think that he, too, was not sure, and hence is willing to reopen the case. Certainly no heart medicine must be given to a patient who has no need of it.

One should not be vague, also, in warning the patient "to be careful." This engenders fear because the patient does not know what he should and should not do. It is better to say, "So long as you can walk ten blocks without any distress and can hurry upstairs, go ahead and do it." The patient should be given the idea that pain and shortness of breath will tell him when he is going too far.

As Dry pointed out, in many cases and especially when the patient is intelligent, the physician does not have to go into all the details of the psychological situation that produced a cardiac neurosis. All he has to do is to satisfy the man that his troubles are due to the situation he is in, and that he is not seriously ill; then he will get better.

Always one must avoid vague statements. An intelligent patient wrote me one day: "My cardiologist told my home doctor that I had 'a little cardiac condition.' What does that mean? How bad is that?"

We physicians are often inclined to regard physical overexertion as the greatest danger and to forget that mental excitement can also do great harm. I remember a farmer, suffering from angina pectoris who, for months, got along well by stopping physical labor. Then he decided to sell his farm. At the auction, when he saw his fine horses going for a fraction of what they were worth, he became so upset that he died.

Paul White (1927) and L. A. Conner (1927) wrote well on methods for rehabilitating patients with heart disease.

Prognosis. Whether a patient ever works again after he has had a coronary occlusion depends, of course, on the amount of damage sustained, on the amount of good muscle left, on the amount of courage and lack of fear that the patient has, and on the optimism of his medical advisers. Much depends also on the character of a patient's work. Naturally, a man who works at a desk can often carry on well, when a day laborer with a similar lesion would have to quit his job. With some persons much may depend on whether there is any disability insurance available.

CHAPTER 20

Psychosomatic Aspects of Surgery, Gynecology, and Obstetrics

PSYCHIC PROBLEMS IN SURGERY

THE WOMAN WHO HAS HAD SIX ABDOMINAL OPERATIONS. A wise clinician is inclined to diagnose a bad neurosis, a psychosis, hysteria, or constitutional inadequacy the moment he learns of more than five abdominal operations. He is the surer of his diagnosis when he learns that none of these operations ever did much good.

I remember once, at a medical meeting, being asked to give a clinic. I asked for a woman with the scars of at least six operations on her abdomen, and the interns in the big hospital soon wheeled one in for me. As I picked up her record in its aluminum binder and showed it to the audience, I remarked that one could just about make the diagnosis from the thickness of the history. The physicians understood, and chuckled; whereupon the woman became violent; she jumped up, crying raucously that she would not be insulted, and ran from the amphitheater. In so doing she strengthened the diagnosis I was making of an unstable nervous system.

On looking over her record, I found that fifteen years before, as a schizoid, sex-fearing girl, she had started training as a nun. But the Sisters soon found her unemployable and dismissed her. With this she began to complain so much of dysmenorrhea that her abdomen was

410

explored and bits of her ovaries were removed, together with her appendix. Because she got worse, the surgeons felt driven to go in again and remove the uterus. Still she had so much distress that they operated again and removed the ovaries. Then she began to regurgitate her food so badly that someone removed the stoneless gallbladder. When this did no good, someone performed gastroenterostomy. This brought on such violent vomiting that someone operated again and took down the gastroenterostomy. During the several years in which this sort of thing was going on the woman spent most of her time in county and university hospitals.

What interested me most in the record were the statements of the surgeons, made before several of the operations. They wrote something like this—"This biologically inferior woman has had hysterical episodes in the hospital and so the chances of helping her are slim. But she has much pain and vomiting, and the roentgenologist thinks he can see something wrong, and so *I am going to give her the benefit of the doubt* and go in again."

My impression was that if in his college days the surgeon had had some training in recognizing psychoses he would have given the woman the benefit of the doubt by *not operating*. Certainly, with better training, he would have known that regurgitation of food in a psychopathic girl is always functional and never helped by any operation. He might have known, also, that operating on the mildly psychotic with the idea of curing their hallucinations of feeling in the abdomen is a waste of time.

The woman who begs to have the abdomen explored. In this chapter I am trying to back up the teachings of all good surgeons who now try to get out of operating on neurotic patients when some internist like me gets to the end of his rope and decides he wants the abdomen explored again. I must admit with shame that I sometimes have talked surgeons into making such explorations. It was against my better judgment but the woman begged so hard for what she felt was her one chance to get well that I gave in.

The psychopaths who love operations. All surgeons know that many a psychopathic woman seems to love operations. Sometimes she thinks she knows which organ is diseased, and she wants it fixed, or perhaps she wants an operation to cure the terrible distress in her head, or she wants an operation to show her family that she was not "imagining her symptoms." Surgeons should remember that occasionally a woman will take refuge in a hospital in order to get away from a husband whom she does not like.

Every surgeon needs to be a bit of a psychiatrist. Every surgeon needs to be a bit of a psychiatrist so as to (1) avoid operating on psychopaths and persons who are poor psychic risks, and (2) take care of those persons who get hysterical or maniacal or depressed after an operation. The surgeon should always note such happenings in the record because they tell so much about the patient. They can warn others against any more operating on that person if it can possibly be avoided.

It helps to note such facts as that a woman kept begging for morphine long after the fourth day, or that she had a man visiting her who was persona non grata to her family, or that she was at swords' points with her husband or his family, or that she insisted on staying on in the hospital long after she was told to go home. Many a time a patient's nurse has obtained for me the secret story of unhappiness which I had suspected but could not get.

One objection to operating on psychopaths is that occasionally one will come back to threaten or to sue or even to shoot. Others, after even a minor operation, such as that of removing tonsils or hemorrhoids, will develop a hysterical syndrome or will go over the edge into a very trying nervous breakdown. Others after an operation will go head-first out of the hospital window.

When a patient is in poor psychic shape, any operation done under local anesthesia is likely to be very upsetting to the nervous system. If an operation must be done, it had better be done under sodium pentothal or a little gas. The person should be unconscious.

Reasons surgeons sometimes operate against their better judgment. When a surgeon is asked why he operated on a certain psychopath he is likely to say that though he recognized that she was neurotic or a bit hysterical, he feared that if he refused to do the work he might later learn that she had been operated on by someone else who had sewed up a kidney or removed the gallbladder and (for a few months at least) had obtained a fine result. A few such experiences, and a surgeon who for a while had been conservative may decide he had better be more radical.

Another reason commonly given by a surgeon who operates on a neurotic person is that the woman was so obviously going to get operated on by someone that he felt he might as well do the job; he felt he could do a good one, and thereby he might save her from losing her life somewhere at the hands of a poor operator.

It is true that many patients, when once infected with the idea that they should be operated on, cannot rest or get back any peace of mind until they have the work done. They keep going from one surgeon to another getting opinions, and although five men may refuse to operate, the fact that one says the work should be done that very day leaves them so uneasy that they are soon up on the operating table.

Such persons are like the young woman I saw once with "shotty breasts" who, when told that she did not need any operation, said, "Take them off anyway; I can no longer stand worrying about them." Or, some persons are like the very worrisome man who got the idea that he should have his appendix out. Although told by several surgeons that he had no indications for the operation, he finally insisted on it to relieve his mind. He said he had to travel a good deal, and he always went in mortal dread of having the appendix rupture while he was on a train!

Should a surgeon be conservative, or radical and venturesome? Many a surgeon is impressed by the fact that, occasionally, after a clinician or two has diagnosed a neurosis, he finds a stone in the common duct, or an ulcer in a Meckel's diverticulum, or a hemangioma in the jejunum, or a posteriorly perforating duodenal ulcer, and cures the patient. Such things, of course, happen, and I have had my moments of chagrin because of them, but the best surgeon is not the man who does forty-nine futile operations in order to succeed with one; the surgeon we physicians all admire and trust is the one who, perhaps, misses operating on one patient with a common duct stone while he saves from a needless operation forty-nine nervous or unhappy or psychopathic persons. All his days this man will be a force for good in his hospital; he will be a good teacher and a highly respected member of the profession.

The great need for a surgeon's trying to place a patient in good hands after he fails to work a cure. It is sad that so many surgeons, when they fail to find anything wrong at an abdominal exploration, deny themselves the pleasure they could gain from putting the patient into the hands of the particular physician in the city or state or country most likely to help. For instance, and this is only one of hundreds of cases I could cite, a fine woman who had drifted into a bad migrainous state because of unhappiness and worry consulted one of the leading surgeons in her state. She told the typical story of sick headaches and a sore colon. After prodding her abdomen he said, "Go out to the hospital this afternoon, and I'll remove your appendix." This he did through a two-finger incision.

As was to be expected, all the woman got out of this operation was a distressing nervous breakdown. When at last she was able to leave the hospital she told the doctor she was worse and asked if he had any suggestions for further treatment. He said, "Take some aspirin." He could have made some amends and given her something for her money if only he had taken the trouble to get her into the hands of someone like Harold Wolff, greatly interested in migraine, but he did not. It was years later that she found a kindly physician who said: "This is a bit out of my line so I will send you to someone who can tell you how to avoid the migrainous spells and how to take gynergen when they come."

Suggestions made by internists to professors of surgery. There are many suggestions which able internists here and there have told me they wished they could make often to teachers of surgery. Following is a list of them.

Have your students better trained to recognize quickly those common neuroses and psychoses and functional troubles which cause symptoms in the abdomen.

Teach them to have all their "chronic" patients examined first by an internist; this would lead to the easy avoidance of so many of the mistakes that now we physicians all regret. If it is dangerous oftentimes for an old diagnostician to make a snap diagnosis and not examine, how much more dangerous must it be for a man whose training was in surgery and not in diagnosis! (Daily I see patients who had an abdominal operation on the basis of a snap diagnosis that I would never have dared to make, and I have spent my life in trying to learn abdominal diagnosis.)

Teach your students that if they feel they must remove a so-called chronic appendix they should do it, not through a small incision, but through a big one, and then they should explore so thoroughly that it will not have to be done soon again.

Teach your young surgeons to face the fact that, especially in the cases of persons past middle age, the removal of a "chronic appendix," *when the patient has not been suffering from attacks of acute appendicitis,* rarely cures anything. (Alvarez: J.A.M.A. *114.*) Remind them that at a big surgical center like the Mayo Clinic, "chronic appendicitis" is looked on as a rare disease, and the diagnosis is almost never made.

Teach your students to keep making follow-up studies so that they may learn quickly if a new operation such as vagotomy is of any value, and, if so, in what types of cases it should be performed.

Try to keep your young surgeons from getting the idea that once they get their hands into an abdomen they can find the cause of a chronic distress. Occasionally they can, but often they will find nothing, simply because the cause of the distress is up in the brain or out in the abdominal wall.

Impress on your students that when they get the abdomen open and find nothing wrong, they should back out and close without performing gastroenterostomy or removing the gallbladder or uterus or anything else except perhaps the appendix.

Keep suggesting to your students that when they open an abdomen and find nothing they say so in their notes dictated at the time. To dictate anything else is to ruin that record so that they cannot ever learn anything from it. For medicolegal reasons they can put down "appendicitis, grade 1," but then when compiling statistics they should always remember what this means. Surgical residents often remark cynically that the more details their Chief dictates about the edge of the liver, the state of the common duct, and the lymph node lying on it, the surer they are that he sensed that he had removed a normal gallbladder!

Teach your young surgeons to give each patient, especially when the abdominal exploration was negative, a copy of the notes dictated at the time of operation. This could be so helpful to a patient with a painful abdomen. It would be helpful, also, to the procession of internists and surgeons who must see and study him later. The report should be so complete and definite as to make further explorations unnecessary.

Teach your young surgeons not to go on exploring an abdomen again and again after it has been well done, especially by a surgeon of national prominence.

Teach your students and keep teaching them that many an abdominal pain is referred out from the brain. They must be taught this so often that eventually they will have no doubts about it.

Teach them that in many cases one of the first signs of a psychosis is abdominal distress.

Teach your young men again and again that repeated air-swallowing and belching, regurgitation, heartburn, epigastric burning, migrainous pains, and hysterical nongassy bloatings (see Chapter 18) are functional troubles which can never be helped by any operation.

Teach your students never to operate on a gallbladder unless there are colics, and the organ is nonfunctioning or seen to contain stones. (A "slowly-emptying" gallbladder is simply filling again with dye reabsorbed from the jejunum.)

Teach that food allergy accounts for some abdominal pains.

Teach that there is such a thing as pseudo-ulcer (see Chapter 18).

Teach your students to recognize more often the gastric crises of tabes or epilepsy or migraine.

Teach them always to lift up and pinch the abdominal wall to make sure that a supposed intra-abdominal distress is really in the muscular wall, and there due to fibrositis or arthritis.

Teach your students always to find out if an abdominal distress is related to the taking of food or to the emptying of the bowel. If not, it is probably not arising in the digestive tract.

Teach your students that surgery cannot be counted on to cure when used purely as a vehicle for psychotherapy (see later on in this chapter).

Teach your students never to chalk up a "cure" until the patient has gone a year without a return of pain. Even then the operation may not have been justified, and the same pain may return.

Teach that in the cases of older persons a flash of pain or distress into the abdomen, especially when it is followed by a rapid loss of weight and changes in character, is probably due to a little stroke.

Teach your students not to operate for adhesions, and not to conclude that because they broke up a few adhesions their operation was justified and did some good.

Teach your students not to remove every myomatous uterus they see, especially if the myoma is not producing any symptoms; teach them again and again that a myoma does not change into a carcinoma; if it were to change into anything, it would be a sarcoma, and sarcoma of the uterus is a very rare disease.

Teach your students not to remove ovaries carelessly, just because they are somewhat cystic.

The surgeon needs to be convinced of the uselessness of certain operations. A big effort must be made by our leading surgeons to *convince* some of their confreres that it is practically 100 per cent useless to operate with the idea of curing such functional troubles as air-swallowing, heartburn, regurgitation, abdominal burnings or flutterings or "butterflies," the sore colon, aches or "hurtings" due to fibrositis of the abdominal wall, functional diarrheas, and pains due to unhappiness or mental strain. Next, our ablest surgeons must try to *convince* some of their confreres that, especially in the cases of highly neurotic or mildly psychotic persons with constant aches, it *rarely,* if ever, helps to stitch up a kidney, or to remove a "chronic appendix," a symptomless myomatous uterus, a slightly cystic ovary, or a "slowly emptying" gallbladder. It rarely helps, also, to anchor forward a uterus, or to break up some adhesions.

When surgeons *are convinced* that a certain operation is useless or almost so they give it up. Thus, today no one need tell a surgeon not to perform gastroenterostomy in the absence of an ulcer or pyloric obstruction. He knows that such an anastomosis commonly causes the patient so much trouble that it later has to be taken down, and hence one cannot hire him to make one. Years ago surgeons had to be warned against fastening up a low-lying stomach or colon, but today hardly anyone does this sort of thing. As time goes on doubtless more and more of the operations that are still being done by poorly trained or underexperienced men will be given up, or tried only in a few well-chosen cases.

The young surgeon who performs operations his old Chief never would perform. It is always disturbing to a fine teacher of surgery to find that some of his old students are performing certain operations which for years he had taught them not to do. They started doing them perhaps (1) because they wanted to convince themselves that really they are futile and unwise, or they found that occasionally they could seem to cure a patient by doing what their old Chief would not do, or when they went on their own they found so many of the surgeons in their community doing these operations that they decided that they might as well get their share of the business. Because the surgeon seldom has the time to "follow up" his patients' careers, he fails to learn how poor the results of some of his operations were.

It is too bad that surgeons commonly remain hopeful about a certain abdominal operation for years after internists have lost all faith in it or have even come to fear it. The trouble is that internists and surgeons commonly do not accept the conclusions derived from each others' follow-up studies. The surgeon thinks the internist is too pessimistic, and the internist thinks the surgeon is too optimistic. Obviously, the two should sit down together and try to agree on the conclusions to be drawn from each patient's letter as it comes in. Does it look as if the old symptoms had remained or returned, or does it look as if the man had derived some or much improvement? If internists and surgeons could ever agree on the interpretation of follow-up letters, they would not have to wait twenty-five years or more for a good appraisal of a particular operation.

A short period of cure means nothing. Surgeons greatly need to remember that a cure lasting even six months may mean nothing. That an operation for a time can appear to cure when it was obviously misdirected and useless was shown me most vividly one day when a woman came with a pain in the right loin, which she said had been relieved beautifully for two months by an appendectomy. The surgeon was pleased and proud, but then the pain came back. A little study showed that what had really been wrong was that her congenitally defective right kidney was a bag full of pus! When this was removed she got well and stayed well. From cases like this, it would appear that for a while the shock of an operation, plus a bit of rest, can cause a person to become so insensitive that pain is not felt. Most curious are those cases in which the same old misery in the right lower quadrant returns *several years* after the removal of an apparently normal appendix.

Surgeons should more often have their cases worked up by a diagnostician. As I said a few pages back, much of the futile surgery being done today would not be done if surgeons would always get internists to work up their more difficult cases for them. For instance, as I started writing this chapter, a minister of the Gospel came in from Chicago. He complained of the classic syndrome of ureteral pain running down from the right loin into the testicle. He had red blood cells in his urine, and in the scout roentgenogram, a stone was easily visible just above the right ureteral meatus. From there one of my urologic friends has since fished it out through the bladder.

Now, this may seem incredible, but three weeks before I saw the patient, one of the surgeons in this minister's congregation removed his

innocent appendix! I tell this story only to show what can happen
when a surgeon operates without examining the patient or apparently
even listening to his story! If this minister's disease had been a psychosis, or an acute meningitis, or a bad diabetes with some distress in the
abdomen, I fear his appendix would have come out just the same.

I know that many a surgeon, after years of experience, is clever at
snap diagnosis, but no matter how good he is, every so often he is
bound to be very wrong, and then probably his mistake could have
been obviated by even a cursory examination of his patient, or by the
taking of a short history.

One of the greatest advances would come if surgeons were all to give
up the practice, now so common, of *rushing* a patient to a hospital to
be operated on within a few hours of the first interview. There is
nothing so certain as this to insure the performing of needless and
futile operations.

**On being sure that neuroses and minor psychoses can be wholly
responsible for abdominal pain.** What is much needed in medical
and surgical practice today is a strong, unwavering conviction that
neuroses, minor psychoses, and cerebral arteriosclerosis, all by themselves, can cause abdominal distress and pain. Acute meningitis in
children can present the picture of an acute abdomen. Many a painful
abdomen is due purely to the fact that the person is suffering from
melancholia. Physicians will admit all this as an academic fact, but,
like me, they sometimes waver when confronted by a woman who for
long has suffered from abdominal pain and who is demanding that
something be done about it. Certainly, all internists and surgeons must
know that often one can explore the abdomen of such a woman, and
one can even do this four or five times without finding anything to account
for her pain and perhaps some fever and diarrhea. One can almost
eviscerate the woman, and one can cut all the nerves leaving her abdomen, and still she can have her pain.

These are facts that all of us must keep remembering, and always
we must cling to the faith that is in us that abdominal pain can arise
in the brain.

**A few questions that would prevent the making of many mis-
takes.** The surgeons of this country could save themselves an enormous
amount of futile operating if only in every puzzling case they were to
ask the patient just two questions. One is, "Are you happy?" The
answer to that would reveal many situational neuroses which are producing the whole syndrome. The second question is, "Is this pain or
discomfort in your abdomen related in any way to the taking of food
or to the passage of feces or flatus or to the taking of an enema or
a laxative?" If the pain is not related to any part of the cycle of di-

gestion, and if it is not made worse or better by the taking of food, or the emptying of the colon, one can assume that there is no lesion in the digestive tract. This conclusion is much strengthened if the patient says that between spells of abdominal pain he can eat and digest anything. Then, further questioning may show that the pain is a psychic one, or one of arthritic or fibrositic origin, out in the abdominal wall, or it is an equivalent of migraine or epilepsy. In women with a pain low in the abdomen a good question is, "Is this pain made worse by menstruation?" If it is not influenced by the engorgement of the pelvic organs that comes every month, it probably is not originating in the pelvic organs.

The surgeon cannot trick a man into getting well. As I wrote in Chapter 1, one cannot count on curing permanently a psychopathic person by operating and telling him that the cause of his disease has been found and removed. Theoretically, this stratagem should work well, but in thousands of cases it does not. I think the difficulty is that after the operation the person still feels the old distress. I, too, would still complain if, let us say, when I had a scratch on my cornea, which made me think I had a bit of dust in my eye, the oculist were surreptitiously to put a bit of dirt on his instrument and, after touching my eye, enthusiastically show me the black speck. I would not be satisfied because I would still be feeling something in the eye; I would say, "You got one speck out, but another is still there."

May the hands of teachers be strengthened and upheld. This chapter has been written with the hope that it will strengthen the hands and support the idealism of all those many young surgeons who are now coming out into practice with a great desire to do only the best, the most honorable, and the finest type of surgery. May it strengthen the hands, also, of those many older surgeons and teachers of surgery who, with much wisdom gained through the years, are now trying hard to raise standards of surgical training, licensure, and practice. This chapter will not be pleasant reading for some surgeons, but, then, they are not at all likely ever to see it. They will be too busy in the operating room!

The surgeon's need for sympathy and kindliness and tact. If there were space I could write another chapter on the need a surgeon has for sympathy, kindliness, and tact in dealing with patients all the way from the first meeting to the last good-by. There are so many things a surgeon can do at the start to inspire feelings of confidence and hope and security. When the patient arrives at the hospital there is much that can be done to give rest and to remove fear and tension, and next morning there is much that can be done to bring the patient relaxed to the operating room. After the operation there is much that can be done to relieve pain and discomfort and anxiety, and there is much that can be done to relieve the anxiety of the patient's relatives. I have known surgeons with great technical skill who wondered why their practice grew so slowly, and why their patients did not seem at all grateful. The answer was that they handled their patients like inanimate objects and made them feel that what happened to them was of no concern.

One of the finest things a surgeon can do is to tell people quickly whether or not cancer was found and whether or not it was removed. The surgeon generally feels that he should put this off indefinitely, or at least until the patient is well over the operation and strong enough to "take it," but a hundred patients have told me that this idea is wrong. The person with a great fear of cancer wakes from the anesthetic with two questions tearing at his mind: "Was cancer found and if so, is it all out?" To put off answering these questions greatly distresses the patient and commonly causes him to dislike the surgeon ever afterward. Even if the news is bad it is better to tell it right away; if it is good, surely it ought to be told immediately.

I remember the agony of a young woman who told me that for three days she had tried without success to find out what operation had been done on her father and whether the feared cancer had been found and removed. No one would tell her anything or show her any kindness. No wonder many people hate physicians.

The surgeons who do cosmetic work or rehabilitation work are particularly in need of skill in handling patients and keeping up their morale.

PSYCHIC TROUBLES OF THE WOMAN WHO GOES TO A GYNECOLOGIST

As every physician knows, some of the women who go frequently to a gynecologist have more troubles in their mind than in their pelvis. The abler type of gynecologist who still finds time in which to talk to his patients will soon tell the woman that there is nothing significantly wrong with her uterus or ovaries. Then he will go on to draw out a story perhaps of unhappiness with the husband or resentment against him, or bad early training by a sex-hating mother, or great fear of pregnancy. Or the doctor may note that he is dealing with an unaffectionate, touch-me-not sort of a schizoid woman.

Unfortunately, today many men doing gynecologic work feel too busy to stop and talk with their patients. As I write this I have just received a letter from an old friend who tells me that she so wishes she could talk to her gynecologist about some fears she has, but he goes rapidly from one to another of the several rooms in his suite, in each one of which lies a woman who has been undressed and placed on the table by a nurse. In each room he glances at the brief history taken by the nurse, examines the woman, and then dictates a note as to what he found in her pelvis. In the case of my friend, he was out of the room again before she could ask the questions that were bothering her. And he is probably the ablest of the gynecologists in his large city.

Obviously, when a man practices in this way, if he finds in the pelvis a uterine myoma or a so-called cystic ovary he is likely to send the woman right out to the hospital for an operation. If he would only sit down and chat with her he might learn that all her symptoms are due to psychic strain or to resentment over something her husband had done.

Illustrative cases. I remember a woman, previously well and happy and affectionate, who started going from one gynecologist to another, complaining of painful intercourse and aches and pains in the pelvis. After much treatment with hormones, and then a cervical dilatation and curettement, a surgeon advised exploration of the pelvis and hysterectomy. As soon as I saw the couple, I noted signs of resentment in the wife, and soon I got the story that all the trouble had started when the husband had confessed that, while at a convention, he had drunk too much and had passed out. On waking next morning he had found himself in a cheap hotel, with his wallet gone, hairpins on his pillow, and no memory of the events of the evening. Fearing that he had been exposed to venereal disease, he refused to touch his wife until he was assured by physicians that he had escaped infection. The wife never forgave him, but after I made her see that her pelvic troubles were the result of anger and the desire to punish, she stopped complaining, and that was the end of her illness.

Another case of this type was that of the young woman who was making her husband very unhappy over their sexual life. For a while after marriage she had been a fine bed-fellow, but then she changed, and in the middle of intercourse, she would begin to cry and to push the husband away. Gynecologists examined her but found no sign of disease. I soon learned that her trouble began when she found that her mother had cancer of the breast. The girl then felt it unseemly that she should be enjoying herself with her mother so ill; and besides, she had an idea that if she denied herself, the Virgin would turn a more sympathetic ear to her prayers for her mother's recovery. Later, when the mother had been operated on and had recovered, the girl was well.

I could tell many stories of women who, marrying without love, soon began to complain about intercourse and a sore pelvis. Some put up with things fairly well until they fell in love with another man. Others, originally well enough satisfied with the husband, later became resentful at things that he did. On the occasions when the woman wanted intercourse all went well, but when it was the husband who wanted it, the woman complained of vaginal pain. With or without conscious intent, she often succeeded in punishing the man and in keeping him from getting much pleasure.

It is a wonder that there is not more trouble of this sort when one realizes how many women are born somewhat schizoid, unaffectionate, poorly sexed, unresponsive, sickly, poorly developed physically, without enthusiasms, without much love or capacity for loving, and often with a prosaic or unpleasant husband.

An occasional woman has told me that soon after marriage she was so disgusted with sex that she told her husband to seek sexual gratification with other women. She would not mind just so long as he did not bother her. Other women have told me that sexual frigidity ran in their family, affecting the mother and two or three daughters. Others have wondered if their trouble might be due, at least in part, to the fact that in their girlhood the mother kept talking about the repulsiveness and nastiness of sexual intercourse.

Unfortunately there is many a woman who married without love, simply because a man kept asking her or because she was tired of supporting herself or because she craved a home and security and someone to eat meals with. Many such a woman married a man who was much older, and perhaps without any of the instincts of a lover; perhaps he was not even a good companion. Naturally, under such circumstances, the woman's sexual life was not happy. In other cases the marriage went well at the start but soon the husband got to drinking or gambling or chasing after women, and eventually all the love the wife had was driven out of her.

Seeing that such things are happening often, and seeing that they can lead to trouble with intercourse, it would seem that every gynecologist should be asking many of his patients, "Is your sexual life happy?" And "Are you in love with your husband?"

Problems of painful intercourse. Frank (1948) reviewed the problem of painful intercourse as complained of by 349 patients. In 114 cases the trouble had existed from the beginning of marriage. In 17.5 per cent of the 349, no pelvic abnormality could be found. The important point was that 54.8 per cent of these apparently normal women were neurotic. Even among those with some organic pelvic disease, 24.6 per cent were highly nervous. Dickinson and Frank both concluded that the psychic factor was the essential one in at least 25 per cent of the cases of painful intercourse. As Frank said, one of the first things a physician should do is to find out if the patient wants to be cured. If she does not, and the husband is willing to accept the situation, it is best to leave the patient alone.

When a woman is complaining about intercourse I always try to find out (1) if to begin with she was normal enough, psychically and physically; (2) if she was in love with the man when she married him; (3) if she enjoyed intercourse at first or after a period of adjustment; (4) if once she did enjoy intercourse, when did the change come? and (5) why did it seem to come? Did she lose her love or get resentful over something? Did the change come after a child was born? Sometimes a woman with but little love for her husband or little interest in intercourse will leave her husband's bed after the first pregnancy. She will largely separate herself from him, and she may even move into the child's room and stay there.

The fear of pregnancy. There must be untold numbers of women who, if only freed from the fear of pregnancy, would enjoy intercourse and be glad, also, to give pleasure to the husband. Perhaps their religion forbids the practice of contraception; the man's salary may be barely enough to keep the family going as it is, and hence, during intercourse, the main thought the woman has is that the coming of an extra child would bring economic disaster. In such cases the man may withdraw or he may use a condom and, in either case, leave the wife unsatisfied, tense, and wakeful. Often, therefore, the gynecologist can cure the woman only by fitting a diaphragm or otherwise helping her with her problems of contraception.

Hormones seldom help. In most cases of sexual frigidity the injection of hormones is not likely to do much good. If a woman is menstruating each month she probably has all the ovarian and pituitary hormones she needs, and it is hard to see why the giving of more should do any good. Occasionally, one hears of a woman who had more sexual interest after large doses of estrogens, but in most cases the effect was only temporary.

So many of the women who complain of dysmenorrhea and are now given many "shots" of estrogens cannot be helped by such medication. Many are constitutionally inadequate, and their bodies are poorly made. In many cases irregularities in the menstrual cycle are probably due to abnormal behavior in the hypothalamus.

Emotions and menstruation. There is no question that emotions have much to do with disturbances in menstruation. T. A. Ross believed that painful menstruation is often of nervous origin. I have been impressed by the fact that after a psychic shock a buxom woman of thirty-five may never menstruate again. Student nurses often suffer for a while with menstrual irregularities due, perhaps, to the excitement of a new life in new surroundings. On the other hand, many a girl with menstrual difficulties gets well when she marries or when she goes

to live in a new place. Dunbar (1946) quoted a good-sized literature
on the dysmenorrhea of the mentally disturbed.

Most of the women I have seen with a severe premenstrual nervous
storm have had a poor nervous ancestry, and that, I think, was their
main trouble. Some of the girls who raise Cain with each menstrual
period need to be taught some stoicism and self-control. I have seen
them behave well when taken out of the home and away from the
influence of a too sympathetic or easily dominated mother.

Leukorrhea of psychic origin. In the cases of many tense nervous
women a so-called leukorrhea appears to be due purely to an oversecretion
of the glands in the cervix and at the mouth of the vagina. In these
cases the secretion contains no pus and no trichomonas, monilia, or
pathogenic bacteria. Dunbar (1946) gave a number of references to
articles about this type of leukorrhea. The vaginal glands in these cases
apparently respond excessively just as do the sweat glands and sebaceous
glands of the skin when they are stimulated strongly by a too active
brain. It is possible that in some of these cases the secretion is stimulated excessively by erotic thoughts or a too erotic life. An intense
type of woman once complained to me that when stimulated by the
affectionate touch of a man her vaginal secretion was so profuse that
it ran down her leg.

Mental and physical distresses that follow hysterectomy. As
every physician knows, a hysterectomy sometimes has a distressing
psychologic effect on the woman. Much depends on her nervous heredity, her age, and the degree to which she is desirous of having a
child or more children. Occasionally the operation will greatly lessen
her sexual interests and feelings, but if she is a loving person, the loss
of her ovaries may have little effect on her sexual life. Occasionally,
and this is curious, the operation puts an end to the husband's sexual
interest in the woman, and this may be very distressing to her. Fritz
Wengraf (1946) has written about these problems. Many women dread
hysterectomy because they fear it will make them coarse, fat, hairy,
and unsexed. Actually, if they do not overeat they need not grow fat,
and certainly there is no need to fear getting coarse.

L. A. Emge tells me that when he decides that he must perform hysterectomy, if there is no reason for haste, he puts off the operation for
a while, until he can have several interviews with the patient. During
these visits he studies her as a mental risk; he answers all her questions about what may happen during and after the operation, and he
drives out fear of the procedure and its results. The woman then
comes to the operation with a minimum of anxiety, she knows her
surgeon as a friend, and she has confidence in him. She knows that if

she loves her husband and has always been a good bed-fellow, she should remain one after the operation.

On needless hysterectomies. Doubtless a good many of the hysterectomies being performed each day in the hospitals of this land are unnecessary and unjustifiable. We physicians have always tended to get a wave of enthusiasm for a certain therapeutic procedure, and then, for some years, we overwork it. I need only mention the days when every man was supposed to part with his teeth; later came the rage for tonsillectomy, and later, almost every man who saw a surgeon was supposed to part with a "chronic" appendix. Today, every woman with a little myoma of the uterus is likely to be sent to the hospital for a hysterectomy which she does not really need.

In a remarkably frank article, Norman F. Miller (1946), distinguished gynecologist of the University of Michigan, showed that a considerable percentage of the hysterectomies performed even by good surgeons (idealistic enough to report their work, good and bad, to Miller) were probably unnecessary. Miller obtained reports on 246 hysterectomies performed mainly in 1945, in ten different hospitals in three midwestern states.

In the 41 per cent in which the woman's complaint had been bleeding, the hysterectomy may well have been advisable. But in 17 per cent there were no symptoms(!) and in 14 per cent the symptoms were nervousness, headache, or backache, almost certainly not produceable by a myomatous uterus. In 50 per cent the preoperative finding was a somewhat enlarged fibrotic uterus, and at operation myomas were found in 43 per cent of the cases. One wonders how many of these myomas were symptomless and harmless. The remarkable fact was that in 31 per cent of the uteruses the pathologist could not find anything wrong, and in 16 per cent more he could find only some probably harmless endometrial hyperplasia! In fairness, of course, to the surgeons, it must be noted that a few of these 47 per cent of normal or almost normal uteruses were probably removed incidental to the removal of diseased tubes (these were present in 13 per cent of the 246 cases), or to the treatment of endometriosis (3 per cent), or of prolapse (2 per cent), or of carcinoma of the ovary (a few cases).

One in six of the women was operated on in spite of the fact that she had neither symptoms of pelvic disease nor palpable disease in the pelvis! Evidently in these cases the abdomen was explored with no more than a hope that something could be found there that could be taken care of. And then a normal uterus was removed! If this sort of thing is being done in the practices of surgeons fine enough to cooperate with Dr. Miller in this study, what must be happening in the practices of some other men of a less idealistic type?

Dr. Miller might well have gone on to say what a tragedy it is that so many thousands of women today are losing the uterus simply because it has on it a little knob of muscle about as harmless as a knob on a potato. In most cases the woman has never had any symptoms that can be ascribed to the myoma. She never flooded, and her blood is in good shape. Why, then, does she get operated on? Because the surgeon scares her badly by telling her that if the myoma is left, it will probably become cancerous. I feel sure he is not justified in saying this.

Obviously, a myoma can turn only into a sarcoma, and sarcomatosis of the uterus is a very rare disease. I do not remember ever having seen a case. Dr. Kernohan, pathologist at the Mayo Clinic, tells me that he can hardly remember having seen one. Dr. L. A. Emge tells me that in the course of a study of 5,000 removed uteruses he found only two that were sarcomatous. Certainly, then, a surgeon is not justified in threatening a woman with sarcomatous degeneration of her myoma. Obviously, it is far more dangerous to remove the myoma than to leave it in.

Perhaps some surgeons will now argue that a myomatous uterus is more subject to invasion by carcinoma, but my experience of forty-five years is much against this idea. For many years I have been advising women with symptomless myomas to keep them, and I cannot remember a case in which the subsequent coming of a carcinoma made me regret my decision. Of course, many patients went home and I did not hear from them again but quite a few were seen repeatedly during the course of twenty-five years.

Naturally, I always recommend removal of a rapidly growing myoma, and in many of these cases I have seen so much improvement in health after the operation that I have suspected that the patient must have been poisoned by some fraction of degenerating protein.

Always, before ordering hysterectomy for a little myoma, the surgeon ought to make some effort to find out if the patient is suffering from a situational neurosis or perhaps a mild psychosis. If she is, he had better put off the operation.

Disturbing psychic changes that go with menstruation. Altman, Knowles and Bull (1941) made a fine study of the psychic changes which accompanied a few sex cycles of ten mature college women. I suspect that these distresses are most likely to be severe and demoralizing in the cases of women who have a poor nervous inheritance and a tendency to psychosis.

Vaginismus. Vaginismus, or marked spasm of the vulval muscles, which interferes greatly with intercourse or makes it impossible, is seen in many schizoid girls who recoil from sex and any contact with men. When a physician examines them these girls contract the adductor muscles of the thighs; they make a great fuss and some become hysterical. As one would expect, in such cases, the cutting of muscles about the mouth of the vagina is not likely to give complete relief. The vagina may still be too tender and too full of spasm for comfortable intercourse. I have seen some young women of this neurotic type who could not enjoy intercourse even after the vagina had been well dilated by the delivery of a child. Commonly one cannot find any anatomic reason for the soreness. In some of these cases fear of intercourse or of being hurt may have something to do with producing the syndrome.

The nervous and mental troubles of the menopause. A nervously stable, quiet, sensible, and perhaps insensitive type of woman can go through the menopause without distresses of any kind. On the other hand, the highly sensitive migrainous type of woman can have very trying hot flushes for ten years or more, and the woman with a poor nervous heredity who has always tended at times to be depressed, or who has become mentally upset at her periods, is likely to have a stormy menopause with perhaps an involutional melancholia. A few women of this type have to be put into an institution. The problem is complicated because so many women are troubled at this time of life by unhappinesses of various origins, such as widowhood, the departure of children, loss of a husband's affection or sexual love, or loss of a feeling of being useful and needed. Other women get into trouble because, about this time, a hypertension becomes bothersome or cerebral arteries begin to plug up.

Strecker and Palmer (Oxf. Med.) stated that when a woman of fifty goes into an involutional melancholia, one can usually learn from the family that she has always been of a rather rigid mental type. She perhaps was always more than usually stubborn, secretive, and opposed to change; she may have been self-sacrificing in a martyr-like way, bigoted, or overly conscientious. She may have had feelings of guilt, or she may always have been moody and unable to play and have fun. In other words, she may always have been mildly manic-depressive; and hence it was easy for the menopause, together with some arteriosclerotic changes in the brain, to send her over the edge into a frank melancholia.

Treatment for the menopause. Some of a woman's troubles at the menopause, such as the flushes, can be helped by estrogens, either of synthetic or natural origin. I usually order 0.5 mg. of stilbestrol a day. Some women can be helped by psychotherapy. Unfortunately, few physicians realize how distressing strong flushes can be to a highly sensitive woman. They may wake her out of sleep every half-hour or so and may make her throw off the bedclothes or jump out of bed. She may be so wet she has to change her nightgown. Every little while throughout the day a flush may come, causing her to perspire and to feel alternately hot and cold.

Such a woman may be upset psychically so that she turns on her husband and accuses him of infidelity and what-not. The poor, puzzled, or outraged man then needs help from the doctor. He may say, "It is so hard now when my business burdens are so great to have my good companion of the years turn on me and blame me for all her troubles. It is hard, after years of a happy sexual life, to have her now turn me out of her bed or to act so unreasonably and suspiciously." The man can often be helped by being shown that it is mental disease and not cussedness that is wrecking his peace. In the worst cases much may be accomplished with the help of institutional care and shock treatments.

THE PSYCHIC PROBLEMS OF THE PREGNANT OR PARTURIENT WOMAN

There are many psychic problems that assail some pregnant women, and the able obstetrician should be prepared to cope with them. For the normal, happily married woman who wants children and who has a husband who also wants them, the coming of pregnancy may be pure joy, but for other women who are perhaps unmarried, or not well balanced, or who do not want children, or are afraid to pass on to them some mental disease or physical defect, or who cannot afford them, or who have a husband who strongly objects to an addition to the family and perhaps demands that an abortion be performed, a pregnancy can bring much unhappiness and strain and indecision.

Occasionally, a woman will spend the nine months of gestation worrying for fear the child will be "marked" or defective, physically or mentally, like some of the forebears. In other cases, under the impact of pregnancy or parturition, the woman's hereditary predisposition to a psychosis will be brought out. In rare cases there will be problems, also, of keeping the husband from straying during the months when the woman is ailing, vomiting, unattractive, and perhaps unaffectionate.

In many such cases the wise and kindly obstetrician should be helping the woman with her psychic problems, keeping up her morale, answering her questions, and driving away her fears.

During some pregnancies, of course, there is terrible nausea or vomiting which can wear the woman down. Of late a number of men have been claiming that the vomiting of pregnancy can be relieved by psychotherapy. Dunbar gave many references to the work of such men. Some forms of hyperemesis can perhaps be helped in this way, but it is doubtful if other forms ever will be. Usually the writers give no hint as to how they give their psychotherapy. I would hate to tell a poor vomiting woman that she wasn't terribly nauseated, or didn't need to vomit, or could stop it. I fear she would want to hit me with whatever blunt instrument came to hand!

Recently, there has been talk of carrying women through parturition with the help mainly of encouragement, reassurance, and psychotherapy. There is no doubt that some women who are sensible, stoical, and without worry will have their children without much fuss, while others who are full of fear and have little self-discipline will put on a tremendous show. Perhaps they suffer more because of their shrieks. There is no question that some women who believe strongly in Christian Science will go through parturition without complaint.

Read (1949) reported a series of 516 consecutive labors in which a sustained effort was made to carry the woman through without anesthetics. He started educating his patients early in pregnancy. Much encouragement was given, and great efforts were made to drive out all fear. During labor the women were encouraged to be stoical and to keep themselves under control. Without fear, the woman should not become so tense, and this should facilitate relaxation of the pelvic floor. Read stated that in 90 per cent of uncomplicated births, his patients refused analgesia or anesthesia, preferring to have the joy of *conscious childbirth*.

CHAPTER 21

Psychic Troubles with the Eyes, Ears, Nose, and Throat

DIFFICULTIES DUE TO A TIRED OR DISORDERED BRAIN. Every year the internist sees many persons who complain of a difficulty with vision or a discomfort in the eyes which they say no oculist has been able to relieve. Usually the person says he has been getting one new pair of glasses after another, but none of them has helped. One wonders why some oculist did not stop the procession and tell what was wrong. It is hard to believe that they were all so stupid they did not know. A few questions would have shown them that the trouble was not in the eyes but up in a tired or disordered brain. What such a patient has is some sort of a fatigue state or nervous breakdown. Put him before the test letters and he will read them all right; he may even have a 6/5 vision. His trouble is that he cannot concentrate well enough to read along comfortably; or he cannot, for long, take in what he reads. He finds himself going back over the same paragraph again and again, getting little out of it, or forgetting what he did get. Or the lines may seem to run together and get fuzzy; perhaps his muscles of accommodation quickly tire, and he will say that he cannot focus well.

That the trouble is in the brain can be seen from the fact that when someone tries to spare the man's eyes by reading to him, his ability to take in and remember the material is not good, and he soon has to ask the reader to stop. Curiously, if he persists in trying to read, he may get cramps in his abdomen. Most convincing is the statement that blind persons, when very tired, have similar distresses in their eyes when reading Braille with their fingers. Certainly in these cases the difficulty must be in the brain.

The physician should recognize the syndrome in a moment, and then should warn the patient not to go on as he is, without stopping for a rest or for some psychiatric treatment. Many a physician has said to me: "You know, that failure of my eyes to work well was one of the first of the symptoms that should have told me that my brain was getting very tired. Sometimes after a few days of rest I would be able to read again, but soon my brain would tire and I would be back where I was before."

Whenever I want to know how tired a patient is or how deep he is in a nervous breakdown I ask if he can read. It is a very good sign when he can.

Headaches due supposedly to eye strain. Many headaches are supposed by physicians to be due to eye strain, when a glance at the person's concave glasses would have shown that this was very doubtful. There cannot be any strain on the muscles of accommodation when the patient is near-sighted.

The interesting and significant fact is that many persons who have a big error never have a headache, while others with almost perfect vision get into trouble as soon as they try to use their eyes. The coming or not coming of a headache usually depends on the condition of the brain rather than of the eyes. Some distresses can be due to strain in the external muscles of the eye which maintain binocular vision, but such imbalance can easily be found and corrected by the oculist.

I went for the first thirty-five years of my life needing prisms and suffering from a tremendous hyperopic astigmatism, only partially corrected. With great ocular strain I read day and night, and I never had a headache. I did not have even a third of normal vision until I was fifty-five, and yet, the only time I ever had difficulty in reading was when, after years of overwork and then an attack of influenza in 1918, my brain for a while became too tired to take things in. Always I could easily make out the letters; it was their meaning which I found hard to keep taking in. In those days I could read an article in a newspaper but I could not even start on a long article in German. If only I had known enough then to stop and take a vacation as soon as I found myself almost unable to read, I could have saved myself a year of suffering.

Floating specks. Many nervous and apprehensive persons, when they slip into a nervous breakdown, become much concerned about floating specks. Because in these cases the oculist, on looking into the eyes, does not see anything unusual in the way of floating opacities, it will be obvious to him that the person has become alarmed over those specks, often on the front of the cornea, that anyone can see at any time by looking at the sky.

The scotoma of migraine. Occasionally a worrisome person will come in, much concerned over having experienced a typical migrainous scintillating scotoma. He may fear that he is going blind, or he may have gotten the idea from some physician that he had the beginnings of a brain tumor. I have seen many such persons who were not immediately reassured and told what their trouble was, even by the oculists whom they consulted! It is hard to believe, but a well-to-do woman had her brain explored surgically for a typical scotoma!

The scotoma begins usually with a blurring or confusion of vision. After a minute or two, on closing the eyes, the person can see a bright spot much like that produced by looking at a strong light. This spot gradually becomes a zigzag line which bows outward to one side or the other. It zigzags like a snake fence; it pulsates rapidly (not with the heartbeat), and sometimes it is bordered by bands of color. Usually in about twenty minutes the line fades, and in twenty-five minutes the vision is clear again. During the time the scotoma is present it is hard for the person to read, but usually he can do it. In the cases of many men, after the scotoma clears there may be only a feeling of fatigue.

Fortunately, one can always reassure the person who is worrying about such a scotoma; hundreds of them can come in a lifetime without the person's ever losing acuity of vision.

Ocular troubles due to hysteria. Hysterical persons can have all sorts of visual disturbances, including temporary blindness of one or both eyes. There is the so-called tubular vision with its apparent marked narrowing of the visual fields.

The wise physician will always suspect a psychic disturbance of vision when he sees a patient wearing heavy dark glasses indoors where they cannot be much needed, if at all. One should become suspicious, also, of a marked photophobia, perhaps with blepharospasm, with a normal cornea and conjunctiva and normal vision. A bilateral ptosis of the upper lid recently acquired is suspicious, especially when the patient, in his effort to see, does not wrinkle his forehead. Suspicious, also, is a marked mydriasis in one or both eyes.

The hysterical person may tell the oculist of fantastic symptoms which do not correspond with any known ocular lesion. He may complain of such things as transient blurring of vision, a difficulty in focusing the eyes, some doubling of vision, or an aching in the eyes. He may be blinking frequently, and usually he will not gaze steadily at a certain point when told to do so. He may resist the efforts of the doctor to open his eyes. The answers he gives to questions will not be clear-cut or consistent, one with another. A common functional disturbance is a defect in convergence. Major hysteria of the eyes is much more common in military than in civil practice.

Wetzel described a number of the tests that can be used to fool the malingerer who maintains that he cannot see. The electroencephalograph can now be used for this purpose because when a person can see, the record changes when the eyes are opened and closed. Rarely a malingerer will put something into his eyes to keep them inflamed. H. M. Traquair felt that with neurotic persons one can oftentimes learn more by blocking out one eye with the help of a strong convex lens than with more complicated apparatus. The secret of this is that the patient does not know that he is seeing with only one eye, and that, his supposedly blind eye.

The hysterical disturbance of vision is never a hemianopsia as it so commonly is with organic disease of the brain. With the help of prisms one can make the hysterical person who thinks he is blind in one eye see double. Evidently he could not do this if he had vision in only one eye. Sometimes the flashing of a strong light into the "blind" eye will cause the person to blink.

Hysterical anesthesia of the conjunctiva is said to be rare.

In soldiers unilateral blindness has been noted in association with loss of hearing, taste, and smell on the same side.

There is an excellent symposium on ocular psychoneuroses recorded in the Transactions of the Ophthalmological Society of the United Kingdom (Vol. 64, Session of 1944, pp. 24-60, published in 1945). There, Davenport stated that he thought that most of the patients with an ocular neurosis give themselves away by certain types of behavior even before the oculist can start examining them. They reveal a certain type of personality and perhaps an exaggerated fear of blindness.

Blinded soldiers commonly worry much about their inability later to find women and to be attractive enough to them. With good reason, they fear that blindness will interfere greatly with their sexual life. They will find it difficult even to locate a house of prostitution unless they have a friend who will guide them to one.

Wing Commander J. H. Doggart pointed out that especially in the cases of psychoneurotics there can be a terrible panic at the mere thought of losing sight. Fear then grips the man. Hence it is that the oculist must at all times guard his tongue so as to avoid throwing his patient into a panic.

In Army practice, the diagnosis of an ocular neurosis should be made right off, and then the patient should not be hospitalized and overexamined. In an Army hospital, nervous patients are too prone to acquire a lot of new symptoms from the man in the next bed.

The oculist should never give new glasses as a placebo. He can help the patient immensely more by explaining to him why his eyes are not comfortable or not working well. With sympathy and kindness he should explain the mechanism of a neurosis and should keep insisting that there is nothing organically wrong with the eyes. It is bad to tell a nervous patient to stop reading so as to "save his sight." He should, instead, be encouraged to read as long as he can do so without discomfort.

Ocular neuroses seen in civil practice. In civil practice nervous eye symptoms are mainly those of headache, eye-ache, "ocular" fatigue, sensitiveness to light, and floating specks. The way in which a patient tells his history can tell much to an alert oculist. Davenport believed that about half of the persons seen by an oculist could be helped by a psychiatrist. Obviously, the oculist must treat most of them himself.

Glaucoma. Inman stated that many oculists believe that emotion can bring on an acute attack of glaucoma. Schoenberg and the discussers of his paper also were satisfied that flare-ups in the course of glaucoma can be associated with periods of anxiety. Hemorrhage into the retina might possibly follow strong emotion.

The care of the blind. Wittkower and Davenport (1946) gave good advice in regard to the psychologic care of the blind. These people dislike pity. Every person who has to deal with the blind should read the last two pages of the article by Wittkower and Davenport. The oculist would do well to read, also, all books by persons who have struggled with the problems of blindness, like O'Brien's story, *Memoirs of a Guinea Pig* (1942), Borghild M. Dahl's *I Wanted to See* (1944), Alice Bretz' *I Begin Again* (1940), Helen Keller's *Story of My Life,* Karsten Ohnstad's *World at My Fingertips* (1942), or Robinson Pierce's *It Was Not My Own Idea* (1944).

Cataracts. The kind-hearted oculist will have to puzzle over how much to tell a person about a beginning cataract, or how frankly to discuss the question of eventual blindness. Naturally, he should always be as optimistic as he honestly can be.

Psychic problems of persons with a squint. Persons with an uncorrected squint may be disturbed mentally because of their shame over the deformity. All such persons should have their eyes straightened if it can possibly be done.

Other persons who may be troubled are those who are disfigured by marked exophthalmos. An operation has been devised to help them.

NERVOUS TROUBLES TREATED BY THE OTOLOGIST

Some of the discomforts that persons feel in their ears are due purely to nervousness or to too keen a sensitiveness. Thus, I remember a woman who, with a rising blood pressure, began to hear the rhythmic whirr of the pulse in her carotid artery where it passed close to her internal ear. Any medical student or intelligent lay person should have been able to make the diagnosis, but for months she went from one aurist to another getting expensive treatments. Finally she wrote asking me for the name of someone who would really help her. Since she wouldn't accept my long-distance suggestion as to the diagnosis, I sent her to the professor of otology in a university in her state, hoping that from him she would get an honest opinion. She did. He said there was nothing wrong with her ears, but, with little knowledge of psychology, he greatly weakened the effect of what he had said by giving her some ear-drops! Doubtless experience had taught him that patients are often dissatisfied if sent away empty handed.

Dizziness. As I showed in Chapter 12, much of the dizziness that is blamed on the ear is not due to any disease in that organ. The person still can hear perfectly, and he responds normally to the tests of labyrinthine function. What he has is usually not a true vertigo but a feeling of uncertainty, of poor balance, or "top-heaviness," or wooziness, or a fear of falling. Often these feelings come with fatigue, or with a nervous breakdown, or a tiny stroke. They are common in persons suffering from migraine, hypertension, cerebral arteriosclerosis, neurocirculatory asthenia, an epileptic inheritance, or the menopause.

Hysterical deafness. As is noted in the chapter on hysteria, men under great nervous strain, as in war, will sometimes go deaf. The problems of diagnosis and treatment of such deafness are discussed in Chapter 16 on hysteria. F. Chavanne (1901) wrote a large book on hysteria and the ear. Much information on the effects of the mind on the ear is to be found in Dunbar's book (1946).

A fine study of psychogenic deafness was made by Lt. Col. N. A. Martin (1946), who had a large experience with this disease during World War II. He said the otologist can often suspect what is wrong, just from the story of the way in which the deafness came. It probably did not come when a shell burst nearby, but a few days later at the hospital. This makes the diagnosis. The results of repeated tests with the electric audiometer are likely to be variable and inconsistent, and there will be no sign of disease in the labyrinth. The several tests that have been used to reveal malingering have not always proved helpful. Now it is stated that if the person can hear, noise will change the "sleeping" electroencephalogram.

Fifteen per cent of the 1,500 men admitted to the Hoff General Hospital were studied under pentothal sodium for a possible psychogenic deafness, and under treatment appropriate for hysteria, 12 per cent of these apparently deafened men regained their hearing. Helpful diagnostically was the fact that in several of the cases there were other hysterical manifestations, such as corneal anesthesia, tubular vision, glove anesthesia, speech defects, or amnesia.

The greatest help was obtained from questioning the patient during light narcosis. The physician kept asking questions, and eventually the man started answering them, showing that he was hearing all right. As he came out of the narcosis and found himself conversing with the doctor, he realized that he was hearing and hence must have good ears. A few of the men, however, when they found that they were hearing, stubbornly went back to their deafness.

The hysterically deaf should always be studied psychologically, so that the emotional blocks and conflicts can be unearthed and discussed. With this there will be less chance, after a cure, of the man's slipping back into deafness or some other hysterical state.

The neuroses of the deaf. The wise otologist should sometimes discuss with a deaf person the mild paranoid psychosis that he is likely to fall into if he does not get a hearing aid and learn to use it. He will become suspicious that persons are talking about him, and he may become solitary and irritable. It takes much effort to talk some persons into purchasing and using the new helpful apparatus.

A good book to place in the hands of the deaf is Mrs. Heiner's merry volume entitled *Hearing is Believing.* She tells how at first, though very deaf, she refused to think of using a hearing aid. Later, when she got it, she was so happy and enthusiastic over her ability to hear that ever since she has been dedicating her spare time and energies to helping other persons to adjust to the idea of using the new apparatus.

As L. W. Coleman has said, a doctor's interest in psychosomatic medicine must not blind him to the possible presence of organic disease. For instance, after a mastoidectomy, a boy sometimes vomited and thereby got out of going to school. When a Rohrschach test suggested an abnormal personality, the boy was disciplined. Later everyone had a red face when it was discovered that the vomiting had been due to a brain abscess secondary to the infection in the ear.

NERVOUS TROUBLES OF THE LARYNX

Occasionally one will see a nervous woman who is whispering. Sometimes one can learn that she lost her voice during a period of psychic strain, and sometimes one will suspect that the trouble is a sort of expiation for feelings of guilt. Oftentimes the trouble came after the death of a loved one. In the Bible one reads of persons who, under stress of emotion, were stricken dumb. Perhaps the woman shows a hysterical lack of interest in her predicament. She may have come to see the physician about some other symptom, and she will not care to join in any efforts to get back her voice. I remember a woman who said she knew why she was whispering but she did not wish to do anything about it.

As in all such cases, it helps to find out what the woman was doing when she lost her voice. According to Clerf and Braceland (1942), the hysterical woman loses her voice suddenly and completely, and then largely accepts the situation. The neurasthenic who complains of hoarseness says it came gradually, and usually he has a lot of other discomforts that bother him. Hysterical soldiers will sometimes become mute.

It is always helpful in these cases to have a laryngologist look to make sure that there is no weakness of the muscles that move the vocal cords and no roughness of these cords. Clerf and Braceland advised that the laryngologist ask the patient to cough because in cases of hysteria the cords still can meet in the midline. It may help to find some anesthesia of the fauces and a loss of the gag reflex, because these are often symptoms of hysteria.

Many a patient with this trouble has been made to talk again quickly with the help of encouragement or hypnosis or perhaps a little faradic stimulation of the skin of the neck. As the woman is made to talk again, every effort should be made to find out why she became mute, so as to help her with her mental problem. Perhaps the inability to talk is getting her out of some unpleasant situation, and the doctor should then know what this is. As Ross, Braceland, and others have said, if the doctor tackles the problem at all, he ought to be prepared to go on with it until he can really help the person to get well and stay well.

Some persons suffer a little break in their voice when under strong emotion. Thus, Theodore Roosevelt, when he was going to tell a funny story, would break into a falsetto.

The younger the patient, the more likely he or she is to be suggestible and to respond to the authority of the physician. It is perhaps easier for a laryngologist to work the cure because he is looked on as the expert in his field, and if he says that the patient can talk again, he or she may do so. Much can be accomplished with tact and kindness. Browbeating will not work so well.

Simple encouragement or the method of Ross will work in most cases, but in some cases there will be no response. Then the doctor may have to use hypnosis or narcosynthesis. Sometimes a patient cannot *afford* to get well: He or she needs the illness, and then it will be hard to cure. Thus, at the end of World War II a young woman was due to travel to a seaport to meet her husband on his return from the front. She developed aphonia and could not go. Questioning showed that during her husband's long absence she had fallen in love with another man.

It was then obvious why she was reluctant to meet the husband and face a painful interview.

In these cases no drug should ever be applied locally by a laryngologist. Such treatment would have a bad effect, and might fix the neurosis in the larynx. This would make the treatment more difficult later for a psychiatrist.

The hacking dry cough. A few persons for years will have a dry hacking cough especially when they talk to strangers. This represents a habit-spasm or tic. I have known a few persons who could not say more than four or five words without stopping to cough. Others have to stop to take a breath.

It is probable that in many cases of troublesome cough for which no cause can be found, help could be given by efforts at educating the person not to give in and cough every time the tickle comes.

In Chapter 16 on hysteria there is more on the use of speaking exercises in the treatment of nervous aphonia and mutism.

NEUROSES OF THE NOSE AND THROAT

Davison (1945) concluded that 36 per cent of his otolaryngologic patients had purely functional troubles, while 22 per cent more had functional troubles in addition to some organic ones. A valuable point he made was that persons with functional troubles in their nose usually have other symptoms of nervous origin, such as insomnia, pruritus, a dry cough, palpitation, air-swallowing, headache, or a pain or a tight feeling or a burning in the head. Others are troubled by dizziness or buzzing in the ears, a fear of deafness, a bad taste in the mouth, a burning tongue, or globus, or choking feelings.

Many of these persons are too conscious of the throat. Many suffer from a red granular mucosa at the back of the pharynx. This area is covered with little granulations consisting of adenoid tissue. About all most rhinologists give for this is lipoiodine, two tablets of which can be taken each day. Often the throat feels too dry. Sometimes, when the nasal mucosa is too dry, the rhinologist will prescribe a spray of hydrocarbon oil.

Many persons complain that when they lie on one side in bed the nose plugs up on that lower side. They should be reassured and told that this is almost normal; it is the result of a vasomotor change.

Few physicians realize how many of the persons who go to nose and throat specialists complaining of chronic sinusitis and a postnasal drip have no sign of local disease.

Day after day, at the request of nose-conscious patients, I have to send them to rhinologists, but soon I get the expected report that the roentgenograms of the sinuses showed no opacities and there was no pus in the nose or the sinuses. One can often rule out sinusitis simply by asking the patient to show his handkerchief. If, toward the end of the day, it is clean, he is not likely to have much of a sinusitis. If a man has several handkerchiefs in his pockets, all full of pus, then, of course, he has a bad nose or a bad bronchitis. Sometimes one can recognize the wide nasal bridge and the nasal voice of a man with an old pansinusitis. In some cases it helps to learn that what the man is hawking out with such effort each morning is not pus but mucus or a jelly-like material; this shows that there is no need for anxiety about the condition in the sinuses.

Many a time, after the rhinologists at the Mayo Clinic have been unable to find any signs of disease in the nose of a man with some form of a nervous breakdown, I have later received a tart letter from him saying that after much searching he found a doctor who located pus in his sinuses and operated and cured him. But in many such cases I have learned later that the man did not stay cured; he went on suffering from his great feelings of fatigue.

The person who loves to hawk and spit. In many cases questioning will show that the man is too greatly worried about his nose; he hawks so hard and so long because he is a perfectionist who likes to have his body clean and just so. Perhaps each morning he spends twenty minutes washing out his nose and putting drops in it. He may fear that if he should swallow any of the nasal secretion it would poison him or injure his stomach and then his brain. Obviously, it cannot poison him or bother him in the least because it is a harmless substance which will be quickly digested in the stomach just like so much soft-boiled egg.

Often the man is fearful that he is getting "catarrh." I am not sure exactly what he means by this, but fifty years ago this word was much feared by laymen, and this dread was fostered and built up by venders of patent medicine. According to them, catarrh could spread to the stomach and the whole body. Such ideas are still influencing the thinking of many persons, and catarrh cures are still being advertised in the newspapers.

Many fussy persons must be exhorted to stop washing the nose, or putting in drops, or hawking by the half-hour, or using an inhaler. Often, by their constant efforts at treatment, they keep the nasal mucosa irritated.

The hawker who is psychotic. Occasionally, when I see a man who hawks unusually hard and noisily for half an hour each morning, I will find on talking to him that he is a psychopath who is obsessed with the dangers of leaving a little mucus in his nose, or swallowing it. He does not need a rhinologist so much as a psychiatrist. One such man I saw a while ago was sure that any mucus he might swallow would poison his brain and upset his reason. When I asked him why he was so sure of this he said his sister had gone insane because of the same sort of catarrh that he had! She, too, had been a terrible hawker in her day, trying always to keep her nose clean, but "eventually the mucus got her!" The more I talked to the man the clearer it became that he was as psychotic as his sister. He told me that he had been treated strenuously by many internists and rhinologists, none of whom had ever seemed to suspect that he was "not right in the head." He came to me as a gastroenterologist, hoping that I would at least protect his stomach from damage. I doubt if my assistants saw anything peculiar in him or his case; they had never been trained to recognize his disease.

The chronic sniffer. Many persons keep constantly using nose-drops or benzedrine inhalers until their mucous membranes are injured. Today quite a few persons keep sniffing at an inhaler every few minutes. Fortunately, in recent years, the finest type of rhinologist has stopped operating on these persons, and has tried to reassure them and to get them to leave their noses alone.

The person with an overly reactive or "vasomotor" nose. Many of the persons with what looks like an allergic nose, and more or less constant distress from it, are a bunch of nerves, and too sensitive. The nasal mucosa and its vasomotor nerves are overreactive just like the rest of the person, and much treatment by rhinologists and allergists can do no good. As Kraines (Arch. Otolaryng. *33*) said, the nose may run because of nervous influences, and it can suffer from paresthesias.

The nasal mucosa is highly subject to vasomotor influences, and some persons have noted that their symptoms can be brought out by emotion. Perhaps their mucosa blushes or blanches as the face does. Since there is a connection between the nasal mucosa and the sexual organs, some women sneeze when sexually excited. The relation between the nose and the sexual organs was well known to the old Greek and Latin poets.

Harold Wolff and his research colleagues have recently published a book on the effects of emotion on the nasal, pharyngeal, and bronchial mucosas, showing how greatly the amount of secretion varies with nervous tension. The nasal mucosa can either shrink or become engorged with certain emotions. T. H. Holmes, H. Goodell, Stewart Wolf, and H. G. Wolff (1949) reported on some of the secretory storms which affect the nose when certain persons are subjected to emotional strain. Lester Coleman watched a woman develop severe vasomotor rhinitis shortly after marriage to an alcoholic man. She got well when she escaped into a hospital.

Supposed colds. Thousands of persons who say they are constantly catching cold, especially when exposed to the least draft, really haven't a cold, they have only a vasomotor change in the nose. That is why, with a little codeine or a few doses of an antihistaminic drug, they can get well.

The allergic nose. There are millions of persons whose nasal troubles are allergic in nature and due to the inhalation of pollens or dusts. These persons have a mild form of hay fever. For instance, when I was a boy working in a library I got sensitized to book dust. As a result, even today, if I take down an old book or rustle some papers on an untidy desk, I am likely to start sneezing, and my nose may run for a few minutes.

More rarely, a nose may be disturbed by the person's eating some food to which he is sensitive. Or his nose may become stuffy at night because of its proximity, perhaps, to a wool blanket.

Treatment. Years ago, some rhinologists kept operating on sensitive noses again and again, removing ethmoid and sphenoid cells until all that was left was a large uncomfortable and evil-smelling cavern. Fortunately, one now sees little of such surgery. Today it is likely to be performed only in a desperate effort to cure a nervous breakdown, a minor psychosis or a depression, or the sequelae of an unrecognized stroke.

Today the overly sensitive nose is likely to be treated with antihistaminic drugs or desensitizing injections of histamine.

CHAPTER 22

Psychic Problems Noted
by the Dermatologist
and the Urologist

DERMATOLOGY

PERHAPS BECAUSE IT IS the organ that covers the body and presents itself to the onlooker, the skin with the blood vessels in it is particularly sensitive to emotion. We all know how violently some persons blush when embarrassed, or how red an angry man's face can get. Many of the changes that appear with anxiety, tension, anger, shame, and embarrassment take place, of course, in the blood vessels. Others take place in the sweat glands, the sebaceous glands, and in the muscles that erect the hairs. As a result, the anxious or tense person often perspires too much, especially in the palms of the hands; he may suffer nervous chills with waves of gooseflesh, or he may complain of too great a greasiness of his skin. Other nervous troubles are changes in the circulation and structure of the skin which result in acne rosacea, neurodermatoses, edemas, and giant hives. There may also be angiospasm, such as that which produces Raynaud's white, cold fingers.

The skin of some persons tends to break out when they are tired or nervous. Klauder described a number of cases in which a skin lesion appeared right after a psychic shock. There are young women who get a small boil on the chin almost every time they menstruate.

Every physician knows how unhappy some adolescents are over a bad acne. The ugly pimples come just at the time when the boy or girl is most interested in winning attention and love. One hope that can usually be given such a youngster is that the disease will probably be gone by the age of twenty-two years.

Some women are much distressed over the disfiguration of nose and cheeks that goes with the butterfly lesion of acne rosacea. A few have to suffer because of an ugly port-wine mark. Others are unhappy because of superfluous hair on face or arms or legs.

On the production of skin lesions by emotion. There is a large literature on the production of skin lesions by mental impressions or by hypnosis, and the dermatologist often has to deal with psychically produced giant urticaria, marked dermographia, and neurodermites. There are many stories of nuns and others who, by concentrating their thoughts on the wounds of Christ, managed to produce hemorrhagic lesions on the backs of the hands and feet. Dunbar (1946) brought together much of this literature. Some of it is suggestive, but it is doubtful if proper precautions were ever taken to rule out a factitious origin of the lesions. During the experiment the girl's hands and feet were not encased in plaster of paris, as they should have been. According to some writers, hemorrhagic lesions have been produced by hypnotic suggestion, but others deny this (Klauder: 1936). According to Dunbar, the most extensive survey of the subject of neurodermites was made by W. D. Sack for Jadassohn's *Handbuch* which was published in 1933.

C. H. Rogerson (1939) listed as skin diseases that can be influenced by the mind, erythemas, eczema, prurigo, alopecia areata, vitiligo, scleroderma, dysidrosis, factitious excoriations, herpes, lichen planus, and psoriasis.

Itching, of course, is often of psychic origin or due to strain or unhappiness. Many a sensitive school nurse has suffered all day from an itchy scalp after seeing lice on a child's head, and many a person in a theater has suffered all evening because of a "psychic flea."

Itching of the anus and vulva is a disease rarely seen in persons who are not highly sensitive and a bit neurotic. Some are unhappy in their sexual life. Hunt (1936), who studied 300 cases of pruritus vulvae, felt that in only eight was there sure evidence that the psychic factor was the only one at work. In many other cases it was contributory.

Many sensitive and worrisome persons suffer from a burning in the epigastrium, a burning which is almost certainly a paresthesia out in the skin. Others suffer from a sort of hallucination, such as the feeling of ants crawling over them.

Excessive or unpleasant perspiration. Every clinician should know well the person who gets a cold wet palm whenever he has to shake hands. A few persons have their life made miserable by such sweating, so much so that they welcome a cervical sympathectomy. A case was recently reported in which giving banthine worked a cure. Other persons perspire excessively from the axillas or elsewhere, when tense or overworking or nervous. The man who is writing rapidly may have perspiration pouring out of his right axilla. John Stokes has called attention to the fact that the person who perspires excessively because of emotion can be bothered with the excessive growth of dermatophytes. It is said that a woman suffering from the flushes and sweats of the menopause can have an extremely annoying case of athlete's foot.

The sweat brought out by unpleasant emotion may have a very strong odor, and it is particularly foul smelling in the cases of some insane persons. Many a time I have been led to the diagnosis of a mild psychosis or hysteria or a psychotic ancestry because of a peculiar type of unpleasant body odor. Such odors sometimes are very distressing to everyone concerned.

Other effects of emotion. According to Klauder and to Marshall and Freeman, there are many authenticated cases of persons who have quickly turned gray from fright, and I have had many patients tell me that they knew of persons who had done this. Sir Arthur Hurst published a picture of a man whose hair stood on end with fright in World War I. Curiously, it stayed that way! Barney Ross, the prize fighter, told me that after staying in a shell hole until all the men about him were killed, his hair turned white. He found it white a few days later when he was able to see himself in a mirror.

There are a number of writers who claim that the popular idea that warts can be charmed away by psychotherapy is true.

In many cases a complete loss of body hair is supposed to be of psychic origin, and I have seen a few cases in which, because of the person's peculiar personality, this might well have been the case. In the last case of this type which I saw, the woman, who had a poor nervous system to begin with, had twice attempted suicide because of jealousy. In another case I could find no reason for the phenomenon.

The dermatologist has to be on the lookout for skin lesions produced and kept open by the patient. Usually, in order to be sure of the diagnosis and to heal the lesions, all the doctor need do is to put the affected hand or leg in a cast.

Urticaria. In my experience, small hives are likely to be due to the eating of some food to which the person is sensitive, but giant urticaria is more likely to be due to some heart-breaking experience or some worry or indecision. I see cases of giant urticaria in which the home physician should have let the skin tests go and instead have asked about a psychic shock. In a few cases I have been unable to get a history of unhappiness, but this does not mean that it was not there.

The studies of John Stokes. John Stokes has for years been emphasizing the effects of the mind and a neurotic constitution on the skin. (See J.A.M.A. *105.*) He listed as conditions much influenced by the mind: acute exudative neurodermatitis, flexural neurodermatitis, the prurigo of Besnier, lichen simplex chronicus, the rosacea complex, and neurogenous pruritus. He pointed out that the persons who are prone to get neurodermites were born with a tense, unstable nervous system. In addition, they are usually trying to carry too heavy a load of responsibility, or they are struggling with the problems of an unhappy marriage or an unhappy job. Many of these persons have a psychotic ancestry, and they can usually be recognized in a few minutes after their history has been taken. Some are highly sensitive and allergic.

As Stokes said, many persons show their nervous tension not only in their skin but in other parts of the body. They may suffer from hay fever, asthma, vasomotor rhinitis, migraine, and hyperthyroidism. Many are troubled because they feel caught in a trap (see Chapter 8); others feel overwhelmed, just thinking of the work that is piled up waiting to be done; others live in conflict with someone, including themselves; others feel defeated, or feel that they can't stand some "last straw"; others feel useless, passed over, or put upon and abused by someone.

Other students of emotion and the skin. Steven Rothman (1945) made a fine study of the mechanisms through which the mind can influence the skin and published a useful bibliography of the subject.

Mittelman and Wolff (1939) did much research to show that usually emotional stress is accompanied by a decided fall in the temperature of the skin of the fingers. The maximum drop observed was 13.5 degrees centigrade. With sustained stress, the hands may take on a temperature pretty close to that of the environment. An intelligent patient of mine with Raynaud's disease has noticed that flare-ups always come when she is under great mental or emotional strain. The trouble began when her husband suddenly died. Another one of my patients, widowed twice, had severe attacks of white fingers with each bereavement.

Walsh and Kierland (1947) found that some persons with neurodermites could be helped by psychiatric treatment. As they said, a neurodermatitis may show itself as single or multiple itching patches of lichenified skin, or there may be what looks like an atopic dermatitis or an exfoliative dermatitis.

Ideas on treatment. Stokes once wrote out a list of some of the things that the physician can do to help a tense nervous patient with neurodermatoses. The doctor should be optimistic and should give some hope. He may have to bring a psychic problem to the surface so that the patient can look at it frankly. The doctor may help by pointing out that time solves a number of problems for those who know how to wait. He should teach serenity and the need for more peace and relaxation. He should teach the need for avoiding conflicts, and the giving up, perhaps, of a constant striving toward some unattainable goal. If anxious enough for a cure, the tense patient should let up on himself a bit, and give up some of his ambitions.

When a patient feels his itching coming on, he can help himself by not getting all excited about it. He will do better if he shrugs his shoulders and says, "Hello, old boy! Back again? Sorry, I'm too busy to bother with you now." Stokes always wanted to know about the sleeping habits of his nervous patients. Many who are sadly in need of sleep putter about until one or two in the morning, doing nothing that is important. This fact can tell the physician much that he needs to know about an individual. For many tense women, an afternoon nap is very helpful.

Stokes has shown that even in the case of an organic disease, such as syphilis, the physician must pay attention to the psychic side of the therapeutic problem. He must combat the horror and mental distress and must help the person to carry on and have faith that some day he will be clean again. Also, in his delightful article on scabies among the well-to-do, Stokes showed how many psychic problems arise in the handling of patients with even a disease caused by mites burrowing through the skin. If it can be avoided, the patients should not be made to feel ashamed and humiliated. It is good to "save face," and hence the physician should be tactful. I will never forget the horror of a well-dressed man whom I saw when I was first out of college. When I showed him that his "eczema" was due to lice in his waist band he rushed out of the office and never returned. Perhaps today I would be more tactful about the matter.

Some patients who are distressed over a disfiguring rash on the face will feel much better if it is covered over with the preparation Covermark.

Women with superfluous hair should be urged to have it removed. Some shave every day while others put on a piece of adhesive plaster and then yank the hair out with it. The electric needle can be bad if it leaves scars and pits. Unsightly nodules and hairy moles should be removed, and this can be done easily with electrocoagulation. When a disfigurement can be removed in a few seconds it is foolish for a woman to keep it and go on suffering shame because of it. Elsewhere in this book I tell of a woman who recovered from a bad neurosis when she was induced to part with a lot of hair on her face.

Pruritus ani or vulvae might be treated best by an internist, a dermatologist, a gynecologist, a proctologist, and a psychiatrist all working together.

Acne of the face and shoulders can be helped by looking for and finding some food such as chocolate to which the patient is sensitive. Overeating may be bad. Some youngsters can help themselves by quickly expressing every comedone as it forms. In this way infection can be avoided.

THE NERVOUS PERSON WITH UROLOGIC TROUBLES

The urinary frequency of the worried. The commonest urinary complaint of nervous persons is that they are running to the toilet every twenty minutes. If, as almost always happens, they are doing this during the day and not at night, and if they have a clear urine without a pus cell, the probability is great that the cause of the trouble is nervousness or worry. Often it is an inability to make a decision about something. In men and also in women it can be due to an intensity of effort over some task such as writing. In children, great frequency can be due to excitement, such as that attendant on going to a birthday party or a wild western movie.

The irritable bladder or urethra. Women, and especially neurotic women past middle age, commonly complain of a frequency of urination, mainly during the daytime, associated with some burning and perhaps pelvic discomfort. The catheterized urine will be sterile and it will contain no pus cells. In these cases, after cystoscopy, the urologist usually reports a chronic urethritis, grade I, but advises that it be left alone because the more it is treated the worse the woman is likely to get. If the woman were not so sensitive she would not experience any symptoms from the little change in the urethra. Oftentimes all her troubles appear to be due to her nervousness and hypersensitiveness.

If a man or woman says there is frequency at night the physician will want to find out if it is an urge to void that wakes the patient or if it is a nervousness that causes the waking. Once awake, a restless person may feel that he or she should go and void, even if the bladder is normal. In some cases it is essential to ask if there is complete relief for from three to ten minutes after voiding because this is consistent with the diagnosis of interstitial cystitis. If there is no relief at all, the trouble may be a pure neurosis.

Occasionally, in these cases one can find that the person's trouble is that, on the advice of someone, he is forcing himself to drink much more water than he needs, or at dinner time he drinks too much milk or beer or coffee. If he goes without much fluid after 4 P.M. he may not have to get up to urinate.

In some cases of irritable bladder I have had excellent results from giving from one to three 5-minim capsules of santal oil. This can soothe the bladder. After taking the oil a woman may be able to go on an auto ride without having to stop at every third gas station.

Many women past fifty years of age keep complaining of urinary frequency and distress. Perhaps a few bacteria of a saprophytic type will be found in the bladder urine, but there will be no pus, the blood sedimentation rate will be low, and there will be no sign of the woman's being made toxic by the slight infection. Under treatment, such a woman may get worse rather than better, and then sometimes the wise urologist will advise her to leave the infection alone and try to put up with the annoyance.

In the old days gynecologists and urologists used to operate on urethral caruncles but today few men fuss with them.

The "dropped kidney" and the "Hunner stricture." A considerable number of the neurotic or mildly psychotic patients seen by the internist because of an ache in the loin have had a kidney stitched up for ptosis. Usually after a while it is found to be low again. Probably it has to be low because it has to move downward when the liver does. But even if it is not as low or as movable as it was before the operation, the ache is likely to be just as bad as it was before. Furthermore, if one takes a good history one often finds that the ache came when the woman (the patient is practically always a nervous woman) was cast down by some sorrow or great strain, such as that which goes with a divorce.

Often, also, cross-questioning will bring out a number of facts such as that the "pain" is not pain but a dull ache or misery that is forgotten when the woman is busy over something. Also it is so constant that it almost certainly is of the type that is due to a psychic cause. Sometimes it extends along all one side of the body, thus suggesting a slight thalamic syndrome such as I have discussed in Chapter 12. Usually there is no relation between the ache and any distress on urination. The factors that make the ache worse are usually fatigue, such as comes from shopping too long or standing too long. Lying down commonly helps, apparently not because the kidney goes up into place but because the woman relaxes and rests. This is shown by the fact that if she remains harassed over something, the rest will not help.

Other important factors in making the pain worse are annoyance, anger, worry and, particularly, mental depression. A little questioning will sometimes show that the woman has some manic-depressive forebears, and she has a cyclic temperament. When she is in a blue spell she gets the "pain in her kidney."

Many of the women suffering from loin aches have been treated for months for a supposed Hunner stricture in a normal-appearing ureter. This has been dilated every week or two. I do not remember ever hearing of a patient being cured in this way, although I have seen some who said they get temporary benefits. In these cases my urologic colleagues at the Mayo Clinic rarely can see anything wrong with the kidney or ureters. They argue that if there were a chronic or intermittent stricture of the ureter there should be some dilation of the pelvis of the kidney, and in these cases none can be demonstrated. Furthermore, with the roentgen rays, the dye-containing urine can be seen to run out and down the ureter normally. I can remember two cases in which an operation on the ureteropelvic junction helped, but in them there was dilatation of the pelvis of the kidney.

I think if psychiatrists could examine all of the patients now being treated for a "Hunner stricture" they would conclude that all or most of them are nervous sufferers with a psychic ache.

It helps in the diagnosis of such a case to keep the woman in bed for a few days to find out if, with the kidney "up in place," she still has her ache. When it does not clear up, I have little faith in the diagnosis of ptosis.

I remember a powerfully built former champion athlete with an unexplainable "severe pain" in the left side of the abdomen. It was thought to be due to disease in the left kidney or ureter but at the Mayo Clinic nothing wrong could be found with the urinary tract. Curiously, he thought he was helped occasionally by a dilation of the ureter. What I thought threw light on the diagnosis was the fact that later the man returned with a hysterical "tumor" made by the contraction into a ball of the lower half of his right rectus muscle. I relieved this in a moment by doubling him up. I then suspected all the more that his old pain had also been hysterical in origin.

Enuresis. Enuresis is a problem which probably concerns the psychiatrist or the geneticist more often than the urologist. I doubt if there is much a psychiatrist can do in the way of curing the condition. Alexander Levine (1943) studied 150 men with enuresis and concluded that it is a manifestation of a deep-seated disturbance in personality. Many of the men suffered from somnambulism, nightmares, nail biting, and nervousness. For the most part they were immature, maladjusted, and emotionally unstable persons. Usually there was psychopathy in the family. A lack of security seemed to be an important factor. In many cases the home had been broken up.

What seems most probable to me is that enuresis is just a manifestation of a poor nervous heredity, and a child might suffer from it for years in spite of the best of environment, a good home, and loving sensible parents. As I have said, the hereditary defect in neurones which affected the grandfather's cerebral gray matter may now, in the grandson, be affecting some center low in the brain, or perhaps one low in the spinal cord.

SEXUAL DIFFICULTIES IN THE MALE

As I said in the section on cardiac neurosis, there are certain parts of the body, such as the face, the heart, and the organs of generation in which the coming of any disease is likely to be particularly disturbing and alarming to the patient.

On cheering the person who has contracted gonorrhea. The urologist often needs to be kindly and fatherly when treating the man or woman who is overwhelmed with shame and worry over a gonorrheal infection. The person should be assured that relief can eventually be attained. Fortunately, today, a cure can usually be obtained quickly. When the disease is slow to clear up, the person must be told that eventually the germs will die out.

Sometimes the prostate gland gets infected, and then the man, if worrisome and sensitive, may be the worse for much massaging. The wise urologist will stop the treatment when he begins to see that the few pus cells in the prostatic fluid are not causing the symptoms, and that the massages are producing more depression than they are worth.

Often the urologist must explain that gonorrhea is not a generalized infection like syphilis; it will not destroy the man's sexual power, and it will not injure the children he may conceive. The doctor may have to explain the big difference between gonorrhea and syphilis; some men think they are variants of the same disease.

More discussion is needed, of course, when a man has a double epididymitis and greatly fears being left sterile. Similar problems arise when a girl gets gonorrhea with extension into her tubes.

Always the wise and kindly physician will be ready to discuss the person's worries, and to explain the situation in simple words. Often, when cured of gonorrhea, a man must be told again and again that he is all right; that the cultures for gonococci are negative, and there is no further indication for treatment. Many such a man who still feels some discomfort may have to be told that he will do better to put up with it than to go on trying by local treatment to get rid of the last vestige of it.

The man who has contracted syphilis. Doubtless often the urologist still is the first specialist to see the man who has gotten a chancre, and often he should take a little time to explain the situation and to give reassurance. Many a sensitive person, on learning that he or she has syphilis, is almost ready for suicide and is in need of encouragement.

In quite a few of the cases I see, the man has to be told again and again by the syphilologists that it is very doubtful if he ever did have syphilis. In such cases all four of the usually used tests (Kline, Kahn, Hinton, and Kolmer-Wassermann) for syphilis will be negative, and even the most sensitive ones, such as the Kline and Hinton, will fail to show those slight changes that commonly persist after even a good treatment of syphilis.

Worries of the man who must submit to prostatectomy. The urologist should often reassure the man who must undergo a prostatic resection; he should tell him that he can be just as potent after the operation as he was before. Fortunately, today, the transurethral resection is not a thing to be greatly feared as were the old operations.

Perineal or testicular aches. As R. E. Cone wrote, many of the aches and pains for which a urologist is consulted are psychic in origin. Such pains do not spread as organic pains do, and they may move around in an erratic way. Many are felt in the perineum or in the testicles. They may tend to come when the man is under strain, or they may follow intercourse. The man may forget them when he is busy. If he concentrates his worry on his penis or testicles, these organs will ache all the more. Often an experienced urologist can guess in a moment what the trouble is when he sees how worried and anxious the patient is. Perhaps the aches or burnings or tinglings followed an old gonorrheal infection and are now due to worry over it. As Cone said, to treat a sexual neurosis, as is now often done, with prostatic massages and instillations of silver nitrate into the posterior urethra can only make matters worse. What the man really needs is a kindly talking-to.

Nocturnal emissions and masturbation. Young men by the thousand are still much upset and worried over nocturnal emissions and masturbation, and then their future health depends on their getting quickly into the hands of a sensible physician who will tell them that emissions are signs only of good health, an actively functioning prostate gland, and continence. He will tell them that the desire to masturbate is a sign of health and normalcy and nothing to worry about. The boy who never is tempted to masturbate must have something wrong with his body or his mind. He should be told that Kinsey has found that almost all boys masturbate at some time to get rid of the great nervous tension that builds up because of continence.

Sometimes it is helpful to explain to the boy that the great fear of the supposed evil results of masturbation was built up years ago by those well-intentioned people who hoped to scare young boys out of the practice, and quacks who hoped to scare them into their "museums of anatomy" where they could be fleeced.

It may help the religiously trained boy to have pointed out to him that the Bible has nothing to say about masturbation.

Curiously, even ministers and teachers seem to be ignorant of the fact that onanism is not masturbation. What Onan did was to follow the old Hebrew injunction to have intercourse with his widowed sister-in-law so as to "raise up seed to his brother." In other words, he was to help get an heir for his brother, someone to carry on the family name and worship. What angered the priests of Israel was that Onan took the fun but slid out of the responsibility; he enjoyed the intercourse but "withdrew" and "spilt his seed to the ground." He did not want to beget and bring up an extra child. Doubtless many boys would be less concerned about masturbation if they only knew that the Bible does not say that hell fire is waiting for them if they yield to the temptation.

A loss of interest in sex, perhaps with impotence. Most men tend to lose interest in sex as they grow older, and as a result, the graph of frequency of intercourse is a straight line slanting downward with advancing years. According to Kinsey, by the age of sixty most married men are having intercourse only about once a month. Some few men are so young for their years that they want it much oftener than this. Much depends, also, on the amount of work a man is doing and the amount of fatigue he suffers. On a vacation he is likely to be much more active sexually. If the wife, also, is overworking and tired, or if she is sickly, or frigid, or sexually anesthetic, or if she has had a hysterectomy or entered the menopause, or if she is unloving or threatening a separation, the man's libido may fade almost to the vanishing point.

Some few men lose sexual interest by the time they are forty, and if then the wife does not care much, they quit. Many women patients have told me that their husband never did care much for intercourse; he never seemed to enjoy it much. Perhaps he never enjoyed anything in life very much, or intercourse may have left him very tired or weak or nervous. I suspect that a man who in early life has little sexual interest will be more likely to quit when he is forty than will the man who originally had much interest and desire. With but little sexual drive a man will not keep going so long. In the cases of other men, much may depend on the affection and the sexual desire of the wife. If she loves intercourse he will oblige her occasionally, but if she hates or fears intercourse, or if early she gets fat and loses her attractiveness, he will quit. Perhaps with a younger or more loving partner the man would desire intercourse more often and would be much more potent.

Some men quit sexual intercourse early in life because they are frail, or intercourse makes them jittery and tense and sleepless, or they are somewhat homosexual, or their health was injured by gonorrhea, syphilis, alcoholism, or dissipation, or they are definitely depressed, or they can feel little love for the spouse, or for anyone, for that matter.

If the wife has died or has left the man, and he has to get along with strange women for whom he has no love, he is still more likely to become rather impotent or to give up his sexual life. He may also have to cope with occasional fears of venereal infection, discovery, or blackmail, or he may have religious scruples and feelings of sinfulness over what he is doing, or he may have to stop to put on a condom. Many a middle-aged man cannot use a condom because, while getting it on, he loses his erection.

The more refined and esthetic the man the more easily he can lose his erection with some little annoyance or disgust or fear, or a feeling that the partner is not as feminine or clean or affectionate as she might be. Or she may say or do something that annoys or upsets or disgusts him. Even very potent and promiscuous men will sometimes suddenly find themselves impotent for some such reason. A fear of getting the woman pregnant or getting caught in a paternity claim may temporarily inhibit the man.

To illustrate: An Army officer returning from a tour of duty looked eagerly for his wife at the railroad station. Not finding her there, he was disappointed and upset. He got to wondering if she really loved him. By the time he got home he thought that he had excused her perfectly, and he was delighted to see her, but when he got into bed he found himself impotent. Evidently the subconscious resentment had taken control of his autonomic nervous system. Another man who came as a patient had always been potent until he became engaged. Going as usual next night to see his old mistress, he felt guilty and ashamed of himself, and as a result he was impotent. This so took away his confidence that, later when he married, he was impotent with his bride.

A religiously inclined man was highly potent with a beautiful second wife until, one night he failed completely, and failed again on subsequent attempts. After much questioning, I got from him the story that he had been thinking how his first wife had died in childbirth and had left him desolate. He had blamed himself for her death. The thought then struck him that if he impregnated his new wife he "might kill her also with his lust." Another man, always potent with his usual sexual partner, failed dismally when she remarked that she had gone to see the doctor about a vaginal discharge. He wondered what it might be due to. Another man, middle-aged and well-to-do, had been going with a young woman, and having no sexual difficulties. One evening she told him some things which led him to suspect strongly that she had given her favors also to a young and impecunious artist. He then became impotent because of the fear that if the boy got her pregnant she would lay the blame on him.

A young man who had always been perfectly potent married a girl athlete who, although beautiful, was somewhat mannish and with but little gift for affection. To his astonishment and distress, he could never get an erection with her. Later, I learned from her two sisters that their husbands, also, had been largely impotent with them. Evidently there was something peculiar in all three of the sisters. Several sensitive men have told me of a lack of potency when they tried to have sexual relations with a bisexual type of woman. Even though she was physically beautiful, there was some repelling influence there that caused the man to be impotent.

A man, always highly potent, was told that he needed a transurethral prostatectomy. Worrying much for fear that it would leave him impotent, he promptly became that way. When told by the urologist that he could put off the operation for several years, he was elated and promptly found himself potent again. As has been well known since the dawn of history, a man who loses potency with an older woman, will often regain it with a younger and more attractive and cooperative partner. A hereditary tendency to depressions will also destroy potency. I have known impotent men who had been treated by several urologists, all of whom had failed to note that their patients were almost ready for an asylum.

One would think that urologists would know these things well, and of course they do, but still patients such as those whose troubles I have just described tell me that when they went to a specialist for help, all they received were examinations and local treatments. They were not given time in which to tell their secret story of mental trouble, or they did not know its importance and it was not dug out of them. The urologists excuse themselves by saying that, in their busy day, they do not have time to stop and practice psychotherapy. It does not seem to them to be their job, and moreover, they were not trained to do it. It would seem, then, that they ought to take time to send these patients to some sensible psychiatrist who, in half an hour, could get the all-important story.

Obviously, every middle-aged man who becomes impotent should have a good general examination to rule out a number of diseases, and then a neurologic study should be made to rule out neurosyphilis or some other disease of the spinal cord and brain. In some cases the spinal fluid should be studied, as well as the functions of the urinary bladder. Occasionally one sees a tabetic with normal knee jerks and a normal Wassermann test.

In some cases a nervous breakdown, a depression, a small unrecognized stroke, a mild attack of encephalitis, or years of alcoholism will do away with a man's sexual interest and power. Alcohol commonly stirs up a man's sexual desires and takes away his inhibitions, but, unfortunately for him, it often diminishes his potency.

Always, of course, one must think of disease in the pituitary, thyroid, or suprarenal glands, and one must make the tests needed to find such disease. It may help to estimate the basal metabolic rate and the titer of the 17-ketosteroids.

In my experience, about the only type of person who is helped by the injection of androsterone is the eunuchoid, boyish person who has never shaved and who has testicles the size of lima beans. He needs the hormone. Doubtless the reason it rarely works in the cases of normal-appearing men is that they already have all of this hormone that they need. Their trouble is in the brain and not in the glands. In some cases the hormonal treatment will work well for a few weeks, due to suggestion, and then the results cannot be duplicated with more injections.

Often a wife will complain of a man's impotence and will beg him to go to a urologist but he won't do anything about it. He is satisfied to let things go as they are.

As I said, it is sad that urologists so seldom have time to treat these troubled men properly. It would be wonderful if, instead of cystoscoping them, they would sit down with them for a chat to find out what the mental trouble is. Sometimes perhaps, they should talk to the wife. She might have avoided all the trouble if, when the man first failed to get a good erection, she had been patient, sympathetic, and encouraging, instead of disappointed and sarcastic.

Premature ejaculation. The man who complains of premature ejaculation usually has what one would expect, and that is, greatly exaggerated reflexes. The fellow's nerves are on a hair-trigger. In my experience, in the worst of these cases the man has epileptic relatives and some dysrhythmia in his electroencephalogram. Such men are at all times very irritable and tense. They are epileptics without the fits. A physician once told me that he cured his tendency to ejaculate prematurely by smearing his glans with nupercaine ointment twenty minutes before intercourse. This somewhat anesthetized the nerve endings. It would be interesting to see what dilantin (1½ grains) and mebaral (1 grain) would do for some of these men.

Other worries. Somewhat psychopathic men may worry much about such things as a small penis or small soft testicles, or testicles that they think hang too low, or an occasional glueing together of the lips of the meatus due to a slight nocturnal emission, or a crooked stream. In the old days when the quacks advertised much, many young men worried about "lost manhood" due supposedly to spermatorrhea or the constant loss of sperm in the urine. Fortunately, one seldom hears of this complaint any more. If now I were to hear a patient complain of it I would go carefully into the question of his sanity.

In the old days men used to worry much over sexual excesses in their youth. Today some may still fear that they overdid things a bit, but they do not seem to worry much about it.

The male menopause. Lately one hears much about the male menopause. I am not sure that there is such a thing comparable to that of the woman. Certainly it is hard to think of a male menopause at fifty when one finds men of sixty-five and seventy still enjoying inter-course once or twice a week. I have talked to men past eighty who said they still enjoyed it about once a month.

What does happen in the cases of many men around forty-five or fifty is a flare-up in sexual interest and activity. Just why this comes it is hard to say. In some cases it seems to be due to a loss of interest in a fat or unpleas-ant or somewhat frigid wife. With the sexual life at home unsatisfactory or ended, the man may start looking around for something better. Perhaps he realizes that he never did have a sexual life that was beautiful or idealistic or satisfactory, and he would like to experience it before his powers fail. Perhaps he reads of the raptures of a perfect sexual life and would like to see what they are like.

Perhaps the man has achieved financial success or some degree of eminence, and then many women easily fall for him or go after him. Perhaps he wants to try a partner more attractive than the one he had to take when he was young and poor. Perhaps his potency is failing with his wife and he wants to see if it is his fault or hers. Certain it is that big executives around the age of forty or fifty often get into mis-chief.

Usually about all the physician is likely to hear about is the man's difficulties in getting and maintaining an erection. Sometimes he has to be reminded that if he would only settle down with one woman he would get accustomed to her, and then he would stop having trouble getting an erection or ejaculating prematurely.

The sexual excesses of the old arteriosclerotic. Occasionally one is consulted by the sons of an old man who are much upset because he has had such a flare-up of his sexual desire that he will take one or two prostitutes to a hotel room for a spree of several days. I suspect that in these cases the arteriosclerotic destruction of higher centers in the brain leaves the man in the grip of lower animal-instinct centers. He then does what an animal would do, without any judgment or good sense or shame to keep him straight. Lawyers have told me that they see cases like this; they are called in to see what can be done to save the family fortune from dissipation.

CHAPTER 23

Psychosomatic Problems of
Several Different
Specialties

THE ORTHOPEDIST

POST-TRAUMATIC, OFTEN HYSTERICAL, TROUBLES. Many of the persons who go to an orthopedist are suffering from nervous strain or hysteria or combinations of the effects of an injury and some hysteria or compensation neurosis (see Chapter 16). Hence it is that in few fields of medical practice is there more need for good clinical judgment and wide experience. In difficult cases, the orthopedist needs to take a searching history; he needs to size up the patient, and often he needs to talk to his or her relatives and friends. Much on compensation and post-traumatic neurosis is to be found in the chapter on hysteria.

Of all the patients hospitalized in one year in Luck's (1946) orthopedic section, 11 per cent had psychologic problems which were either the sole cause or the most important contributing cause of their disability. Of the orthopedic troubles seen in an outpatient department over 25 per cent were predominantly psychogenic in origin. One should always suspect a psychogenic factor in producing a painful joint if movement does not much influence the pain. Furthermore, what the patient may first call pain may turn out, on careful questioning, to be only a feeling of tension or pressure or fatigue.

Often the trouble is apparent when the patient limps in. As M. S. Henderson of the Mayo Clinic says, many children get curious limps and ways of walking, and then, when nothing physically wrong can be found, one wonders if the trouble can be purely hysterical in nature. This suspicion will be strengthened if questioning of the parents shows that the limp followed some strong clash of opinion, or served to get the child excused from some chore. Then, perhaps, with a few concessions to the child's wishes and a little encouragement, the walk will become normal again.

Adults, also, will walk into the office with curious gaits and muscular contractions. Some of the postures assumed can immediately be recognized by the orthopedist as hysterical in nature, and then he may quickly cure, or perhaps, better yet, if there is a neuropsychiatrist handy, this expert can cure the contraction and find out why it came. The psychological cause should be treated so that the trouble will not soon come back in the same or some other place.

Some patients will tell of an accident or of some doctor's belief that he found signs of a broken neck or a broken back. The big point to bring out often is that the contraction or weakness or change in gait came, not at the time of the accident, but some time later, perhaps when someone suggested that it might pay to sue and get something out of an insurance company. As I say in Chapter 16, the diagnosis can often be made easily and in a few minutes, *not by examining,* but by getting a detailed history which shows that the patient walked away from the accident with hardly a bruise and certainly no limp. A twisted neck is a favorite symptom of such persons.

It is worthy of note that farmers, skiers, and horsemen, when they get injured, rarely get a neurosis, perhaps because there is no industrial compensation to try for. As Henderson has said to me, when in doubt about a compensation case, the orthopedist will do well to withhold his opinion until he has had good consultations with, let us say, an internist, a neurologist, and a psychiatrist. Nowhere in medicine is there more need for the combined wisdom of several men.

A wise physician will sometimes feel like saying to a bedridden patient, "Your trouble is nothing but hysteria; you get up out of that bed; you can walk as well as I do." But the doctor hates to "get tough" in this way because it would be most embarrassing if it were to turn out that the patient really did have an injury to his spinal cord. And so, as Doctor Henderson says, the older a man gets the kinder he is likely to get. Through the years, whenever Henderson thought a patient's main trouble was a compensation neurosis, he advised the insurance company to settle quickly for a lump sum. That is usually the best way out for everyone. In Denmark doctors found that over 90 per cent of the patients with a traumatic neurosis recovered promptly probably because the custom there is to give a lump settlement. In

Germany, where the money used to be handed out on the installment plan, only 9.3 per cent of the patients recovered.

So often, if the first orthopedist who saw the patient were immediately to recognize a "compensation neurosis" and *be sure of it* from the history and the appearance of the contracture, he might get the patient to accept a hundred dollars and let the matter drop. If, however, for several months several doctors keep hospitalizing the man and examining him and getting more and more roentgenograms made, the bills keep mounting up until any settlement made has to be a big one. Then, if the man sues, a sympathetic jury is likely to ignore all the evidence against the fellow, and the result is a big verdict in his favor.

Henderson has said that often an orthopedist might be able to cure a chronic complainer, not by saying that there never was much wrong with him, but by promising a cure and then manipulating the painful joint under an anesthetic or injecting some procaine around it. To be cured in this way the patient must first be tired of his complaint, and then he must have some such little operation in order to save face and avoid criticism from his family and others.

Another thing a wise orthopedist must do occasionally is to say, "This physiotherapy has gone on too long; we must stop it." Then he must get a good clinician to investigate to see why the patient has not recovered. I remember one such case in which a woman had gone on complaining bitterly for months after a fracture had apparently healed well. Then the orthopedist told the physiotherapists that he thought they had done all that could be accomplished. He sent the woman to an internist who soon found that the reason she had not gotten well was that she came of an insane family and was in a depression.

When called to see a patient with a smashed limb the orthopedist, if wise, does not volunteer a bad prognosis. Some men are in a hurry to tell the patient and his family how bad the outlook is. It is much better to wait and see, because oftentimes the patient comes out with a much better arm or foot than anyone had hoped he would get.

It is wise, also, to fight as long as possible to preserve an arm or leg or hand or foot. So many times in a physician's life he has a patient show him a useful hand or foot and say, "Doctor So-and-so was bound he was going to take that off, but I would not let him," or "I got Doctor So-and-so, and he fought hard to save it, and did." Every so often, also, one sees a person who, years ago, was given up for lost with what looked like a sarcoma of a bone; perhaps he had some roentgenotherapy, and here he is, well. I have seen several such cases, and they keep me from offering bad prognoses.

The psychic problems of amputees. Obviously, the amputee has many psychic problems, and sometimes he needs psychiatric help. Every medical school might do well each year to show the film, *The Best Years of Our Lives* to its students, and particularly those surgical students who will some day be performing amputations. The actor in that play, Harold Russell, later wrote a book called *Victory in My Hands,* which ought to be in every hospital library and ought to be read by every orthopedist, rehabilitationist, and physiotherapist.

Amputees can suffer severe pain of a causalgic type. In most cases it apparently is very real and due to curious effects arising in disease in sympathetic nerves. Unfortunately, the way to a cure is often far from clear. W. K. Livingston once wrote a book called *Pain Mechanisms,* summing up what is known on the subject.

Symptoms of a traumatic neurosis. Among the commoner symptoms complained of by persons suffering from traumatic neurosis one finds headache, backache, aching in the limbs, failure of memory, loss of concentration, introspection and brooding, fears and phobias, changes in temper, rapid heart action, vasomotor disturbances, and disturbances of digestion. Often the appearance of the patient is suggestive of a neurosis, as is the way in which he behaves in the office or in court.

An excellent paper on the traumatic neuroses is by Moorhead (1944) who has had a big experience in this field. He commented on the fact that traumatic neuroses rarely follow *severe* injuries. They come more often after minor injuries, and in many cases are the result of suggestion, fear, anxiety, or desire for revenge or financial gain. They develop often from unwise suggestions or actions by interns, doctors, nurses, physiotherapists, lawyers, or others. Curiously, a neurosis will develop sometimes in the case of a person who only witnessed an accident. Recovery usually occurs only after the desire for remuneration has been satisfied. Several men with huge experiences in this field have said that no one with a traumatic neurosis ever recovers while a suit is pending.

Le Vay (1947) commented on the fact that the orthopedist must often take into account psychic effects produced in the patient by his illness. It is hard for many persons to adjust to problems that come with a physical disability. Some few remain ill apparently in order to punish someone whom they hold responsible for the accident or for poor treatment. In handling these problems much depends on the patient's confidence in his physician and on the physician's dynamic influence on him. The nurses and physiotherapists can also have an important influence for good or for evil.

As I point out elsewhere in this book, sometimes one can talk a patient into getting well by hammering home repeatedly the fact that the rewards of getting up and going back to work are decidedly greater than are those of staying on compensation.

The big thing an orthopedist can often do is to insist that a change observed in, let us say, the spine is a congenital anomaly, often seen, and often seen in the cases of persons who have no pain.

Emotional problems of the physically handicapped. Whenever I pass a hunchback I glance sympathetically at his face, hoping to see that he has been able to stand up well to the great strains of frustration, humiliation, defeat, and unhappiness that he has had to experience. I feel so sorry for the perhaps otherwise attractive woman who has gone unmarried because of a short paralyzed leg, a twisted spine, clubfeet, an amputation, too great tallness or bigness, a badly receding chin, an ugly skin, or a sickly appearance. I feel sympathy for the man who is so short that he must constantly feel unhappy about it. Fortunately, quite a few of these persons manage to stay sane and stable and friendly; many earn a good living, and many a one eventually finds a mate.

The best study I know of the mental reactions of a hunchback is to be found in the two beautifully written books by Mrs. Hathaway: *The Little Locksmith* and *The Journals of the Little Locksmith*. There one learns of the sorrows that came when a sensitive girl found that she was crippled and disfigured and would probably have to live a life of loneliness and pain. Another remarkable book of this type is Barbellion's *The Journal of a Disappointed Man*. It is a brilliantly written story of the rebellious feelings that arose in the mind of a gifted young naturalist when he found he was to die in a few years with multiple sclerosis.

A much merrier reaction to crippling was that of Louise Baker (*Out on a Limb*) who, in childhood, had to have a leg amputated. She never wasted any time on regrets. Another optimistic study is that of R. L. Goldman (*Even the Night*) who, in spite of severe deafness and a bad poliomyelitis which paralyzed both legs, became a successful writer, and was happily married twice.

Following is a list of some other hopeful and stimulating books: *Born That Way* by Dr. Carlson, a spastic; Borghild Dahl: *I Wanted to See;* Anne Ellis: *Sunshine Preferred, or the Philosophy of an Ordinary Woman;* Harold Russell (with both hands amputated): *Victory in My Hands;* Noreen Linduska: *My Polio Past;* Betsy A. Barton (crippled by an accident): *And Now to Live Again;* E. E. Calkins (deaf): *Louder Please;* Alice Bretz: *I Begin Again;* Helen E. Heckman: *My Life Transformed;* Dame Agnes G. Hunt: *This Is My Life;* Helen A. Keller (blind, deaf, and dumb): *Story of My Life;* Karsten Ohnstad (blind): *World at My Fingertips;* Robinson Pierce: *It Was Not My Own Idea;* H. V. O'Brien (going blind): *Memoirs of a Guinea Pig;* A. L. Trudeau (tuberculous): *An Autobiography;* Gertrude Hoopes (crippled): *Out of the Running;* Frances Pastorelli (bedridden with heart disease): *Strength Out of Suffering;* C. Y. Harrison: *Thank God for My Heart Attack.*

According to some psychiatrists who have made studies of physically handicapped women, these persons sometimes tend to remain immature. They may become Mama's or big sister's little girl; they may give up trying to attract men; they may give up all hope of a sexual life, and they may wind up with a rather childish and dependent outlook on life.

THE ENDOCRINOLOGIST

I have seen many persons, thoroughly treated by endocrinologists, whose trouble was really a neurosis or mild psychosis or the residue of an attack of unrecognized encephalitis or a little stroke. Many a case of what, at first glance, is taken for ovarian disease is really a case of injury to the hypothalamus. Especially when assays of some of the important secretions show normal amounts, and when thorough dosing with hormones fails to have any effect, the endocrinologist would do well to stop and ask himself if the trouble might not be due to some other disease due perhaps to a poor nervous inheritance. So often a poor mental development is associated with a poor sexual development and severe dysmenorrhea. No one should attempt to be an endocrinologist until first he is a good physician and a good internist with some knowledge of psychiatry. Otherwise his practice may resemble that of a charlatan. He must keep his feet on the ground, and most of the patients who come to him he must promptly send elsewhere.

In cases of disease in the brain, treatment with estrogens and androgens will do no good. To illustrate: A stout, mannish woman was referred to me as a case of mild menopausal psychosis. The hope of the local physician was·that I would know of some new hormone which had not yet been tried on her by the local endocrinologists who had for some time been giving her "shots" of this and that. It was obvious at a glance that the woman must always have been homosexual and odd, and this hunch was confirmed by her brother. Later, it was confirmed by her when she said she knew she had always been eccentric and abnormal. As she remarked one day, "This isn't due to the menopause; I have always been a bit of a screwball like my aunt before me." She had always suffered from dysmenorrhea, and she had always been too masculine and too odd to get a beau. Measurements of the amounts of estrin, prolan, and 17-ketosteroids gave normal figures for her sex and age, and the more I saw of the woman the surer I was that all her trouble was in her brain, and that it had always been there.

In my early years in medicine I often puzzled over the relationship between signs of ovarian deficiency and mild psychopathy. I wondered if the psychopathy was primary or if it was secondary to the ovarian defect? No one could enlighten me. Curious, also, was the fact that in some of the families I knew with a strain of psychopathy running through them, some of the members suffered from a psychosis while others suffered from what appeared to be purely glandular defects such as myxedema or hypo-ovarianism. Later, there came on the market the first estrogens, and then I learned that the injection of these substances into women who showed these related sexual and psychic difficulties seldom restored the victim to good mental health. Gradually, through many years, I have come to feel that in most of these families the apparent endocrine diseases were too built-in to be eradicated by any glandular extract.

Occasionally, of course, the endocrinologist can cure a mild psychosis. Thus, I remember a sad-looking woman with what appeared to be an ordinary endogenous depression not due to any life strain. I was disturbed, however, because I could not get any family history of depressions. Then, fortunately, the woman told me that her sister, when she was once depressed, had been cured by the removal of a goiter. Although my patient had no goiter and showed none of the usual signs of thyrotoxicosis I had some estimates made of her basal metabolic rate and found them to be about 35 per cent above normal. When part of her thyroid gland was removed she promptly got well.

As everyone knows, persons suffering from myxedema can become somewhat psychopathic, and oftentimes in their cases the true diagnosis is missed.

Possible psychic effects on the suprarenal glands. Because of their close relation to the sympathetic nervous system, one would expect a psychic storm to upset the functions of the suprarenal glands, especially when they have been weakened by disease. Possibly the suprarenal glands have something to do with sudden death due to fright or grief. Marañon reported three cases of Addison's disease in which he felt the causation by emotion was clearly established. The probability is that emotion brought out a disease that had been lying latent. Thus, I remember a woman who, after a wild alcoholic party, vomited steadily for forty-eight hours and died. Necropsy showed atrophy of the suprarenal glands.

A useful article on the diagnostic significance of the new hormonal assays is that by Escamilla (1949).

Psychic Disturbances Associated with Disease of the Pituitary Gland

Harvey Cushing described peculiar mental conditions in persons developing a lesion of the pituitary gland. For instance, a man of thirty-eight began to grow stout and drowsy. He would come home and just sit, worrying and perhaps crying and insisting that he was hopelessly ill. Later he complained of feeling lonely; he wanted a light in every room, and demanded that his wife play the piano and sing to him. His trouble proved to be a lesion of the pituitary gland.

Three out of thirty acromegalic women studied showed mental aberrations. These patients had fits of despondency in which they talked of suicide. One of them eventually did commit suicide. Cushing stated that the literature contained frequent allusions to similar deviations in the mental processes of victims of acromegaly. Such psychic troubles could be due in part to the disease of tissue situated so near the brain, and in part to the terrible crucifixion of having to live with so homely and repulsive a face.

HYPERTHYROIDISM AND PSYCHOSIS

It is not surprising that persons whose bodies and brains are poisoned by hyperthyroidism should sometimes be irritable, unreasonable, abusive, or more or less psychotic. Often this fact should be explained to the relatives who, perhaps for years, have been puzzled and hurt by the unpleasant or unfair behavior of the invalid.

Especially in the days before Lugol's solution when surgeons removed the toxin-producing gland without previous treatment of the patient with iodine, some of the women, right after the operation, would go into a maniacal state.

Foss and Jackson once studied 2,500 persons, 1,700 of them in an insane asylum, and concluded that not only does toxic goiter not tend to appear more often in the psychotic, but the common forms of long-lasting psychosis are not found abnormally often in the cases of the goitrous.

The internist sometimes needs all his clinical sense to differentiate mild hyperthyroidism from psychoneurosis or a mild psychosis. For instance, a young woman who was acting queerly at times and who had prominent eyes and a diarrhea was found to have a basal metabolic rate varying from $+18$ to $+25$ per cent. Everyone hoped that the cause of her difficulties had been found, but she lacked many of the symptoms and signs of hyperthyroidsm, and she had a poor nervous heredity. Furthermore, a study with radioactive iodine showed that her thyroid gland did not have any unusual avidity for this element. Subsequent long-continued study of the girl showed that her troubles were psychic in origin, and with rest and psychotherapy she recovered beautifully.

Another way in which the differential diagnosis can sometimes now be made in puzzling cases of this type is through estimation of the protein-bound iodine. Curtis, at the school of medicine at Ohio State University, has found this method a most helpful one.

The person who becomes hyperthyroid because of emotional strain. One would expect to hear at times of exophthalmic goiter following a psychic shock, and actually such cases have been described. Dunbar, in the third edition of her book, abstracted literature on the subject, and Marañon (1921), Mittelman (1933), Conrad (1934), and Lidz and Whitehorn (1949) reported many cases in which the disease followed fright or psychic strain. For these cases the Germans use the term Schreckbasedow, or Basedow's disease due to fright. In **Parry's** first case (1803) the disease followed a fright. It is very questionable, however, if the syndrome always follows psychic strain.

Treatment. It is highly improbable that, once full blown, the disease could ever be cured by restoring peace or happiness. When once marked organic changes have appeared in the thyroid gland it is best to remove surgically much of the tissue. Some men are getting results with thiouracil or radioactive iodine, but these "cures" are often only temporary.

The woman who once suffered from a toxic goiter. It is well to notice when a woman has the scar of a thyroidectomy and then to ask if, before the operation, she was jittery and too warm and toxic. Perhaps the eyes are still prominent. If a woman once suffered from a toxic goiter she is likely still to be very nervous because of the injury that was once wrought in her brain. Usually the basal metabolic rate will be found to be normal. Sometimes the woman's old glandular illness will seem to explain her sexual frigidity.

MYXEDEMA AND PSYCHOSIS

One would expect the slowing-up of metabolism in cases of myxedema to produce mental depression, and actually it is said that 15 per cent of patients with myxedema have some psychotic symptoms. Ziegler (1930) described these psychoses and summarized the literature. His conclusion was that a loss of thyroid function can bring out a latent hereditary disposition to psychosis. Some of the patients become very irritable, some get delusions and hallucinations, others go definitely insane with mania, dementia, or melancholia, or with a marked tendency to suspicion and self-accusation. Often the memory fails a great deal. Usually there is a marked change in the quality of speech; it becomes slow and drawling and monotonous. Hearing and sight are often impaired.

Howard and Woods, of the Iowa state psychopathic hospital, also described the mental derangements seen in cases of hypothyroidism. Some of their patients became depressed and apprehensive, so that the condition could easily be mistaken for an ordinary endogenous depression. Occasional patients showed an irritability and excitement suggesting ordinary mania. Some showed distortions of thought, with bizarre hallucinations and delusions.

Treatment. The treatment, of course, is the giving of sufficient thyroid substance to raise the metabolic rate to normal.

THE GONADS

Troubles due to abnormalities in the ovaries are discussed in the chapter on gynecology and are touched on in several other chapters. Eunuchoid men often seem to be well enough adjusted to life.

OBESITY

Some few obese persons suffer from glandular dysfunction but most do not, and nothing is to be gained from examining them or giving hormones. Their basal metabolic rate is normal and their main trouble seems to be a huge appetite. Many were born to be fat like their huge relatives. They are a variety of the human race. A few are fat because of disease in the hypothalamus.

The only treatment for most of them is a scientifically designed low-caloric diet. Nothing can be done if the patient hasn't the intelligence, the desire, or the will power to reduce and then keep his or her figure.

PSYCHIC PROBLEMS OF THE ALLERGIC PERSON

In recent years many observant physicians have come to see that he who would succeed in treating allergic disease *or what looks like allergic disease* must always be on the watch for psychic factors. Scoffers at food allergy go so far as to say that it is all "in the patient's head." The truth is that allergic sensitiveness is just one form of sensitiveness, and an allergen is just one of the things that can pull the trigger. It is probably true that a man cannot very well be allergic unless he is sensitive to stimuli of many kinds. For this reason I always expect to find many more sufferers from allergy among the nervous children of university professors than among the stolid children of day laborers.

The reinforcing effect of emotion on allergy. Nervousness and fatigue can set the allergic trigger so fine that it can almost go off by itself. It may be, also, that some types of storm, such as those that produce migraine, a mucous colic, diarrhea, giant urticaria, vasomotor rhinitis, or paroxysmal tachycardia can be set off *either by emotion or by an allergen.* For instance, a woman can get an attack of migraine either by losing sleep, getting tired, looking at shining organ pipes or a tessellated floor, or eating some chocolate, and she can get a mucous colic either from nervous tension, catching a cold, or eating eggs.

That emotion can reinforce the action of an allergen is well known to me from my own experience. Years ago, when I ate chicken in my own home it produced only indigestion and a dull headache, but when I ate it at a banquet where I was under the strain of giving the principal address, it was often a violent poison. Similarly, a surgeon friend of mine, when rested after a good night's sleep, can scrub up without any discomfort in his arms, but if he is very tired from having been up part of the night, scrubbing up will cause his arms and hands to swell and to break out with a dermatitis. The necessary mechanism has evidently been sensitized by the fatigue. Many a man has remarked to me that the foods that fill him with gas at home can be eaten with impunity on a camping trip.

The allergist must then always be a student of psychosomatic medicine, and he must always be taking histories detailed enough to reveal either a direct psychic cause or a reinforcing psychic cause for the symptoms, granting that such a cause exists. Curiously, some books on allergy hardly mention this psychic component.

I can remember three women I once saw, one after the other, all complaining of swollen eyelids. All of them had been studied thoroughly by allergists who had all worked hard on the supposition that the cause must be some cosmetic. By going deeply into the history, I found that the lids of the first woman had started swelling on her honeymoon when she had discovered that the physician she had just married was a psychopath, unable to get a practice, and intending to live off her for the rest of his days. The eyes of the second woman started swelling when, shortly before her wedding, her intended changed his mind and expressed a desire to back out; and the eyes of the third woman swelled at a time when she was distraught and trying to make up her mind what to do about an unhappy marriage.

Urticaria. My impression from years of observation is that giant urticaria is more likely to be due to painful emotion and conflict and indecision than to the eating of food. The *little hives* may be due to food.

I remember a choleric nurse who got giant urticaria whenever she lost her temper. Another very passionate woman became covered with big wheals when she fell violently in love with a man and had to decide whether to run off with him or go back to her husband and three little children. A young woman became covered with hives each year during examination week at college. A man suffered greatly from giant urticaria when the promotion he had been promised was given to another man. Interesting in this case was the development, with the mental strain, of insomnia and a remarkable dermographia which went with the hives. Other men got giant hives when they lost a job.

B. Woodhead (1946) has reported cases in which a psychologic approach led to marked improvement in the condition of children with skin diseases. The parent also had to be treated. Stokes, also, has written much on the psychosomatic aspects of allergic skin disease (see Chapter 22 on dermatology).

Asthma. Anyone who has ever dealt with asthmatics knows that at times the attacks appear to be due to nervous strain, tension, anxiety, a quarrel, or too much excitement of an evening. I remember a boy who got asthma whenever his father, in the evening, romped with him, played Indians or hide-and-seek, and sent him to bed all excited. I remember another asthmatic child who got well when his parents promised him they would give up their plans for getting a divorce. Certainly, in all cases in which a child has attacks of asthma, the situation at home should be studied. The physician must look for sources of strain, conflict, fear, and insecurity. It is not hard to understand why these things sometimes set the trigger very fine.

A. T. Henderson (1946) concluded from his study that asthma is rarely due to emotion alone, but emotion can often sensitize the mechanism which responds to an allergen. According to McDermott and Cobb (1939) twenty of their fifty patients with asthma got their first attack because of emotion, and thirty-seven of the fifty had an emotional component in the factors bringing on attacks. More evidence as to the psychic production of asthma was gathered by Mitchell, Curran, and Myers (1947), and Schatia (1941).

It is curious to see how asthma can occasionally be relieved for a time by some hocus-pocus. I remember a chronic asthmatic who was highly sensitive to the goose feathers in his pillows. A short time before I saw him he had been "cured" spectacularly by a quack who exposed his chest to ultraviolet light. The relief lasted a few weeks, and then the wheezing came back.

Dunbar gave a large number of references to the literature on the psychic causation of asthma. She said that Hippocrates noted that the asthmatic must guard against getting angry. I knew a man who got his asthma only when his disliked mother-in-law came to visit him. Sir Arthur Hurst, a chronic asthmatic, used to tell of a day when the brakes on his car failed to work so that he shot down a hill toward an embankment. When at last he managed to bring the car to a stop, he found his wheezing gone! Probably with his fright he had poured a dose of epinephrine into his circulation. Other cases are known in which emotion *stopped* an attack of asthma.

The production of manifestations of allergy with the help of neuromimetic hormones. An observation of interest is that urticarial wheals can be produced by injecting histamine into the skin, and changes that look like those of a mucous colic have been produced in the mucosa of the sigmoid colon by the injection of a choline compound.

Migraine. Some allergists claim that migraine is only a manifestation of allergy but I am sure they are wrong; allergy is just one stimulus that can pull the migrainous trigger.

Syndromes that are confusing. There are a number of curious syndromes that are hard to classify—so hard that for a time the diagnostician may be baffled. He may suspect that the syndrome is due to a storm in the nervous system, but, then again, it may be due to some antigen. In some of these cases an offending antigen eventually is discovered and the patient is cured by its removal from the diet. In other cases both nervousness and an allergen have been at work. Certain it is that the allergist and the psychiatrist should work hand in hand in the solution of their more difficult problems.

PSYCHIC PROBLEMS OF THE TUBERCULOUS

As every expert on the treatment of tuberculosis knows, the patient whose morale is kept at a high level is likely to do better than will the one whose morale has been lowered by discouragement, worry, sorrow, or bad news.

In an excellent article, Coleman, Hurst, and Hornbein (1947) showed how much psychiatric help the tuberculous patient needs at every stage of his illness. At the start the physician should remember that when a patient is being apprised of the fact that he has tuberculosis he is likely to "black out" so that he will seem hardly to hear what is being said. Because of this, it is well to let the man rest over night before starting on a discussion of what has to be done about his disease.

The diagnosis of tuberculosis naturally brings with it the need for big changes in the emotional, social, economic, and family life of the patient. The reactions of different patients are different. Some become dull and apathetic and remain that way for weeks or months. Others face the problem more courageously and optimistically. Much will depend on the personality of the patient and the strength or weakness of that personality, and much may depend on the way in which the person's loved ones rally to his support. The patient's reaction may depend partly on the amount of desire he has to go on living or on the amount of desire he has to work and accomplish things. If the man likes to be taken care of he may cheerfully accept the prospect of dependency with a good excuse to be idle.

The physician should never minimize the seriousness of the disease and should never speak vaguely about it. The illness and all its implications should be described honestly so that the patient can face them fully and intelligently. It is not fair to say, "Oh, you'll be all right and out of the hospital in no time." Obviously, of course, all favorable and hopeful aspects of the individual situation should be stressed. A promise to use some of the new drugs like streptomycin can be encouraging.

Many things will have to be talked over with the patient and decided, such as the matters of financing the long period of rest or of caring for a wife and children, or of terminating an engagement to marry, or of winding up a business. A sanatorium has to be chosen.

When the patient comes into the hospital his reaction to the life there will, again, depend partly on his temperament and partly on the local conditions. As Betty McDonald showed in her book, *The Plague and I,* the patient's morale can be raised by friendliness and humanity shown by the staff, and also by friendliness and good sense emanating from the patient in the next bed. Enforced inactivity may intensify pre-existing emotional problems. Many patients are unable to relax and calm down and rest. They are like the man in the Army who is said to travel ten miles a day in his sleeping bag. Many persons are distressed by sexual hunger or bedeviled by worries over what is going on at home. Letters may not come regularly enough, and many of them may be distressing. Some relatives have curious ideas of what to write to a sick person. I remember a young woman with an apparently healed pulmonary tuberculosis who became ill again and developed a diarrhea which was thought to be due to a tuberculous ileitis. But I drew from her the admission that her troubles started when the letters from her soldier husband became fewer and fewer. Then came one saying that he was so tired of having an invalid for a wife that he was never coming back to her and was taking up with another woman.

Every so often a patient needs to have explained to him just what the physician plans to do, why he wants to do it, and why rest or an operation is likely to work a cure. He should know why the doctors want him to submit to an intrapleural injection of air, or why they want to perform thoracoplasty or lobectomy. Such explanations may have to be given more than once because when talked to, the patient may be too upset to take in much of what is said.

The director of a sanatorium must struggle to keep up the morale, not only of the patients, but also of the assistants and nurses in the institution. Those who come in contact with the sick should have a feeling of devotion to their work and a realization of its great value.

A good book to be put into the hands of the tuberculous is that of Dr. E. W. Hayes, *Tuberculosis as It Comes and Goes.* He could write better on the subject because he had had the disease himself. One of the chapters is written by a patient who tells of the emotions of a man when he first discovers that his lungs are diseased.

The fine specialist in tuberculosis needs to become much of a philosopher and a physician to the soul as well as the lung, one who can keep up the morale and strengthen the patient's will to carry on and to live. When hemorrhages and setbacks come the patient can greatly profit by his help. Often Gerald Webb used to help his patients even by directing their reading and finding stimulating books for them.

The dislike some patients have for admitting they have tuberculosis. There are some persons who need to be talked to about their great reluctance to admit ever having had tuberculosis. Fortunately, matters have greatly improved in the last thirty-five years. Long ago, I knew patients who would as soon admit that they had syphilis as that they had had tuberculosis. Sometimes an overly sensitive person of this type can be induced to take the plunge and get the thing over with. If the doctor can get him to tell his friends that he has been to a sanatorium (they probably all know it anyhow) the constant strain of concealment will be over.

The fear of contagion. In some cases one of the psychologic hazards of patients is their constant fear of giving the disease to loved ones. When a person has had, to begin with, minimal changes in the lungs, and later a fine arrest, with no more cough or sputum, a negative culture for tubercle bacilli in the morning gastric contents, feelings of good health and energy, a low blood sedimentation rate, and never any fever, the physician should reassure him in no uncertain terms, and should try to get him to live a normal life, without fear.

On warning the tuberculous young woman against marriage and childbearing. The physician sometimes has the unpleasant duty of warning a young tuberculous woman about the dangers she runs if she marries and tries to have a child, especially before she has a very definite arrest of the disease. She must be told how great the dangers are. In some cases, if marriage is entered into, it might be well to have the girl's tubes tied.

The question of rehabilitation. Naturally, when the patient leaves the sanatorium and goes out to face life again and the problems of earning a living, he may need help and advice as to what sort of work he can attempt.

PSYCHOSOMATIC ASPECTS OF HYPERTENSION

There is no doubt that at times and in some cases mental strain and strong emotion have something to do with hypertension. I have known hypertensives whose blood pressure shot up 50 mm. or so when they got angry. I remember a widow whose blood pressure used to shoot up from about 160 mm. to 240 mm. whenever she had a stormy interview with her good-for-nothing son who was always trying to break into the trust fund which his father had set up for him.

Although for thirty-eight years I have been teaching the importance of strong emotion in the causation of hypertension, I have little sympathy with the recent efforts of several men to ascribe the syndrome to certain traits and resentments and mental characteristics. I think a man without wide clinical experience and much knowledge of human types can easily overwork the idea. My impression is that the most important factor in the production of hypertension is a hereditary predisposition. Without this, a man can live a most strenuous life with plenty of worry and resentment but no hypertension. With a certain inborn predisposition, worry can bring a peptic ulcer, or with other predispositions it can bring migraine or asthma or giant urticaria. It would seem that in each case there must have been some genes present to determine which disease the individual could fret himself into.

Of late it has become popular in psychiatric circles to describe a certain constitution as characteristic for patients with peptic ulcer or hypertension, but I doubt if this can yet be done. I doubt if the temperaments found in a number of highly neurotic displaced persons seen in a free clinic in New York will be found in a group of husky executives in Detroit, or in a group of Swedish farmers in Minnesota, or Southerners in Mississippi, or of Italians or Japanese or Chinese in California. It will be interesting to see if the psychiatrists who are now analyzing a few hypertensives here and there ever agree on a type, and if this type is different from the supposed ulcer-bearing type.

One reason I cannot accept freely the types proposed by psychiatrists or the ideas of resentment or inferiority that they talk about is the fact, apparently not yet known to them, that commonly one can find any amount of decided hypertension in children, long before they have come up against the strains of life in the market place.

Another reason I have for doubting if psychic strain is the main cause of hypertension is that I have known so many hypertensives who had an easy happy life and perfect health until perhaps their late fifties, when cerebral or cardiac arteriosclerosis began to pull them down. It would seem that if they had long been torn by animosities or fears, they should have shown it in other ways besides the development of hypertension. Certainly I have known intimately a number of hypertensives who were unusually competent, well-adjusted, friendly, and easy-going persons, without any signs of resentments or inadequacies.

Binger and his associates wrote a book on the personality of a number of persons with hypertension. They found as outstanding elements in the character of these individuals exaggerated dependent strivings, submissiveness coupled with stubbornness, feelings of weakness and defenselessness, suppression of hostility, fear of injury, and emotional detachment. There seemed to be an inefficiency of the patterns of defense against anxiety, and a weakness of the repressive mechanisms. There was also a restricted social life, inhibited sexual development, and a tendency to failure of heterosexual adjustment. Very wisely, Binger and his associates did not conclude that all hypertensives are like this. If they had, I would have enjoyed showing them a number of two-fisted, hard-driving business executives and self-made millionaires, old hypertensive patients of mine, who were anything but fearful, repressed, or inhibited. One of these men for years dominated one of the toughest unions on the San Francisco waterfront, and another fought his way up from being a stevedore to being the owner of many ships.

Harold Wolff concluded that the person with essential hypertension has a personality which is the resultant of divergent drives: He is a tense person, poised and calm; one who has all the reins in his fingers, but who finds that the task requires constant alertness and readiness to spring into offense. Evidently all such studies can have little value until they are made on much larger samples drawn from the several racial groups in this country and in other parts of the world.

Probably all the physician needs to know about the psychosomatics of hypertension is that if a patient with type II or a dangerous type III hypertension wants to go all out to help himself he should quit the strenuous life and either retire or seek an easier and quieter employment. Perhaps the patient will then say to his physician, as Clark Gable did in a recent movie, "You mean that I can live if I cease living!" This sums up the situation perfectly, and I sympathize with the man who prefers to go on living as he has always lived. I suspect he has much on his side of the argument.

Treatment. When a man comes in much upset over the discovery of a hypertension, and especially when it has been making his heart somewhat irritable, often all one has to do to make him happy is to tell him that there are four types of hypertension with different degrees of severity and danger to life. He may be fortunate enough to have type I, which may never bother him, and may not even shorten his life. One can tell him of some of the many men and women who have lived comfortably for forty or fifty years with a hypertension grade I or II. I often tell of the man whom I have been watching now for twelve years with a systolic blood pressure of 220 mm. of mercury. As yet, he hasn't developed any symptoms! In women, hypertension grade I or II, even when the systolic pressure is over 200 mm., commonly is symptomless, and without much menace for the patient's future.

I have little faith in the drugs that are used to lower blood pressure. Potassium thiocyanate appears to be the most effective of the lot, but it is toxic, and a number of persons have died because of its use. Some died even when the concentration of the drug in the blood appeared to be within safe limits. There is no evidence that its use lengthens life. I do not like the use of phenobarbital because it tends to dull the person.

Lumbar sympathectomy seldom does much good when performed after the age of forty years, and at the Mayo Clinic it is only a rare hypertensive who is permitted to have this operation after the age of fifty years. It probably should not be performed unless it has been found that with bed rest and the giving of barbiturates or tetra-ethyl ammonium chloride the pressure can be decidedly lowered. Even then the operation may do but little good.

Peet and Isberg wrote that there is no good evidence that splanchnicec- tomy beneficially alters the course of hypertension or prolongs the lives of patients with hypertensive cerebrovascular disease. It is hard to tell how much the operation does in the way of lengthening life. Smithwick thought he had proved that his operation decidedly lengthens life, but clinicians working with the same material were not so optimistic. The men at the Mayo Clinic have little faith in their ability to help the patient with the malignant type of hypertension, and this is sad, because he is the man who most needs help.

PSYCHOGENIC RHEUMATISM, OR ACHING OF PSYCHIC ORIGIN

It is said that Paulus Aegineta remarked some 1,300 years ago that sorrow, care, or passion could bring on a bad attack of arthritis. I re- member a woman of fifty, previously healthy, who within twenty-four hours after her husband's death became crippled by arthritis. Another woman I saw developed severe arthritis when her daughter contracted an unfortunate marriage. Doctor Cecil has said that when one of his arthritic patients returns with a flare-up, his first question is, "What happened to upset you?" In 1932 Millard Smith noted that in fifty-two of 102 cases of arthritis the disease flared up after "a depleting and unbalancing ex- perience." Many backaches in nervous women appear to be equivalents of fatigue, and the soreness of many a stiff neck is due to muscular tension. In fact, the back of the neck appears to be a region particularly vulner- able to nervous tension. Psychiatrists have noticed that severe backache may be one of the first signs of a depression.

In 1946 Hench and Boland published a fine study of the many soldiers whom they saw during World War II with what was thought at first to be arthritis but which proved after observation to be only a neurosis. These authors stated that psychogenic rheumatism, or the musculoskeletal expression of a tension state, or a psychoneurosis, is one of the commonest causes of generalized or localized aches and pains in the muscles and joints. It may exist alone or it may be combined with fibrositis. Hench and Boland felt that a good term would be "psychoneurosis manifested by musculoskeletal discomforts."

Some 20 per cent of the soldiers sent to the center in Hot Springs, Arkansas for the study of arthritis showed no sign of arthritis. Their aches appeared to be psychic in origin. The main problem of the phy- sicians in charge was usually to rule out fibrositis. Fibrositis responds to changes in the external environment, such as those that go with an approaching storm. Sitting or lying down for a while makes fibrositis worse, and getting up and walking around makes it better. Psychogenic rheumatism is not influenced in these ways. It is influenced more by the patient's feelings of satisfaction or depression, excitement, mental distraction, worry, or feelings of fatigue.

In Army practice it helped the doctor to note that the arthritic soldier was usually docile, quiet, and well behaved, while the man with psychogenic rheumatism was often troublesome and inclined to behave like the neuropath that he was. He complained at great length about everything, and he wanted to take up a lot of the physician's time. Hench and Boland always suspected the presence of a psychogenic rheumatism whenever the pain or ache had been constant, day and night, over the course of years. I, too, have been much impressed by the diagnostic value of this fact, when obtained during history taking. Fibrositic aches come and go.

Often it was helpful to note that the person with psychogenic rheumatism had other nervous symptoms in other parts of the body: symptoms such as numbnesses, tinglings, or burnings, or feelings of weakness, or general fatigue. Such fatigue is worst in the morning. Rest does not help it, except in those cases in which the person, usually a frail woman, feels better when off her feet. Sometimes in cases of psychogenic rheumatism the patient showed symptoms suggestive of hysteria, and this fact was helpful in making the diagnosis.

In cases of psychogenic rheumatism it is significant that it does not help to apply heat or to give massage or to prescribe aspirin. Often the patient says nothing helps.

DIABETES AND EMOTION

Because Cannon showed that emotion can increase the amount of sugar in the blood of animals and man and can sometimes even cause sugar to appear in the urine, it would not be surprising if sometimes the course of diabetes were to be influenced adversely by fright or painful emotion. According to Cushing, Smillie found sugar in the urine of five of fourteen students taking an examination.

It is hard to see why painful emotion, especially if of short duration, should produce lasting diabetes, but clinicians of experience can remember cases in which a severe diabetes appeared immediately after a nervous shock. I remember a previously healthy woman who got a severe and permanent diabetes when she learned of her husband's infidelity. Much evidence, however, makes it probable that such happenings are "purely coincidental."

G. E. Daniels, in 1936-1937, gathered case reports to show that fright or psychic strain can produce diabetes, but later, in 1939, after much study of the literature, he came to doubt his first conclusions. William

Menninger found a close association between emotion and diabetes in only two of ninety-three cases. Weiss and English discussed the subject at some length, and concluded that much against the idea of an association is the fact that the great strain of war did not appear to produce diabetes. Joslin thought he could rule out a psychic causation for diabetes. Highly significant is the fact that during World War I he could find only two cases of diabetes in a hospital center through which 40,000 soldiers passed.

The psychic problems of the diabetic. Naturally, it is a shock for a man or woman to discover the presence of a severe diabetes, but obviously there is only one thing to do and that is to settle down and learn to handle the disease well. The young diabetic can now be cheered with Joslin's statement that today some diabetics are exceeding the life expectation of nondiabetics. The diabetic does not always have to die early from atherosclerosis.

SOME PSYCHIC PROBLEMS IN ANESTHESIOLOGY

Fifty years ago, when I used to give anesthetics for my father in his country practice I decided I never again wanted to have anything to do with a man who said he was going to die on the table; usually he all but fulfilled his promise.

I have known a number of persons whose death on the table seemed to me to have been due to fear of the operation. Before going under, the patient had been abnormally apprehensive and perhaps desirous of backing out. In most cases the death came with the first few whiffs of the anesthetic, and in a few it came just before the anesthetic was started!

When one sees a few such cases one feels all the more that the wise anesthetist and surgeon should do everything possible to cut down on preoperative fright. In the worst cases it would be well if the patient could be anesthetized in his room, perhaps while he was still woozy from a barbiturate. Today he often has to go through the surgical department, usually without his wife or someone who could help him keep up his courage. Then he may have to wait an hour or two. After that he is ushered into the operating room where he may see many frightening sights. Then he is strapped down on the table. This strapping alone is very frightening to many persons. It may be almost unbearable for a man or woman subject to claustrophobia. Recently I talked to a surgeon who, when he had to be operated on, absolutely refused to be strapped down. Fortunately, today, anesthesia is often started with pentothal sodium which spares the patient the fright of having a mask clamped on his face or of having to breathe a strange gas.

The anesthetist and the surgeon should always be well apprised of the fact when a particular patient is much afraid of the operation and fearful of dying under the anesthetic. Oftentimes this fear is due to the fact that a relative or friend died in this way. I remember a very nervous and apprehensive physician who had to have a colostomy made. He kept telling me that he expected, after the operation, to balloon with gas and die. Immediately after he returned to his room, his pulse shot up to 130, and it stayed that way until three days later when he died. Necropsy showed nothing to explain the death, and hence I have always suspected that it was due purely to fright.

I think that fifty years from now a visitor to operating rooms will find many precautions being taken to protect the patient from alarm and fear and bad impressions. Perhaps some of the old ideas of Crile in regard to anesthetizing the patient unknowingly in his room will be brought back and used.

For many persons, a spinal anesthetic is a very distressing experience and perhaps in the cases of very sensitive persons the introduction of the needle should be started only after the patient has had a little sodium pentothal.

Many highly sensitive and nervous persons, when told that their short operation can easily be done under a local or block anesthesia, will beg to be "put out completely." And they are right. The strain of lying there, knowing what is going on and expecting any moment to feel a terrible jab of pain, is very hard on some persons, and I have seen some cases in which the ordeal was followed by a nervous breakdown. In many such cases, sodium pentothal is the ideal anesthetic.

One thing the anesthetist should often do is to assure the worried patient that he will not feel a thing. Many persons have a great dread of being conscious of pain but unable to move or cry out. They must be assured that this will not happen.

CHAPTER 24

*Psychosomatic Problems
of the Child*

THE SUBJECT OF PSYCHOLOGY in pediatrics is so enormous that no one could do justice to it in a chapter; one finds it hard to know what to put in and what to leave out.

Every good pediatrician must, to a large extent, be a psychiatrist because not only are many of his little patients full of nervous and mental problems; but commonly they are being spoiled and upset by childish, foolish, quarreling, undisciplined, or psychopathic parents. Several persons in the family may then be in need of psychiatric advice, and unless the doctor can somewhat reform the parents he cannot help the child.

Obviously, the busy pediatrician cannot always stop to spend the time he would like to spend on such work, and sometimes, in the worst cases, he must try to get the parents and the child into the hands of an expert on child guidance. Sometimes the best thing he can do is to induce the parents to read some helpful books on the handling of children. The all-essential point in many cases is that the physician recognize quickly that the symptoms of his little patient are nervous in origin and due to a bad situation at home.

Every pediatrician should be a philosopher and an understanding wise counselor. So often he must warn parents that their behavior is wrecking the nerves and the health of their children. Often he must talk to them as once the prophets of Israel talked to their people. Like Nathan before David, he must say, "Thou art the man" (II Samuel 12:7); in other words, "It is you who are at fault."

Often, he must face seriously the problems of a child who is behaving badly and perhaps psychotically or criminally; perhaps the youngster is late in getting over bed wetting, or he is stuttering, or having tantrums, or not developing mentally, or is having serious conflicts with his teachers at school.

As Clifford Sweet has said so truly, "All in medicine who are worthy of their calling must have an interest in their patients which goes beyond the mere use of technical skill and the material rewards therefore, but the pediatrician must have genuine emotional, I might say spiritual, attachment to children—a concern for their welfare which will always cause him to accept generously as a considerable part of his rewards the consciousness that he has contributed to life at its beginning."

Children show certain characteristics from infancy. Anyone who knows anything about children knows that from the first month of life they are individual and different. Some are good, pleasant, lovable, affectionate, and easily handled. They need little correction or admonition, and they respond quickly and well to what they are told. They fit happily and easily into the family circle, and they show no unpleasant or vicious traits. They walk and talk on time, and they stop wetting the bed when they should. Later they become good students at school, liked by their teachers and their schoolmates.

Other children give trouble from the start. Gessell says they can be recognized at eight weeks. They may show great determination to dominate and run the mother, and early they may learn some trick, such as that of breath holding that frightens her into subjection. Every so often a child will have a tantrum and perhaps strike the mother or bang his head on the floor. At times he will be rebellious, disobedient, belligerent, unamenable to discipline, sullen, highly destructive, or cruel to any kitten or puppy that gets into his clutches. A little later he may be attacking his playmates, stealing, lying, and throwing stones through the school windows. He may be insolent and incorrigible, and later he may join the worst gang in the neighborhood.

In between these two groups of children are others who are acting badly, mainly because of the association with stupid parents or ones who are such poor disciplinarians that they are incapable of gaining the respect or liking of the child or of giving him any sense of security. It would be an unusual child who could grow up happily or normally in the company of some persons. I can think of persons who are too rigid in their ways, or who show no affection, or who are too quick to punish and to punish severely.

The need for good training of children. There is a tendency in many quarters today to let children do as they please, never curbing them or demanding obedience or courtesy to others. To me this course has always seemed very foolish; it fails to help the child in learning to live easily and comfortably and happily in this world; it commonly tends to make a little pest of the child; it adds greatly to the parents' strain in living with him, and it adds much to the strain the child experiences in living with himself and others. I have no use for this new practice of letting children grow up as they please; I am sure it is wrong.

As I look about I see that the most important lesson everyone, young and old, has to learn in this world is how to get along comfortably and happily with his fellows. For many a person this is a hard thing to do, and for some the lesson seems unlearnable. It is so difficult for many to outgrow the original tendency of the little child to grab all the toys in sight, including those of a guest, and then to slap the guest when he tries to get back a toy or two. It is hard for some to learn, also, to overcome the early childish reluctance to see the guest get a little of the ice cream, or, later in life, to see the guest win an occasional game of some kind. It is hard to learn to stick to the rules and not to insist that these be changed when one is losing. It is hard for a child to learn not to set up a howl for mother when a little hurt is sustained or when he is being worsted in some contest.

Since a child must learn these lessons some day, if he is not eventually to be disliked and shunned as a pest and a boor, I think he ought to be helped to learn them early. I think the parent who does not quickly train his child to be a gentleman is derelict in his duty *to the child;* he is being most unkind to him. Why should he want to run any chances of bringing his child up to be a selfish "stinker," without courtesy, and without respect for the rights and feelings of others? Why not raise him to be a likable child with nice manners; why not, with good manners, make his path through life easy? Surely the young man or woman with lovely manners has a tremendous advantage in this world and is much more likely to be happy. One advantage of a child's learning at home to be polite and thoughtful is that later, when he grows up, his good manners will be part of his nature—they will never seem to have been put on for the occasion.

Why not teach him in the first few years of life to so respect the rights and personality of others that when he marries he will keep the love of his wife and make her happy? Why not teach him to be such a square shooter that some day he will be respected and well liked on the athletic field, and later, he will be a fine respected executive in some business? Why not so bring him up that he will never be trying to grab what does not belong to him?

So often, when I have gone into a home, I have marveled at the lack of thought the parents were taking for the future of their youngsters. The mother would give a command to a child and then show no concern when all he or she did was to look at her contemptuously. Perhaps at dinner a child in his high chair kept kicking the underside of the dining table and jangling the nerves of the guests. The mother, for a time, ignored it, perhaps feeling that the child had a right to do this, a right which must not be denied him; but finally she said, "Don't do that." The child, sizing her up shrewdly out of the corner of his eye, just went on kicking. Then the woman either threatened, stupidly and futilely, perhaps to call a policeman, or to send the child out in the street alone to be an orphan, or she did nothing and let her guests suffer.

How much more fun it is for a guest to go into a home where the children are a joy, where they are friendly, well behaved, respectful of their elders and considerate of their comfort. When I see such children I think of an excellent proverb that is often heard in southeastern Europe, "Better that early a little bottom be spanked than that later a big back be flogged." Or, I think of a great headmaster who, patting his German shepherd dog, said, "If I had let Judy run wild and do as she damn well pleased as a pup, she'd be a vicious, savage beast today. You can't develop leaders by letting them do as they damn please when they're boys. If nothing else, we're training boys here at the school to be less obnoxious."

Children need training and they need discipline, but naturally the discipline should not be too strict or tyrannical or *meddlesome,* and it should never be vindictive or cruel. Instead of commanding, the parent can always request a service politely, much as he would do with an adult, but then the child should be trained almost in infancy to honor these requests quickly. The requests will be few, but early in the child's life the parent will see to it that the habit is acquired of complying quickly with them.

As soon as the child can understand and reason it should be made clear to him that most of the things he is asked to do are much more for his own training and his own good than for the parent's convenience. He should also be given the idea that it can be a joy to help his parents and to be useful in the home, a real member of the family.

If a child is not taught obedience and respect for his elders at home, he is likely to be a hellion at school, and that will not help his progress there.

So far as possible children should be treated as adults, and with the same courtesy. Obviously, this will be done only in homes in which the parents are well bred, courteous, and self-controlled. It will not be done where the parents are violent, quarrelsome, psychopathic, or alcoholic.

Parents so reduce the strain on themselves when they teach prompt obedience. I often think how much strain and trouble and wasted time mothers could save themselves if, especially in the early years of their child's life, they were to teach quick obedience. For instance, a devoted and too complaisant young mother may be having a terrible time because, when called at lunch time, her boy will not come in from play. When he finally does arrive he wants to be cajoled for half an hour before he will eat. Perhaps, then, one day his grand-mother arrives to take over while the mother goes to the hospital to await the arrival of another baby. The first noon, when the grandmother calls the boy for luncheon and he does not come, she says, "All right, if you do not come you will get no food until supper time."

Accustomed to his mother's futile threats, the boy goes on playing. Finally, an hour later, when he does come in, he finds that the dishes are washed and put away and he must wait until supper for his food. He cries and wheedles, but grandmother will not be drawn into any argument; she is sorry, but adamant. Next day, when the boy is called for luncheon he comes running. Thus, in one day, the grandmother has made a change which, in the next two weeks, will save her endless trouble. What is more, the boy, respecting her as a strong character, will now behave much better with her than he did with his mother. He did not think much of the mother because she was weak and he could run her. Now he tries to "shine up to" the grandmother and to in-gratiate himself with her.

To my way of thinking, one of the greatest stupidities of parents is their constant threatening of punishments which they rarely administer. They just keep calling "wolf," until the child is contemptuous of their futility. Another miserable trait of mothers is to threaten long-winded and complicated punishments which they would not have the heart or the time or energy to carry out. The punishment would be too great a nuisance; when a child disobeys or defies a parent the matter should be settled immediately.

Discipline makes it easier on the child's nerves. Too few people realize that good discipline saves wear and tear on the child's nervous system. It relieves him of a lot of needless fussing and wheedling and arguing. It gives him a sense of security; he knows what to expect and when to expect it. Less is left to his indecision and his whims. With many parents the child never knows that to expect. One minute he gets too rigid a discipline and the next too great an indulgence, and so he never knows where he stands.

On avoiding head-on conflicts with children. As Spock (1945,

1946) has said so wisely, parents should not keep asking a child if he would *like* to go to bed or would *like* to have a bath or would *like* to have his supper. They should simply say it is time now for supper or a bath or going to bed. Often when a child does not want to do something like going to bed, resistance can easily be overcome, not by a head-on collision and the exertion of authority, but by a game. A doll may have to be bathed or put to bed, or the child may be enticed into a race with the mother or another child to see who can get upstairs and into bed first.

Small children are fortunate when they are put to bed early. They get needed rest, as does the mother. She also gets a chance to visit with her husband as she used to do before the children came. Next day she is a better mother for this rest.

So often the wise mother can avoid a conflict of authority simply by waiting a bit or by being playful. Children so love play that it is hard for them to stay in a bad humor when the mother is full of fun. Thus, if a mother must get a sickly undernourished child to eat when it prefers not to, she can usually induce him to get down a bowl of mush by playing a game. Perhaps little dabs of jelly are put here and there on the mush and these are undermined, or the picture on the bottom of the dish is uncovered with much interest, or two children see which one can finish his food first in order to uncover the bottom of the dish.

It would be so helpful if only mothers would learn not to "start something" unless it is very important So often they say "Come here" to a child who is intent on some job or game. A wiser or even a more courteous woman would have left the child alone until he had finished. It is very important, however, that once the mother has made a reasonable request she should see to it that the child complies immediately. It is very bad to let the child get away with disobedience, especially of the contemptuous type. The wise parent, of course, will not pick a time for a conflict of wills late in the day when the child is tired, irritable, sleepy, or spoiling for a fight.

The need for recognizing the fact that curiosity and great activity are highly desirable in a child and never punishable. One of the great sorrows of childhood comes from the fact that most mothers do not seem to know that the healthier a child is and the more intelligent and likely to succeed in this world, the more active he is, and the more likely to get into everything so as to examine it and perhaps pull it apart.

How wonderful it is when a mother sees that such curiosity is not naughtiness and that it should not be punished or even reprimanded. So commonly, when a mother comes into my office with a boy of six and he starts exploring the room as any normal child should, she starts saying, "Don't go near that" and "Don't touch that." I always say, "No, let us be very grateful that he is curious and eager to explore. It would be such a tragedy if he were apathetic or too stupid to look about him. No, let him explore all he likes. He is not a 'bad' child; he is a good child. Let us thank God that he is so venturesome that he is likely to get into things."

Dr. Gibbons, my wise old professor of pediatrics, used to tell fussy mothers that the only perfectly behaved, quiet, unexploring, never-dirty-or-rowdy Lord Fauntleroy little boys hat he had ever seen were tuberculous! If only mothers could learn that, and keep thinking of it every day, they and their children could be so much happier. If wise, a mother would have a lot of toys in the house of the type that the child can take apart and put together again. He could then work off his energies on them.

The wise mother is not always saying "Don't." As the child grows older and wants to go on Scout trips or to picnics the wise mother should not always be saying, "No, you can't go," simply because she would worry if he went. Under such circumstances, to say "Yes" can save her much time and strain, because when she says "No" the child, to get his way, has to wheedle and wheedle until eventually she becomes worn down, and perhaps has to give in. This is bad also, because later, when for some good reason a request *must* be refused, the child will keep begging and fussing for hours. If all reasonable requests were granted immediately, then, "Noes" would be accepted without much, if any, question, and the child and parent would be saved much wrangling and ill feeling.

As Clifford Sweet has said, if we train a girl to get what she wants by being a pest or having a tantrum, why should we be surprised if, later in adult life, we find her controlling her husband or her family with exactly this technic?

On the need for lavishing love. One big secret in the handling of children is to lavish love on them so that they will always feel secure and never have to worry as to whether they "belong." The things that they make should be admired and, whenever possible, they should be praised for being helpful. The normal child dearly loves to be helpful and to have some small part in a family enterprise. His help should be welcomed and appreciated even when he gets in the way.

One of the saddest features of human life is that so many persons have never had the feeling that they belonged, either in the home, the school, or the company in which they worked. No one ever told them that they were liked or looked on as a valued member of the group. The loving parent need not be an overindulgent one who does nothing but give, give, give. He or she will let the child have the joy of taking some responsibility and doing some kindnesses, too. One of the thrilling events of my life came on my sixty-fifth birthday when I received, from a loving seven-year-old grandson, 50 cents with which to go to the dime store and get myself a present. With great effort and much thought, he had saved the money for me in his little piggy-bank!

Incidentally, it is good for a child to be allowed to earn a little money. It teaches him the value of it. Early in life he should be allowed to go to the store to spend what he has earned and saved, without any advice or admonition.

The most stupid thing a parent can do is to threaten a child with being sent away or turned over to a policeman. Moodie (1940) states in his fine book that some of the worst behavior of children appears to be due to their frantic fear that they may lose one or both parents or their home.

On the wise child who, as he grows up, learns the wisdom of conforming. One hope many troubled parents can cling to when they are having trouble with a willful or difficult and perhaps only child is that, if he has a high I.Q. and is sane, he will probably reform as he grows older and sees that the selfish and discourteous behavior which he gets away with at home brings only contempt, dislike, disapproval, ostracism, or a beating-up in the school yard. Because of this, many a spoiled brat grows up into a fine man. A few summers in a good camp will often straighten out Mom's badly spoiled pet. In camp he so craves the approval of his teachers and "the gang" that he quickly learns to be "a good fellow." If he does not show any desire to gain the approval of the group, the outlook for his future is bad. Then an expert on child behavior should be called in to see if the youngster is headed for a psychosis.

The dangers of too much coddling. Many children, and especially only children, are hurt by too much coddling. They never are allowed to learn self-reliance. Perhaps, also, they get the idea that they must always hold the spotlight at home. The minute they lose it, as when someone comes in to visit, there is likely to be a tantrum or feigned illness or an attack of pseudostuttering.

The teaching of some stoicism. I know a home in which the boys and the girls were brought up in the same way. When, in their early years, one of them fell and skinned a knee and cried, he or she was first comforted and kissed, and then, if there was too prolonged a wailing with an appeal for sympathy, he or she was told to stop: that that was enough crying for that particular amount of pain. As a result, today, thirty years later, the girls in this family, when subjected to pain or illness, behave with the same stoicism and self-control as would be shown by their brothers, if similarly afflicted. Such stoicism would be a wonderful thing for many of the whiney women whom we physicians see every month.

Transference of parental anxieties to the child. Many children are made overly anxious because their parents are so alarmed over every little ailment and mishap. The parents are chronic worriers: dreaders of infection, or drafts, and of many foods, and if they do not look out, they will train their children to be like themselves. When a child in such a family is ill he may get worse because he sees the parents are almost out of their minds with anxiety. The physician who is called may also say unwise and alarming things, such as, "We'll have to watch that heart" or "He may never be able to run or swim." The child is not supposed to note such things, but he does, and oftentimes it does him harm for the rest of his life. As I tell some parents, "If some foundation were paying you to perform an experiment to see if you could turn a normal child into a hypochondriac, you could not be going at the project with more skill or pertinacity."

It is an unfortunate child who is early given the idea that health is a precarious thing. He is taught that he must always be taking tonics or vitamins, and that to avoid blood poisoning every least scratch must be quickly daubed with some disinfectant.

The child in an unhappy home. It is hard on a child to have to live in a home where the father does not provide enough food or comfort, or where there is constant fighting, or where one parent is psychopathic or alcoholic or cruel or overly rigid or religious. Occasionally, it may seem to the physician that a divorce would be a lesser evil than having the child brought up in a home where there is constant quarreling and even physical violence.

Oftentimes the neurosis of a child is made worse by the jeering and persecution of older brothers or sisters. One day a quiet reserved woman explained that she had had six brothers who jeered at her ideas until, like a turtle, she retired into a shell; to avoid criticism she said little. Many a patient has told me of great cruelties, mental and physical, inflicted for years by an older and decidedly sadistic brother or sister who, perhaps, kept saying, "You are so ugly and unattractive you will never get a beau or hold a husband."

It is terrible, also, when a child hears often that he was not wanted and not welcomed when he came into the world as "un petit accident." Many a patient has told me that he had often heard his mother telling how distressed she was when she found herself pregnant with him, or how disgusted she was when she found he wasn't a girl. As a result, he never felt he "belonged." He was always lonely and unhappy.

The child who fears the parents will get divorced. Occasionally one sees a schoolgirl who is much upset because she fears her parents are going to get a divorce and break up the home. Thus, I remember a plumpish, pretty girl who, within a few months, while at boarding school, lost 40 pounds in weight. When no physical cause could be found for this by the several physicians who examined her at the school, she was sent to the Mayo Clinic. We soon drew from her the story that her illness started when she became much distressed over the news that the mother and father were contemplating a separation. When, for the child's sake, the parents decided to call off this plan, the girl promptly recovered. A little later I saw another girl with the same story. Another girl got nocturnal attacks of asthma when she feared that her father and the mother whom she adored might get divorced.

The lesson to be learned from all this is that when children fall ill with curious syndromes it is well sometimes to find out if their sense of security has been knocked out from under them.

The dangers of too much religion. As I noted in Chapter 14 one of the great trials of childhood comes from over-religiousness in the parents. It never occurs to many good people that a healthy, normal child cannot possibly enjoy sitting still in church three or four times on Sunday, and he cannot possibly be interested in the average sermon on the fine points of sectarian dogma, or on the cleansing of souls by "the blood of the Lamb." It is curious that most adults cannot remember what they liked and did not like when they were children. Many misguided parents try to scare a child into being good. It is doubtful if this technic ever works well, and the process certainly can do great harm.

Many children today are rebellious because the parents are too strict with them and keep trying to bring them up according to the mores of fifty years ago. In countless homes children keep saying, "But, Mother, they don't do that any more!"

The "difficult child" who is hard to manage. In a series of 1,000 consecutive cases of children seen in the former Institute for Child Guidance in New York City, the following difficulties were listed in order of frequency: negativism, temper and tantrums, lying, failure in school, nervousness, enuresis, fears, excessive fantasy and day-dreaming, stealing, disturbance of sleep, masturbation, truancy, finicky behavior about food, oversensitiveness, defects in speech, late thumb sucking, show-off behavior, excessive jealousy, timidity, sex activity, trouble in reading, bullying, and cruelty.

Many "bad children" doubtless are a bit psychopathic and are headed for trouble in later life with neuroses or minor psychoses.

The child who won't eat. Most children, at some time or other, worry their parents half to death by not wanting to eat. Usually the situation is made much worse by the parents' obvious anxiety and fussing and fretting. Often, if the mother would only leave the child alone and say nothing he would start eating again. He may be enjoying the fuss that is being made over him. If his behavior were to be ignored he would soon get hungry and then he would want to eat. Thus, one day, a mother who was anxious over her boy's unwillingness to eat, and who was always fussing at him, was called out of town. The father then paid no attention to the boy at the table, and perhaps as a result of this, he almost immediately started eating second and third helpings.

Convulsions in children. It is now strongly suspected that the fever convulsions of children are often equivalents of a convulsive disorder in some of their forebears. The physician will, of course, be particularly concerned about such convulsions when there is a history of epilepsy in the family. It may be helpful, then, to have an electroencephalogram made to see if dysrhythmia is present. Children sometimes suffer from an unrecognized petit mal. Much excitement will sometimes produce a convulsion in a highly sensitive child.

The backward child. The backward child should always be studied with care to find out what the trouble is, and if it can be remedied. The intelligence quotient should be estimated. A very bright child may refuse to study at school because he is so bored over the poor quality of the teaching. He may dislike the school and his teacher, and he may see that much of the teaching is stupid and useless. Some gifted children, when transferred to another school or another room where the teacher is wiser, more sympathetic, and more interesting, will immediately quiet down and go to work.

Occasionally a child who is thought to be backward is really only hard of hearing. Other children get into trouble at school because they are near-sighted and cannot see the blackboard. Some children have difficulty in reading because of a peculiarity of the brain. Others who are mentally retarded find the going so tough at school that they give up and quit trying. They need to be put with children of their own mental level so that they can compete with them on an equal footing.

The cretin should, of course, be recognized promptly. Sometimes the defective child should early be placed in an institution so as not to wreck the health and morale of the mother and perhaps the health of other children in the home. Parents need to be told that the dull or badly handicapped child will be more comfortable and happy among children of his own type.

Parents should be made to see that if a child is backward it is cruel and utterly stupid to punish him or to try to shame him into working harder. He cannot do better. If a child has an I.Q. below 70 he is mentally defective. In school some children with a low intelligence will get by well enough because of an ability to memorize their lessons.

In studying what is wrong with a backward child it may help to measure separately the several faculties of memory, reasoning, judgment, and ability in language. It is said that a marked scatter in the values obtained with these four tests should suggest the beginnings of some mental disorder.

The late bed wetters. Parents can begin to worry about a child's bed wetting if he keeps it up past the age of three or four years. It is well known that bed wetting runs in families. According to McGuinness from 30 to 40 per cent of bed wetters have bed-wetting forebears. As I was writing this, I saw three sisters who wet the bed until the ages of sixteen, seventeen, and nineteen, respectively. There was much psychosis and feeblemindedness in their ancestry. It would seem evident, then, that not all of the trouble is due to feelings of resentment against the mother, such as are now being talked about by analysts. It seems more probable that these children have inherited some difficulty in developing in the nervous system those reflexes which control the bladder during deep sleep.

Most of the writers who have studied enuresis agree that the parents should not be unkind to the unfortunate child; they should not punish him for having a wet bed, and they should not concentrate all his attention on this one problem by offering big rewards for a good night.

Occasionally the taking of a child out of the home for a while will stop the habit. If put with other children in a hospital the child may make a big effort to merit their approval. Sweet (1946) thought that enuresis must be treated by the education of both the parents and the child. It interested him to note that in both sexes the practice is often discontinued just before marriage. This would suggest that it might have been discontinued some time before.

Levine (1943) found that most of a group of enuretic Navy recruits had suffered from somnambulism, bad nightmares, and nervousness. They were usually immature, maladjusted, emotionally unstable, and insecure. Usually there was much psychopathy in the family. According to Michaels the enuretic often shows an abnormal electroencephalogram. Others have shown an abnormal cystometrogram and a too violent reaction to distention of the bladder. For the best hints as to treatment, see The Practitioner, 1950.

Masturbation. Now that the researches of Kinsey and his associates have shown that almost 100 per cent of boys masturbate at some time, and that the usual prohibitions of parents and church have no effect, it would seem best for parents not to get excited about this habit. No well-informed person today believes that masturbation a few times a week does any harm to mind or body. The child who masturbates several times a day is usually below par mentally to begin with.

Interest in sex. Parents get excited often because a small child shows an interest in sex. Perhaps a boy exposes his sister and examines her to see how different she is from him. Such innocent curiosity is so natural and harmless that one wonders why parents should get so concerned and alarmed over it.

The great importance of giving a child what he needs when he needs it. As a child becomes adolescent and aware of sex, the wise and kindly parent will do everything possible to help him or her to be socially attractive and well dressed. Dancing lessons should be provided because skill in this art is such a social asset. If teeth are ugly, or a nose has a big hump, or ears are sticking out, these defects should quickly be corrected, even if it takes most of the family savings.

As the boy or girl starts going out in the evening the parents must act in a trustful manner. They might as well, because if a child wants to get into mischief, he or she cannot be kept from it. Fussy mothers who demand that the children come home long before parties or dances break up should keep remembering that a youngster can get into just as much mischief before 10 P.M. as after that.

It is highly important that the parents find out what the present-day mores are, and then let the child conform to them, unless some of them seem too foolish and too wrong. This would put a stop to much wrangling at home and would lead to better relations between parent and child. Kindly and wise parents will, also, not only allow but encourage the children to give parties and dances in the home, and will suggest that at times they bring home a chum, perhaps to share a meal or stay for the night. It is much better that a boy's friends meet in his back yard where there is a handball wall, a basket-ball basket, or a little clubroom, than that he be out with a gang or hanging around a pool hall. It is wonderful for a boy to have at home plenty of "things to do with." I think it better often that a father buy such things for his children than that he put the money in the bank.

Especially when parents have a bright boy of the type who wants to build a radio set or fit out a little laboratory they should stay close enough to him so that they will always know what it is that he wants tremendously and could use to great advantage. Then they should get it for him if they can possibly do so. It will mean more to him then than anything can mean to him later, and it will be a splendid investment.

Truancy. The child who objects to going to school has some good reason for this, and immediately this reason should be ascertained and something done about it. Often a new school or a new teacher will work wonders.

Undescended testicles. The boy with undescended testicles should be operated on before his playmates have a chance to jeer at him and to turn him into a hermit and a misanthrope who hides his shame. In many cases a surgeon can bring the testicles down, anchoring them for a while to the fascia of the thigh, and then moving them into the scrotum.

The spastic child. The spastic child can be a terrible problem to himself and the family. The tragedy often is that he is bright. Many parents could be helped by reading the book by Doctor Carlson, a spastic himself. He called it *Born That Way;* Doctor and Mrs. Carlson now run two schools where spastic children are trained. With expert care they can be helped. As Mrs. Carlson once said to me, when afflicted children arrive at these schools they seem comforted to find that there are many others like them, suffering in the same way, and being helped.

The highly nervous child. The highly nervous child can usually be recognized at a glance. Often he is thin and frail looking, and he may be sniffing or making grimaces. He may suck his thumb late, and he may bite his nails. He may seem older than his years. He may show considerable anxiety, and he may be restless, and may find it hard to take a nap after luncheon. He is usually a poor sleeper and he may suffer from nightmares and night terrors. He may wet the bed late; he may get excited and frightened easily. He may be much afraid of thunder, or of the dark, or of dogs. He may be very subject to infections and may often be ill with a fever.

The psychotic child. It is known today that prodromes of schizophrenia and manic-depressive psychosis show up early in childhood, and it is well that such diseases be quickly recognized because, with good care, something may perhaps be done to help the situation. Certainly with bad care the child is likely to be doomed. The great problem is to differentiate ordinary nervousness, naughtiness, badly spoiled behavior, or frantic behavior due to feelings of insecurity, and the vicious or antisocial behavior of the psychopathic child.

Violence on the part of a child must always be looked on with anxiety because it may indicate a beginning psychosis. A violent child may be extremely active; he may suddenly strike out at people; he may become abusive, and he may have outbursts of temper. Without provocation he may strike his mother, or he may get down and bang his head on the floor. He may be much more than ordinarily destructive. He may walk in his sleep, he may wet the bed late, and he may be unmanageable at home and at school. He may be a liar and a thief, and if caught, he will either be sullen or he will show no concern over his predicament. Sometimes one can tell from a glance at the sullen or evil-looking child that he is mentally abnormal and probably headed for a life of crime. He may early run away from home. He is likely to be horribly cruel to any small animal that comes within his reach.

Some children have depressions which are recognizable. A schizophrenic child may seem, at first glance, to be unusually good, well behaved, and studious. But, as Jelliffe and Adolph Meyer have emphasized, these children are impractical; their minds seem to be turned inward and taken up with meditation. They may revolt against imposed regulations and requirements, and they may be subject to fits of abstraction when they become very irritable with the family. With strangers they may be unusually amiable, or they may be abnormally sensitive and suspicious. They have a love of abstractions and an aversion to tackling the daily jobs of life.

As Jelliffe said, one of these traits alone might not indicate much, but when a number of them are found together, the physician should become anxious. Another early sign of trouble is a tendency to solitariness. A boy with a beginning schizophrenia may like to take long walks by himself. Usually he is not much interested in other children, or in children of the opposite sex. A psychopathic child may not do well at school because he does not concentrate. His thoughts are off in the clouds. Some psychopathic children are overly fearful; they see ghosts and are terribly afraid of the dark.

The child who suffers from hysteria. There are quite a few children who suffer from hysteria, so many in fact, that the pediatrician must constantly be on the watch for them. They may become mute, or develop paralyses, or limps, or they may just take to their bed for a while. Seabrook tells in his book, *No Hiding Place,* how one day, as a boy, for no reason that he could see, he told his mother that he had a pain in his "stomach"; he went to bed and remained there for several weeks. It was the first of several fugues or flights from life which Seabrook was to have, until eventually he committed suicide.

The handicapped child. As Spock has pointed out, the most important thing in handling the handicapped child is that the parents treat him as if he were normal. They must try not to be self-conscious about defects, and they must not be so ashamed of him that they constantly keep hiding him from their friends. They must try never to add to his consciousness of his defect and his shame over it. There are many persons in this world who have succeeded eminently in spite of a decided physical handicap, and the child can be told about them.

Every parent of a handicapped child should read Mrs. Hathaway's remarkable book, *The Little Locksmith,* to see how her devoted parents, because of their New England reticence, failed to help her while her back was caving in and she was becoming a hunchback. They could not bring themselves to talk of it, so they said nothing, and she went on suffering the tortures of utter loneliness and a lack of information.

While being always loving with the defective child, the parents must not overprotect or overindulge him. They must not let him get away with rudeness to others, meanness, laziness, or an unwillingness to do his share of the chores about the house. Neither must they be too critical of him. Certainly they must not take out on him their disappointment in him. I have had many a physically handicapped man tell me that his father never made any effort to conceal from him and others the disappointment he felt over the sort of defective that had been assigned to him in the way of a son and heir.

Books that can help parents in handling their problems. Fortunately, many good books on child psychology have been written, and every young pediatrician should be reading and rereading some like those of Spock (1945, 1946), Moodie (1940), Aldrich and Aldrich (1938), and Weill (1940). Spock's book is splendid and full of homely wisdom, simply expressed. Every young mother should own a copy. It can now be obtained in a 25-cent edition. Such books can do much to help troubled parents and to save the time of the pediatrician.

Treatment. In trying to help children whose parents are at fault, the physician will have to be tactful in his criticisms and exhortations. Otherwise they will only feel hurt and inclined to turn against him. Sometimes it is well to write out instructions or advice because the people, while in the doctor's office, will be so upset that they will not remember what they are told; they will get things all mixed up, and they may become angry at the doctor because of things they thought he said or implied. In the worst cases one or the other parent may have to be helped by a psychiatrist. As Dr. Clifford Sweet has emphasized, sometimes a young father must be told of the great need for his spending some time with his children, for making friends with them, for playing with them, and for binding them to him with bonds of love and sympathy. Just providing for their food and physical comfort is not enough. If a man craves the love of his children he will have to earn it. As a fine pediatrician once said to me, "I so wanted the love of my children that I always, to a large extent, kept wooing them much as I kept wooing my wife."

It is highly significant that in a number of the child-guidance clinics the physicians in charge have wound up spending 95 per cent of their time trying to put sense into the parents. As a result, they spend only 5 per cent of their time on the children!

Part VI

Treatment

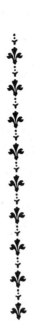

CHAPTER 25

The Tactful Handling
of the Nervous Patient

THERE IS GREAT NEED TODAY for much study of the art of handling nervous patients, so that when they get a diagnosis of a functional trouble they will not feel hurt, ashamed, outraged, let down, or somewhat cheated, and so that they will not just move on to find a new physician who will give them more tests and a diagnosis more to their liking.

In big clinics, where the internist is interested mainly in diagnosis, and where most patients leave for home after their examination, many are told little more than that there is nothing the matter with them, and then they are dismissed. This, of course, disappoints many, and often they have good reason to be puzzled and unhappy. *If the physician had only spent a little more time in explaining the situation he could have changed a disgruntled patient into a satisfied one.*

For instance, a pleasant intelligent man of sixty-nine years came in to say that in his youth he had contracted syphilis, and in the years that followed he had had much treatment. He wanted to know if he needed any more. A syphilologist, after finding a plus minus Kline, a 2 plus Kahn, a doubtful Hinton and a negative Wassermann, tested the spinal fluid and on finding this normal, told the man to "forget it," and showed him to the door. But the man remained puzzled and upset and did not want to leave. He came back to ask why, with a positive Kahn test, he should not be getting more treatment. The physician he had seen sent out word that there was no more that needed to be said.

Fortunately, another man in the department agreed to talk to the patient, and in a few minutes sent him away satisfied. He told him that, from experience gained with thousands of cases, experts felt that when a man was sixty-nine, and had had adequate treatment, and when he had no symptoms, and a normal spinal fluid, he was safe; in the years of life that were left to him he was not likely to get either tabes or paresis, and so he should not be bothered with more treatment. The doctor told the man, also, what he did not know, and that is that in countless cases, even after the best of treatment, some of the blood tests will remain slightly positive.

The unwisdom of saying only, "There is nothing the matter." As I watch able young physicians at work I think one of their worst faults in handling nervous patients lies in their tendency to dismiss with a curt statement to the effect that the results of all the tests were negative and hence *there is nothing the matter*. They forget that even if a man's organs are essentially sound, the fact that he is miserable and keeps going from one physician to another shows that there is something wrong with him. The patient senses this, and says, "But still I am sick; and I have pain."

Many a physician thinks that when he tells a woman she is all right she ought to go home happy, and hence he is annoyed or impatient or even angry with her when she refuses to go. What he fails to see is that although when one is ill it is reassuring to be told that all one's essential organs are sound, it is terribly disappointing not to be given any hope of relief for one's headache or pain or diarrhea. What is to be done about that? The doctor often says, "Oh, forget it," but this may be a stupid and cruel thing to say: A woman cannot forget a diarrhea that has put an end to her social life and is now threatening her ability to earn a living. And this is true even if the diarrhea is due purely to anxiety or nervous tension.

It is no wonder some patients get panicky when told there is nothing wrong. Each successive doctor who fails to find "the cause of the illness" frightens them that much more, and leaves them the more fearful that they have some dread disease unknown to science, and hence are beyond the reach of medicine and surgery.

The need for finding out exactly what type of neurosis it is. The most important thing for a physician to do when the findings are negative is to try to determine exactly what type of functional disease the person has and just how the symptoms are being produced. Usually this has to be done with the help of a good history.

There are many ways in which, let us say, an indigestion or abdominal distress can be produced, and the treatment that is good for food sensitiveness is useless for tabagism or the abdominal quiverings due to anxiety. Similarly, there are a number of ways in which a pseudo-anginal pain can be produced (see Chapters 5 and 19).

I cannot emphasize strongly enough that *a physician's diagnostic work is not done when he reports negative findings;* often it should then be just beginning. For instance, a young colleague asked me to see a woman who, when told that her eighteen-year-old son had nothing the matter with him, had refused to go home. As the doctor said, he and the woman had finally become so angry at each other that there was no use in his trying any more to reason with her.

I found a woman who was panicky, and like some panicky persons, she had become angry and aggressive. As she said; she was scared because on borrowed money she and her boy had come some 1,500 miles; she had received nothing for her money; the boy was still in pain, and she did not dare return home and face her husband empty handed. I calmed her down and made friends with her in a few minutes by saying that I understood perfectly that she was on a spot; that I sympathized deeply, and that I would not think of making her go home until I understood better what the boy's pain was due to, how it had come, and how it might be cured.

Going over with the woman the record of the very thorough examination that had been made, I told her in simple speech what the many tests were for and pointed out that all of them had shown that her boy's internal organs were sound. Hence we could not blame the pain on an ulcer or inflammation anywhere and so would have to find the cause in some strain or worry.

The boy, the son of a day laborer, was obviously not very bright; he was an unusually awkward fellow, who might not have done well even at digging a ditch. But the father had wanted better things for him, and so had sent him to a school for barbers. On his return home, the boy had worked a few days and then had begun to suffer so much from stomach-ache that he had had to quit. I took the lad off by himself and asked him why he had quit. He said he was "scared to death" of botching each man's hair-cut or nicking him with the razor and then having to face his wrath! He said he knew he did not have what it took to be a barber! He was awkward, and he hadn't the right personality. He wanted to work in the mill, but when he said this, his father got angry. All that stood between him and his father's disappointment and wrath was his stomach-ache. Accordingly, I wrote as tactful a letter as I could to the father saying that the boy had always wanted to work with him, that he could not be happy and well until he did, and that I strongly recommended that he be given a job in the mill. I also wrote to the boss asking that he give the boy a chance. With this the boy cheered up and lost his pain. When I explained to the mother how the anxiety of being "caught in a trap" made some people ill, she understood; she had sensed that the boy was worried and unhappy, and she had tried to get her husband to see this. She left for home in a friendly mood, apparently satisfied with the diagnosis and the proposed treatment.

The case just described can show how, several times a day, a few minutes spent on going to the roots of a problem will make all the difference between sending a patient away dissatisfied or even angry, and sending her away pleased and helped and friendly.

The handicap of the physician who dislikes nervous patients. One great trouble in practice is that many a physician does not like the nervous patient; he gets annoyed at her (it often is a woman), he tends to argue impatiently with her, or to flare in anger if she questions anything that he says. He may become impatient if she keeps coming back with more questions. Often he cannot believe she is suffering as much as she says she is, and he shows it. He dislikes listening to her long and poorly told history, and so he gets her out of the office as quickly as possible.

Typical of the attitude of some physicians toward nervous persons with a constant tendency to illness was the response of a doctor when one of his patients, a fine woman of fifty, but one commonly filled with aches and pains, called him on the telephone. She was staggered by his peevish, "Oh, for Heaven's sake, you again? *Now* what's the matter with you?" Terribly hurt, she hung up, weeping. Perhaps the physician was glad when she quit him; perhaps he muttered, "A good riddance," even though the woman's husband was president of a big company. But this sort of behavior not only does the individual doctor harm, it does great harm to the whole cause of medicine. As one might have expected, this woman in her anger turned next to a quack who did her a lot of harm. But she forgave him because, as she said, "At least he was sympathetic, and he tried to do something for me."

It might be a good thing if all physicians who do not like "neuros," who cannot be nice to them, and who do not want them around, would hang out a sign to this effect, just as landlords hang out a sign to the effect that families with children and dogs are not wanted.

Actually, it is easy to handle most patients and to get their good will if one will only be friendly and courteous and sympathetic. Most persons appreciate friendliness, and before a smiling face, they soon thaw out, no matter how antagonistic they may have been when they came in. It is hard to be unpleasant to a man who appears to like us, and soon we are liking him. I know of no surer way to build a big practice than to like people.

As a doctor grows older he should become a thoughtful and kindly philosopher. It is all the better if he develops a warm, sympathetic nature. He will be the more convincing with patients if he is a lucid and interesting speaker and a good explainer. It is wonderfully helpful, also, to be a good listener; patients so greatly appreciate this rare trait in a doctor. A constant good humor is very helpful, and a merry jest is often good medicine. Obviously, the doctor must always laugh *with* the patient and never *at* him.

On true politeness. A wonderful gift in a physician is what the French call, "politesse du coeur," or the real, genuine, and unassumed politeness that comes from a kind and gentle heart. A gentleman will never willingly hurt the feelings of anyone.

So often a woman tells me of her distress or humiliation when some physician put a question to her in some apparently sarcastic or unpleasant way. It made her feel as if she were in the wrong, or stupid, or not in the right office; it made her feel on the defensive, and as if she ought to be ashamed of being ill and complaining about something.

In some of these cases I think the physician was without malice, and he hurt without realizing what he did. For instance, a consultant often gets a woman all upset right at the start by asking her brusquely what she is doing in his office; who referred her, and what gave her the idea that she had the disease that falls within the scope of his interests. He makes her feel as if she were a book agent who had forced her way in. Perhaps, if he had only taken the trouble first to establish friendly contact with her and had quieted her agitation, and then had asked his questions, or had asked them in a less impatient or aggressive or peevish tone, or if he had asked them in such a way that she immediately understood why he wanted the information for his records, all would have been well.

So often a physician who does not like the looks of a patient will ask his questions in such a way as to humiliate or outrage. At many a consultation I have been greatly embarrassed on hearing this sort of thing, and then feeling the electric tension in the atmosphere that had come between two persons who in a moment had taken a great dislike to each other. Both were angry, and it was all so unnecessary.

Recently a fine business executive with a bad torticollis said to me, "I so hate to go to neurologists about this because I soon get the feeling that they think it is all imaginary and due to the hell I have been through with my insane wife. Perhaps it is due to that strain, I cannot tell; but supposing it is, how can I get over it, and what can I do to help myself? I need help and not poorly concealed contempt."

The need for a good rapport. How wonderful it would be if always before a physician started talking to a patient about his illness he would establish a happy and comfortable rapport. By this I mean a harmonious relationship, a sympathetic contact, a good meeting-ground of understanding and common experience, a discovery of an ability to speak and think in a common language of the heart. With a good rapport the rest of the interview becomes pleasant and easy.

There usually are many ways of establishing rapport, and often only a few friendly words are necessary. To give a few examples: Let us say that a patient comes in from California. I often stop then to say that, being a native-born Californian myself, I am always particularly happy to see people from that state. I talk for a few minutes about the city or town from which the patient comes, or I find that we have some acquaintances in common, and then the rest of the interview is easy. Or, here comes a patient from South America. Perhaps I soon find that his grandparents came from my father's province in Spain and, especially if he has traveled through Spain as I have, we are soon old friends with a bond between us. Or, here comes an anxious woman of sixty, fearful of what I am going to say and do. I ask her about her grandchildren and get her to show me their pictures. I tell her something of my grandchildren, and soon her fears of me are gone. Or, here comes a farmer, and I ask him what he is raising, and if he had trouble with his planting because of the late spring, and soon we are friends. All this may take a few minutes but it saves so much time later, and besides, it makes the practice of medicine so much more fun. Later in this chapter I show how much it helps a physician if he has suffered from some of the diseases he has to treat, and if he tells patients about this.

The best handler of nervous patients is born for the work. Doubtless, the best handler of nervous and psychopathic persons is the one who is born to the job. Some physicians owe their success in psychotherapy to an unusual and outstanding personality; one that gives them dominance over their fellows. Such a person was born to be a leader. He radiates strength and the feeling that he is in command of the situation before him. As years pass, honesty and integrity and kindliness are likely to show in his face and this gives him much power to heal. Naturally, when gray hair, great experience, and much success arrive, they add to his prestige and his healing skill.

Many another man, however, even with a small unimpressive body and mediocre talents can soon have a huge practice and can be successful in healing nervous persons if only he is patient, kind, sympathetic, and understanding. I remember two friends of mine who were such patient listeners that they seldom finished their afternoon office hours until nine o'clock. They were never hurried, and thousands of persons loved them for this trait.

Although gifts of character are very important in psychotherapy, skill can be acquired by the man who is willing to study and to learn the art from others. I know that I have received much help from the writings of masters in this field. Some physicians say snippy things about the man with a good "bedside manner." They assume that with such skill he must be a bit quackish or insincere. This is not the case. Many of the doctors with the best bedside manner are among the ablest and most respected in the community.

The need for liking people. Obviously, the physician who can most easily succeed in helping nervous and worried patients is the one who likes people of all kinds, makes friends with them in a minute, and gets along easily with them. We humans tend to like the person who obviously likes and admires us. Conversely, we dislike anyone who looks down his nose at us, or who is critical, arrogant, or unsympathetic. Many a time I have heard a fine college-educated woman say, "That doctor outraged me because he talked down to me as if I were a child or a fool."

I admit that there is not much to like about some patients, and what with their endless fears, their constant begging for more tests, and their efforts to get in ahead of their turn, they are a trial to the flesh; but *if one is to handle them at all,* one had best do it in a friendly way. The doctor should try not to be annoyed, because annoyance is hard to conceal.

Everyone knows the three little monkeys who see no evil, hear no evil, and speak no evil. There is another one, not in the group but he should be there, because he is the most important one of all; he is the one who *thinks no evil.* If a physician thinks no evil about a patient he is safe, and he will seldom have much trouble with him. I often tell my graduate students that since most of us humans are poor actors it is not much use making believe we like patients: The only sure way to their hearts is through *really* liking them. Nearly always one can like something about a patient. Always when a person is so annoying, unreasonable, and perhaps insulting that one wants to knock him down and literally kick him out of the office, one must stop and remember that he must be psychopathic or he would not be acting that way. A true physician will never allow himself to get angry with a man who is not sane; the fellow is sick and not responsible for his "orneriness."

The need for courtesy. There is every reason why a physician should be courteous to patients in all his dealings with them. He should remember that it is an iron rule in many stores that the customer must always be treated with courtesy and his statements accepted, even when it is obvious that he is in the wrong.

Fortunately, in this country there is little of the feeling there used to be in Europe that a physician is a superior being who has a right to

be boorish or unpleasant. But even in these United States there is many
a doctor who walks away without answering when a patient, or a relative of one, anxiously asks him a question.

We physicians should never question a patient's statement of fact,
only his interpretation of the fact. We would do well to say, "I do not
doubt that you have pain, but I doubt if it is due, as you think, to the
sedative I gave you last night to help you sleep." Sometimes a physician
and his patient must disagree, but then the physician should either see
the patient's point or else try to win him over with good reasoning;
he must not just beat him down with the club of authority. Many physicians get angry whenever what they say is questioned. This is unwise
because often the patient's objection is a good one, and it may even
invalidate the physician's diagnosis. I tell further on in this chapter of
a time when only my stopping to listen to a woman's correction of a
mistake in her history saved me from making an awful blunder.

**The handicap of the physician who is unable to sympathize be-
cause he never was ill.** The physician who has always been strong and
well and without a nerve in his body or any tendency to worry is terribly handicapped when it comes to handling and treating the highly
sensitive, overly reactive, congenitally worrisome, and sickly little woman
who rarely has had a comfortable day in her life. He cannot see why
a person like her, without anything demonstrably wrong, should have
so many distresses and complaints, and as she tells her story it may be
impossible for him not to show incredulity and dislike.

What such a man much needs in order to make him over into an
understanding, sympathetic, and more kindly physician is some long
illness or a nervous breakdown. He needs to know what it is to lie
awake half the night with nerves all on edge, perhaps painfully conscious
of an irregular heart action, or of waves struggling over a gas-filled
bowel. He needs to know what is to fear a lingering death, or to fear
that funds will be exhausted before recovery can come. He needs to
know what it feels like to have great pain and to have to beg for morphine from interns who think he is only a whining "neuro."

The doctor must know that certain persons suffer in bizarre ways.
Some highly neurotic and hypersensitive women tell such a weird and
apparently improbable story of suffering that the average physician is
likely to disbelieve the tale and therefore to feel contempt for the teller.
The woman, on the defensive and watching the doctor's face for the
first signs of disbelief and disgust, is likely to sense quickly what he
thinks, and immediately then she becomes angry and combative and
ready to leave in a huff.

The only possible way in which a physician can handle such a patient
and help her is to *know* that some persons are so sensitive that they *can*

sense a storm coming twenty-four hours before it arrives or they *can* get a skin eruption from the amount of chlorine in the city water. If the doctor knows these things he will not get contemptuous; he will maintain sympathetic rapport with the patient, and then he may help her.

When inclined sometimes to disbelieve something a highly sensitive woman tells me, such as that she cannot get to sleep because of the ticking of her husband's watch in the next room, I say to myself, "Hold on; would you be contemptuous of your dog if he could talk and tell you how troubled he was by the all-permeating smell of the people who used to live in the house long before you moved in?" Of course I would not. I'd believe the dog unhesitatingly. Actually, there are some people whose five senses are much keener than those of their fellows. Some persons with a keen sense of smell suffer because of it. They suffer acutely in a crowded elevator on a hot day; they can hardly wait to get out, while others do not notice anything wrong. One evening I watched Helen Keller thrill as she touched the side of an organ. I touched the organ but could feel only the stronger vibrations. A blind connoisseur used to take delight in feeling the texture of an ancient Chinese vase; I could feel only smoothness. Because of these differences in sensitiveness no physician should ever feel contempt for the man or woman who can experience sensations which he himself cannot experience.

The help that comes from sharing one's experience with patients. When a woman comes into the office much afraid that I may become impatient and contemptuous because she keeps breaking down and crying, I usually put her at ease in a moment by saying what is true, that after my influenza in 1918 I had several months of misery from a fatigue state with much nervousness and insomnia. From personal experience I know all about "nerves," and hence no patient need ever feel apologetic when telling me of his or her nervous troubles. My experience helps, also, when it comes to treatment. Often a patient says, "Since you obviously came out of that spell with such good health, perhaps I can, too. You just tell me what you did to get well and I will follow your course to the letter."

In practice it has helped me tremendously to be able to tell patients with migraine or a sensitive colon or a tendency to fatigue that my highly nervous mother bequeathed me all these troubles, and so I know about them and have great sympathy for anyone who suffers from them. So often, with this one statement, I turn an angry or disgruntled patient into a friendly one who is anxious to hear how I solved the problems of avoiding sick headaches and mucous colics.

Similarly, the expert in tuberculosis often grips his patients to him in a friendly way by telling that he once spent a year in a sanatorium. Obviously, not all physicians have had such helpful experiences, but

those who have had them ought more often to use them as aids in helping patients similarly affected.

I think that often a patient finds more comfort in talking to a layman
who has shared his disease than he finds in talking to a physician who
has learned of the trouble from books. Hence it is that when he finds
a one-time-patient and a physician in the same person he is happy.

The physician helps best when he is an optimist. In handling
worrisome and easily frightened persons the physician is most successful
when he is naturally optimistic, cheerful, and reassuring. Sensible people will like him this way, and for years afterward they will keep coming
to him whenever they are alarmed or ill or in trouble.

Some physicians needlessly get themselves disliked by giving bad
prognoses even when they are not asked about the future of the disease. Others unwisely go to the opposite extreme and tell people
the minute they come in that they need not worry, and that all
will be well. A patient with any sense will resent this because he will
doubt if the physician has as yet any basis on which to form such a
judgment. The doctor may, of course, start reassuring as soon as he has
taken the history. Often then he can say, "This is the typical story of
a nervous trouble which I know well, and one which should never bring
you to any bad end." Or, after palpating a nodule in a breast, he may
say, "This should be removed so that you can be safe, but it feels so
much like a benign cyst that I am not much worried about it." Patients
are usually grateful for such immediate encouragement which may enable them to start sleeping again.

**The need for the physician's ready willingness to revise an
opinion.** Many a time a patient will question an opinion or a pro-
nouncement, and then, instead of getting angry and impatient, we physicians must stop to listen and, in the face of new or amended facts,
to change our diagnosis. I remember how, once, after I had told a
woman with attacks of severe abdominal pain that I wanted her common duct explored, she stopped in the doorway and said, "But, doctor,
the attacks which I am getting now are different from the colics I had
before my gallbladder was removed. The pain now is centered in the
left side of my abdomen; it is much more agonizing, there is much more
retching, and this type of storm is not well relieved by morphine."

This conversation took place toward the end of a tiring day; there
still were patients waiting, and the last thing I wanted then to do was
to stop and go over that story again, but it had to be done. Evidently,
during several previous consultations, my assistants and I had not obtained a good enough history. And so I sat down again and in a half-
hour of cross-questioning I drew forth a story of a gastric crisis type
of attack. I found, also, that she had had a few curious falling spells,

and next day, on sending her for an electroencephalogram, I got the report of a decided dysrhythmia. She was put on dilantin, and the terrible spells that for years had wrecked her life stopped coming. The lesson from this is that we physicians must never be impatient or angry with the person who says, "But, doctor, I don't think you got my story quite straight; I had this same pain long before that last operation." Always, then, we must sit right down and patiently go over the history again.

We physicians must never take out on the patient our disgust because we cannot cure. One of the saddest features of our medical practice is that at times we physicians yield to a human trait, and when we are stumped diagnostically or therapeutically, we get angry with the patient rather than with our lack of knowledge of disease and or inability to cure. Obviously we should never do this; we should really be kinder than usual to the patient whom we do not know how to help.

The importance of the first visit of the patient to the doctor. For many a woman it is a fearful ordeal to go to a new doctor. She is so afraid that he will be brusque, or that he will quickly shut her up and dismiss her before she has had a chance to tell her story. She may be afraid, also, that if he is snappy or impatient she will break down and cry. Because I know of these fears, always at the first interview, I try quickly to put a nervous woman at her ease.

I like to reserve at least a half-hour for the first interview, and I may take more time if the patient gets into a communicative mood and starts telling about sorrows and tragedies and follies and sins. I will not then want to shut her off because, if I do, I may not later be able to get her to talking freely again. It is a good thing at such times to ask the secretary and nurses not to telephone or interrupt. As a much-traveled patient with a nervous problem once wrote, after seeing my friend Dr. Harold Wolff, "At last I have found the neuropsychiatrist for whom I have for so long been looking. Just think, he listened to me for an hour, during which time the telephone did not ring and no assistant came in. Now I have had a hearing, and at last someone knows my problem well enough so that he can give me a worthwhile opinion."

T. A. Ross used to say that the first interview is the most important one because the patient's satisfaction or dissatisfaction with it often decides whether he or she can ever be helped by that particular doctor.

I realize fully that the busy physician who now does not see how he can ever give more than ten minutes to any one patient can only shake his head at the thought of anyone's giving an hour. It is sad that the physician with a large practice hasn't much time for psychotherapy, because, without such time, he cannot be of much use to his hundreds of nervous patients. Obviously, also, a psychiatrist, giving a half-hour or an hour to each patient, cannot see many patients in a day, and there-fore his fees must be large; too large for the resources of many persons.

The physician need not always give a definite diagnosis of organic disease. It is unfortunate that there seems to be an ancient tradition to the effect that to every patient the physician must promptly give a diagnosis, and usually a diagnosis of some organic disease. Ac-tually, there is no reason why the physician should always feel that he should quickly give a diagnosis. In many cases no definite diagnosis can logically be made, and certainly not at the first interview. I see many persons with indigestion and abdominal pain the exact mechan-ism of which I cannot explain. Sometimes all I can say is, "Take a rest, and make sure that the distress is not due to the eating of some food, and if you are not soon on the road to recovery let me see you again."

Often when at a lecture, I remark that sometimes I tell a patient that I cannot make a diagnosis, a young doctor will come up and say that while it may be all right for someone with my gray hair to say this, it would never do for him to admit such ignorance. And my answer is that even in my youth I commonly told patients I did not know what was the matter. Often when the person was intelligent he did not object to this. He said that if, after the careful examination I had given him, I did not know what the trouble was, he would stay with me until I did know. In some cases I called a consultant to help me, and in other cases I told the patient what was true, and that was that if I knew any physician in all America who I thought would recog-nize the syndrome I would send him to him.

On a physician's deterioration if he fails often to tell the truth. One of the most important reasons why all of us physicians should avoid placebos of diagnosis and why we should keep telling patients all of the truth that they can understand and face is that only in this way can we keep growing intellectually; only in this way can we go on learning medicine and becoming ever better diagnosticians and consultants.

The dangers of talking too much or too little. As I pointed out in Chapter 8 it is easy for the talkative doctor to put more fears and neuroses into a man than he came in with. Hence the doctor should never think aloud around his patients. Once he puts a hurtful idea into a worrisome person's head he may have to labor for months or years to get it out. It takes wisdom to know what to tell and what not to tell a patient; and what one can tell safely to an intelligent courageous person one cannot safely tell to a scatterbrained, pathologic worrier or coward.

Many physicians, after experiences in which they got themselves into endless trouble by talking too much, become cautious and too taciturn; when questioned they grunt and walk away. But, I think, this is poor practice.

The need for explaining to a patient what is to be done or what has been done. If a physician would only take time to explain to his patient what needs to be done, or what was done, or why it was done, and what it showed, things would go much more smoothly. If a patient of mine needs a gastroenterostomy, a gastric resection, or a cholecystectomy I quickly draw a diagram to show how the operation will be performed. Once I was interested to see how easy it was to sell a gastroenterostomy even to a devout Christian Scientist with a painful duodenal ulcer which had produced a marked pyloric obstruction and gastric stasis. When he came in he said he wished it understood that he would never be operated on. I replied that that was all right. But later I showed him in his roentgenograms the blocked pylorus and the big dilated stomach full of fluid which could not get out. I asked him what he would do if he knew a wicked fairy had tied a piece of tape around his pylorus. Surely he would not then think of using diet or medicine or prayer on that. Wouldn't he immediately get a man to go in and cut the tape? "Yes," he said, "I see the problem now; it is a purely mechanical one. Get me a surgeon and tell me what hospital to go to." I remember another case in which, when I drew a diagram and explained the problem to the woman's Christian Science practitioner, that sensible man said to his patient, "Go ahead and be operated on." The doctor should explain things like this not only to the patient but often to his wife or other relatives. Then the family will help and not hinder the doctor's efforts at treatment.

The need for telling patients the truth. One of the big questions in medicine is, should one tell a patient of the presence of cancer or other serious disease? In the early years of my practice I tried lying and I tried telling the truth. I soon had so many unhappy experiences with lying that after that I insisted on telling the truth. After forty years I am sure that the truth is easier on most patients and more satisfying to them. It is much better for the physician. With truth he is more likely to gain and keep the trust and liking and friendship of the patient and his family.

This does not mean that I insist on telling every patient all I know about him, especially when I am not asked, or when my information is not desired or can do no possible good. But when the patient looks me in the eye and asks, "What did you find?" I tell him. I dislike guessing as to how long a man will live, and I will usually refuse to do this. I will do it only for a businessman who has to know how much time he has in which to put his house in order.

If a wo.nan goes under an anesthetic hoping that she will have only a small nodule removed from her breast, and later wakes with the whole breast and her anterior thoracic muscles gone, why should the surgeon worry her badly, perhaps for days, by saying nothing? Why should he put her off when she asks what was found, or why should he lie to her and tell her she is all right? Why should he lie to her when, at the same time, he tells her family the truth, and they then break down and cry as they try to talk to her? Why should he lie when the patient is likely soon to hear a nurse talking to an intern about her cancer? And why should he keep lying to her when later he orders a course of roentgenotherapy and tells her to return in four months for a check-up? People are not such fools that they cannot see why such treatment has been ordered.

In my experience patients are very grateful when the doctor promptly tells them the worst and answers all their questions. They are so relieved to find in the doctor a friend with whom they can talk frankly and who will treat them honestly, like an adult, and not like a child who cannot be trusted to "take it."

Families commonly tell me that I must not tell the patient the truth, but I refuse to take cases on this basis. People often fear the man will commit suicide, but I have been telling patients the truth for over forty years and I have yet to see one who even attempted suicide because of it. Most people take the news bravely and without much emotion. Curiously, I have seen more violent emotional storms on those occasions when I was able to tell a woman that she did not have the cancer that she had been fearing! A few, then, for a few minutes, have collapsed or become hysterical.

Often one of the hard things the physician has to do with badly frightened persons is to convince them that he told them the truth when he said that all the tests showed nothing wrong. Naturally, since the patient knows that most physicians believe that it is their duty to lie about cancer or other serious disease, he has no faith in what he is told. Why should he have? He may have no faith even when he is shown the reports that came from the laboratory man, the roentgenologist, and the men who made the special examinations. Sometimes the only thing that works is for the physician to leave the records on his desk and to go out of the room. Then the patient may grab the history and read it.

Often I explain to the patient that since he is paying me for an opinion I feel morally and legally bound to give him an honest one. I tell him I see no reason why he should not sue me if I give him a false report for his good money. Ross, Sadler, and others have come out strongly for the telling of the truth to patients. As Ross said, uncertainty is far more distressing than certainty.

In consultant practice the physician often gets into much embarrassing trouble because of medical lying. For instance, a woman comes with great pain in her spine, a bad cough, and her chest full of fluid. A year before, her breast was removed at home, and she was told that the lesion was benign. If now I tell the patient what her trouble is, as I have to do if I am to help her at all, it is likely to make bad feeling, first, between the patient's family and the surgeon, and then, between the surgeon and me. He will think that I ought to have protected him by keeping up the deception, but I couldn't have done so even if I had tried. Lying is an uncomfortable business, and it seldom fools anyone or does any good.

A while ago I had a case that showed well the futility and stupidity and undesirability of lying. A fine able businesswoman of forty had been operated on. The home surgeon, finding a mass of adhesions in her pelvis, decided the trouble was probably cancer, and closed the abdomen. He ordered radiotherapy; he told the patient that all was well, and told her devoted sister what he feared. But the patient one night in the hospital read her history, so she knew what had been found. When the two sisters arrived, they each took me aside alone and urged me under no circumstances to tell the other the truth. Neither wanted to worry the other. I brought them together and said, "Why, when you both know the truth, do you keep up this deception? You who are such devoted chums, why not now discuss your fears and problems frankly as you have always done in the past?" With this they embraced affectionately, and for months afterward they kept writing to thank me for having helped them to share the burden and carry it together. They were so much happier without the old loneliness.

On keeping the door of hope open. I always try to leave the door of hope open for the apparently condemned patient. I tell of some of the cases I have seen in which either the diagnosis was wrong or else for years the patient's body fought the cancer cells to a standstill. Perhaps one in fifty patients with inoperable cancer lives on for years. Also, the patient must keep hoping that out of some laboratory a cure will come in time. Whenever possible, radiation should be used to slow the growth of the malignant cells, to relieve pain, and to give hope. It so helps the patient and the family to be doing something. If the physician does not do something the patient is likely to get into the hands of a rapacious quack. Today, many men with cancer of the prostate gland are getting estrogens, and women with cancer of the breast or pelvic organs are getting androgens, and some are being helped.

When severe pain comes, the patient should have plenty of methadon, dilaudid, demerol, or even morphine; whatever is needed to make life bearable. Better even a little habituation than months of agonizing pain. Devoutly religious relatives who fear that the loved one's life may be shortened by the giving of sedatives should be told what is true, and that is that relief of pain lengthens life.

In handling patients a physician needs a good memory. The wise physician will always avoid asking the patient anything which he could learn from the record. Many a time 'a woman has told me that she left her old doctor because so often he asked her what medicine he had given or what he had done or told her. The woman did not like a doctor who could remember so little about her case. The secret of success often is to have good records and then to consult them. If a patient comes back after a year or more, the wise physician, before the interview, will quickly glance over the old record. Then he can talk intelligently about the old trouble, and the patient will feel complimented and happy.

Often I find I need a long memory when dealing with several members of a family. I have to remember who told me what and who does not know what. For instance, the mother may not be supposed to know of a disastrous "affair" one of her daughters had. One sister knows about it, but another who is religious and a bit prissy has never been told. Naturally, the patient does not want the story written down in her record, so I carry the secret in my head, perhaps for years.

In many cases the physician must never tell where he got certain information, or he must not even let on that he has it. A hundred times I have had to work hard to draw out of a patient information that I had already obtained from some member of the family, and in some cases I *never* was able to get the confession from the patient; to this day he or she does not know that I know. To reveal it would cause bitterness in the family, or much hurt to one or more persons who, in their efforts to help the patient, put great trust in my abilities to remember and to keep silent.

The need for talking to patients in plain English. As I say repeatedly in this book, especially in view of the fact that many patients tend to misunderstand what is told them, we physicians must try always to explain our diagnosis, prognosis, and treatment in the clearest possible speech. Often, I am sorry to say, we drop into our usual medical jargon and use long Latin words, or abbreviations which mean nothing to a layman. We may tell a laborer that he has CNE, or that his NPN was a bit high, or his KUB (kidney, ureter, and bladder) roentgenogram was negative, or his EKG showed a left ventricular preponderance!

Often when I get a new assistant, I find it hard to figure out what his abbreviations mean; they differ so much in different hospitals. At consultations, I have even heard men of national prominence using such slang. Commonly, we doctors try to cheer a patient by telling him his trouble is "functional." Dr. F. C. Redlich, told of asking twenty-five of his more intelligent patients what they thought "functional" meant. Three out of four did not know. For that matter, even we physicians are somewhat hazy as to what it means, as I learned when I tried to define it in Chapter 2.

I doubt if many physicians realize what an advantage a man has in practice when he can talk to his patients so simply that he can be understood. Often this makes all the difference between failing to help and please a patient, and succeeding in helping and winning to lifelong friendship the patient and his family. When a sick man understands his problem and is satisfied that the correct diagnosis has been made, he is so much happier and so much easier to handle and treat.

On taking a moment to show interest. Many a physician grips his people to him with bonds of affection by showing that he is interested in them and concerned over their problems. For instance, some devoted pediatricians, before retiring for the night, will telephone to several anxious mothers to make sure that a sick child is doing all right. Or an internist will write a patient to find out if he is recovering well. Such signs of interest are exceedingly gratifying to patients; the memory of them is treasured and never forgotten.

On being nice to the patient who is not satisfied. Human nature being what it is, it is not easy for most doctors to be patient and kindly when, after a man is dismissed, he returns to say that he is not satisfied and would like more tests, or a consultation with someone else. Usually in these cases, unless there is some good reason for denying the request, it should be acceded to. If the patient can and will pay for tests or consultations it would seem as if he should have all he wants. The only patients to whom I hate to give more tests are (1) those who, I feel sure, do not need them *and cannot afford them,* and (2) those who, I fear, will return later to say angrily that they will not pay for them because "they did not show what was wrong."

Occasionally a patient is right in asking for a more extended study of his case. The physician with much clinical wisdom may be satisfied that a "fever" is a nervous hyperthermia, or a pain is functional in nature, and in most cases he will be right. But he must remember that in a few cases he will miss a carcinoma of the pancreas, or a gallstone in the common bile duct, or a gastric crisis due to an atypical tabes. Hence it is that when a patient is anxious to have everything done that can be done, he should have it. Our self-love should not enter into the matter. Too often it does.

The wisdom of the physician who welcomes consultations. Innumerable physicians make the big mistake of resenting requests for consultations. As I often say to a young colleague, "Why should you want to hog all the responsibility and get all the blame when things are going badly with a very sick patient and the family is suggesting that you call a consultant? Why not let a consultant share the blame, if blame there must be, or credit if it should turn out to be credit?" One of the great advantages of clinic practice is that the several men in the group are constantly calling each other in consultation and are gladly turning over many a patient to some colleague who is better trained to handle the particular problem.

I often think of the wisdom of a physician I once knew who, with a very poor primary training in medicine, built up and held for half a century the biggest and one of the most wealthy and distinguished of all practices in a great city. The way he did it was, in all puzzling or important cases, quickly to call good consultants. They usually gave him the diagnosis and told him how to treat the patient, and then he danced attendance. Although he never learned much medicine, people loved him and swore by him.

On acknowledging mistakes. One of the finest and hardest things a physician can often do, and one that will win him the respect and liking of many a patient, is freely and quickly to admit having made a mistake or having missed something. Some physicians try to brazen the thing out, but especially when it is perfectly obvious to everyone that the doctor missed a toxic goiter or a carcinoma of the colon, and the patient has been well ever since its removal, nothing can be gained by blustering.

Oftentimes, when a patient comes back to tell how he got cured elsewhere, if his physician can be nice about it, he will please the man, and he may win back his good will and patronage. Through the years I have made it a practice to thank such patients for telling me of their experiences after they left me and went elsewhere. As I say truly, if only I could hear what happened to all of my patients after they left me, I doubtless would many times be ashamed and distressed over having missed the diagnosis, but oh, with all that experience, how much better a physician I could be! Even when I question if the "chronic" appendix removed was as diseased as the surgeon thought it was, I keep these doubts to myself. It does no good to express them. Without any help from me the patient will soon find out whether the operation was curative.

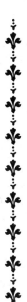

CHAPTER 26

The Art of Convincing
A Patient That His
Troubles Are of Nervous
Origin

As EVERY PHYSICIAN KNOWS, most nervous patients hate to accept the diagnosis of a functional trouble, and they may even get angry when they see it coming. Hence it is that the doctor who would sell the idea of a neurosis must learn the art of convincing persons who do not want to be convinced. He must study this art all his days, learning to use those arguments that have proved most helpful in past experience and to avoid those that usually have fallen flat or bored or produced antagonism. In this chapter I bring together many of the arguments and explanations that, through the years, I have found helpful and effective in my practice. I think this the most important chapter in the book because it can so help a man in his practice.

Much of a physician's success in preparing patients to accept the diagnosis of functional disease will depend on his skill in history taking and diagnosis. Physicians today do not realize sufficiently that in many cases the only way in which to please a disgruntled patient, to make friends with him, to satisfy him, and to really help him is to know medicine so well that one can quickly see what the diagnosis probably is, and then draw out the significant history. As this is done the patient may see why he is nervous, why he gets his attacks of distress, and how he might avoid them.

To illustrate: Let us say that a consultant in a clinic is asked to see a woman who is much dissatisfied with the diagnosis of "a functional indigestion." All he may have to do, perhaps, is to recognize at a glance the typical bright eyes, attractive face, and trim build of a migrainous woman. Then, quickly, he will bring out the story of her headaches, which she hadn't thought to mention, her hypersensitiveness, her tendency to fatigue suddenly, and her tendency to get into trouble when she tries to get too many things done in a hurry or at one time. As he does this the woman will begin to see her illness in its entirety, and will begin to understand it and herself as she never did before. Her fears of the distressing spells will drop away from her, and in their stead will come confidence and a desire to work toward a new and happier life. With this will come gratitude to the physician for the help he has given.

I remember a tense, keen, hypersensitive diplomat who went from specialist to specialist much worried about a distress in his lower abdomen and rectum. Most of his physicians had realized that the trouble must be functional in type, but, stopping there, they had left him unconvinced and unhelped. I was puzzled as to the exact nature of the syndrome until, with considerable effort, I unscrambled his long complicated story, and made one fact stand out clearly; namely, that he would get a mucous colic whenever he had to speak in public or give a dinner or dine out. As he came to see this clearly, and as he remembered that his attacks started coming in his boyhood, he saw that the syndrome, long-lasting as it was, could not possibly have been due to a cancer, as he had feared. He saw at last the psychic origin of the spells, and with many expressions of pleasure over the solution of his problem, he departed. So long as he knew what the spells were, he would not fuss about them; he could stand them.

Another illustrative case is that of an elderly man who complained of a burning distress in his abdomen. When it came suddenly one morning, his physician rushed him to a hospital with the diagnosis of an acute ulcer. After this the man kept going from one gastroenterologist to another until he was disgusted with diets and antacids. Noticing that he was talking more out of one side of his mouth than the other, and using his right hand clumsily, I soon brought out the story of a slight stroke with some loss of memory, complete loss of ability to work, and a loss of ability to write legibly. When I asked him if, in the first spell, he hadn't wondered if he was having a little stroke, he said yes, that was exactly what he thought he was experiencing. He thought he was about to die. He said that, ever since, he had been disturbed because no physician had seemed to think of this possibility. He had wanted to talk to them about it but had not dared. As a result he had been left with a feeling of great loneliness and isolation. He was very grateful because I had broached the subject and then had gone on to answer all his questions. I cheered him much by telling him that he might live for years before he got another little shock.

The big point I want to make is, how could I have helped this man if I had not recognized the slight signs of a cerebral thrombosis or if I had not known that such little strokes can cause distress in the abdomen? No amount of reassurance would have done a particle of good unless I had satisfied the man that I knew exactly what had happened to him.

An unmarried, highly intelligent secretary of forty had been going from physician to physician complaining of abdominal distresses and getting diagnoses and treatments which never satisfied her. Gradually, as I took her history, it became apparent that for most of her adult life, her troubles had come in spells lasting a few weeks, during which time she would be depressed and barely able to keep at work. Although, as this story was drawn out, she began to see her problem more clearly than she had ever seen it before, I doubt if she would have accepted my diagnosis of a manic-depressive temperament if I hadn't gone on to find out which side of the family had bequeathed her this curse. Soon she was telling of her formerly brilliant uncle who had ruined himself by periodic drunkenness. When I suggested that he too might be manic-depressive her eyes were suddenly opened and she said, "That is right; now I see it all. One day when I was telling uncle about my blue spells he said, 'Yes, dear, I know all about them; I have them and that is why I drink; in my spells of terrible mental suffering only alcohol gives me some relief.'" With this opening of her eyes, the woman became satisfied with the diagnosis: It seemed to her so logical. At last she saw that it was during her spells of depression that she had most of her fatigue, weakness, indigestion, gas, and aches all over.

As I said, in innumerable cases the physician who wins the patient's confidence does so largely or only because he shows that he knows the disease well. As he draws out and clarifies the essential story which the patient did not know how to tell, he unrolls the picture of the illness in its entirety, together with the inciting causes of many of the acute episodes. Let us physicians never forget that *as a prelude to psychotherapy there is no substitute for a good knowledge of medicine and diagnosis.*

It might be noted that in this series of cases just described, the patients did not need or expect much treatment after they had come to see what was wrong with them. Cheerfully they went home to make the best of life in spite of their handicap.

"Could it have been that?" To me one of the most remarkable things in medicine is the fact that even highly intelligent patients often fail to see the relation between the coming of great strain or unhappiness and the coming of their ill health. They do not see the relation between flare-ups of anxiety and flare-ups of discomfort. Often, after I have induced a woman to tell of some great sorrow that preceded her nervous breakdown she has asked, "Could it have been that?"

For instance, an intelligent woman did not see any connection between the coming of her insomnia and her discovery that her fiancé was going out with another girl. As she went through one big clinic after another, getting examined, she made no mention of her mental anguish. Another woman did not see any connection between the coming of indigestion and nervousness and the discovery that her husband was a bigamist; still another did not see the close relation between her mucous colics and her crises of indecision as to what to do about an unhappy marriage. Another, unhappily married to a traveling man, had noted the relation between her attacks of diarrhea and her husband's home comings, but she still continued to go from physician to physician getting prescriptions and diets.

The sensible woman, when she sees that really it "is that," generally goes home satisfied either to get out of her unhappy situation or else to acquiesce and adjust better to it.

The need for explaining what the physician means by "nervousness." One of the worst handicaps a physician has in dealing with a fretty woman is that, when he talks of nervousness, he and she are not thinking of the same thing. What the physician means is that either the woman was born with a tendency to hypersensitiveness, tension, and worry, or that she has been worn down by overwork, strain, sorrow, or illness. The doctor may admire her as a fine, able, sensible person who has kept going bravely in spite of much suffering, but to her the label "nervous" or "neurotic" means that she is silly, flighty, hysterical, imagining her symptoms, or enjoying ill health. Naturally, then, she is hurt or angry, and she protests that she really is a calm, sensible person who meets emergencies well.

Even after forty years of studying the art of getting such women to see what I mean by nervousness, I still can go wrong and get one of them angry. I watch the one before me, and if I see signs of annoyance and unbelief I hurry on to explain that I do not mean any of the things she thinks I mean. I often use myself as an example, pointing out that although outwardly I am my calm and good-natured father, inwardly I am my tense, migrainous mother with a digestive tract highly reactive to emotion. I remind the woman that it is possible to be calm externally and seething inside, and later she may say that this is certainly true in her case.

An essential point is that some persons are so constituted that emotion upsets the functions of the bodily organs, while other persons are not bothered in this way. For instance, I was once impressed by the different reactions of a man and his wife as they watched their daughter close to the jaws of death. Both of them were calm, with their emotions under perfect outward control. The wife had always been much more worrisome about the children than the husband had been, but in the face of this great danger she was able to eat three square meals a day and to sleep at night. The man suffered with severe abdominal pain and such frequent regurgitation and belching that he could not eat. He was unable to sleep, and he suffered from diarrhea. He had a great sensation of being seriously ill. Evidently his autonomic nerves were much more inclined to upset his body functions than were his wife's. This weakness in the husband was naturally not to his discredit; it was only an accident of inheritance.

I often find it necessary to point out to intelligent patients that there are many actresses and singers who vomit or have diarrhea for much of the day before a performance. There are persons who have diarrhea all day if they are to take a train, and there are businessmen who suffer from nausea when on their way to close a deal. There are women who vomited when their beau proposed, and mothers who, during World War II, vomited when an aviator son unexpectedly dropped in from the skies. Everyone knows of persons whose stomach "ties up in a knot" or who get palpitation after a fright, or who blush or blanch, or get a lump in the throat or a dry mouth, or who faint at the sight of blood. Others get a distressing feeling of contraction in the pelvis if they hear of someone who grasped the blade of a knife and got cut, or of someone who fell on a sharp spike. Some persons get tied up in knots inside while watching circus performers or even football players. Darwin spoke of thrills running up and down his spine when he was under emotional strain.

When a woman is reminded of these known distresses due to *acute* emotion she may be the more willing to believe that *chronic* emotion, such as is represented by her constant worry or resentment, can produce similar symptoms. The physician can go on to point out that great sensitiveness to emotion is seen much more often in the cases of gifted, well-educated, and charming persons than in the cases of stupid, ignorant, and stolid persons. If a woman is bright and wide awake, one can remind her that she owes much of her social charm to the very sensitiveness and reactiveness which now cause her headaches and her indigestion.

With these nervous patients one must keep insisting that there is no question about the *existence* and the *realness* of the symptoms: This is not doubted or questioned, it is only their *mode of production* which is under discussion. Vomiting due to nervousness is just as real as that due to sea-sickness, and diarrhea due to fright is just as real as that due to castor oil, and yet in neither case is there any organic disease in the abdomen.

Often I help a patient to understand what I am trying to tell her by speaking of those many women who get headaches when tired, as after shopping or coming in from an auto trip. No one ever thinks of cutting into such a woman's head to find the cause of the ache; everyone knows it is "just a headache" or a "neuralgia." And after fifty years of such headaches, the woman may still be healthy and getting stout. Obviously, the cause must have been a "functional" one, or the woman would long ago have come to some bad end. As I often say, "You appear to have the same sort of ache in your abdomen that your mother had in her head."

The need for emphasizing that it is no disgrace to be nervous.
Often the patient must be told repeatedly that it is no disgrace to have a neurosis, and no disgrace to have parents or grandparents who were neurotic or even a bit psychotic. No one is likely to accomplish much in the fields of artistic endeavor unless he is sensitive and even a bit neurotic. A tranquil, unemotional pianist is not likely to thrill an audience. A writer cannot sell his books unless he has a vivid way of seeing and feeling and describing things. And if a man is an unusually vivid character—keen, wide-awake, highly sensitive and responsive to emotion, if he thrills over a symphony, a poem, a picture, or a beautiful sunset, then occasionally he will have to pay the price in mental and physical suffering. Tschaikowsky would never have produced the *Symphony Pathetique* or *None But the Lonely Heart* if he had not suffered loneliness so poignantly. Keats would never have written his exquisite poems if he had had the body and nervous system of a wrestler. As Cobb has said, the elimination from the world of all neurotic persons would cause inestimable loss to the world of art, science, and the professions.

The need for explaining the effects of emotion. It is often helpful to point out to a patient with indigestion that some persons, when they see or fear something disgusting about their food, will begin to vomit, or they will get sick after just seeing or smelling the food. This shows that the trouble is all due to the mental impression. Other persons will vomit and be ill if, after eating, they gain the impression that the food was spoiled or bad. For instance, Montaigne tells of a girl who was told after a dinner that she had eaten baked cat. Her disgust was so tremendous that she became very ill. Actually, a practical joker was only teasing her, and she had not eaten cat meat. Another example of emotion affecting the body is that of the medical student who faints on seeing his first operation, or the soldier who falls down at sight of a hypodermic syringe.

What the physician might learn if he were to visit for a day in the patient's home. Hundreds of times when a woman has protested that she didn't know what she was doing that she should not do or what was bothering her, I have said that if I could only visit in her home for a day or two I could probably learn most of what I needed to know about her, her bad habits, and her annoyances. As I showed in Chapter 4, occasionally, in such cases, I have been able to go into the patient's home, and in a few minutes I have seen the things that were causing most of the trouble.

The importance of explaining why some nervous spells come out of a clear sky. As I show in Chapter 9, one of the most important things a physician can sometimes do is to explain to a patient why some of his distressing attacks come out of what appears to be a clear sky. A woman who is having nervous storms will protest that often one will come at a time when she has no extra strain and when she is feeling well. She may admit that for weeks she has been under stress, but still she cannot recognize any exciting cause for some of her storms. She may even claim that she is not a nervous person in any sense of the word, and in this she may be backed up by her relatives. Why, then, should she be having her spells? Unless this question is well answered, she will not be satisfied.

As I said in Chapter 9, many a nervous syndrome is not due to poor thinking, *at least at the moment* when the symptoms came. The "storm" may be an equivalent of migraine, or of epilepsy, or it may be due to the nervous instability of the menopause, to disease in some gland of internal secretion, to hypertension, or to the coming of a slight cold. Other storms may come with some tide in the chemical processes of the body, or they may be due to an injury to some nerve center by a neurotrophic virus, or by a thrombus in some small artery of the brain. Other storms may be due to the outpouring of neuromimetic chemicals into the blood, and others may be due to an allergen, breathed in or eaten.

In many a case the patient can be helped only by the taking of a history so good that it will show what the cause of the trouble is. In other cases the cause can be found only if the patient keeps a record of happenings and of drugs taken or foods eaten before each storm. Oftentimes, by keeping a record of sleepless nights, fatiguing events, or emotional crises occurring just before a "storm," the patient will learn what the triggers are.

Oftentimes one can help a patient by pointing out that if the trigger gets set too fine by some strain, tension, or fatigue, it will be tripped without obvious cause. On the other hand, if, with rest and relaxation, the patient gets the trigger set coarsely, it will rarely go off, and then only with a strong stimulus.

The great usefulness of the idea of energy spreading away from an overactive brain. One of the best and most helpful explanations I know of for much of the jitteriness, tension, and distress experienced by hard workers is that when, for a time, the brain has been very active, excessive and unwanted energy spreads away into the autonomic nervous system, there to play tricks with normal organs in thorax, abdomen, and skin. For instance, many an author has told me how, when he is writing rapidly, he urinates every twenty minutes; perspiration runs out of his right armpit, his heart speeds up, his temperature goes up a degree, and he feels tension in the back of his neck and in his jaws. He may remark, also, that when he works in the evening his brain gets so "lit-up" and active that he cannot turn it off. Then if he does not take two sleeping tablets he cannot get much rest. Every hour or two he may be waking and having to sit up a while. Similarly, a man who has made an after-dinner address is likely to be "lit-up" and unable to go to sleep. If he isn't "lit-up," he probably hasn't made a good speech!

That the insomnia and nightly distresses of brain workers is due to this overactivity of the brain is shown by the fact that when on a vacation they sleep soundly all night. The tense nervous man with a duodenal ulcer often seems to sleep with part of his brain actively at work, and this may well account for the excessive night secretion of hydrochloric acid in his stomach.

The importance of the idea of nerves playing tricks. One of the most useful ideas that a physician can present when trying to get nervous persons to see what is happening to them is the idea that their autonomic nerves are playing miserable tricks with their perfectly normal heart, stomach, bowel, bladder, or skin. I have discussed this idea in Chapters 9 and 15.

The next question is, why are the autonomic nerves playing such tricks? There are several possible reasons. One is that an overworked and overactive brain is sending out waves of energy. Many of these waves probably arise in an irritable or erratic hypothalamus. Perhaps in the particular patients this organ at the base of the brain and the associated autonomic nerves were unstable from birth, or they may have gotten on edge and unreliable in their behavior because the patient has worked too hard and become too tired. The centers in the hypothalamus seem often to be erratic in their behavior much as they are in menopausal women with hot flushes. In such women a tiny thermostat at the base of the brain appears to have been thrown out of good regulation for a time, and as a result one minute the woman feels too hot and the next, too cold.

Many a man will feel much reassured with such an explanation. He will feel that at last he has an answer to questions that have long been troubling him. At last he can see why it is that with organs so sound he can still be so uncomfortable. When he understands how this is he will the more readily listen to the physician when he tells him of things that he can do in order to get well.

Cannon's idea of flight or fight mechanisms. Some intelligent patients who are having many conflicts and who suffer from resentments and antagonisms may be helped by hearing of Cannon's idea that when faced by great danger, animals pour out into the blood epinephrine which can be of help to their bodies in either fighting or running away. In the fight or flight, the substances are used up, but in civilized life they are not used up because the man does not run and he does not fight with his muscles. He fights with his bank account or a series of telegrams. Hence it is that, for a while, the epinephrine remains in his blood and causes his heart to misbehave or causes him to feel nervous and trembly.

As Wolff has pointed out, these defense reactions were devised for *sudden* emergencies. When the neuromimetic hormones are poured out for only a few minutes they cannot do harm, but when, through *long-lasting* resentment or anxiety, they are kept pouring out day and night for months, they can do harm to a number of organs. Elsewhere in this book I tell of a man, so enraged over a bitter family lawsuit, that he developed poisons in his body and went down hill and died.

The vomiting or diarrhea that comes at times with fright may be like that of an animal which, when it sees an enemy approaching, suddenly empties its digestive tract, perhaps so that the body will be lighter and in better condition for flight.

The advisability of showing a patient the significance of greatly exaggerated knee jerks. When, as often happens, a nervous woman has knee jerks so exaggerated that when one tendon is tapped both legs fly up and perhaps she jumps all over, I think it helpful to point out that with such violent reactions to stimuli, she must often suffer. She will jump when the phone rings near her or she will scream when she finds that someone has come quietly into the room and is standing beside her. If only she could live for six months so quietly that those knee jerks could get back to normal, she would be a happier and healthier woman. I once wrote an article on this group of persons with a hyperactive knee jerk (Alvarez: 1945). I found that almost all of them were suffering from diseases in which nervousness was an important factor.

The need for explaining the curse of hypersensitiveness. Often, as a woman goes through her tests, the physician will note that she is abnormally sensitive. She complains too much when a fold of skin is lifted up and pinched a little, or she says a rectal examination is very painful. She blinks at the open window, and she is distressed by sounds and smells. She should then have pointed out to her the fact that she has to suffer if only because so many impressions are beating in too heavily on her brain. Because of her hypersensitiveness, stimuli which would go unnoticed by most persons or would cause them only slight discomfort *will be felt by her as pain*. Much of this sensitiveness is inborn, but some can come because of fatigue.

A woman's teen-age children may love to have the radio blaring all evening while they do their homework, but to her, after a few minutes, such noise becomes almost unbearable torture. The migrainous woman is especially likely to suffer in this way. She is tortured by glaring lights, clattering sounds, and strong odors. In a smelly restaurant she cannot eat. She suffers on getting into a crowd, and at a tea, much cross-talk confuses and disturbs her.

It may help to give her the physiologist's idea of a lowered threshold of sensation. Better, perhaps, would be the idea of an irrigation ditch with its boards which are lowered or raised as water is needed or not needed in side ditches. Then the woman can see how much more comfortable she might be if by rest, saner living, and better mental hygiene, she could raise the threshold of sensations and thus shut out from her consciousness many of the stimuli which now torture her. It is well to show her that when her threshold is too low she may become conscious even of goings-on in her body which are normal. Thus, she may feel her heart beating or she may hear the throb of the internal carotid artery as it passes through the bony canal near her ear. She may feel waves of contraction in the muscles that erect the hairs of her skin. Some few persons can even feel nauseated and sore all over when a storm 200 miles away begins to move toward them. Others get so tired just from holding themselves in that they feel as if they could jump out of their skin, or shriek at some person who is irritating them.

In the cases of these hypersensitive persons, just the impact on the brain of the stream of vivid sensations which is constantly coming in from the outside world seems to be enough to produce fatigue. Perhaps this is one reason why these people get particularly exhausted on a journey or in a museum or at a concert where they must take in thousands of impressions.

The occasional need for explaining to a patient how a pain felt at the periphery can be produced somewhere at a distance or even up in the brain. Before the physician can get a woman to accept his ideas about the production of her pains up in her brain he may have to remind her that if she cracks her "funny bone" at the elbow she will feel a burning pain, not there, but in the last two fingers of the hand. The doctor may use, also, the simile of the lineman who, on the edge of town, climbs a pole to call in. "Central" will then assume that he is speaking from some distant farmhouse which has always in the past corresponded to that wire. She will have a mental picture of him out in the country. For this reason, when there is some irritation of the cut end of a nerve in an amputation stump, the man complains that his nonexistent toes are twisting and hurting him. Obviously, a distress which is originating in the stump is referred by the brain out to the old periphery.

Distresses which originate in a troubled brain are also often referred out to the periphery, as when an oversympathetic mother, whose pregnant daughter is in labor, gets pains in her pelvis. Many persons, as they hear of some accident and perhaps especially an accident in which a child falls and is impaled on a picket fence, will feel distress in the crotch. Elsewhere in this book I describe the cases of two girls who got a pain in the face when confronted suddenly with a sight that greatly shocked them.

The physician can go on to remind his patient that when she is seasick there is nothing wrong with her stomach. The whole trouble comes from too much stimulation of nerves in the balancing mechanism in the inner ear. The fluid in the little "spirit levels" keeps swishing back and forth. The storm produced by this goes to the brain and is thence projected down into the abdomen. Persons who have had a stroke will sometimes feel pain projected into the face, the thorax, or the abdomen.

When a person is troubled by sciatica or a nerve root type of pain, one can often show him in the roentgenograms of his spine the bony excrescences about the points of emergence of the affected nerves. He can readily see, then, why with these nerves irritated, he can have pain in his thigh or the muscles of the thoracic or abdominal wall. This idea of projected or outwardly referred pain is one of the most important ones that many a patient can be given. As I point out in other chapters, there are many psychically produced aches which can quickly be recognized because of their constancy and their lack of association with digestion, urination, or exercise.

Explaining why the patient got pain in a certain spot. Often a patient will ask, "But why, if this trouble is due to nervousness and fears, did it pick on only my right loin, or my heart, my stomach, my colon, or the nape of my neck?" The answer is that this is the nature of functional disease; it hits one person in one place and another person in another. Some persons are hit all over so that they ache everywhere. Many are conditioned to suffer pain in a certain area because of their fear of a certain type of illness. Thus, if they fear a family tendency to heart disease they are likely to get distress in the precordium, while if they fear cancer of the liver they may get an ache in the right upper quadrant of the abdomen.

The production of symptoms by the concentration of attention on an organ. Sometimes it helps to explain to a worrisome and overly imaginative woman that if she concentrates her attention on her heart or her colon she can soon experience an ache in the region. She will be like the worrisome man who, after illicit sexual intercourse, gets the idea that he has been infected with a venereal disease. For days he may go through an agony of apprehension during which time he will feel that the penis aches and burns as if it had been severely bruised. Finally, as the period of incubation passes and fear goes, he gets well.

This sort of anxiety probably accounts for a number of the aches so commonly complained of in the precordium, in the perineum of men, and in the pelvis of women.

The need for explaining what is meant by "functional" and "organic." As I point out in Chapter 2, there is often great need to make a patient see what we physicians mean by the words "functional" and "organic." We commonly use these words in talking to people, forgetting that they mean little or nothing to them. Perhaps a good way of making a patient with indigestion see what we physicians mean is to remind him that many a patient with severe abdominal pain has had his abdomen opened and explored carefully without anything wrong being found. *Apparently the cause was not where the pain was.* Another example I often use is that of headache. Many women have headache almost every day of a long life without any demonstrable cause, yet they do not come to any bad end.

In such cases the cause of the pain was not any *local* disease or certainly not any *local disease that could be identified with the naked eye.* It is conceivable that there may have been chemical or microscopic changes in the tissues which gave pain, or there may have been microscopic changes in the nerves. One can remind a patient of the great pain felt in certain forms of fibrositis in which the roentgenograms show no changes in the bones making up the joints. Fingers which for years have been stiff and painful may still look perfectly normal. They will not be deformed. There is certainly something wrong with them but it is not anything that can be seen with the naked eye.

One of the worst pains I ever experienced was in my hands as I was thawing them out after freezing them a bit in a blizzard at 10 degrees below zero. Although the pain was almost unbearable, the hands looked perfectly normal. A person who has been stung by a black widow spider may suffer terrible abdominal pain but, if by mistake, he has his abdomen explored, nothing wrong will be seen. The pain is probably due to the effect of the spider's venom on some part of the nervous system. Another good example of a functional trouble is that of the abdominal pain that some persons have when subjected to great emotion.

The all-important point is that one can have severe pain with no gross local lesion to explain it. When I think of all the myriad possible microscopic and chemical causes for pain I am inclined to wonder, not that the surgeon so often fails to find gross disease to explain pain, but that he finds it as often as he does.

The need for showing that the patient with a functional trouble can suffer more than does one with organic disease. Often, when a woman is told that her pain is probably functional in nature, she replies that it can't be because it is so troublesome and so constant. But she is wrong. I often tell of two women who once came into my office. The old mother, with a big cancer of the stomach, said she was not ill; she had no pain. It was the daughter who was in great pain and vomiting steadily. What was the matter with her? Only sympathy for her mother and fright on hearing what was wrong!

I point out, also, that the very fact that the ache is so constant suggests that it is functional rather than organic in origin. Distresses due to organic disease such as cholecystitis usually are present for hours or a day or two and then go away for weeks or months. The pain of arthritis, fibrositis, or peptic ulcer tends to come and go. There is no question that functional pains are often very distressing and disabling. A great sorrow or a nervous breakdown can be much more distressing than a broken leg, and much harder to cure.

Showing a person that he is much too ill for the amount of disease he has. Oftentimes one must try to get a person to see that he is much too ill for the amount of organic disease he has. For instance, a woman came in pathologically depressed, crying, and all to pieces nervously because of a buzzing in an ear. I had a hard time getting her to see that 90 per cent of her illness was due to her lifelong tendency to get depressed and terribly worried about any little thing that ever went wrong with her body. Because of this, my job with her was not so much to treat the buzzing as to get her to see that by her depression and her carrying-on she was wrecking her life and the happiness of her husband and her children. Fortunately, with great effort I at last was able to lift her spirits and get her to go back to living again and to putting up with some buzzing.

The need for gentleness and skill in taking away previously made diagnoses and some medical beliefs of patients. Chronic complainers sometimes have a lot of firmly held ideas about medicine in general and their health in particular, and because of this, they tend to clash with some of their physicians. A woman will say that $\frac{1}{10}$ grain of codeine will make her deathly ill, or that the chlorine in the city water is causing her skin to break out, or that the amount of milk in a piece of bread is giving her migraine. Such ideas may or may not be true, but in order to get and keep the patient's liking and trust it is best not to show any immediate sign of disbelief. Later, perhaps after the woman and the physician are on a friendly basis, if he thinks it necessary, he can try to show her that another interpretation can be placed on her observation.

We physicians must not treat contemptuously a patient's cherished ideas such as that he has a torpid liver, too much acid in his system, intestinal autointoxication, or a badly dropped stomach. We must not pooh-pooh immediately the diagnosis a patient brings with him. He may be very fond of it, and he may like the kindly doctor who made it. Perhaps we can say, after a while, that this diagnosis is not now adequate to explain the symptoms, and that, with the appearance of new symptoms, another explanation has become more probable.

The patient may feel that his new physician has no right to differ with the ones who went before unless he has examined at least as thoroughly as the others did. This, of course, is not a fact. What the patient does not know is that after ordering all known tests and getting the reports, a poorly trained internist can easily make a wrong diagnosis, while a keen old country doctor, after one glance at the invalid and a question or two, may make the correct one.

Always, when taking away a placebo of diagnosis, we physicians should be tactful, and *we should give some explanation why a brother physician held the opinion he did,* and why now a new diagnosis seems more nearly right than the old one was. For instance, if a constitutionally frail, neurotic woman comes with a diagnosis of brucellosis and no signs or symptoms of it, except perhaps a so-called fever of 99.6°, one can first point out that most tense nervous persons run a temperature of 99.6° in the afternoon. One can tell of Kleitman's two girls who regularly, after seeing an exciting movie, got a rise in temperature of a degree or more. One can tell of patients who get a temperature of 102° when much worried, or of university students whose daily temperature of 100° or more has now been running for years and still appears to be normal for the individual. One can point out that all bodily measurements range up and down around a central point, and hence normal temperature is not 98.6° but something between 96° and 100°.

After explaining in this way the little rise in temperature, one can go on to say that doubtless a year ago the attending physician had reasons for believing that the patient had brucellosis, but if she had it then, she apparently has now recovered from it because her blood no longer reacts to the germ, and she has no sign of the disease. Besides, perhaps one can remind the patient that she has been frail and sickly for twenty-five years, and she cannot have suffered from brucellosis all that time. By talking in this way one does not confuse or outrage the woman, and one does not undermine one's position in her estimation by attacking the reliability of a physician whom she may have come to like personally, even if he did not cure her. One must remember, also, that she will much prefer his positive diagnosis of organic disease to the new rather negative and unpleasant diagnosis of constitutional inadequacy.

Always when we physicians must differ with a patient we can do it in a courteous way: not with the lie direct but with a "possibly there is another explanation" technic, or "since the day when your physician told you that, medical science has advanced, and today we seldom make that diagnosis." A good example of the problems involved in straightening out a person puzzled by conflicting diagnoses is to be found in the case of a worrisome woman of forty-five years who, alarmed by the "get examined-for-cancer" drive, went to a surgeon for a check-up. He said she had a tumor of the uterus and must immediately have a hysterectomy. Horrified, she went to an internist who curtly said, "You have no tumor," and dismissed her. Only more puzzled, she went to another man who said, "Yes, you have a tumor but I see no need of operating." The next man said, "Yes, you have a tumor and I'll take it out tomorrow." The next said, "You have no more tumor than I have."

One can imagine the state of mind she and her family were then in, and how difficult had to be the task of giving her back her mental peace. Finding that what she had was a small myoma of the uterus, I explained that many doctors would consider this as harmless as a wen on the back of the neck and would therefore refuse to dignify it by the name of tumor. Others would call it a tumor, but would not operate on it; others would call it a tumor and would want to operate on it because of the remote chance that some day it might become malignant. Since, in my experience, that chance is very small, I thought she should leave it alone. She went off apparently satisfied, but of course if she ever started shopping around again, as she probably did, we can be fairly certain that she eventually consented to an operation as the only thing that would restore her peace of mind.

The patient who is very devoted to a physician who overtreats. Often, when a woman tells proudly of all that a certain physician did to "pull her through" and save her life it may sound to other physicians like senseless and meddlesome overtreating or much unnecessary surgery, but it would be useless to tell the patient this. She hasn't the medical knowledge that would enable her to see what really was **done**

to her and that she recovered *in spite of* much very bad treatment. For instance, a woman was heard bragging about her small-town would-be surgeon who, she said, had taken four hours to remove part of her uterus! As was to be expected, she got peritonitis and later pneumonia. With "wonderful skill" he filled her with every known antibiotic, and eventually "saved her life." With all the complications, she was in the hospital three months! In her eyes her doctor is a wonderful man, and whatever he says she now believes. Such devotion of a patient to a physician is beautiful, and it should not be disturbed.

Explaining why findings, even when correct, may have no significance. Often one has to try to get a patient to see that although what the home doctor reported was there all right, this could not explain the illness. For instance, many a patient with diarrhea of a functional type says that amebas were found in the stools. But since several courses of emetin and arsenicals failed to help, one can be fairly certain that the amebas, if really present, were not the cause of the frequent bowel movements. In order to put this idea over, one must explain that thousands of persons in the tropics have a bowel full of amebas and no symptoms from them. It is hard for a woman to believe that without any symptoms, she can have a large myoma of the uterus, or many gallstones, or a peptic ulcer. In Chapter 7 I discuss the many findings that often have no significance.

The value of showing patients that a physician has some clinical knowledge and can recognize many diseases without tests. In these days when laymen and, I am sorry to say, many physicians regard tests as everything in diagnosis, I find at times that a patient looks on me largely as a broker or middle man to whom he has to come when he wants an order for tests. It does not seem to occur to the man that a physician should be able to diagnose many diseases without tests, just from the clinical picture.

Sometimes a patient will even resent the fact that the physician recognizes the nature of his trouble after asking a few questions. I suspect then he is angry largely because he does not like the diagnosis the physician made and hopes that with tests he may get one more to his liking. A woman who knows in her heart that she has inherited the family psychoneurosis usually feels this way. She may say, "I won't have a neurosis; give me anything but that; go on making tests until you find something else!" A man who knows he has had a stroke may try with the help of many tests to get a pleasanter diagnosis.

Oftentimes I doubt if I can sell a woman my diagnosis unless I can get her to see that after forty-five years of dealing with the sick I ought to know some diseases at a glance or at least after hearing what the symptoms are. In trying to explain this, I will say to the woman, "If you were to hear a child coughing violently in a peculiar brassy way, and then if you were to hear it whoop and see it vomit, what would you say it had?" "Whooping cough." "Of course, and you would be sure of it without any tests or roentgenograms. You'd be sure of it because you had seen that group of symptoms many times before. Well, then, why can't you see that I, too, must know many illnesses at a glance just as you know whooping cough?" This argument sometimes helps.

Once, when confronted by a woman who would not believe that I could recognize her menopausal depression from looking at her and talking to her, I turned to her husband, an old floor walker, and asked him if, when a woman came into his store, he could tell if she was just looking around, or waiting for her sister, or hunting for something she needed to finish a dress. He said, "Sure, I can tell in a minute." Because this man had spent his life in sizing up people, he could see that in my line of work I, too, must have learned to appraise people and to make many diagnoses at a glance. Unfortunately, it was hard to get his wife to see this; her life work apparently had not prepared her for the idea.

Obviously, a young physician just out of college cannot trust to his first diagnostic hunches as safely as can his Chief who has been seeing patients for thirty or forty years. What I have tried to do in this book is to show that (1) as rapidly as possible a doctor should learn to diagnose many diseases from a good history and some shrewd observing, and (2) as he grows in experience he should trust more and more to these hunches. Often they are correct when the results of tests are wrong or misleading.

Withholding the diagnosis until the reports of tests are all in. Because the nervous, much-doctored woman so fears the diagnosis of a neurosis, it is best not to start the first interview by telling her that this is what she has. This may enrage her, and, worse yet, it may cause her to fear that she is dealing with a physician whose mind is so closed in regard to her case that even if he were to find organic disease he would not report it to her. She fears he will not be big enough to admit that his first hunch was wrong. What she is looking for so desperately is a physician who will not notice her jitteriness and overemotionalism, but will feel, as she does, that there must be organic disease somewhere in her body, disease which he will hunt for determinedly until it is found.

Because of this, there is much to say for the rule that a physician should never give even an intimation of his opinion until the results of all the tests are in. Patients like this way of doing things, and it can save the physician embarrassment in case, during the examination, serious organic disease should show up. Unfortunately, there is a bad feature of this type of examination and this is that it tends to confirm the patients in their view that the physician is pretty much a passive know-nothing who makes his diagnosis purely by tests. It leaves them, also, with the bad idea that neuroses are to be diagnosed only through the exclusion of organic disease. If they believe this, then when no organic disease is found they are likely to conclude that it would have been found if only more tests had been made. For this reason, when a patient comes in with an obvious neurosis, I like to show that I know what is wrong, and I like to say that I do not expect the tests to reveal anything serious. I may go further and say that even if, let us say, some gallstones should be found, their presence could not account for the migrainous woman's nervousness and her headaches. I want her to see that I am diagnosing migraine because I know the syndrome well, having seen it a thousand times before.

My other objection to leaving the diagnosis to the last minute is that in my type of practice in a clinic to which practically all of the patients come from a distance, it is bad to wait until perhaps closing time on Saturday, when the patient's main concern is catching the plane for home, to tell him that the results of all the tests were negative. I may not then have enough time in which to explain the situation, answer all arguments, and sell the idea of a neurosis. Hence it is that often, *in my type of practice,* I think it well to start right off preparing the patient for a disappointment and for the likelihood that he will get a diagnosis other than the one he hoped to get.

The reader may say, "But why don't you keep the patient around longer? After traveling far to reach you he surely ought to be willing to stay a few days for treatment." Doubtless he should be willing to do this, but commonly he isn't. The businessman wants to get back to his appointments; the farmer wants to get back to his animals, and the woman wants to get back to her baby or her daughter's graduation, or someone's wedding.

In many cases it does help to prepare the patient for a diagnosis of "functional" disease. For instance, a man from South America told me on departing that he was the more easily convinced of the correctness of my diagnosis because, two weeks before, when he walked into the office and started shading his eyes from the light, I got a hunch and quickly drew out the story of his migraine. Then I told him that I did not expect the tests to reveal anything significantly wrong. Later, when the results did turn out to be negative, he was prepared and did not become incredulous, dissatisfied, or disappointed and inclined to go elsewhere to find someone who would give him more tests.

Naturally, in other types of puzzling cases, on the first day the physician cannot hazard much of a guess as to the diagnosis. He may suspect the presence of organic disease, and he then will want to search through the body for it. I dislike the type of practice in which, with the case being worked up by an assistant, the senior physician does not see the patient until the last day. I like to meet the patient when he comes in, and I like to take some of the history. I like to plan the examination, and I like to keep seeing the person every other day as the reports of the tests keep coming in. Then, if necessary, I can alter the plan of study. For instance, if the patient with a pain in the right loin is found to have red blood cells in his urine, I will want to study his kidney before I give him the gallbladder dye and especially before I put barium into his stomach and bowel. I like to keep seeing the patient in this way so that (1) I can get to know him better, (2) after a few interviews I may get the important history of psychic strain, and (3) during these interviews I can be practicing psychotherapy.

Admitting that even the patient with a neurosis must be well examined. It is well to say to the nervous person, "Yes, you are right; the nervous man or woman is not immune to serious organic disease, and so I shall see to it that you have a careful and thorough examination." I remember an elderly woman suffering from severe epigastric pain who had always been a psychopath and a chronic complainer and who had recently suffered a little stroke. Her physicians wrote that with this background her pain had to be functional, but actually a little study showed that she was dying with a carcinoma of the pancreas!

The explanation for feelings of great fatigue. Often one cannot get the confidence and cooperation of a patient until one has helped him to see why he, whose body appears by all the tests to be healthy, can feel so tired and weak and without any ambition or joy in life.

I often start by telling a patient that I spend my days examining persons like him who complain of fatigue and lack of feelings of "pep" and good health, and that rarely can I find any cancer or focus of infection. Often all I find is an inborn tendency to nervousness, plus a story of overwork or great strain.

Often I have to point out that many tired persons have a sort of nervous breakdown, and then I go into the story to find out if the patient before me has one, and if so, how he came by it. Only if I can satisfy the patient that I know what I am talking about, and only if I can show him how the trouble came, can I hope to convince him or help him.

The reader is referred to Chapters 8, 13, and 15 for more help in understanding nervous breakdowns and fatigue states and depressions.

A patient may have to be reminded that a body kept under great strain should eventually complain or break down. Many a man with a nervous breakdown finds it hard to see why one should have come to him. Then the physician must go back over his history, perhaps with the help of the wife. Oftentimes she is vehement in stating that for years she kept warning him to slow up: that trouble was surely coming to him if he kept on overworking. Finally, he got to the end of his rope and collapsed. Until one can get the man to admit the truth of this story there is little chance of getting him to stop looking for organic disease, and instead, to take a rest.

The need for explaining why the patient broke when he did. After some argument a patient may admit that he overworked for years, and probably had a breakdown coming to him, but he may still be unconvinced because he cannot see why he cracked up when he did. He may maintain that at the time he wasn't under any unusual strain. Perhaps he says he was under a much greater strain six months before. Often the physician cannot answer this objection. He might, perhaps, if he knew all the facts of the man's emotional life at the time. Too often the patient withholds the essential information. For instance, I remember a man whose breakdown was inexplicable until the wife told me that for a time he had been spending his nights gambling and losing large sums of money which were not his to lose. A woman eventually confessed that when she cracked up she was winding up an unhappy love affair; another had been going through a crisis of religious doubt, and another had been suffering panics of fear over her child's tuberculosis.

Sometimes a person who has overworked for years will one day collapse, much as if he had had a little stroke. It is conceivable that he had one in the night, especially when the breakdown came just after a loved one died. Or the patient may have had a slight attack of encephalitis. Often the break comes when the sudden death of a relative or business associate unnerves the man and makes him fear that he will go next. Occasionally a sudden unexplained nervous breakdown is due merely to the working out of a hereditary tendency to a psychosis.

In the case of a constitutionally inadequate woman who breaks down soon after she starts teaching or after she marries or bears her first child, her protest usually is that she cannot be constitutionally frail because, for the first twenty years of her life she was well. The answer is that this is the common story, and there is nothing strange about it. One body cracks after twenty years of strain and another after sixty years or eighty years. It depends on the sort of materials that went into the individual at the time of conception (see Chapter 13).

The need for explaining why a rest cure did not help. Often when one tells a woman that she is in a fatigue state and can be helped only by a good rest she snaps back that she had one and it did no good. Then she cannot be helped until this fact is explained to her satisfaction. Often one finds that the period of rest was too short. Perhaps all a worn-out mother of several children got was a two-weeks' so-called vacation. As I say then, "After your twenty years of over-work and strain you cannot expect to appease an outraged Mother Nature that easily and quickly."

Another common reason for the failure of "a rest" to help is that, although the woman was not working, she was not resting. Perhaps she went on fretting and stewing and worrying, or she failed to get help-ful sleep. Or, although she went on a vacation she took her worry and her unhappiness along with her. Perhaps she took along an un-loved husband who made her the more tense and upset because he was cooped up with her in a hotel room with no office to escape to. The unmarried woman, on her own, and particularly the woman who works in an office to help support a family, may have received no benefit from a vacation because she kept worrying about the expense, or kept won-dering if she would go broke before she could get well enough to go back to work, or kept wondering what her beau at home was doing.

I often think of the athletic young woman with severe nervous symp-toms, who got no help from four months of loafing on the beach at Waikiki. Why? Because, shortly after arrival there she heard from a "friend" that her husband was going out with a blonde, and she was frantic to get back to look into the matter!

I often say to a tired, jittery woman who sadly needs a rest that she might get it if, for a few weeks, she could only turn off her worries and her painful thinking much as she would turn off a radio that was blar-ing loudly. Since she cannot do this, it will probably be months before she feels better. So often the annoyances which led to the breakdown go on unabated, and this makes recovery almost impossible. Perhaps it takes all the self-control the woman has just not to strike back in anger at a nagging sister or mother-in-law who does not conceal her conviction that the illness of the patient is all due to her own "foolish-ness." Perhaps her mother keeps saying, "I told you so!"

Commonly when a tired woman is told that what she needs most is a few months of mornings in bed, her answer is, "Why, I couldn't stay in bed even one day; I'd be so restless I would go crazy." And this shows how tense she is and how badly she needs the rest. She is de-pending on constant activity to keep from thinking. She is like a man who, on the verge of delirium tremens, keeps drinking because alcohol seems to steady his nerves. Many women do this sort of thing; when tortured by painful thoughts they try to find relief in great activity— they clean house, they change the curtains, they do the washing, or they dig in the garden. Oftentimes this helps, but sometimes it makes the woman so much more tired that she cracks up.

On showing that much nervous illness is a price paid for civil-ization. Oftentimes when a patient wants a quick miraculous cure he cannot see why he cannot get it. Then the physician must call his attention to the fact that so long as he lives the strenuous and abnormal life that he does, perhaps as head of a large business, with three telephones constantly ringing on his desk, he can hardly expect to get well or stay well. Often I tell such a fellow of the cultured man whom I once found out in the mountains of the West, running a gas station. He told me he had cracked under the strain of a big law practice in New York and had had to give it up. During his two years of simple life he had had neither a headache nor a stomach-ache. He wasn't making much money but what he got was enough for his needs. As I say to many patients, how I wish that they could do this sort of thing. It could do more for them than several operations.

The significance of aches all over. Often one of the best arguments the physician can give a woman who thinks there is something in her abdomen which ought to be attended to surgically is that she has too many aches and pains all over her body. Hardly any of them could be due to a diseased gallbladder or appendix or ovary, granting that she had such a thing. She may have a headache, a pulling in the back of her eyes, a tension in the back of her neck, pains all through her muscles, a backache, soreness in her chest wall, an ache all down one side of her body, and cramps in her legs.

Even a lay person should be able to see that so many troubles in so many different parts of the body are not likely to be produced by a lesion in one little corner of the abdomen. They are probably being referred out to the periphery from a tired or troubled brain. Even good physicians, while trying to make a diagnosis, often fail to note the great significance of this wide scattering of symptoms. Particularly significant may be the fact, also, that the woman has several purely mental symptoms such as a great fear of going on the street, or into a telephone booth, or of meeting people. These symptoms show that there is much more to her trouble than a supposed cystic ovary.

On patiently answering all objections. One of my colleagues with a flair for the vivid phrase once asked me to take over a nervous patient. He said, "I have talked to her for half an hour but she is still in the 'yes, but,' stage!" In other words, he had not succeeded in answering, to her satisfaction, all her objections to the diagnosis he was trying to give her. He hoped that someone else might bring forth arguments and explanations that would convince and satisfy her. This had to be done if the woman was to be helped at all.

Reassuring the patient who has good reason to doubt the diagnosis. One of the most difficult persons to reassure is the man with, let us say, a headache, who feels sure he has a brain tumor. Why is he so fearful? Because a relative, after having been repeatedly reassured, went blind and died with an obvious tumor of the brain. Every time one tries to cheer the man he says, "Sure, they gave my uncle that baloney for months." One can see why the nephew now feels as he does. About all the physician can say is that he has thought of a brain tumor and has looked most carefully for signs of it, and he is satisfied that the neurologists and the oculists have gone far to rule out the presence of one. Often the most satisfying thing one can say is, "If you had had a brain tumor two years ago, when your trouble appeared, the chances are that by now you would have so many symptoms that the diagnosis would be obvious."

Similarly, many a patient with a peptic ulcer will be dissatisfied with the diagnosis. To much reassurance he will say, "Yes, but for a year my mother was treated for ulcer, and then she suddenly went down hill and died of a cancer." Again, probably the best thing the physician can do is to return the patient for more roentgenologic studies and perhaps gastroscopy.

When a man greatly fears heart disease and is told that his electro-cardiogram is normal, his retort may be that he knows of men who dropped dead shortly after being told that their electrocardiogram was perfect. In these cases I think the physician should explain why this can happen. The man who died probably had an anginal pain which was due only to a narrowing of a coronary artery. Until it plugged up and caused part of the heart muscle to die there was no reason why the electrocardiogram should be abnormal; the electric impulse which makes the electrocardiogram was still traveling over the heart in the usual way. The doctor might go on to say that in these cases a good physician can usually make the diagnosis of a dangerously narrowed artery because of the typical pain which comes on exertion. If a man has no symptoms of a narrowed artery or of a failing heart, he need not go in fear of sudden death.

Answering the argument that patients diagnosed as having a functional complaint come back later with organic disease. Many a patient, when told that the results of all his tests were negative, remains dissatisfied. He fears that in a year or two he will come back to be told, "Sorry, we made a mistake; apparently you had a cancer; we missed it and now it is inoperable."

Unfortunately, mistakes can happen, and every so often the ablest of internists will be saddened to hear that with all his testing he failed to recognize or to view with concern a few signs that pointed to the presence of a carcinoma of the pancreas, a brain tumor, a duodenal ulcer, or a beginning encephalitis. The most hopeful thing I can tell a person who fears such an oversight is that some studies have been made to see how often such mistakes are made, and the evidence indicated that when histories are well taken and examinations are thorough, oversights are not common.

In 1934, Macy and Allen reviewed the records of 235 patients who returned to the Mayo Clinic for reexamination on an average of six and one-half years after a diagnosis had been made of "chronic nervous exhaustion." The symptoms complained of by most of these patients had been nervousness, headache, fatigue, palpitation, bloating, belching, soreness of the abdomen, constipation, eructation of food, vague distresses, insomnia, emotional instability, and feelings of depression.

In 85 per cent of the cases no organic disease had appeared during the interval. Some 9 per cent of the patients returned with organic disease, but in all but a few of these cases this was something like cancer which, because of the time interval, probably started to grow a long time after the patient was at the Clinic and given his clean bill of health. In the remaining 6 per cent of the total number of cases the organic disease discovered might conceivably have been present at the first examination and responsible for the symptoms then complained of. In three of these fourteen cases the disease was encephalitis, in two it was hyperthyroidism, and in three, tuberculosis.

Interestingly, in all but four of these fourteen cases, organic disease had been so strongly suspected from the history that it had been looked for with special care, but the little evidence that had been found had been deemed insufficient to warrant a diagnosis. In only a few, then, of the 235 cases did it seem highly probable that there had been an oversight in diagnosis which could have been avoided if more care had been taken or if the patient had been urged to come back in a few months for reexamination. Doubtless there were other such cases in which the patient never returned to Rochester. Unfortunately, this was not a follow-up study with a 100 per cent coverage.

A similar study of 354 cases of "functional indigestion" was made in 1938 by Wilbur and Mills. Some seven years after the first examination they found that 85.6 per cent of these patients who returned for a check-up were still without signs of organic disease. In this series the commonest disease that had been missed was peptic ulcer. The mistake was made usually because the roentgenologist could not see the suspected lesion or any puckering of the duodenum.

These studies are encouraging. They are the more encouraging when one remembers that by the time most persons with chronic and puzzling disease have reached a consultant they have had a number of examinations and some have had a surgical exploration of the abdomen. When the results of all these examinations are negative, and *especially when the symptoms are typically those of a neurosis,* the chances are large that organic disease has not been missed and is not present. As I often say to a patient, "If, as you say, several able physicians have examined you thoroughly and have told you that your trouble is a neurosis, is it not possible that all were right? Might it not be a good idea now to accept their diagnosis and to follow the treatment they advised? You might give it at least a short trial!"

The use of stories in explaining things. I could not practice medicine without the help of many illustrative stories. The physician should remember that all able influencers of men, like old politicians, are always driving home their points with the help of a good story, and especially one that quickly paints a vivid picture. Christ did most of His teaching with simple parables or stories, which ever since have greatly influenced the speech and thinking of mankind. A homely story easily reaches the understanding of everyone; it makes a point vividly, and often more convincingly than would any amount of argument. It is likely to influence the person's behavior. On the other hand, an abstract statement is hard to grasp; it is likely to go over the head of all but the well educated, and it may not convince or influence even them. For instance, often when I am trying to talk a patient out of an operation which I think would be worse than the disease, all I have to do is to quote the Chinese who say, "Don't call in a tiger to chase away a dog."

The wise physician, much of whose work each day is that of a teacher and influencer of behavior, will do well, then, often to tell illustrative stories. They must be very brief (1) because the doctor's time is short and (2) because most sick persons quickly tire; their attention wanders or they start talking. Hence, a story is not good if it takes more than a minute in the telling.

To show what I mean, when I want quickly to show a woman most of what she needs to know about the dependence of migraine on the strain of life, I do not give her a textbook explanation. I just tell her of the sweet old bishop who, inheriting a tendency to migraine from his mother, had a terrible time with it while working his way through college and on up the ladder to the day when he got a fine church, a pastor's assistant, and a smoothly running routine. After this, with his life happy and fairly easy, he went twenty-five years without a headache. At sixty, they made him a bishop, and then, what with overwork and annoyance and strain, the old migraines came back to strike him down every few days. With this story, I quickly show the woman why there is no need for exhaustive examinations of her body, why she will not be cured by the removal of her teeth or tonsils, her gallbladder or her uterus, and why I want her to live more quietly and peacefully and sensibly.

CHAPTER 27

What Can the Patient Do to Help Himself

OFTENTIMES A PATIENT WILL say to his physician, "Well, if my trouble is due to nervousness what can I do about it? Just how can I help myself?" Unfortunately the physician is usually too busy to give much of an answer, and if he did have time and wanted to practice some psychotherapy, he might not know how to go at it. During his years in college no instruction was ever given him in this most important subject. Books have been written on it, many for laymen. All of them contain some good ideas, and thousands of persons are doubtless now getting some help from them. I shall give the titles of a few of these books at the end of this volume. Thousands of persons are getting help, also, from magazines such as Woman's Life, Your Health, and Your Marriage. Today innumerable men and women are searching for suggestions as to how they can become more normal nervously and psychically.

It is hard to write a chapter like this without saying much that may sound trite and schoolmasterish, and yet it seems worth writing. Physicians need help in formulating what they can say when an occasional patient asks for a little advice on remaking his life and getting over bad habits. Too often all the doctor can think to say is "Forget it," which does not help much.

On finding out why one is unhappy. One of the first things a vaguely unhappy man should do is to try, perhaps with the help of a physician, to put into words, clearly, what his dissatisfactions are. As Wendell Johnson says, perhaps when he gets this done and sees what is wrong he will not be so unhappy, or he will see what he can quickly do to remedy what is bothering him.

A good example of the way some persons flounder about mentally is given by Wendell Johnson. On page 248 of his book (1946), he told of a young man who, when asked by the university counselor what his difficulty was, replied, "Why, I can't—that is, I am not . . . , I am not . . . , I am not sure I know. That is . . . , well, a professor of mine, one of my professors, he said that he thought that I . . . , maybe it was that . . . , he feels that . . . , well, that I have trouble expressing what I want to say." What the boy was trying to say was, that his father had wanted him to be a physician; that he had flunked his premedical course, and now he did not know what to do. He was all at sea and did not know how to replan his life.

An artistically gifted young man with a good job in his father's bank was drinking and nearly wrecking his marriage and his life. When asked what he was unhappy about he was not sure, but his wife explained that he had no interest in stocks and bonds but wanted to write plays. Doubtless, if he had had more guts, he could have done what he wanted to do, but he lacked the drive to spend all his spare time in studying and writing. He just went on dreaming of what he might have been, and blaming his father for his failure to achieve happiness.

The world is full of persons like that. They seem to be waiting always for a Guggenheim Fellowship which would enable them to go abroad for study. They forget that many a busy man, earning a good living for his family, in spare time writes or paints or develops professional skill in some hobby. One of America's greatest painters was forced by his family to work in a store, but whenever his father went out on an errand, the young man grabbed his paints, retired to a back room, and went to work. He succeeded in spite of every handicap put in his way.

On trying to improve one's life. The first thing, of course, for many a person, is to face the fact that he himself has been messing up his life; that he has not been living wisely, and that his troubles are self-made. So long as he tries to save his "face," and so long as he blames society, his parents, his wife, people "who had it in for him," or his bad luck, he will not get anywhere.

As Fosdick has said, when the prodigal son went into a far country, he had a high opinion of himself; he thought his mother and father had made mistakes in his upbringing; he despised his industrious brother, who he thought was just a plodding stick-in-the-mud; and he thought he was going to be a traveler, a polished man of the world, and a "big shot." Later, after misfortune had knocked the conceit out of him, "He came to himself," and he had the sense to go back home and say, "Father, I have sinned." Because there are some persons who can come to themselves and say, "I have sinned; now show me what I must do, and I will try to do it," we physicians must be on the watch for them, and prepared to help them.

The first thing, then, that many a man must do is to realize that the job of remaking his life is up to him. The next thing he must do is to *want very much to reform* and to regain health and happiness. Too often he is like the child who said, "I wish I wanted to do that." He would like the results but he will not tackle the hard work. The next thing he must get is faith that with hard work he can do much to help himself and to win through to success. He must resolve, also, that he will keep up the fight for self-improvement in spite of repeated discouragements.

Many an unhappy man wastes endless time and gets himself down in the dumps by repeatedly trying to analyze his failures. He should stop this foolish practice. It is all right to confess his sins once, but that is enough. He must not keep brooding over the mistakes of the past; it is better just to buckle down to work. Let a man live sensibly for a while and then he can see how it feels, and what the new way of life can do for his happiness and that of his loved ones.

If his situation in shop or office is almost unendurable the man should try hard to get out of it. Many a man should quickly get out of a blind-alley job and look for one in which he can work his way up, or one in which he can be happy. Any man who expects to get ahead in this world must constantly be studying his job and preparing for advancement. Many a man who is handicapped by lack of an education could be getting it from correspondence or extension courses. Many a woman, caught in an unhappy marriage, should make up her mind quickly either to get out of it or else to stay in and no longer fret at the bars. Many a single woman, caught in an uninteresting job where she never meets marriageable men, should move to a better job in a better city. It takes courage, but the girl will not starve to death if she makes the move.

In order to reform one must have an inner spark. I realize that most of the persons who need the suggestions offered in this chapter are of a type who will never read them or be willing or able to act on them. Others who might try them would soon backslide and give up. We physicians must keep watching for those persons with a certain spark in them who are looking for help and who much want to get well. Monica Baldwin said in *I Leap Over the Wall*—"If you fail to get what you want it is simply because you have not 'wanted' it with sufficient passion and intensity" (p. 289). Often all a person needs is to be made to see that his troubles are not physical but mental, and that the mental trouble is curable.

Avoiding the wrong turning. Many men drift in this world or remain for years unhappy in a poor job that someone gave them. A wise man directs the course of his life, and when offered one or more opportunities, he chooses the one that will take him farthest along the road he wants to travel. Obviously, he must have a chosen road; he must know where he wants to go. Sometimes he will choose the job with the smaller salary if it will give him a greater opportunity for advancement and soul-satisfying work, and if it will take him in the direction in which he wants to go. I have known scientists who wisely turned down positions carrying two and three times the salary they were getting. Why? Because the new work would have taken them out of the current which was carrying them to success in a chosen field, or it would have taken them out of their beloved research and into an administrative position.

Often, for years after having taken a wrong turning, a man will suffer from regret, and will lose his morale. A few unfortunates, early in life, and perhaps in great need of money, will make the mistake of going to work for an employer with a bad reputation, and then they may be unhappy pariahs for the rest of their days. They can never live down that early mistake. The troubles about helping such persons when they come with a neurosis are (1) that the doctor may not be able to put much sense into them, (2) they may have become bitter at society and not amenable to reason, or (3) there may be no way of erasing the mistake and starting over again.

On stopping to look where one is going in this world, and why. All of us men and women need to stop occasionally to think a bit, and wonder where we are going, if anywhere, and why we are working so hard. A fine book for anyone who wonders where he is going, and why, is Philip Barry's play *Holiday*. It tells of a man, orphaned, who throughout boyhood and young manhood had to work terribly hard just to keep alive and get some education. Then he made a lot of money, and with this he decided to take a holiday in which he was going to sit and do a lot of thinking; he wanted to figure out what life was all about, what goal was worth aiming at, and what accomplishment in life would make him most happy. In the last few years a number of the men who came out of war service have been doing this sort of thing: They have gone to college, they have obtained an education, and they have struck out on a new career.

Living each day in a compartment. One of Osler's best bits of advice was to live each day in "a day-tight compartment," worrying little about the dangers of the morrow and wasting few regrets on the mistakes and sorrows of the past. It would be wonderful if all nervous patients could follow this maxim. Some, of course, *must* worry about the future. The mother with a sick child or the man caught, over-extended, with a big inventory and falling prices, must sleep poorly. But it would seem that everyone ought to be able to avoid the habit of often living over the mistakes of the past.

Sometimes a person can be given the idea of writing off mistakes and thinking no more about them. I often tell patients about a telephone conversation I once could not help overhearing as, in 1931, I sat in the office of a country banker. Evidently, before 1929, a subordinate had loaned money on a group of poor farms which had not paid well. The banker asked his farm expert what it would cost to rehabilitate the properties. When told the figure, he said, "We could never get that much money back, so get rid of the land for anything it will bring, and we'll write off the loss." Then he cheerfully turned his attention to the next problem, and in this way, evidently, he worked all day. As I saw this man make his quick decisions I thought how wonderful it would be if hundreds of my patients could learn the trick; if they could only learn to forget mistakes, and never think of them again except perhaps to vow never to fall into that particular trap again. If only they could learn, also, to leave emotion out of the process. It is painful emotion that causes most of the distress and the fatigue.

"Burning one's own smoke." A fine thing that Osler said was that we humans should all burn our own smoke—in other words, keep quiet about our discomforts and never inflict the long account of them on someone else. Not only would other persons be saved annoyance but we ourselves would be happier and healthier.

I belong to a mountain club whose first unwritten law goes some-thing like this: "Thou shalt never utter the least word of complaint to the management or thy neighbor if, on an outing trip, it rains all day and all night and if then thy sheet of oiled silk leaks and drips water on thy head, or if the pack train is late and thy sleeping bag and thy food do not arrive." For years I went on expeditions with this club. Many an evening found us wet, cold, hungry, weary, and without shel-ter, but never did I hear anyone complain. To grouse was the un-pardonable sin. How wonderful if this idea could be adopted whole-heartedly by many of our neurotic and unhappy patients. It is, of course, the immature childish person who cries and whines when un-comfortable; he did it when he was a baby and he keeps doing it now when he is fifty.

One of the worst habits of hundreds of thousands of men and women is to talk along by the hour, in a monologue, telling again and again in detail and at endless length of their annoyances and hurt feelings, and the injustices done them by relatives, children, neighbors, or employers. Eventually they have to live alone because no one can long stand the endless clatter of their tongues and the endless repetition of already well-known stories. The world is full of such horrible bores. Often they make themselves ill by this constant reliving of unpleasant happenings.

Hoarding energies and making decisions quickly. The asthenic, constitutionally inadequate or migrainous person needs to be exhorted to hoard energy and not waste it on things that do not count. Many persons are constantly spending ten dollars worth of emotion on a tencent problem or accomplishment.

One way in which to hoard energies is to make decisions quickly and easily and finally. Many persons keep reopening a subject again and again long after it was well settled.

Dr. W. J. Mayo once told me that with so many demands on his time each day he avoided doing anything that he did not feel was important. He avoided giving any more time than was needed to a decision.

Many a woman becomes tired partly because of her inability to make decisions. She will wrestle with a problem all night and never settle it. I tell her that a physician has to make important decisions all day: Here a leg must be taken off, and there a breast. A life often depends on the correctness of his judgment and the quickness of his decision. If he can make such decisions about big things she should learn to make them about little things. One thing a woman often needs to do is not to start worrying about a decision long before the question comes up for consideration. In many cases it will never come up and then if she has fretted over it she will have wasted her time. All unimportant decisions should be made in a moment and then stuck to, unless some very good reason comes up for making a change. Many men, of course, are just as reluctant as are some of their sisters to make decisions.

Tackling each job quickly. Many a nervous person needs to learn to face his problems squarely and then to tackle them quickly. The trouble with many neurotic or mildly psychotic persons is that they always put off decisions and slide out of facing difficult problems. They also put off starting on a difficult job. I remember a storekeeper who, at the end of each day, should have sat right down and straightened out his cash. But, hating the job, he would decide first to smoke a cigarette and then he would smoke another. Then, perhaps, he would go out to visit some crony, or he might drop in at a bar for a drink or two or three. Gradually he would get more and more dilatory until he would get to tackling the job around 2 in the morning! After months of this he would drift into a nervous breakdown, due largely to the lack of sleep and rest.

The sensible businessman, on reaching his office in the morning, immediately tackles the hardest problems while his brain is fresh. Quickly he answers his mail and cleans off his desk. He sees his associates and makes all the decisions that can be made that day. Such a man gets much done, and he does it without much fatigue.

Avoiding habits of tension. Most nervous persons need advice in regard to the avoidance of getting tense over everything they do. They must try to learn to work easily, without the tension that comes from trying to go too fast, or to do several things at a time. Worst of all sometimes is a tendency to look ahead at the job, finished, or to work while annoyed over the number of persons waiting to be seen. I remember a physician who used to get demoralized whenever he knew that many persons were in his waiting room. The strain which often wrecked him came not from his work but from his anxiety to keep fairly close to his schedule of appointments. Similarly, I knew a bank teller who would go to pieces nervously whenever he saw several persons in line in front of his cage. His greatest need was to learn to pay no attention to any but the man right in front of his window. Migrainous persons are particularly likely to get tense trying to finish things too fast and to do more than one thing at a time. Many of them are bedeviled by the feeling that a job must be done by a certain time.

Many tense nervous patients have been helped by Stewart Edward White's story of the old mountaineer who used to sit and watch him as he built a cabin in the Sierras. One day, as White was sawing through a log as rapidly as he could, the old fellow said, "When you city fellows saw you just can't wait to get that log sawed in two. Now, when I saw, I just saws." It would be wonderful if many nervous persons could just saw; in other words, if they would just do the work at hand and not worry about when it is supposed to be finished.

One of the best indexes of a person's tenseness is the tightness and soreness of the muscles at the back of the neck. Many persons get their headaches there because of this tension. Often, when such a person cannot sleep, if he would only stop and relax his muscles, he would find that he was so tense that he was holding his head slightly off the pillow. One can relax such tension voluntarily but it is hard to keep it relaxed. Doubtless, many persons are born to be tense in this way, and it is hard for them to do anything about it, but still, they should keep trying.

Jacobson has written books on the art of voluntarily relaxing one's muscles. It would be wonderful to learn the art but I fear most persons cannot do it. It would take constant watchfulness. Especially if the person has a tendency to insomnia he should try to keep his evenings restful, avoiding anything which experience has shown him will produce tenseness. A quiet evening makes for a good night's sleep.

Many persons must try to learn to even sit and *wait* without getting tense. For instance, a lecturer's train was seven hours late and it was very doubtful if he could reach his audience on time. If he had followed his impulse he would have paced the floor like a madman, but wisely he said to himself, "That will not get me there any sooner. All it will do will be to get me into a dither." Accordingly, he opened his brief case, got out some papers, and calmly went to work. Luckily he did, because the train did get him to his destination on time.

Avoiding internal frictions. Much fatigue and nervous illness is produced by internal frictions or conflicts between two parts of a person's personality. One half of him may be good, sensible, kindly, and generous, and the other half may be mean, selfish, unpleasant, mischievous, trouble making, vindictive, soul searching, or too religious. Sometimes a woman will say that she hasn't yet been able to fuse or amalgamate the two natures which she got, one from, let us say, her father's good, fine, religious stock, and the other from her mother's wild, hard-drinking tribe.

Some persons of this type exhaust themselves at times by great contrition over petty or even imagined sins. I like Rigg's way of saying to these persons with a New England conscience that, "One must take one's essential decency for granted!" Sometimes it helps these people to tell them that probably most fine and essentially good persons occasionally do things which are not consistent with the bulk of their character. They have to accept this behavior as common to mankind. Perhaps the patient would be helped by reading Pepys' *Diary*. There he would see the frank confessions of an unusually able and essentially good man who, at times, acted despicably.

Many men and women worry because evil thoughts come to them—perhaps sexual desires, or realizations that the death of someone would bring promotion, or freedom to marry, or freedom from constant care and financial drain. They are horrified at such thoughts, and often they do penance for them. They must be told that such thoughts occur to the best of persons. Sexual thoughts *should* occur to all persons who are normally sexed, and they constitute no sin. The realization that an aged dependent's death would have great advantages is also inevitable; it must come at times, and there is no need for having horrors over it. It is foolish to do penance for it and thus to make oneself ill. No one can blame himself for being struck by a fleeting evil thought; he can be blamed only if he harbors it *and acts on it*.

Sometimes I tell an overly religious person worrying about his peccadilloes and wondering how distressed Heaven is about them, that probably the Lord is so busy with other more weighty matters that He is not greatly upset or concerned. Often I point out, also, that such fretting on the part of an individual is usually a sign of a very selfish and self-centered nature. Usually while a woman is fretting herself sick over some peccadillo, she is being a poor wife and mother, and is hurting an innocent husband and innocent children in a cruel way. She ought to be far more concerned over this behavior—a big fault—than about the little fault. The physician can point out, also, to the man who is terribly concerned over the sins which he thought of committing but didn't, that since St. Peter gives us no credit for the good deeds that we planned but never got around to doing, he will almost certainly give us no black mark for the sins we thought of but didn't commit!

Day after day many a person has to fight against feelings of dislike for others. He has to fight against envies and jealousies, and he has to watch out that he does not show any sign of them or demean himself by acting upon any of them.

All of us would do well to be more tolerant of the inefficiencies and mistakes of others around us. We must try to be more patient, remembering always that sometimes we too forget and make mistakes. Such charity could save us a lot of nervous energy. Women who are much annoyed by the stupidities of a maid should remember that if the girl had half the sense they have she'd have her own home and would not be working out.

Certainly, it would be a wonderful thing if all of us could so keep at peace with ourselves that we could throw all of our energies into our work. Then we would have joy and better health.

Avoiding irascibility. Many persons are too easily angered and annoyed. They are irascible and hot tempered, and they "explode" or "blow up" before they know what they are doing. That a man can hold in if he really wants to is shown by the fact that a salesman practically never blows up in the face of a buyer. Most of his blowing-up is done at loved ones or at subordinates in the office or store. My impression is that a tantrum of temper must hurt the nervous system of persons even when they appear to be callous to the sufferings of those who are "bawled out." The person who is not entirely callous can hardly help but feel disturbed by seeing his victims hurt or sullen or weepy for the rest of the day. Certainly, "blowing his top" can run a man's blood pressure up or it can stir up an ulcer. It can also produce a very troublesome neurosis in a wife or child or business associate.

Many a patient has told me that his physician advised him to let his temper fly so as to get his anger off his chest, but I am sure this is wrong. Surely, self-control is immensely better for everyone concerned. Perhaps, after years of such control, the person will no longer get so

angry at every small annoyance or what he used to think
front. Then life will become much more comfortable for
certainly he will be much more popular at home and in his
will no longer be feared, and I think he will be more healthy

All people, as they grow older, are likely to become irri...... and
impatient, and the wise person watches for this tendency and fights it.
Most aging animals show this increase in irascibility. A young gorilla
or young lion may be a lovable pet, showing much affection for his
owner, but as he grows older he gets ugly, and then he becomes so
dangerous that he has to be kept always in a cage.

Learning to get along easily with people. One of the greatest
arts to be learned in this life, especially by all nervous, irritable, and
impatient persons, is that of getting along easily with people, without
much conflict. Everyone should keep studying and learning this art,
first in the family group, next in the school, and finally in the world of
business. Parents should constantly be praying a little prayer: "May
we so raise these children of ours that all their days they can live easily
and comfortably and happily with their fellows in home and office and
shop and drawing room!" This thought could be immensely more helpful in the long run than the modern one of never interfering with the
personality of the little darlings!

How often one hears it said of some unusual man that he has a
marvelous asset in his affability and friendliness and courteous ways.
Everyone likes him, and hence his path through life is easy. Why then
shouldn't all young persons try quickly to learn to meet people easily,
smilingly, and with friendliness. They should learn to so behave as
never to offend others needlessly.

The wise man should learn to keep out of violent and useless arguments. When some question comes up he will give in quickly on all
unessential points, and especially on all points on which the other fellow
may well be in the right. A person should never argue at length just for
the sake of an argument or to have his or her own way. A woman wanting to go out to a movie will suggest to her husband that they go. He
will say, "All right, dear, if you wish it, I'll take you." Then she will
start arguing with him and protesting, much as if he had proposed to
drag her out into a rainy night against her will. He will answer that
he does not care one way or another, but this will annoy her because
she wants him to beg her to come with him. But he does not realize
that this is her idea, and so they just keep arguing until both are out
of patience and ill humored.

The wise person is not always demanding his or her "rights." The
paranoid person is inclined to do this. The sane person sees often
that to fight for what he feels are his rights will be too costly in energy

and in the esteem of those about him. He will do better to go along
with things as they are and not be a fighter and a nuisance.

The wise person learns always to be fair and generous; he will see
the other fellow's side of the argument and will try to compromise and
meet him half way. The wise man will even prefer to pay a little more
for something than it is worth rather than to make a fuss over a little
money. The wise man will get on amicably with his employers, his
immediate boss, and his fellow workers. Much labor trouble has come
because many bosses are bawlers-out. The man who never bawls out
employees but talks to them quietly and calmly saves wear and tear on
his nervous system.

A sensible person is not touchy, and if he is hurt a bit he will not
show it or discuss it or make an issue of it. The wise man will never
carry grudges or hold resentments. They are too costly in nervous
energy. A kind man will forgive quickly and will never try to pay back
an injury or an affront with another injury. He will not expect much
from others; he will know that their time is taken up with their own
thoughts and problems and tasks. If he does not expect much he will
not be hurt when he does not get much in the way of recognition or
attention or thanks.

Many men lose out in life because of their uncompromising attitudes.
In every organization there are many unwritten laws, and the man who
expects to get along happily and easily and smoothly will not transgress
many of them. When he does try to change a law he will go about it
slowly and tactfully so as not to stir up a hornet's nest against him.

The world is full of men who, because of their great dislike for any
compromise, or any supervision or direction, have to work alone. They
cannot work with groups, or they cannot work for a boss. Much of
the strain on men in organizations is due to the fact that so much that
they work at and plan is subject to review or pigeonholing by others.
Their pet project on which they have worked so hard may be torn to
pieces, or done over, or handed to someone else, or scrapped. The wise
man who must work in a group must learn to take these disappointments
philosophically, even when he feels sure that he was right and his superiors were wrong.

Conforming easily to many rules of society. I was much impressed one day by a statement made by a willful girl of eighteen who
was ill because for some time she had been fighting with her mother.
The girl's complaint was that the mother was always thwarting her
desire to do this or that. She said, "Just wait until I am of age, and
then *I am going to do everything I please."*

After thinking a moment, I said to the girl, "I fear that when you
are grown up you will find that you still cannot, or *you had better not,*

do many of the things that you will want to do. I am of age but there are scores of things that I cannot do. I have no mother to chide me; but if I were to do certain proscribed things, my colleagues who work beside me, or the members of my profession, or my neighbors, or my wife would somehow punish me or make me very uncomfortable. In other words, I *could* transgress certain unwritten laws but the cost to me in discomfort and the loss of the approval and good will and liking of those about me would be too great. And so I acquiesce to the rules and the mores of my community. You, too, will have to learn to do this."

It is best to live sensibly, pretty much as others do, because the world has so many ways of striking back at those persons who refuse to conform, and who try to go their own way. Often the world insists on conformity. This fact is well expressed in the limerick:

> There was an old man of Thermopylae,
> Who never did anything properly,
> But they said, 'If you choose
> To boil eggs in your shoes,
> You cannot remain in Thermopylae.'

This is one of the cleverest jingles ever written because it expresses so well an important truth. The leader and the thinker must always pay something in solitariness and isolation for their originality, but they can make life more easy for themselves by conforming in most fields of behavior.

Avoiding resentments and grudges. The wise man will avoid holding resentments and grudges if only because they can poison him physically, probably with chemical toxins formed in the body. The deepest resentments we humans have are often mixed up with love or jealousy, or with feelings that the loved one has let us down. Such painful emotions are particularly destructive of peace of mind and even of health. As Mrs. Henry Wallace is reported to have said, "I can't bear to hate, it hurts me." I tell people that the hated person goes scot free while the hater is made miserable and ill. Haters should remember, also, that one cannot get happiness by trying to take it away from someone else.

Many husbands and wives are tortured by mixtures of love and resentment. They cannot bear to live apart, and yet they cannot get along when they are together. Unfortunately, when a physician tries to straighten them out, and they promise to reform and get together again, they keep see-sawing back and forth: When one is ready for a reconciliation the other gets to thinking of old hurts; he or she wants to punish a little more, and so the fight goes on.

The wise and big man pays little attention to slights, and if he meets a person who once dealt with him unfairly, he will act as if nothing had happened. He will be on his guard but he will avoid starting any unpleasantness. Eventually his enemy may lose his animosity and may stop trying to cause trouble.

To show how stupid and childish some resentments are, when the car of a certain choleric man got loose on a hill and rolled down and stopped against a bush, he was so angry at it that he borrowed a blacksmith's hammer and demolished the engine! "That would show it!" Another man was even more illogical: While sitting in an outside toilet he was stung by a hornet. Enraged and unable to get at the hornet, he knocked over the little building and burned it to the ground!

Quite a few persons easily and frequently become enraged at some inanimate object like a drawer that sticks or a shade that will not go up. One morning one of my patients, angered because the coffee was bad, grabbed the pot and all the dishes on the table, and threw them out of the window!

Fighting jealousy and envy. Men and women must often fight desperately against jealousy and distrust of those they love. In the case of many persons, jealousy goes on torturing in spite of the fact that it has little, if any, basis. It may help the jealous person to be often reminded of the fact that his suspicions, his accusations, and his spying will eventually destroy the love which he seems to desire so greatly. Sometimes a jealous man needs to be reminded, also, that the most foolish thing he could do would be to spy on his loved one and thereby get proof of her interest in another man. Then he would be utterly miserable, and having angered his wife, he might lose her entirely. Many a sensible man, when in doubt about the love of his wife, refuses to check up on her. He does not want to know the worst.

Innumerable persons are painfully jealous of the people who work alongside them, and some spend much time and energy in efforts to pull down or hold back the more successful of their fellow workers. An official of one of America's great corporations once told me why his company was in serious financial trouble. He said that after their old Chief died there were five able men left near the top, any one of whom might have made a good president. But every time one of these men tried to do something constructive the other four ganged up on him and kept him from accomplishing anything. They spent almost as much time blocking each other as they did on their regular work.

Probably no physician could do much about reforming any one of these men. About all he could do would be to understand the frustration and neurosis some of these men drifted into, with insomnia, and nocturnal attacks of belching, heartburn, and extrasystoles.

Adjusting well to marriage. It is worth remembering that Dr. Tooth, of the British Navy, found that 25 per cent of the 284 invalided sailors whom he studied broke down, not because of the horrors of war, but because of worry over a bad situation at home. It is worth remembering, also, that today perhaps one in three marriages is ending in the divorce courts. As I pointed out in Chapter 11, there are many persons who could never stay happily married with anyone because they are too childish in their behavior. They constantly behave like selfish, willful, and undisciplined children who want their own way, and who will kick and scream (or some equivalent) if they do not get it.

Often I say to these persons, "If you break up this marriage your next one will be just as unhappy and unsuccessful because of your lack of self-control and adult behavior." Usually when a man reaches his third divorce he gets frightened and says, "There must be something wrong with me." And there is! Even if one finds that much of the blame can be put on the three wives, the man must still be culpable. Perhaps he drinks too much or is unable to leave pretty women alone; or, as more than one such man has said to me, "When it comes to choosing a wife I have no sense; I always pick a good-looking devil."

In many cases, even when the spouses behave most of the time in an adult way, the big difficulty seems to have been that one or both had the idea that when a person is once married, there is no need for adjustments in living or for further courtship. Thousands of women today are unhappy because they have a type of husband who goes his way much as if he were a bachelor.

When people who have been much in love are fighting, "rocking the boat," and talking of divorce, they should stop and think of the loneliness and mental distress that may come to them if they break up. One or both may then go into "outer darkness" in which there is no happiness. Some married couples need to be reminded that divorce will separate them only legally. One of the partners may remain dependent on the other, often telephoning for help and advice and comfort.

Oftentimes there would be no divorce if the man would realize how wonderful might be his reward if he would only court his wife a bit and try to show love *in acceptable ways*. I have known many men who were puzzled because when they gave their wife money or some expensive gift she wept. They could not see why she would have been much happier with a little remembrance of an anniversary, perhaps with a rose and a cute note, or an invitation to a chummy supper out somewhere. She so much wanted an occasional vacation together, or more real friendship and companionship and fun. Often a wife is unhappy over her gift because it is something for the house or something that shows that the husband had no idea of what she wanted or loved or was then interested in. Often, also, the wife craves some expression of love in words, or some favorable notice of her appearance or dress.

Unfortunately, most husbands do not realize that efforts toward making their marriage happier could pay richly; such efforts could go farther to produce good mental health than efforts made in any other line of endeavor.

Often the wife is the one most at fault because she is selfish and thinks little of trying to make the husband happy. She shows him little affection; she never thanks him for kindnesses, she runs a poor home, or she does not make him feel comfortable in it; she may not be willing to put herself out to be nice to him or his friends, and she may not make an effort even to look nice for him. (For more on marriage, see Chapter 11.)

Overcoming shyness. Shy persons should constantly be telling themselves that they are much more concerned about how they appear and what they say or do than other persons will ever be about them. Other people are absorbed in their own problems. The sensitive person long remembers his own embarrassing moments, but he promptly forgets the gauche things other people did or said in his presence. Every time, then, that he starts worrying about some slip of the tongue he can say to himself, "The other fellow probably did not notice it, or if he did, he will soon forget it."

The shy person would get along easily in public if he were to spend his time being interested, not in himself, but in the people he meets. Often when he has been silent he says, "I didn't know what to say," or "I couldn't think of anything to say." He could probably have handled the situation very easily by asking the people about him what they had been doing lately that was of interest. They would gladly have told him.

The shy person should keep going out into society and making friends. He should join clubs or groups because to be accepted by them is reassuring and satisfying. Some young men are much helped by joining classes in public speaking. It helps many a shy person to keep appearing in public and doing the things that, at first, are very hard for him to do. In my youth the giving of a paper at a medical society made me physically ill. I had terrible stage fright, but I kept forcing myself to speak in public until, after a few years, I could do it without any distress; in fact, I could even enjoy it.

Often it helps greatly if a shy and unhappy young woman will look in her mirror and accept the fact that she is not a bad-looking girl, and that she has good eyes and pretty hair and a trim body. What then is she doing with an inferiority complex? She hasn't anything to feel ashamed of. If she feels she hasn't enough education let her study hard and get more. I once had as a patient a nice-looking young woman from a poor home who wanted to marry a well-to-do man but knew that she should not because she hadn't enough savoire faire. I induced her to give up her secretarial job and to work for a time as a maid in the lovely home of cultured people. There, she learned much that she needed to know about home making, preparing and serving attractive meals, and being at ease among educated people. Many an unhappy girl would feel like a new person if she would only keep going to a dancing school until she became a graceful dancer.

It is doubtful if the shy, schizoid person will ever entirely rid himself of his curse, but with steady effort over the years he ought eventually to be much more comfortable with people.

Avoiding debauches of emotion. Many persons suffer much from their stormy emotions. They feel disagreements too strongly; they get "all steamed up" over little annoyances, and they make it hard for themselves to live with people.

Unfortunately, much of the overemotionalism a physician sees is inborn and hard to help, but the fact that one sees most of it in women indicates that the men, who presumably also inherited the tendency, are too busy every day to indulge themselves in riots of emotion. If the men can keep themselves calm, the women should also learn the art.

A physician must remonstrate with the woman who keeps going into debauches of emotion over unhappinesses of the past. Some of them spend nights thinking of what they might have done to avoid some accident or illness which injured a loved one. They keep saying, "If only I had not asked my sister to go on that automobile ride," or, "If only I had asked for another surgeon," or "If only I had taken sister to another hospital," and so on and so on.

I remember an old maid who used to spend much of her time after work brooding over her folly in once driving away a fine man who was going to marry her. Having hurt his feelings and puzzled him by ugly behavior during a premenstrual tension spell, she would not explain or apologize, and so he left.

Fighting worry. The man who has good cause for worry often must go on worrying until perhaps his business gets on its feet or a sick wife or child recovers. The man who most needs help is the one who worries almost insanely over fears that he knows are practically groundless, fears such as that of dropping dead, going insane, getting crippled with arthritis, or dying of cancer. A man of this worrying type often carries every type of insurance that he can buy, and still he worries. Every day and all day he is anxious and uneasy and fearful about something.

Obviously, the first thing such a person should do, when he fears ill health, is to get thoroughly examined by a good physician or clinic.

Then, if told he is all right, he should take comfort in the reassurance. He should not keep going the rounds of doctors behaving as if he hoped desperately that someone would reverse the good verdict and confirm his worst fears!

Some persons must accept a certain amount of disability or discomfort. This is much better than demanding bodily perfection, and in trying to get it, submitting to one futile operation after the other. When doctors disagree, the worrisome person had better take the opinion of an eminent consultant rather than that of some man who has had no special training in caring for the disease that the person thinks he has.

Because worry is one of the great causes of nervous illness, fatigue, and unhappiness, every person who is born with a tendency to it should make a big effort to fight the habit. The old advice of our ancestors not to cross a bridge until you come to it is still excellent, as is the Irishman's injunction not "to be afther barking y'r shins on a stuhl that ain't there." As we all know, most of the things we worried about during our lifetime never came to pass.

There are many bad worriers who cannot be reassured because they feel that if the physician found cancer he would lie to them and say he hadn't found anything. A patient might ask his doctor if he would show him the original reports from roentgenologists, laboratory workers, pathologists, and surgeons and would explain their significance. This might reassure him.

A sample of stupid worry is that of the woman of thirty-five who begins worrying for fear that at fifty, when she has the menopause, she will go crazy. Another woman worried because her husband would not worry, and another worried much because her old pain left her! She wondered where it had gone!

Fighting phobias. There are innumerable persons whose lives are disturbed by phobias. These are fears which the person knows to be groundless but which nevertheless are very hard to overcome. For instance, many a woman, during a thunderstorm, has to hide in a closet or under a bed. Others go into a panic at sight of a dog or a cat, or they cannot go into a dark basement, or a dark house. There are able men who cannot go on a journey unless accompanied by their wife, and others cannot walk far from the home unless accompanied by someone.

Probably many of these persons could have cured themselves, if at the start they had forced themselves to do repeatedly what they feared. I sometimes tell such persons of a skittish horse I once had who would shy at every big piece of paper in the road. I largely broke him of this by forcing him to walk back and forth over such papers until he got to know that they were harmless.

A boy of four years, lying in his crib, felt what he thought was a hand touching his back. Turning quickly, he was much frightened to find no one there. Apparently a muscle had twitched and he had misinterpreted the sensation. After that, until he went to college, he could never sleep except with his back to a wall. Then he said to himself, "You big baby, the time has come when you must overcome this thing." For months afterward, it was only with the greatest effort that he could lie for a few minutes with his back to the room, but eventually he won out and lost his fear. Unfortunately, in many cases these phobias are never conquered, largely because of the inability of the patient to fight hard against them. In many cases a bad phobia seems to be an equivalent of a psychosis. Interesting in this connection is the story in Professor William Ellery Leonard's book, *The Locomotive God.* In it, he tells how he could not go more than a few yards away from his house.

Some persons say that the reason they fear to fight a phobia is that when they refuse to do the thing they feel compelled to do, their heart races and their blood pressure seems to go up. They fear then that they may injure themselves. I doubt if they can, and I think it better to keep fighting the phobias whenever they appear. The man who does not fight may soon find himself tied up so tight that he can hardly do anything. Some should seek an able psychiatrist who might uncover the secret cause of the phobia and perhaps then help to clear it away. I say, *perhaps,* because these phobias are not easily helped by psychoanalysis. In the case of Professor Leonard, he felt sure that the underlying cause of his phobia had been revealed, but still he could not walk far from his house.

Fighting the compulsion to run often to doctors. A very worrisome man, full of pathologic fears, must do one thing if he is ever to be cured and stay cured. After he has been well examined by good doctors and told that he is all right, he must quit shopping around for more examinations and more reassurance. I promise him that if he will only consult enough physicians he will surely find a few who are such pessimists and alarmists that they will soon have him all upset and frightened again.

Those many patients who are always getting themselves examined seem to be hoping to find a series of perhaps four doctors in a row who will give the same encouraging opinion. Unfortunately, in most cases, the patient never succeeds in this quest. He may find four consecutive physicians who will say that there isn't much wrong with his heart, but one may hedge a bit, another may give a heart tonic, another may warn against walking upstairs, and another may give a salt-free diet, and with all this the man will be left confused and uneasy.

As I often say to such persons, "A good cardiologist and I agree that there is nothing wrong with your heart, and that all your suffering is

due to fright. Your only hope of health now is to go back to your fine
sensible family doctor who, at the start, was perfectly right in what he
told you. He has a good influence on you, so why not stay with him?
If you go wandering around to other doctors you'll soon be back in the
slough of despond." Sometimes I am tempted to say to the long-
suffering wife, "If you ever catch your husband going to doctors again,
take a baseball bat and hit him hard!"

Many persons who are disturbed by compulsions to count things, or
to go back and see if gas jets are turned off, if a child in his crib is
covered, or if the doors are locked would do well to fight these things.
If one refuses to be dominated by them, one can eventually go free. He
who gives in all the time will soon be a slave to such *folies de doute*.

On always trying to behave as an adult. There would not be so
much for psychiatrists and divorce lawyers to do if everyone would always try to behave as an adult or try to act as if guided by good sense
and not by passion, jealousy, annoyance, or greediness. How wonderful if all persons could take discomfort without whining, could play a
game without insisting on winning, could think of the comfort of others,
could conform always to the rules of polite life, or could accept responsibility, or never become swinish over food or liquor. I remember
once being a bit depressed when some men who were running a fra-
ternity banquet said, "Tonight let us make the fellows buy their own
drinks; if we have free liquor so many will get drunk and noisy that we
won't have any fun at the banquet." What a commentary this was on
the maturity and self-control of a group of better-than-average college men.

The adult tries to keep himself always under the control of his reason.
Many neurotic persons are led most of the time by their emotions. A
man will often know that a certain line of action is wrong or foolish
or likely to lead to trouble or disaster, but if he wants to do the foolish
thing he commonly does it. Many of us use our reason for explaining away our foolish acts and finding excuses for our wrong behavior.
As everyone knows, the wise and sane man always thinks more of future
good than of present pleasure; the childish man always goes after immediate gratification, never caring what this will cost him later.

On thinking of others. Many persons could find health and happiness if only they could learn to think of others besides themselves. They
cannot get well so long as they spend all their time thinking and talking
of their own misfortunes, their own resentments, their own "bad luck,"
their own illnesses, their own symptoms, and their own operations.
Typical is the fact that if disaster or illness strikes down a relative, their
only thought is of how the thing will affect them. Sometimes, then, they
will speak resentfully, almost as if the relative had willfully hurt them

by falling ill. They talk as if he had done it on purpose to plague them or to get out of his responsibilities to them.

Often they are unhappy because they feel lonely, unwanted, and unloved. The trouble is that they do not love anyone; they are not even interested in anyone. Some crave love but they cannot earn it or keep it. They cannot stand listening for more than a minute to someone else's difficulties; they always break in to talk about their own. This, of course, is a human trait, but it is exaggerated in the cases of all highly self-centered persons. Curiously, some of them realize that they have this tendency and complain that they are bothered by it. They will say to a physician, "How I wish I could stop thinking all the time of myself; it is such a troublesome obsession!"

A hundred times in my life, when I have been bothered much by some personal problem and have become a bit depressed over it, I have been lifted up and made happy again by a morning spent with patients: a morning in which I forgot my difficulty as I struggled to help other people with theirs. Perhaps other troubled persons could be helped, much as I have been helped, by getting interested in the troubles of others.

The dangers of being self-centered. I fear, however, that the markedly self-centered person will never help himself much. He cannot see what is wrong with him, and if he did, it is doubtful if he could make much of an effort toward reform. Some of the worst of these persons are somewhat psychotic, and others, after years of self-pity, self-indulgence, and the constant feeling that others must always defer to their wishes and consider their comfort, are set in a mold of selfishness. It would never occur to a woman of this type to think of the likes or preferences or needs of others near her. She who has been spoiled and given into for half a lifetime by an indulgent spouse or family comes to expect deference to her wishes as a right. She may feel little gratitude to those who serve her, and rarely if ever will she express thanks. She may even complain that her husband and family have not been devoted enough or kind or sympathetic enough.

A book which shows well the insidious dangers of becoming corrupted by illness is that written by Madame France Pastorelli (*Strength out of Suffering,* a translation of *Servitude et Grandeur de la Malade*). Kept in bed for years with a bad heart, she tells how she had constantly to fight the temptation to be selfish and to ruin the life of her daughter by chaining her to her side. Other books that can help intelligent patients in adjusting to illness are listed at the end of this volume. They were all written by persons who knew what they were talking about because they had suffered and had fought their way up out of a morass of ill health.

Some women who are fundamentally good and sensible, after months of illness, can drift into selfish ways, but with help they can reform. All the doctor has to do is to show them what they are doing to themselves and others. Some will then be kinder to the husband, and others will help themselves by getting some outside interests. A childless woman with some financial means will perhaps help with the care of nephews or nieces, or she will adopt a child, or she will take more interest in good works in her community. A woman who for years was a mass of aches and pains wrote me later that she had cured herself by bearing a child. Now she is too busy caring for her little girl and loving her to think of her own body. I know other women who gained weight and lost their pains and much ill health when they forgave their husband for some peccadillo and settled down to be kind and thoughtful and loving again.

On avoiding loneliness. The world is full of lonely and unhappy persons who have no absorbing purpose in life and are of little use to anyone. They would feel so much better if they would only find some person or group whom they could help and who would greatly profit by their help. I remember a widow who was lonely and unable to make enough money to keep her little daughter with her. She had to send her far away to live with relatives. One day she took the position of nurse to the sick wife of a wealthy man. Finding the home in a mess, with no one to run it, she took hold and in a few weeks had everything going smoothly, with another nurse and some servants to help her. The man was so grateful that he gave her a fine salary and sent for her child to come and live with her in a little apartment in his big home.

Many another woman who is now lonely and unhappy could help herself by finding, as this woman did, someone who much needs help. I once practically cured a well-to-do, unmarried, unoccupied, and bored woman who for years had been going from one psychiatrist to another. I got her to take over the care of a family in which the one wage earner, a frail girl, was breaking under the strain. The woman got so interested in the job of rehabilitating this family that she stopped thinking so much about herself, and soon she went back into a useful life. In other cases I have watched a lonely woman rehabilitate herself by moving from a lonely apartment into a room in a home where there were children whom she could help and grow to love.

It is sad that thousands of wealthy but lonely men and women do not know the pleasure they could get from using some of their money to give education and opportunity to gifted youngsters in their city who haven't the means with which to support themselves while studying for an advanced degree.

The unwisdom of paying too much for having one's own way. Occasionally the physician can save a marriage by pointing out, perhaps to the husband, that he is paying too much for his demand that, let us say, the house be ultraneat or quiet, or that the wife and children be punctual at all times. Perhaps the wife and children are trying hard to conform and to please, but they are uncomfortable and fearful, and their love for the man is evaporating. The man should then stop to ask himself if the thing he is fighting for is worth all that it is costing him. Is he not paying too much for it? Sometimes, when he comes to see the matter in this light, he mends his ways.

Similarly, a woman may be controlling her husband and forcing him to do what she wants. Or, she may subtly be punishing him because of some resentment she feels; she may be having her way all the time, but, oh! at what a price! She may be trading *little things* for all her husband's old love and affection and companionship. He may go on living with her but no longer as one who loves. Few persons think often enough of the cost to them of always getting their own way.

On not trying to run the lives of those about one. One of the worst curses of humanity is the conviction of many persons that they know what is best for all their relatives. They think they can and should run the lives of those about them, or they should constantly be guarding them from harm and ill health. In winter they keep telling others when to wear overcoats and mufflers and overshoes.

Parents, of course, are inclined to keep telling children what to do long after these children are grown up, and after some years, the children start telling their parents what to do! I have often said that some day, when I retire, I am going to found a much-needed "Society for the prevention of cruelty to aged parents by their loving and oversolicitous children." Too often children gang up on an aged parent, and with the help of physicians, take away his pipe, his evening highball, the food he likes, his salt, his meat, and his daily stroll around the neighborhood. I say to them, "What if you should lengthen his life by six months? The price is too big, and besides, he does not want to trade his comforts for a longer life."

The wise and kindly person will never try to run the lives of those about him; he will not strangle other people with supposed kindness or "that form of constant persecution that goes by the name of love." All aged parents, trying to live independently, should read that delightful story, *All Passion Spent,* by V. Sackville-West.

One of the worst motives for this type of constant persecution is the feeling many persons have that every Sunday and always they must see to it that those they love get ready for Heaven; that is their terrible responsibility, or so they think.

Fighting the habit of being sorry for oneself. Many a woman must fight the bad habit of feeling sorry for herself. She must avoid the martyr complex. It is hard on the martyr and very hard on those about her. Often if she would look about she might see that her situation was not such a bad one. Perhaps she is a bit infantile in her thinking.

Perhaps the woman, at fifty-five, is very sorry for herself because her children have married and gone away. They tend to forget her, or they do not write often, or her husband is too busy to give her much time, or she has hot flushes. She could help herself if she would stop complaining and stop looking for sympathy. Instead, she should try to get out and live more richly and usefully; she should direct and lead her own life, and find things to enjoy.

I am often tempted to remind the woman who is distressed because the husband does not do much to entertain her that in the marriage ceremony the man promised to love and cherish, but not to amuse!

Developing a better mental hygiene. The man who wishes better mental health should often be cultivating better mental hygiene. He should not only work hard but he should set aside sufficient time out of each day or week or year for sleep, rest, recreation, and some play. Some men can overwork terribly for years and stay well, but others cannot.

Vacations should be so designed as to be restful. The test of a good vacation is that it sent the person back home in better shape for work and life. Some persons get little out of a vacation because while away they play harder than they usually work.

Today innumerable persons stay up too late at night to no useful purpose. They just putter around. They could be so much better off if they would only go to bed around ten each evening.

Of late, more and more city dwellers have been curing their neuroses by becoming commuters. Moving to the country, they live a simpler and quieter life, with less company, less liquor, and more sleep. Sometimes a marriage that in the city was breaking up becomes cemented again when, in the country, husband and wife spend evenings and week ends together.

The need sometimes for acquiescing. Sometimes the only way in which one can help a frail and sickly person is to stress the value of acquiescence. This was the idea that Trudeau gave to many a patient suffering from tuberculosis. He said that sometimes "the conquest of fate is not by struggling against it, not by trying to escape from it, but by acquiescence." What he meant was that the man with tuberculosis who refuses to rest and face the limitations imposed by his disease is likely to finish himself off. He must acquiesce and, at whatever cost, must take the long rest that is essential if he is to recover. To kick against the pricks and to refuse to face the facts is likely to bring disaster and death.

Similarly, the asthenic, or the constitutionally inadequate person, or the person with a very irritable bowel or frequent migraines can often be helped to a happier and more useful life if he or she can be taught this lesson—to stop looking for a complete cure, and instead to try to live sensibly and patiently with the handicap, and to accomplish what is possible with the amount of strength that is available. The person must learn to "take it" and to carry on.

As Mrs. Dorothy Cottrell said so well, the turning point in her life came the day her old family doctor told her bluntly that her polio-stricken legs were not likely ever to carry her around. For years, specialists and her family had had one idea and that was to make her *walk* again. But her doctor said, "Why not learn to live a full life sitting in your wheel chair?" With this, a great light broke over the girl, and she started out to live a normal and useful and happy life—from her chair. She won out when she acquiesced.

The need for accepting a certain amount of failure in life. Some men are unhappy and suffering from a neurosis because they are so dissatisfied with the amount of success that has come to them. This success may be so great as to cause the man to be envied by his fellows, but he is not satisfied because he wanted something else or something more. Here, perhaps, is a teacher of music in a large city. He has many pupils and a good income, but he is unhappy because, in his eyes, he is a miserable failure. He set out to be a concert pianist or violinist, and after years of practicing many hours a day, he acquired a good technic. But there was no fire in him; he could not thrill an audience; he could not "put himself over," and so he had to fall back on teaching.

A sad sight in this world is that of an unusually able man who, because of the lack of some one quality, or the presence of some harmful mental quirk, barely missed eminence. The fact that once great success was almost in his grasp, or the fact that he knows he has a spark of genius in him, makes it so hard for him to bear mediocrity. I know a man who can make a magnificent portrait in oils, but only from a photograph. He hasn't any originality, and hence can only copy the work of others. If Nature had given him a stronger personality and a greater artistic sense he could have been a great success.

It is hard to help or give cheer to such a person when he cracks up. He knows too well that he failed in what he set out to do, and that failure can never be explained away. Often he is the more upset by seeing the great financial rewards that keep going to ignorant men much less gifted than he, but men who, with some gift of the showman or the charlatan, caught the popular fancy of the moment and cashed in.

On staying social. One of the best things many persons can do is to try to be more social and to get more friends. A man should learn the value of taking time to cultivate and hold good friends. He should remember that the hermit is likely to get queerer and queerer. The man who is social and friendly is usually sane. The mildly schizophrenic man may never, in his lifetime, invite a person to his house.

I remember a schizoid young woman who was very lonely and unhappy until I induced her to become a leader in the social activities of her club. First, I had to convince her that she was really a sweet person whom people would like if she would only let them know her. Her new habit of sociability made her popular, and popularity brought her the joy in life that she had so missed and so wanted.

A woman who often needs advice to stay social is the widow who was much in love with her husband. Since his death she may have built a wall about her, a wall through which even her relatives can hardly penetrate. She would do better to stay social and try to be useful in the world and kind to many troubled persons like herself.

Older persons need to keep up the habit of seeing their friends, and as these old friends die off, efforts should be made to make new ones.

On trying to stay mentally young. The man who remains young is the one who is always looking toward the future. He is greatly interested in his work and in improving his knowledge of it. He is always reading and studying to improve himself. His mind is avid for new ideas. He has many interests. Usually he has one or more hobbies. Even when he is retired at sixty-five he is looking forward to the fun of doing many things that he never before had time to do.

The value of creative work. One of the best things one can do with some nervous and worried persons is to try to get them into some creative work. As a badly worried minister once wrote from a psychopathic hospital, so long as he was busy making things in the sanatorium workshop, he forgot all about his supposed unpardonable sin. And gradually, as he kept at work, he got well. Few things give a person more joy and satisfaction in life than creative work. The woman who sews, makes a dress, crochets, knits, weaves, or paints derives much satisfaction from what she sees forming under her hands, and she is much less likely to develop a neurosis than is her idle sister.

One sad feature about the work of most factory mechanics today is that it is not creative; they do not have the joy of making a cloisonné vase or an ivory carving as an Oriental workman does. The American workman spends his days watching a machine or assembling some part of a mechanism. The human need for making things in their entirety can be seen in the recent great multiplication of basement workshops. Such shops are good for many men, and a home loom or knitting needles are good for many a woman.

Today in most institutions for the treatment of persons with psychoses

there are workshops. In some places these shops are designed ju
keep the patients busy and to get their minds off their worries, bu
other hospitals they are designed to give a handicapped man a trade a
a means of livelihood after he recovers and goes out into the worl
again.

One must not expect much attention from others. Men and
women need to learn not to get upset when others do not treat them
with the consideration, deference, tact, and kindness that they desire.
Many a mother who is upset when her children do not write should
remember that when she was a girl she was not exemplary in writing
home. Millions of persons who crave praise for what they have done
should remember that they rarely give enthusiastic praise to anyone.

Unfortunately, in this busy world where everyone is interested in his
own affairs one cannot expect much from others. If one does not expect
much, one will not be hurt when it does not come. Instead of demanding praise and attention, a person would do well to stop more often
to say a kind or appreciative word to someone.

The avoidance of overconscientiousness in work. A helpful idea
for many persons might be that of trying to do much of the day's work
automatically, without conscious effort, great deliberation, or fear of
making a mistake. One reason some persons break down is that they
are so fearful of making a mistake. For instance, a young woman working as a chemist in a war plant broke down because of her pathologic
fear of making a mistake and thereby hurting her country. She got into
the habit of staying overtime to repeat each analysis, and even then,
she kept fearing that some of her results might be wrong.

At the close of each day when the person goes home he should try
hard to leave his business cares at the office or in the factory. He should
see that to err is human, and that no one can ever hope to be perfect.
If he has done his best, that is all that can be expected of him. With
this he must learn to be content.

Avoiding paranoid attitudes. Some persons need to fight against
their natural tendency to look on the acts of other persons as directed
against them. They should keep remembering that the chances are that
the person who seemed to speak pointedly meant no harm, or what
appeared to be a slight was only a bit of absentmindedness.

Fighting the fear of insanity. Many a person with a poor nervous
heredity and a tendency to a psychotic type of tenseness and worry is
frightened every so often by the feeling that he is about to lose his mind.
Usually these persons can be given reassurance and comfort, especially
if they have reached their forties or fifties without cracking. After talking to the patient and sizing him up an experienced physician may be
able to say that a man who has been so sane for so many years is not

likely to change now. If he had been born for a crack-up he would probably have had it long before.

Perhaps the physician will be optimistic because the patient is so intelligent and has such good insight. In some ways it is encouraging that he *fears* insanity because many men while going insane do not appear to know it. They may accuse those about them of being the unreasonable ones. It may help the patient to know that thousands of persons who have remained sane have feared the coming of insanity, especially at those times when they have been very tired or feverish or unable to sleep.

The patient with psychotic relatives should remember that he may be one of those in the family who did not inherit the curse, or, if he has inherited a little of it, it is only a tendency, and he may never go on to become insane. He should know that most of the children born to a psychotic person will not be psychotic unless the spouse is also psychotic or comes from a psychotic stirp. Often the physician can say, after studying a patient, "It looks to me as if you had missed the curse entirely." In other cases he can say, "It looks as if you had already received your small share of it. Your neuroses and mild phobias and eccentricities represent your part of the inheritance; take comfort now in the thought that you were allotted no more of it. What you have is bearable, and by practicing better mental hygiene you may make it even less troublesome." Many of the persons who for years have been full of worry can be much reassured by such an opinion.

Avoiding the selfishness of confessing. Many a time, when talking to a patient, I have found that his or her trouble dated from an unfortunate confession that almost wrecked the happiness of the spouse. Sometimes the confession was of a peccadillo or of an unfortunate mistake made in youth. The impulse to tell came with a desire to purge the conscience, but this was selfish because it wrecked another's happiness and peace of mind. Always the person with a desire to confess should stop and ask himself, "Am I purchasing peace for myself at great cost to someone else?" He or she might remember, also, that the resentment or hurt of the other person can later some day boomerang back on the confessor.

A woman sometimes asks me if she should confess to her fiancé or husband that once during high-school days she had a love affair with a few sexual contacts. I say, "No; what good could that do? Why hurt your man or give him a club with which to bruise you some day when he is angry?" Or a man will want to know if he should tell his wife that once in his ignorant youth he suffered from gonorrhea. Again, what good will that do? He was well cured long before he married.

One of the worst habits of an older man on a second honeymoon, perhaps with a mature widow or divorcee, is to assume that she is such a "good scout" that she will not mind hearing of his old "affairs" and sexual sins. Later, when the woman's hurts and jealousies and distrusts crop up to nearly ruin the marriage, the man may wish devoutly that he had kept his mouth shut. Other men will talk of their infidelities after their tongue has been loosened by several cocktails. After that they may have to live for years with a resentful and ever-watchful wife.

The need for becoming frightened at the sight of growing bad habits and mental rigidities. It would seem that the man who finds himself becoming irascible and uncontrolled ought to be as worried about it as he might be were he suddenly to realize that he was becoming habituated to morphine. The abyss yawns, and a wise man will scramble back up and away from the edge as fast as he can.

A man should be alarmed if he finds he is becoming set in his ways, overly conservative, and unable to change, or to respond to the helpful suggestions of others. He should become frightened if he finds that when talking, he monopolizes the conversation, or gets on one topic and talks violently about it all evening, or brooks no argument about some pet idea of his. He will then be a bore, and his friends will begin to avoid him. He will become lonely and perhaps unemployable. Unfortunately, few men can note the coming of these changes in themselves. A wife may repeatedly call attention to them, but usually she cannot help much.

We men and women must all fight rigidities if only because in time we are likely to get so that if anyone asks us to vary our routine in the slightest we will get irritable or flustered. A wise man will avoid saying such things as "I *never* do this or that," or, "I *never* would try this or that." One should not tie oneself up in rigidities.

What the alcoholic can do to help himself. The man who drinks in sprees or even drinks too much every night is usually very hard to help. If he goes on the wagon, he is likely to fall off again whenever he gets tired or distressed or discouraged over anything. As noted in Chapters 14 and 15, alcoholism is a sign of something decidedly wrong with the personality. Some of these men are mild manic-depressives; others are troubled by feelings of inadequacy and failure. This is well shown in autobiographies of drunkards. It may help an intelligent alcoholic to read some of these books and thereby to understand himself better.

Maine (*If a Man Be Mad*) tells that by the age of twelve he already had built up a fictional existence for himself. Early he started building up a defense against fear and insecurity. "Neither my parents nor my teachers could ever know me. I couldn't meet responsibility." By eighteen he was a chronic alcoholic. "When drink was in me I feared no consequences but those of being without a drink." He fought to reconcile a dream world with the actual world, and he lost. He came to feel a terrible loneliness. He had to drink "in order to break through and talk to people." But his wild talk frightened them, and so he took to drinking alone. He could not stay in one place because of a feeling that "guilts would accumulate." One "alibi" was that he feared to be cured because he might "end up as an average and dull individual!" It is important to note that it was only creative writing that could keep him sober for months. But when his first novel was rejected by a publisher, back he went to the bottle.

This remarkable book is filled with descriptions of such mental torture that one does not wonder that the man drank; he felt he had to escape the pain of being different from other people, unable to talk to them freely, and unable to share their joys. Even when women loved him devotedly he could not take and keep this happiness: He still had to run away and get drunk. Many of these persons will suddenly run away and start drinking when everything in life should keep them from it: business success, a fine home, a lovely wife, and adored children. Only an insane urge could possibly compel a man to give up everything in life for a bottle that will only make him swinish and sick and utterly miserable.

Every chronic alcoholic should be studied by a good psychiatrist because sometimes when the underlying mental distresses are brought to light, something can be done to help the unhappy victim. An alcoholic once said to his psychiatrist, "I see now that I've been a fraud all my life; I never knew it before. I used to think I was interested in people but that wasn't so. Thus, when my own mother was ill my only thought was, 'What will happen to *me* when she is gone?'" The patient said later that after his treatment, he began sometimes to think of other people besides himself. He felt easier when with other alcoholics because he did not feel hostile to them, and he did not fear that they were hostile to him.

There is many an alcoholic who has been helped by the organization known as Alcoholics Anonymous, and oftentimes a physician will be wise to turn his patient over to them. Obviously, the man must want to go to them for help. He would do well first to read their book which is well written and most interesting. Then, if he is willing, he can be brought into contact with the local branch of the organization. Their main address is P.O. Box 459, Grand Central Annex, New York, 17. Their technic is to send help to a man when he is tempted to go on a spree. If he will call the Center they will immediately send out some man who once was a heavy drinker and hence knows all about the temptation and the suffering.

Alcoholics Anonymous maintains that before a man can be helped he must first give up pretending that he can "take it or leave it." He must admit freely that he is a chronic alcoholic and that without help he cannot "leave it." He must admit that he needs help, and he must ask for it. He is the more likely to get well and stay well if he becomes a helper of others. This helping of others is a great secret of the success of Alcoholics Anonymous. The members are taught, also, to put themselves in the hands of God. The association claims a recovery rate of 75 per cent.

CHAPTER 28

Help a Non-Psychiatrist
Can Give a Nervous Patient

SOME OF THE THINGS A non-psychiatric physician can do to help those many nervous persons whose problems are fairly simple are discussed briefly in this chapter. I am thinking now of the nervous, the tired, the frail, the overworked, and the unhappy. In the next chapter I shall discuss the problems of those more troubled persons who need the help of a sensible and kindly psychiatrist.

Because this book was written for fellow non-psychiatrists I shall talk mainly about the types of patient they and I see and what we can do for them in the half-hour or less that we can give each one of them during the course of a busy day. Obviously, a general practitioner or an internist, with all the people he has to see, can seldom go deeply into the mental problems of any one patient, as a psychiatrist commonly does. The doctor will do well if he probes deep enough to see how the patient fell ill and what his or her *immediate* problems are.

As I showed in previous chapters, the physician must (1) try to learn if the patient has a psychic trouble; (2) learn what it is; (3) satisfy him that the diagnosis of a neurosis is correct; (4) perhaps take away "organic" diagnoses and placebos given by other physicians; (5) give understanding, confidence, and new hope; (6) perhaps sell the idea that it would be more fun to be well than sick; and (7) sell the idea that the patient must do most of the curing.

Methods of simple psychotherapy. Much of psychotherapy is practised almost unconsciously as the doctor takes a good history, examines
the man thoroughly, and assures him that no serious organic disease is
present. Perhaps he just shows him that he has a mild, and not a serious, form of hypertension or diabetes or arthritis and hence will not
suffer much or be cut down in his prime. Often he needs only to show
that the abnormality found has no great significance.

Help will be given by listening to the patient and giving mental catharsis. Much help can be given by explaining how the symptoms came.
Then there may have to be encouragement to carry on, reasons given
for making the effort, and helpful advice given about living life better
and more usefully and more sensibly.

In most cases the physician will have to depend on his ingenuity and
good sense to know what to do about the psychic problem unearthed.
From his wisdom and philosophy and experience in life he must decide
what advice it is best to give.

The physician commonly does not realize it when he is working as a
faith-healer, and the patient does not realize it when he is being cured
by psychotherapy. He does not note that he got better as he told the
story of the disaster that hit him and made him ill, or that he got well
when he was examined and told that the results of his tests were negative, or when the physician made some reassuring remark, such as that
his own father had extrasystoles most of his life and lived happily
into old age.

Perhaps the patient suddenly understood the nature of his disease
when the doctor drew out the fact that the shock of a brother's sudden
death brought the first symptoms, or the patient became cheered when
he found that the story of "colitis" which he had thought was so rare
and puzzling was really a common, well-known one, or he was cheered
when he saw that his new physician felt no great concern over his
illness.

On changing the name of a disease. As I was writing this I was
interested to see how easily I "cured" a woman who came badly frightened over pains around her joints. She was frightened because her
mother had for long been crippled with rheumatoid arthritis. When I
found a low sedimentation rate and no changes in the woman's joints,
I said, "You have fibrositis and not arthritis. You need never be
crippled or deformed." With this she was overjoyed. As she said later,
"Here I am, going home with my same old pains, but practically well
because I have a nicer diagnosis."

Similarly, one can often send a man home happy with a hypertension
simply by telling him that there are four types of the disease and he has
only the fairly harmless type 1. Or one can send a diabetic away

happy simply by showing him that he has the mildest form of the disease which should never shorten his life.

Psychotherapy starts when the patient hears good things about the physician. Often the most important part of psychotherapy starts when the patient hears good things said about a physician. A woman will meet a former patient who raves about "her doctor" and tells of the cure he worked for her. Then the family physician is questioned and if he knows the consultant and expresses admiration for him and his skill, the woman will go to him with the stage set for a helpful interview.

The doctor's office has psychotherapeutic value. A patient will be helped if she likes the appearance of the doctor's office; if she likes his attendant, and if the waiting room is full of well-dressed persons. All this will reassure her and make her feel that the physician must have had some success in his work.

More psychotherapy will emanate from the physician's appearance and demeanor. Much may depend, next, on the patient's first impression of the physician. It helps much if the doctor makes a good first appearance, if he greets with ease, and if he is friendly and kindly and looks as if he were able and interested. A woman wrote one of her physicians: "From the moment I met you I felt safe. Some inner feeling told me, 'Here is a doctor who feels deeply and sincerely, both with and for his patients, and both within and outside of his medical practice.' Soon you sent me to the particular specialist I needed for treatment of my rare disease, and again, the minute he started examining me I felt I was in the right hands. He so evidently knew what he was doing; he examined me more carefully and skillfully than anyone had ever done before, and I was confident then that I was going to be cured."

The ideal psychotherapist, and for that matter, the ideal physician, is born and not made. If the gods who presided at his birth were generous one will find him with a well-built body, an impressive face, and good, frank, and kindly eyes. He will be the sort of man whom people like and trust and to whom children quickly go. He will be the sort of man to whom all his relatives turn in times of trouble and sorrow. He may be the type of man whom most women like and trust and go to for guidance. He may be the type of man who can take the hand of a hysterically paralyzed girl and with a word of command have her up and walking again. He may have the God-given gift of sensing what helpful words to say to troubled patients. People like much the doctor who is human, informal, and easily approachable. Such a man will quickly establish rapport with his patients, and he will do this often even with eccentric and difficult characters. I have known a few physicians who could take a hostile, resentful, and distrustful patient who had just had a "run-in" with an assistant, and in a few minutes have him or her "eating out of his hand" and looking on him as an old and trusted crony.

Naturally, this sort of thing is more easily done by the older physician who has "arrived" and become a bit of a philosopher, but I have seen it done sometimes by a young physician in his twenties who happened to have been born with a friendly or impressive personality. There are some men who probably can never hope to have any success in psychotherapy because they haven't the right personality and cannot develop it.

It would seem best that a psychotherapist be well integrated and well-adjusted himself, but I have seen a few odd characters who could help others of the same stripe.

A doctor is fortunate if he has much vitality, energy, enthusiasm, optimism, forcefulness, and some eloquence. He also should have endless patience, constant good humor, and idealism. According to Osler, he must have a quality of imperturbability, and must never give the appearance of being flustered or unable to cope with a situation.

The handicap of the physician who is impassive, uninterested, and unsympathetic. Many a patient today complains that his doctors have shown no interest in him as a human being. As he went through a clinic he greatly resented being handled like an animal or some inanimate object.

Medicine is more than a business. Some physicians say, "I handle my business like any other. The patient comes, I treat him; he pays me, and he goes. He and his personal problems do not interest me a particle. I cannot see why they should." In a way the doctor is right. There is no law against practising that way, but as Osler used to say, that is not the practise of medicine as Hippocrates conceived it. He looked on it as a *calling:* a sort of religion—a profession—and never just a business. *It should be an affair of the heart as well as of the head.*

When trying to lift people up and help them and make them change their ways or accept some unpleasant diagnosis or treatment, the physician needs strength of character and sometimes intensity of feeling. He must feel strongly about things or the patient will not feel any answering response such as might stir him to effort. If a physician says, "If you were my brother I would want this treatment to be carried out" the patient may say, "Yes, I see you feel that way, and so I will surely follow your advice."

In the treatment of, let us say, tuberculosis or ulcerative colitis, one physician will say impassively to his patients, "There is no specific treatment for your disease. You will just have to rest and hope for the best." In the hospital he will make his rounds every day as if it were just a job to be done, and, as a result, many of his patients will do poorly. Another physician will stride cheerfully into the patient's room, radiating strength and enthusiasm. With real interest he will ask how the patient feels and he may even go on to talk about personal or home problems. Perhaps a woman is worried about things at home or about letters that have not come. Each patient will feel that this doctor is concerned about his or her problem. Each day the doctor will be delighted and encouraged if the patient's temperature has dropped a bit, or if there is a gain in weight, or if there is a little less sputum, or less diarrhea. His hopefulness will be communicated to the patients.

In hospitals and clinics one can watch the two types of physicians at work: one taciturn and uninspiring and the other dynamic and hopeful; and one can see how many more cures are worked by the enthusiast.

The art of saying the right thing. Some physicians have the gift of speaking pleasingly, convincingly, and helpfully, and some gradually learn to do it. Ross used to express his gratitude to a certain Dr. Williamson who, he said, had taught him much of what he knew of this art. I think it very helpful for a doctor to write many medical papers because in doing this he organizes his thoughts, he thinks up the best arguments, and he learns to express them well and logically and briefly.

A man can be fairly safe in being friendly and sympathetic, but he must guard against being maudlin or sugary. Many seriously ill persons dislike a lot of sympathy, and they are enraged at Pollyannaism. They do not like it when someone feels sorry for them or tries to quiet them with platitudes. All physicians and psychiatrists would do well to read the books written by the sick and crippled to see what they hate to hear and how they hate to be treated.

Avoiding platitudes. The physician will do well to avoid platitudes, such as "It might have been worse," or, "Be grateful that you have enough money to get by on." In my youth, a woman, after a crippling stroke, took a great dislike to me because of my efforts to cheer her. She taught me a lesson which has served me well ever since. I did not then know that there is no solace for the utter misery felt day and night after a stroke of a certain type, and I did not realize that all the woman wanted of me was relief, not talk. Since I could not give relief, I should not have annoyed her with platitudes.

It is a particularly cruel thing to talk platitudes to an unfortunate girl caught in one of the traps such as I describe in Chapter 8. If she cannot get free, where is she to find happiness or health? Under such circumstances what can a physician say that will help? What can one say that will really cheer a young woman who has just lost an adored fiancé or a devoted and much-loved husband or a first-born son? What can one say that will lessen the woman's terrible and constant torture? I do not know and I doubt if anyone knows.

The person who has suffered can cure best. Occasionally one can help a person facing an ordeal or going through a great sorrow by putting him or her in touch with another fine person who has been through the same experience. I remember a woman, suddenly faced with the need of an operation for cancer of the colon, who was frantic until I got another woman, who five years before had passed through the same ordeal, to talk to her. Then she was comforted and able to go ahead. Another lovely woman, when staggered by the news that one lower limb would have to be amputated because of a sarcoma, was helped, not by my words, but by those of another amputee who had had the same disease and had survived for ten years. Fortunately, I saw him passing my office door a few minutes after the woman reeled under her blow, and I got him to talk to her.

This idea of getting the once-sick and now-cured to help the sick is well used by Alcoholics Anonymous. A doctor who has never experienced a great craving for alcohol and hence knows nothing about it might easily talk to a dipsomaniac in such a prissy way as to gain his contempt and dislike. But when another dipsomaniac comes to help, that is different; here is a man who has been through the hell many times and knows what he is talking about.

It is for these reasons that the physician most likely to cure certain patients is the one who has suffered from their disease. For instance, the physician who once had tuberculosis can easily cheer a patient with this disease, or the one who has suffered from migraine can the more easily help women with a sick headache.

So often when a woman comes to tell of a severe food allergy, she is fearful that I will say it "is all in her head." And how relieved she is the minute I say, "Don't feel apologetic, for years I suffered from severe food allergy; I know what it is."

Curiously, oftentimes, a nurse, a physiotherapist, a druggist, or a layman who has suffered as the patient has will be able to cheer him much more than can his physician. I think this is because the physician, back of his desk, seems so remote and so removed from common humanity, or the patient feels that it is a doctor's business to be optimistic even when he has no right to be. A nurse seems closer to the hoi polloi and therefore more to be trusted by them.

Fortunately, as a physician grows older, if he has long watched his words and studied their effects, he should get more skill in helping troubled people, in lifting them up, and in putting them on the road to health.

On inviting confessions and effecting mental purgation. The confessional which works so well in the church would work well for many of our patients if only we physicians would more often use it.

The desire of many persons to confess is great. Thousands of patients will gladly tell their story to a sympathetic physician (1) perhaps to just confess and purge the soul; (2) to get a problem straight in their minds; (3) to see if the physician will be horrified at them, and (4) to get his advice as to what to do and how to get out of a difficulty.

Many persons struggle for years with some psychic problem or some unhappiness without ever daring to confide in anyone. Often there is no one with whom they can talk. In such cases a sharing of the secret with the doctor will help tremendously.

The most remarkable result of mental catharsis I ever saw came in the case of a woman who complained of severe long-lasting insomnia with resulting emaciation. After listening to her story and finding that these troubles dated back to the beginning of an unhappy marriage, I told her to make a definite decision as to her long-contemplated divorce and then to see me again. A few months later she returned looking wonderfully well. She said she had started to sleep and eat and gain weight the day she had seen me and had decided that she would not give up her home but would accept her prosaic husband as he was.

Is the cost of good diagnosing and good psychotherapy prohibitive? Many a physician has said to me, "You doubtless are right, and many patients need psychotherapy, but I can't afford to take the time to talk to them: I have to earn a living." My answer is that during my many years of practice I have always stopped to talk to my nervous patients about their life problems; I have always charged moderate fees, and I have always earned a living. I made a living even when in San Francisco I was spending more than half of my day in a research laboratory.

In order to keep doing good work in internal medicine a physician cannot see more than a certain number of patients every day. In difficult cases he cannot make a correct diagnosis without spending much time on the problem. I know how hard it is to keep a rapidly growing practice within limits. When a doctor begins to feel enslaved by his job and worn down by the strain of overwork he must decide which one of several courses he is to follow. He can (1) shorten the time spent with each patient and thus give each one only a few minutes. This is a poor type of practice, and one that will result in the making of many mistakes. (2) He can put up his prices so as to scare many away. But this is not a happy solution. The nicest patients to deal with are often those with little money, and besides, big bills often anger the rich. (3) He can employ assistants. This will add much to his financial burdens and responsibilities and it will not be entirely satisfactory, but it seems to be the best way out of the dilemma.

Another thing a too busy physician might do would be to refuse to accept as patients those fussy and stupid neurotics who will keep demanding more and more tests and more and more time. Often he will recognize this type of person at the first interview, but how to get rid of him with any degree of politeness? One trouble is that so often, after the man has used up a few hours of time, he will go away disappointed and perhaps angry. Many a time I have felt like giving such a man some money to go elsewhere! I know one nationally eminent physician who protects himself from certain people whose cases he feels are not worth undertaking by demanding a large fee in advance, but this is not a happy or dignified way out of the situation.

The physician who does not spend enough time on diagnosis spends endless time on futile treatments. Obviously, the physician who does not spend enough time on a patient to make the correct diagnosis later spends an aggregate of hours on futile treatments—futile because they are designed to cure a disease that is not there.

Typical is the story told by Weiss and English (1949) of a boy of nine years who, because of a snapshot diagnosis of organic heart disease, cost his parents some $6,000 in fees to private physicians, and then cost social agencies in the community another $4,000 for care in hospitals and for examinations in clinics. Actually, all the boy had was a cardiac neurosis which was cured by a few visits to a psychiatrist. I remember the frail constitutionally inadequate man who had undergone ten abdominal operations for an ulcer which apparently he had never had.

On not giving placebos. Often the physician who would cure a neurosis must not hand out medicine. It would be like giving a wheel chair to a man with a hysterical paralysis. As I have said elsewhere in this book, if a doctor tells a man that he has a neurosis he must not greatly weaken his statement by giving medicine appropriate for an organic disease that the patient fears he has.

On the need for taking away diagnostic placebos. In many cases no physician can do anything with psychotherapy until he has resolutely taken away the several diagnostic placebos which other doctors have given the patient. As I pointed out in Chapter 26, this taking away must be done tactfully because otherwise the patient will be confused and perhaps angered.

The physician must be practical in his advice. The sensible physician will hesitate to advise expensive measures of relief until he has inquired to see if the patient can afford them. I remember a woman with arthritis who was treated so strenuously by an able consultant that, after some improvement, she began to get worse again. What had happened was that she had begun to have horrors over the size of the bills that were being run up.

The need for talking to relatives. The near relatives of a patient should often be talked to at some length. They must understand the problem and must be taught to think of the patient as ill and not just mean and unreasonable and cantankerous. They can help much by keeping their tempers and perhaps not exhorting the patient "to snap out of it." In some cases, as when a mother of a family becomes psychopathic, they can help much by, for a time, carrying some of her burdens.

The patient should face facts. Often the most important thing in treating a patient with functional troubles is to get him to face the facts as the physician sees them. So long as he goes on insisting that some organic disease be found, and so long as he refuses to face the possibility that he might be ill because he is a constitutionally frail person, or one who has inherited bad nerves, or has been under great strain, or has been living foolishly, little can be done for him. He will keep going from one physician to another getting placebos of various kinds or getting himself operated on. He cannot get well until he is willing to accept what an experienced physician tells him. Often he argues and argues until his doctor feels like reminding him that he is behaving like a man who, when caught in a dangerous lawsuit, keeps telling his wise old lawyer how to handle the case.

Most patients' problems are simple. My impression, gained from thousands of interviews with nervous patients, is that most of their problems are simple. A glance at the person's face and a few minutes of listening to the story and I may feel sure that I am dealing with a born neurotic and worrier. A few more questions and I may learn what the recent sources of unhappiness and strain have been. At the patient's place of work there may be fatigue, financial worry, a choleric boss, feelings of insecurity, or unhappiness over insufficient remuneration; at home there may be a nagging wife, or a hard-drinking husband, a trouble-making relative, or a defective or wayward child. Obviously, one can get at these essential facts without making any extensive psycho-analysis. The things that most commonly produce nervous illness seem to me to be usually hereditary tendencies to neurosis plus recent worries and strains.

Myerson, in his very practical book, *The Nervous Housewife,* and Ross and Gillespie taught that the great bulk of functional nervous disorders are of such simple origin that they can hardly interest a professional psychiatrist; they are too simple for him. Riggs, Weir Mitchell, Richard Cabot, Peabody, and others felt the same way. Ross thought that most of the patients he saw could be helped by any kindly and sensible practitioner, and as he said, this is fortunate because the great bulk of these patients will always have to be cared for by non-psychiatrists.

All that is needed to help most patients is ordinary sensible advice. As I read the literature of the psychiatrists I am distressed to find some of them speaking disparagingly or even contemptuously of such "superficial" analyses. I think they are wrong; they ought to be glad to see that in this land of ours there are some physicians who are learning to recognize the common neuroses and to treat them.

While it is true that the ordinary physician's efforts to cheer a worried patient are designed mainly to tide over the situation, still they often give satisfactory results which last for years. For instance, when a man comes with great fear of cancer of the stomach, and the doctor has him roentgenoscoped and sends him home reassured and happy, he has done a good job. A psychiatrist may complain that he has not gone to the root of the trouble to see why the man was so anxious, but actually, some internists do inquire, and they do find why the man fears cancer and what precipitated his acute fright. Usually it was the sudden death from cancer of a relative.

Doubtless a psychiatrist could go much further to dig out all sorts of curious facts about the patient's early life and his ways of thinking, but as Ross used to say, how much good would that do? Would it stop the man from being a worrier over every little thing? I doubt it. The man's wife would probably say, "You'll never stop him from worrying; he'll always do that just like his mother before him."

There is a big place in medicine for "superficial" analyses. At least, in the cases of neuroses, their results are much better than those of the appendectomies, hysterectomies, and operations for adhesions now being dispensed by way of treatment.

Reassurance. Reassurance must be given with strength and sureness, without doubts, reservations, and hedging. A physician is never going to cure neuroses unless he is positive when he says that the examinations showed nothing wrong. If he hedges and straddles and tries to keep a line of retreat open in case things go wrong, the worried patient will never be cured.

It often helps a worrisome patient to let him see his laboratory and roentgenologic reports. I like to explain the meaning of each test. For instance, I explain that hemoglobin is the red coloring matter of the blood, or that a normal blood urea suggests that the kidney function is adequate. If the patient has a low blood sedimentation rate I explain briefly why this is reassuring. If the patient is worried about a little change found in his electrocardiogram I may explain that it is like his baldness: It came with age, it is not exactly normal, but it need cause no concern.

Obviously, the best psychiatric treatment for the much-worried patient is a thorough examination. Next in helpfulness is a convincing explanation of how all the symptoms complained of can be produced by nervousness. It may be helpful, also, to show the patient that the doctor knows the disease well because he has seen it a thousand times before. Most helpful often is a consultation with a good specialist who is an authority on the particular disease under consideration. His reassurance, if well done, will do more than anything else to satisfy the patient and put an end to his worries.

As everyone knows, often when the worry is gone the symptoms are bearable. For instance, a husband whose chronically ill, migrainous wife had been reassured, wrote a year later to say that she was much better. He said, "To be sure, she has not been free from discomfort, but she has been free from the old paralyzing fear of her spells which used to make our days miserable. Now, when a nervous storm begins to grumble within her, she recognizes it for what it is; she eases up on her always too busy program, and soon she is all right again." Every physician must try "to cure sometimes, to relieve often, and to comfort always."

Often I am surprised when accidentally I discover what the person is terribly worried about. I hadn't even thought of it. To illustrate: A woman with a neurofibroma in the neck was having horrors fearing that it would produce insanity! Perhaps some doctor inadvertently had put the idea in her head.

Cheering the patient who has a good heredity. Before starting treatment, especially of a person whose story suggests a trend toward psychosis, I like to find out what his nervous heredity is. If it is good I have less fear for him than if it is bad, and I feel more justified in reassuring him.

The cure that comes in a moment. Many a time, after a chat with a patient, I have been impressed with the fact that he or she left for home without even asking for a prescription or a bit of advice. For instance, a big husky farmer had come to the Clinic several times with an arthritic ache in his left loin. When examinations failed to reveal anything else, I asked him what he would do if I were to assure him that he had no ulcer or cancer or anything that would ever "turn into something." He reached for his hat and laughingly said, "I'd say, 'To hell with it.' " And off he went, happy.

The need for inspiring faith and hope. As every good physician knows, one of the best things he can do for many nervous and worried patients is to inspire them with hope that they can ultimately get well. This is so important because (1) it removes fear which is so injurious to health, (2) it puts to work healing forces, and (3) it causes the patient to do many things to help himself. The best physician is often the greatest inspirer of hope. In all cases of doubt it is best to be optimistic because many an apparently hopeless illness eventually clears up.

On helping a person who is facing death. The kindly physician can often help the person who is facing death from an incurable disease. Usually some little hope can be given. The diagnosis could be wrong, or radiation or some drug may help, or a new and effectual drug may come in time. Some persons with malignant lesions go for many years without a recurrence, and this is something to hope for. Even more remarkable is the fact that an occasional person suffering from cancer appears to fight the disease to a stand-still so that he lives on for years.

Often the patient is glad to be able to talk frankly to someone about his future and to get answers to his questions. With a hopeless cancer will he have to suffer much pain? (Probably some.) If he does, can he safely take opiates? (Yes.) How long will it be before he is incapacitated? (Perhaps months.) Is his disease contagious so that his family will catch it? (No.) Should he sell out his business? (He must decide.) Should he talk frankly with his wife? (Yes.) Should he keep working as long as he can? (Yes.) Should he try an operation, when it appears hopeless? (Probably no.) What about quacks? Do they ever cure? (No.) After being turned down by able physicians should he spend his savings in a search for a cure, or should he leave what money he has for the education of his children? (Better leave it.) These are some of the questions that may be asked if the physician is kindly and willing to spend a little time answering them.

After talking with the patient it often helps to talk to the family. I often say to an old couple, "You two have gone through forty years of travail, sorrow, and joy, hand in hand, sharing everything; now when one of you has to go down through the valley of the shadow, why shouldn't you go through that also, hand in hand? Why should you be lying to each other, and making believe you do not know what the loved one has? That can give rise only to loneliness." For more on this subject see Chapter 13.

THE TREATMENT OF FATIGUE

Naturally, before attempting to treat a fatigue state with psychotherapy or rest the physician should have a good idea as to the cause. Patients with obvious organic disease should be treated appropriately, and those with a depression should, if possible, be turned over to a psychiatrist.

It is the man or woman who has overworked or lost sleep or carried burdens that were too heavy who can be helped by a rest. Some can be induced to take a vacation, or to rest more each day, or to sleep longer each night, or to go to bed earlier, or to take a nap during the day, or for a time to work shorter hours. Some men have to face the need for changing their work or giving up some ambitions or pulling some irons out of the fire.

Many men in a small business greatly need a clerk or a partner. For instance, the owner of a one-man drug store works long hours and seldom gets any rest. Many physicians on call twenty-four hours out of each day are terribly overworked and need to get an assistant or a partner. Often a man who owns a small business will say that he never had a vacation.

On getting some rest at home. Some persons who cannot take a long vacation can sometimes catch up on rest by spending Saturday afternoons and Sundays on a couch. An executive, when tired out and unable to take a couple of months off, may help himself by, for a time, spending only mornings at the office. He can answer his mail, confer with his department heads and subordinates, and then go back home for a rest or out to the club for golf.

The tired mother can often get straightened out by spending mornings on her bed and getting a nap every afternoon. While resting in bed she may be doing some mending, sewing, writing, or darning of socks. It is wonderful how much help can come from stretching out for hours in a semirecumbent position. Obviously, most helpful to a tired woman would be the getting of some help with the housework.

Before she will consent to rest she may have to be made to understand that she is not being "lazy" but is really helping her family. I often say to such a woman that, for a time, the neglecting of her household duties would be the most conscientious thing she could do. I may have to point out, also, that especially if she has children to take care of, her good health is her husband's greatest asset. What on earth would he do if she were to become incapacitated?

Oftentimes I have to say to the woman, "You who so want to be a fine wife and mother, can't you see that when you get as tired, irritable, and upset as you are now you must be a poor wife and mother? You cannot be otherwise. You will be upsetting your children and making them tense and nervous. If you keep going until you crack up, you will cost your husband much more money in the end." Sometimes, then, the woman will be convinced and will try to get a rest.

Especially when a woman is frail and inclined at times to break down, it is important that the husband be taught to do something about the situation as soon as he recognizes the signs of an impending crack-up. He should try then quickly to get his wife away for a rest before she goes over the edge. This is true, also, when the wife has a somewhat psychopathic personality. She should get out of the home for a week or two whenever she finds herself getting highly irritable and ugly and inclined to "fly off the handle." It would be wonderful if she could get away and get control of herself *before* she has a pitched battle with her husband and before she gets her children all upset.

A Weir Mitchell cure in a sanatorium. There is no doubt that for some nervous, thin, and troubled women a Weir Mitchell type of rest cure in a sanatorium can work a beautiful cure. Many a time I've seen my old preceptor in medicine work a miracle of healing in this way. Much of the cure was due to rest and the getting of better sleep; much was due to taking the patient out of a disturbing environment at home; some was due to the putting on of needed weight, and much was due to the enthusiasm of the physician and his unconsciously practiced psychotherapy. Ross tells us that after some years of getting good results with Weir Mitchell cures, he lost some of his faith in the procedure, and with this loss his treatment was no longer so effective. This made him think that the good results he had obtained before must have been due largely to unconscious psychotherapy.

Unfortunately, it is difficult to find a place in which a rest cure can be carried out well. One would like to have a quiet, well-run sanatorium with a good kitchen and nurses who have some sense about not waking every patient at 5 A.M. Usually a nurse feels that she just has to go in at daybreak to wake the patient and wash her face or take her temperature! The patient is barely asleep again when at the back door of the hospital the garbage man starts pounding each can as he empties it, and at 6 o'clock a man starts polishing the floor of the hall with a noisy machine.

Because of such noises around a sanatorium, the rest cure may better be carried out in the home of a devoted sister or mother. It is almost impossible to carry it out in the patient's home, especially when there are children about. The door bell and the telephone are ringing constantly or at intervals; a peevish child sets up a howl, or a servant comes with some annoyance. Never for a moment does the mother feel free from responsibility. Unfortunately, a rest cure outside the home is not available to most women because of the expense; and if the woman is worrying about expense the "cure" is not likely to work.

In order to fatten a thin woman the food should be concentrated, with plenty of calories, and it should be attractively prepared. It helps at first to have a tactful nurse who will encourage the patient to eat. To avoid the tendency to dawdle over the food it may help to insist that the patient get all the food down within fifteen minutes. Even if she complains of feeling stuffed, she should be encouraged to go on eating. After a while appetite comes, and the stomach accepts the burden of food. During the first few days it may help to give the woman 10 units of insulin twenty minutes before each meal. This may give her the appetite she needs.

It is useless to try to fatten a nervous woman if she is much disturbed over some unhappiness. So long as she is distressed and worried she will not gain. The foot of the bed should never be raised because there is no need for it; it only causes discomfort. It is better not to give purgatives but to relieve constipation with a daily enema of warm physiologic salt solution. Usually the large amount of food taken in a fattening cure tends to prevent constipation.

While the patient is in the hospital, symptoms may appear which will enable the physician to recognize organic disease. Or the nurse may discover what the annoying factors are which caused all the trouble. She may get a story of unhappiness which the doctor could not get. Incidentally, if the nurse should start "rubbing the patient the wrong way" she should immediately be taken off the case. Far better no nurse at all than one who chatters so incessantly that the poor patient feels like screaming.

Physical therapy, exercise, and massage. Occasionally one sees a neurotic woman who, months or years before, perhaps after a slight accident, drifted into a state of constant illness. Oftentimes she can be lifted out of the illness by a good course of physical therapy carried out by a cheerful and encouraging woman who will build back the strength of flaccid muscles and will loosen up stiff and painful joints. In this way I have seen some chronic invalids put back into a normal life again. Massage gives a woman something to look forward to each day; it gives hope, and it brings her each day under the influence of the cheerful therapist and perhaps the doctor.

Many other patients who go to internists complaining of backaches, sacroiliac strains, or tension in the muscles at the back of the neck can be helped by baking, massage, and the modern types of diathermy.

Developing a hobby. Many a woman with a bored and difficult husband on her hands evenings and weekends might solve her problem by getting him a camera and a basement darkroom, or a basement shop, a potter's wheel, or a garden. There are books and magazines on hobbies, showing what can be done.

Treatment with drugs. One of the commonest practices today is to give all nervous patients, and even the depressed ones, a dose of phenobarbital three times a day. There is no question that sometimes this makes the person less tense and more comfortable, but in other cases it does harm because it adds to the gloom, feelings of dullness, or lack of "pep." It would seem better practice, when giving a sedative, to prescribe that it be taken only when the person has a jittery few hours or a bad day. Then it might be well to give a drug that has a shorter action and less of a tendency to produce a hangover than phenobarbital has. Phenobarbital is one of the longest acting of all the calming drugs, and hence when it is taken every day its action may be cumulative. Another drug which is commonly prescribed in large doses and without proper supervision is sodium or potassium bromide. When taken every day in good-sized doses this drug accumulates in the blood, and every so often one sees a woman so full of bromine (usually over 50 mg. per 100 cc. of blood) that she has a mild psychosis.

Often a better sedative is bromural which is an alpha-monobrom-isovaleryl carbamide. It comes in 5-grain tablets. Only rarely does it produce a bromide rash. It helps persons who are jittery.

A physician, who once felt he had to live always in a mental sanatorium because of a constant jitteriness with feelings of impending disaster, discovered that by taking nembutal several times a day he could be perfectly well. He went back to work and for over ten years now he has been handling a good practice. He takes about 10 grains a day and feels no desire to increase the dose. He is pleasant and wide awake and is a fine useful member of his community. This is a most interesting case in that it shows what can sometimes be done with the help of a barbiturate. It shows, also, how safe barbiturates can be; it shows that there need be no habituation and no mental or moral deterioration. I know another physician who, because of insomnia, has used barbiturates practically every night for thirty years. He has never felt any desire to increase the dosage, and when on a vacation when he can sleep naturally, he never has any desire for the drugs.

There is many a tense nervous man who says that one cocktail before dinner will relieve all his jitteriness and his abdominal distress. For him a little alcohol is good medicine. I wonder if a small dose of nembutal might not have the same effect.

There is evidence that myanesin (tolserol) or thenylene will help patients to relax. They are said to allay anxiety without clouding consciousness, and this, of course, is what we physicians want.

Before I see them, most of my nervous patients, and especially those who have mucous colics or abdominal distress, have been thoroughly dosed with belladonna. Most of them report that the drug did not help. One would expect this because the medicine was given with several ideas in mind, all of them probably erroneous. One idea was that the person's troubles were due to spasm in the bowel, and it is doubtful if this was the case. Another idea was that the spasm would be relaxed by the belladonna, but experiments on the bowel of men and women with balloons passed through fistulas show that belladonna and the other new synthetic relaxants have little effect, and what they do have is of too short duration (a few minutes) to be of clinical value. The third idea was that belladonna would block parasympathetic impulses, and this it does not do. It may weaken them but it is doubtful if it could completely block them even if it were given in large, toxic, and discomfort-producing doses. Physicians forget that if they could give enough belladonna to block all parasympathetic influences on the colon, the patient would probably have no power of accommodation in his eyes, his heart would be racing, his mouth would be so dry that he would be miserable, and he probably would have a mild psychosis with disorientation.

The physician should always remember that granting that he could get a drug that would disconnect autonomic nerves, he could not expect it to disconnect the nerves from one organ without disconnecting them from all organs, in which case the patient might go into shock or even die. Actually, some of the new nerve-blocking drugs such as dibenamine have at times worked so efficiently that they have produced alarming reactions.

New drugs are constantly being discovered and tested, and it is possible that some of the new ones will be found helpful to nervous persons. For insance, dramamine (50-mg. tablets) is now relieving many sufferers from car-sickness, air-sickness and sea-sickness, and it is helping many persons who suffer from nausea.

According to Bennett (1946), estrogens do not cure involutional melancholias. They can, however, be very helpful in calming menopausal flushes. Thyroid substance will, of course, help the woman with definite hypothyroidism.

The mildly depressed person can sometimes be helped by a tablet of benzedrine or dexedrine or desoxyn. This may wake him up much as he might be waked by a big cup of coffee.

THE NEED FOR FIGHTING INSOMNIA

In the case of many a nervous, tired, worn-out patient the surest way back to health is through the getting of more sleep. The person who lies awake half the night cannot feel well next day and cannot get anywhere in his efforts to recover from a nervous breakdown. One of the first things, then, that many a nervous person can do is to go to bed earlier. Today thousands make the mistake of sitting up late. They say, "Why go to bed when I cannot sleep?" But they are wrong. They would be better off in bed resting, even if they did not sleep right away.

Many persons will never sleep much so long as they spend their nights going over the day's problems, worrying, and trying to plan for the future. Others might sleep better if they could get over their *fear* of insomnia. The physician can help them by assuring them that insomnia can be endured for years, without its bringing death or insanity. Some persons, instead of fretting and tossing around, would do well to turn on the light and read a while until they get sleepy.

Older persons should be warned not to drink much water or milk or other fluid late in the day. It will only get them up at night. Some older persons would sleep better at night if they did not drowse so much during the day.

Some persons need to be reminded that when they think they have lain awake most of the night they probably have been drowsing much of the time. Many a person in a hospital who is sure he had no sleep was snoring every time the nurse looked in. Many a spouse knows that the mate sleeps a few minutes and then wakes for a few minutes and does this all night.

A few persons who suffer from gas and indigestion during much of the night ought to go without supper a few times to see if then they can have a more comfortable night. If not, food is not the cause of their restlessness. If, however, after fasting they sleep well, each evening they can experiment with one food after another, keeping a record, until they know which ones give trouble and which do not.

The need for a sedative. Many persons with insomnia need help from drugs. They could get to sleep without them, but they might have to wait until 2 A.M., and that would mean that they would be sleepy next day. If the person had nothing to do next day, this might be all right, but usually he or she has to go to work, and work needs a wide-awake brain. Under such circumstances, I think a person must take something that will bring sleep quickly. In other cases a person, without the help of a drug, sleeps fitfully and is awake much of the night. With the help of a mild barbiturate sleep would be deeper; there would be less waking and the periods of waking would be shorter.

There are times when a person can sleep well and other times when he cannot, and then is when he needs help. There are times, as when a man has to give an after-dinner address or attend a long evening committee meeting, when his brain will be "lit-up." Then it will not quiet down for hours, and that is when he needs a sedative.

Often, within ten minutes after turning out the light, a person who has long suffered from insomnia can tell whether he is going to be able to get to sleep. If he sees that his brain is too wide awake and his muscles too tense, he had better take a pill. Sometimes a man can read until he is sleepy and then if he lies down quickly and turns out the light, sleep will come.

Many laymen and even some physicians fear soporifics and think that they are habit forming, but in my experience, they are not. True habituation with euphoria, or a running-up of the dosage, or withdrawal symptoms have been reported, but I have not seen the syndrome. In forty-five years I have seen perhaps a dozen persons who were taking barbiturates to excess, but they had all had a psychopathic personality to begin with. Every one of them was able to stop the use of the drug instantly and without symptoms of withdrawal; their only complaint then was that without help from *something* they could not sleep.

Two types of insomnia. There are two main types of insomnia—one in which the person on going to bed has difficulty in getting to sleep, and the other in which he or she wakes, perhaps around 4 o'clock in the morning, and cannot get back to sleep again. For the first type of case, one can prescribe either a short-acting or a long-acting drug. Often all that is needed is something to get the person calmed down. The commonest drug used in this country appears to be phenobarbital, but this has the disadvantage of having a long action-time, so long that there may be some hangover in the morning. Milder and shorter acting are drugs like seconal and adalin (carbromal) or bromural. Some persons can get to sleep with ¾ of a grain of seconal; others need 1½ grains. Adalin is so mild that an insensitive patient may have to take 2 or 3 tablets. Nembutal works well for some persons in doses of 1½ grains. It is too strong for others. Carbrital, a mixture of carbromal and nembutal, sometimes works well.

For the person who wakes at 4 or 5 A.M. one must give a short-acting drug, and my favorite is bromural. For a sensitive person even half a tablet will work in a few minutes, and its action will be over at seven when it is time to get up.

If a person has some pain at night, such as that due to arthritis, one may have to combine a barbiturate with aspirin or phenacetin or acetanilid.

When barbiturates work wrongly. The neurotic woman and the woman whose nerves are terribly on edge will often be unable to take barbiturates. She is so keyed-up that the drug works wrongly; it makes her feel wild and manic, and it may cause bad nightmares. Her brain is so irritable that it takes a big dose of any drug to calm it down. In such cases repeated doses may eventually bring sleep, but before this comes the patient has to go through an unpleasant stage of mild mania. In many such cases, and especially in the cases of psychotic persons and alcoholics, the physician will have to resort to the use of chloral and paraldehyde (see the next chapter). In some cases benadryl or some other antihistaminic will work well as a soporific.

On the need for separate beds or separate rooms. There is many a nervous and often sleepless woman who greatly needs the physician's help in talking the husband into letting her have her own bed or her own room. In their youth two people are likely to sleep so soundly, or when they wake are likely to fall asleep again so quickly, that they can share a bed. It is good when they can, because it gives them more chance for a display of that affection which brings them close together at the end of the day and heals psychic hurts. But as the two grow older, one or both may get to snoring loudly; or one or both may develop insomnia, or one or both may toss about or have to get up seceral times to urinate. One or both may develop individual habits of wanting to read or to go to sleep or to wake up at strange times early or late. After the menopause, the woman may be waking every little while with a flush, and wanting to kick off the bed clothes. Then it may become highly important that the couple have separate rooms. Often the husband objects because he looks on this as the first sign of a loss of romance or the break-up of the marriage, but if his snoring is causing the wife to lie awake hours each night, and if this is a big factor in causing her nervous illness, he ought to be wise and kind and give in.

Similarly, if the wife's need for rising several times at night to care for a feeble-minded or asthmatic child or a senile mother is breaking into the man's rest so that next day he cannot work well at the office, she must give in and let him have a separate room.

On getting an eye shade to help the patient to sleep. Many women, and especially those migrainous ones whose eyes are very sensitive to light, could help themselves greatly by buying or making an eye shade much like a domino mask but without holes for the eyes. Such shades are to be found in drug stores. With one, the patient can more easily get a nap, or she can sleep later on a summer morning, or she can sleep on a porch, or she may not wake when at night her husband turns on the light.

Good ear plugs are much needed today to shut out disturbing sounds but as yet I have not found a good type.

Difficult interviews. In some cases the patient is so quickly outraged at any intimation on the part of the physician that the trouble is even partly psychic in origin that no doctor will want to bother with him. It is too ticklish a business, and too likely to end in bitterness and mutual dislike. In dealing with such persons the physician must have great control over his temper and great patience. If he wants to help the man he must keep insisting that he is not questioning the fact that there is pain or that the man is a highly intelligent fellow; he is only trying to say that from long experience every wise physician who sees him will sense that he is a pathologically hypersensitive individual with a peculiar personality and many neurosis-building factors in his life. Certainly the man has all the set-up for a neurosis, and any physician who would treat him without thinking first and foremost of a neurosis would be a fool or an incompetent or an evader of the issue. There could, of course, be also an organic lesion but this has been well looked for and apparently excluded.

Sometimes I remind the patient that he came to me for an opinion because he had heard I was competent and experienced. I then had him thoroughly examined by an able neurologist and perhaps other able specialists. All of us feel the same way about him—that his troubles are of psychic origin. If he cannot believe this and does not want to accept it, that is his privilege and right. But he hasn't a right to be angry with us any more than we have a right to be angry with him. We ought to be able to part amicably, with an admission on both sides that there is a chance that the other one is right. Sometimes if a physician is sufficiently kind, urbane, and self-controlled he can keep the peace with such a person, or he can eventually gain his trust and liking, and with this can greatly help him.

I must admit that in the worst cases I feel like bowing myself out; it is so hard to do anything with a hurt, incredulous, and perhaps angry patient who cannot see that a neurosis is the most logical diagnosis that can be made. As patients have said, "I told the neurologist that I deeply resented his diagnosis and his apparent dislike of me, and his answer was that he didn't like me, and so we parted company." It is most unfortunate for both patients and physicians that occasionally they must have such interviews.

The need for consultations, especially in difficult cases. As I read books on psychiatry I look in vain for an adequate discussion of the fact that often, even when it is obvious to any keen physician that the patient needs psychiatric help, this cannot be attempted until a study has been made by a number of able specialists. I say "able" because these men will have to bring to the task an unusual amount of good sense and clinical wisdom, such as can be acquired only in the course of thirty or forty years of practice. They must decide wisely whether there is some organic disease present which either cannot be cured or can be relieved by an operation.

For instance, a nervous and anxious woman came complaining of pain, numbness, tingling, weakness, soreness, and slight edema in a leg. She was obviously an emotionally unstable person, and what with a divorce, a slight automobile accident, and an insurance problem, she had all the "set-up" for a bit of hysteria. I thought she belonged primarily in the hands of a psychiatrist, but first I had to rule out organic disease in the spine, abdomen, and pelvis, and in the bones, muscles, arteries, veins, and nerves of the extremity. After a general examination designed to rule out such things as a primary anemia, syphilis, marked hypertension, metastatic carcinoma, a tumor in the pelvis, an aneurysm of the iliac artery, or Paget's disease of the tibia, an expert on arteries and veins and lymph channels was called to see the leg; an orthopedist looked for signs of a slipped disc, a neurologist looked for signs of disease in the brain, the spinal cord, or the local nerves, and an expert on arthritis gave an opinion as to the presence of an atypical fibrositis or arthritis.

Interestingly, when all the examinations had failed to reveal any alarming disease, the woman felt much better. I talked over with her the psychic problems that had assailed her before and after her divorce; I talked her out of bringing a suit for compensation, and with all this, her worries were so well dispelled that she went home satisfied and willing to put up with what little discomfort she had in the leg. This case showed, as others often do, that sometimes the ordinary medical handling of a patient is sufficient to cure, and then the time of a psychiatrist is spared for the helping of patients who need him badly.

Another example of the extremely difficult problems presented at times is that of the middle-aged widow who, while riding with friends, was involved in an auto accident and received a blow on her pelvis and spine. There was always a question as to whether much physical injury had been sustained. Most of the doctors who saw her thought the roentgenograms were "negative," while a few thought they saw signs of a crack in a pelvic bone. At any rate, a year and a half passed and the woman was still unable to get out of bed. Some orthopedists thought there was still some abnormality in the spine, while others could see no reason why she should not get up and go to work. Some gynecologists thought there might be some injury to the pelvic organs, while others could find no sign of any. Several internists thought the disability was all out of proportion to the amount of injury sustained, granting that there had been some. Certainly, the neurologists could not find any sign of an injury to the spinal cord. Finally, with the running out of all funds for her support, and with some physical therapy, she got up and went to work.

In this case a psychiatrist could have pointed to many facts suggesting a compensation neurosis, but in the face of diagnoses of organic disease made by good specialists, I doubt if he could have been positive enough or convincing enough in his psychotherapy to work a cure. Besides, the woman was in no mood to accept psychotherapy, and I think if anyone had ever even hinted that the accident had been a minor one she would angrily have shown him the door.

Another case that illustrates the problems under discussion was that of an unmarried woman of forty years, an executive secretary, who was referred with the diagnosis of a slipped lumbar disc. She complained of pain down one thigh and leg which could conceivably be due to pressure from a disc. But what impressed me much was the fact that the night she arrived she was in an agitated depression, terribly restless, talking of suicide, and unable to sleep even when given large doses of sedatives. I was impressed, also, by the type of long story she told of unwise overwork, engagements to marry that fell through, and mix-ups with some poorly chosen friends. She apparently had a poor nervous inheritance and an unstable nervous system, and one had to suspect that most of her illness and pain was arising in her troubled brain.

The few signs of nerve injury that could be found by the neurologists were in one lower extremity, and for a few days they were impressed by them. But, then, it was discovered that this limb had been slightly injured by poliomyelitis in childhood and thereafter had been weak and uncomfortable. Because of (1) the woman's temperament, (2) a normal spinal fluid, and (3) no roentgenologic signs of a slipped disc, orthopedists and neurologists and internists agreed that an operation was not indicated, and any exploration of the spine would be unwise. But the girl promptly went to a great university medical hospital where she was operated on. This left her with such pain that she had to have several more operations in an effort to get back to where she was before. The lesson is that in cases of this type the fact that a person has poor materials in her nervous system and no definite signs of local disease should warn surgeons not to begin operating. Even if they should find local disease and remove it they are not likely to work a cure.

Just as we clinicians ought often to be consulting with psychiatrists, so they should sometimes be consulting with us. For instance, a middle-aged man who began to have severe constipation was induced by a friend to see a psychiatrist. Learning of his marital infelicity, the psychiatrist promptly diagnosed an unwillingness of the patient to give up even fecal matter to the wife, and started treating him for this. Finally, the man went to a clinician who, in a minute, found a big carcinoma of the rectum. I know full well that we clinicians often order operations for patients who are suffering only from insanity. The one important point we must all agree on is that all of us, psychiatrists and non-psychiatrists, must often meet in consultation; we must help each other and protect each other from mistakes.

The need often to stop treating one spot and to treat instead the whole patient. One of the most important things a consultant must often do is to call a halt in the constant treatment of some aching organ or spot and insist instead that the whole patient be treated. Oftentimes a long series of examinations, strenuous local treatments, and perhaps oft-repeated operations have reduced a woman to such a nervous state that she cannot even tell when she is free from pain. In such cases the wise doctor will say, "We will never get anywhere treating that one spot. Our only hope of relieving your distress must lie in improving your general health so that you will not be so full of misery all over." Perhaps he can explain what is meant by raising the threshold for pain.

To illustrate: A frail girl who had broken under the strain of managing a good-sized office was getting three bad migraines a week. She was treated for a year by the best internists in a large city. They gave her many drugs; they drained her sinuses; they removed her appendix, they cauterized her sphenopalatine ganglion, and they gave her many injections of this and that. Nothing helped until a physician discovered how trying her job was. He got her family to take her on a long vacation, and on her return she got an easier job in a happier environment. With this she was almost well.

Helping the person who is running a race between getting well and going broke. One of the hard things a physician has to do sometimes is to try to help the person who, after breaking down nervously so that he cannot work, faces the problem of getting well before he goes broke. Naturally, if he worries much about the situation he is not likely to get well, but under the circumstances, it is hard not to worry.

Every so often I see a school teacher who has broken down under some strain and is rapidly using up the sick leave that is coming to her. It is hard to help her when she lies awake night after night, wondering if she can get well in time or if she should stay out for a semester and use up her savings. Sometimes an aunt will put up enough money for a few months, but even with this, it still is a race between recovery and the exhaustion of the aunt's purse or patience.

In these cases the physician may help if he can get the person to see that there is only one thing to do, and that is to refuse to worry, and instead to get the maximum rest and peace of mind. If the patient is uncontrolled enough to go on fretting and doing the things that produced the breakdown, he or she cannot hope to get well.

Some persons are likely to be incurable. By nature I am an optimist, and I like trying to help people, but experience has taught me that some persons I almost certainly will not be able to help. When I recognize one of them I hate to go ahead and waste time. The person may make no effort to reform, or probably he *cannot* make much of an effort; certainly he cannot make any *lasting* effort. He may not even listen to me as I talk; he keeps breaking in to tell me what someone once diagnosed, or what someone once gave in the way of medicine. He will not remember anything of what I told him or he will get it all twisted.

When a patient will not listen to me as I talk, I am reminded of what a trainer of monkeys for a vaudeville act told Darwin. As I remember the story, the trainer said that if the price of monkeys was a pound, he would offer the animal seller five pounds for a monkey he would choose after briefly interviewing a couple of dozen in the store. When Darwin asked him how he could tell so quickly which monkey was going to be trainable, the man said it would be the one that looked at him and paid attention. He could not teach a monkey anything if it would not pay attention!

If the reader will turn back to Chapter 8 on persons who are ill because they feel caught in a trap, he will see why many of them are incurable. There is no way of setting them free.

There are many patients who cannot see (1) that a disease can be functional in nature, (2) that its cause can be a bad nervous inheritance, or the strain of living, or an irreparable injury to the nervous system such as that left by a little stroke, or (3) that a cure cannot be expected so long as unhygienic or unhappy conditions continue.

Many persons cannot conceive of a cure being worked largely by themselves; their only idea of treatment is something that comes out of a bottle or an operating room. They never heard of psychotherapy, and the idea of getting well with that is not among those which make up their country's medical folklore. As a result, often when I am faced by a neurosis in an elderly and unintelligent immigrant to our shores, I feel almost hopeless. I doubt if I can make her understand what I want her to do. I feel the same way when an ignorant woman starts telling me of all the things various quacks have done for her. She and I have such different ideas about medicine that there is little use in our talking to each other.

I remember a constitutionally inadequate, always sickly woman who got by fairly well until her husband, fed up with her complaining, deserted her. On going back to work in an office she soon broke down, and had to fall back on the grudging charity of relatives. One surgeon then stitched up a kidney, and another removed her stoneless gallbladder. Before these operations she could do some work, but afterward she could not. When I saw her she could not see why I did not give her some medicine that would promptly cure her, and she went off disgusted with medicine in general and me in particular. She was amazed at my ignorance and incompetence!

It is hard to cure a neurosis that has been present for years. A good physician will commonly see in a few minutes that a patient's many complaints must be largely or entirely psychic in origin. Often he will be almost certain that the whole syndrome is hysterical. But, after the patient has been ill so long it would be hard to prove this or to get the patient to face or accept the suggestion. He or she has been treated too long for organic illness. There may be a substratum of organic disease, but after several operations it is now impossible to mark the limits of this. The chances are that the patient started with an inborn tendency to neurosis; she got one, and now years of illness have fastened on her habits of complaining and dependency. Perhaps by now she hasn't even much desire for recovery.

Occasionally a person like this will be cured by a quack of some kind, or by some magnetic and enthusiastic physician, or an Elizabeth Barrett will be cured when her Robert Browning comes along. Occasionally, one can get an Elizabeth Barrett well by building up her strength through physical therapy. I have seen several women who, after being bedridden for years, were gotten up and back into life by the efforts of a good physical therapist. Some chronic invalids get·well when their money is gone, or when either a supporting or a disturbing relative dies.

On trying to remake a personality. We physicians are always talking about making over a defective personality, but I wonder how much of this sort of thing we can do. I wonder how far the patient cares to go along this line. Certainly, in many cases, one can soon see that a man is not going to make any great effort to make himself over. Perhaps he would like to be well, but he has no stomach for the long course of self-discipline and training that would have to be undergone before he could recover. He is much like the clerk who would like the boss' job but will make no effort to train himself for it, or he is like the child who said, "I wish I wanted to do that!"

One of the most foolish things a physician can do is to try to cure a person against his or her will. In my youth I used to attempt this, but I finally learned that all I got for my pains was dislike. Sometimes even now I try to sell a nervous or hysterical woman the idea that she would have much more fun out of life if she were to get well, but I fear this is often a waste of time. If the woman does not take kindly to the idea, and if, for some reason or other, she wants to keep her neurosis, I let her go.

Thorner told of an able woman trying to help her uneducated husband to take correspondence courses. Finally he got angry and said, "Can't you see I like to be the way I am? I'm not smart as you are. I'm not interested in your books or in bettering myself. I'm satisfied as I am." Many persons when being "uplifted" doubtless feel as this man did.

That something can be done in the way of remaking people's lives is shown by the fact that every so often a physician will get a letter from some woman whom he saw a year or two before, saying that she is now a new person because of some talks they had. She says she went home and pulled herself together, conquered some bad habits, gave up some resentments and some efforts to dominate others, ac-

cepted some discomforts and distresses, and got practically well. I
have known a number of such cases.

It is sad that some persons, when they are made to see clearly that
something they are doing is causing their illness or the illness of a
loved one, seem unable to make the change which would bring them
health and happiness. For instance, I remember a fine minister who
had spent all his savings trying to cure his wife's severe migraine. He
admitted that she was probably right in saying that she would be well if
he would only start writing his next Sunday's sermon by Wednesday. It
was her worry over his tendency to put off this all-essential work that
threw her into a headache. He adored her, but since he was a born
procrastinator, he went on as usual, and the wife wound up a wreck.

Even after a person has become, so to speak, converted by the doctor and has gone up to the "mourner's bench," his difficulties are far
from over. Naturally, bad habits of thinking which have been built
up through half a lifetime are not going to be conquered overnight.
A woman who has been in a sanatorium for months under the care
of a good psychiatrist may come home feeling well and determined
to keep the peace and behave sensibly, but with the first annoyance
she may "blow up" again and blame her husband for all her troubles.
This is only human, but if she has profited by her course of psychotherapy, this time she will quickly quiet down: She will not sulk for
two or three days as she used to do, and she will not try to punish
the husband for her sins.

Shaking a patient out of his or her complacency. Often I find it
necessary, when a woman seems too complacent about her illness, to
shake her by saying, "Look what a mess you have made of these last
thirty years of your life; you will probably have to live another forty
years; do you want to go on like this until you are seventy, sick, full
of misery, and unable to have fun?" Usually the patient says, "The
Lord forbid: I could not bear the thought of living this way for another forty years. That frightens me; it would be awful. All right,
then, tell me what I must do and I will try to do it."

Why cannot some people learn? One of the worst handicaps of
the neurotic or psychopathic person is his or her inability to profit
by repeated sad experiences. A hundred times a woman may see that
every time she loses her temper she gets a terrible attack of migraine,
or alienates still further an adored husband, or gets a crop of giant
hives, but still, with every little annoyance, she "blows up." These
persons are feebly inhibited. They are like a diabetic who goes on
eating candy when he is going blind or a chain smoker who is losing
his legs because of sclerosing arteries. Such a man belongs, of course,
in that large group of persons whose immediate desire is not blocked

by the sureness of future punishment. Such persons are not curable by physicians.

The help a patient can obtain from religion. There are some patients who can be helped through religion and the efforts of a spiritual advisor, and the good physician will use such help whenever he can. In a few cases, when I have found a patient torn by religious doubts, I have sent him to his priest, his minister, or his rabbi. For many years now, some able ministers have been studying psychotherapy, and with its help they are aiding many troubled parishioners. Harry Emerson Fosdick, the late Rabbi Liebman, and Monsignor Sheen have all written helpful books on developing character and attaining peace of mind and soul.

Religion is sometimes used as a means of escape. Men and women who feel incompetent to handle their own affairs may ask God to take over and do everything for them. For a while after joining some group of persons who preach that one should turn to God for every decision, a person may feel better and happier. Persons with a religious trend can, of course, get help from prayer. Probably in order to get anything out of prayer a person must pray intelligently, knowing well what he wants and how to ask for it. A man will do well probably to ask only that God *help him to get* what he wants. Many ministers say that the supplicant has to make some contribution in the way of intelligent desire and effort. I love the old prayer which says, "Oh Lord, I ask you not to favor me with good things: just tell me where they are and I will go and get them."

The influence of sex. In this chapter I say little about sexual troubles. There is no question that sex often is a factor in producing neuroses, and when the sexual life is unsatisfactory there is likely to be some unhappiness. But as Myerson used to say, most of the highly nervous, sickly persons who came to see him were too tired, weak, apprehensive, worried, bored, selfish, or fearful of poverty, illness, unwanted pregnancy, or loss of employment to be greatly concerned with sex. My impression is much the same, and I must say that I think the Freudians overdo the matter of sex as a cause of the neuroses.

As I wrote this, a keen, attractive, ex-businesswoman of forty-two came in. Her nervous troubles began two years ago, when, in order to put her girls through college, she had married a well-to-do but crude sort of man. Now the couple is constantly fighting and she has been asking for a divorce. What interested me was that with all her dislike of the man she has no complaint to make about her sexual life; that is satisfactory. She and the man are incompatible only mentally and socially, and it is only his lack of culture and refinement that bothers her.

Instruction in contraceptive technic. It may seem odd to some physicians that instruction in contraceptive technic should be included in a chapter on psychotherapy, but often it is highly important. Much of the friction between some couples arises from the reluctance of the wife to have intercourse, and this may be due to the woman's great fear of pregnancy and the economic tragedy that this would usher in. If interrupted coitus or coitus with a condom is leaving the woman unsatisfied and upset, she should be fitted with a diaphragm. Occasionally, religious objections to contraception must be discussed.

The restoration of a happy sexual life can go far to help both the wife and the husband, especially when, with the giving up of intercourse, the husband starts straying, or the wife thinks he must be straying when he is kind enough not to "bother" her.

The unwisdom of some trends in psychiatry today. An important point that has been emphasized by Ross and others is that the man who is not well trained and well experienced in psychotherapy had better not try to pry too deeply into the minds and motives of certain patients. He can do serious harm. Thus, I knew a man with a functional illness who, on several occasions, was greatly helped by an able specialist who, after a thorough examination, assured him that he did not have the cancer he feared. Then one day the specialist suggested that the patient consult a psychiatrist. He consulted someone who called himself a psychiatrist who apparently accused him of something awful, because in a few days he committed suicide.

Some psychiatrists have been saying that the reason men with an active ulcer drink milk every two hours is that in their infancy the mother denied them the breast. Now they are showing their resentment. This, to me, seems very silly because while busy with his mind on his work, a man with an ulcer will suddenly feel his pain. One moment it wasn't there and the next minute it is there. The man then drinks milk simply because he knows this will bring him relief. That it is not just milk that he wants is shown by the fact that if this liquid is not handy he will eat crackers or take some antacid. These things will satisfy him perfectly just so long as they relieve his pain. Also, the day the ulcer stops hurting, the man loses all interest in milk or anything else between meals.

Today I am happy to find that some of the leaders of psychiatry are warning their students to go slow on fantastic interpretations. For instance, in the Minneapolis Graduate Course (p. 55) Rennie said, "I feel very strongly that the important thing is not to jump to conclusions about personality structure but rather to approach every patient with open-mindedness." Dr. Romano went on to say that a psychiatrist might see a patient with hypertension and say, "Aha, hypertension is related to rage, hence I have to find out what this man's resentments are and then show them to him. That may not be right. One has to be honest enough to get the data as they come, and not to make premature judgments, or be biased by what may prove to be an unsound hypothesis." I say, "Amen; there spoke a wise man and a good teacher."

It is good to find Franz Alexander saying so wisely that "our theoretical abstractions . . . require constant critical revision . . . regarding conceptual precision and clarity. This is particularly true in our young discipline in which theory has been prematurely developed into a consistent system, and has tended to become dogmatic and rigid." Alexander might well have gone on to say that anything that has become dogmatic and rigid is a religious faith and has no resemblance to anything scientific. Freyhan (1947) has accused certain psychiatrists of practicing a narrow religion and not a science. As he said, in this religion as in most others, a heretic is immediately cast out and excommunicated. So far as his old group goes he is through, and his name is never mentioned again in their writings.

Another psychiatrist wrote, "The greatest need in psychiatry today is for a constant skepticism on the part of every student of the subject. Every statement of his teacher must be scrutinized and questioned. The student must keep asking always, 'How did the teacher know that, or did he know it?' "

It is interesting to learn of psychic shocks in childhood, but one wonders how often the unearthing of these things works a cure or improves a defective personality.

The physician must often feel his way. In many of the sections that follow I will say little about *details* of therapy because commonly the treatment needed is obvious as soon as the cause of the illness has been established. In many such cases, the patient himself sees what he must do in order to help himself, or he sees as well as the physician does that under the circumstances little can be done or needs to be done for him. In other cases the doctor can quickly suggest what would be best to do. In still others he will have to feel his way, using what human wisdom he has.

The occasional need for searching for psychic traumas in the patient's early years. At times, of course, even a non-psychiatrist will want to go back with the patient over his early life and experiences to find a cause for some neurosis or phobia. For example, a fine, well-educated, nice-looking young woman came complaining of a nervous diarrhea. She soon confessed to much suffering from a marked inferiority complex which had always plagued her, especially in her dealings with men. It was easy enough to point out to her that she had little logical reason for feeling inferior. She was a woman with more than average good looks and intelligence and ability.

This reassurance helped a bit but I then went back with her into her childhood and got the story of a sadistic mother. The father, an able man, displeased with the lack of culture in his wife, kept telling her that in his youth a "baby face" had tricked him into a stupid marriage. The wife got even by telling her daughter that she, too, was no good, and would never be able to hold a man. She kept saying this until the girl came to believe it. She believed it so fully that several times she was all set to marry a cripple so that she would not be likely later to be deserted. Often I have found that a girl like this, with an inferiority complex, was confirmed in it by a sadistic devil of a brother who, for years, kept telling her she was ugly and unattractive.

Sometimes, when the physician talks over these old psychic scars with the patient, the trouble becomes less distressing, and more easily combated.

The unwisdom of immediately telling the patient what he is thinking and why. As Hinsie has so wisely said, it is a mistake for a physician to start *telling* a patient what he thinks and what motivates him, and what nervous trauma he has had in his infancy. No scientist would think of doing such a thing. He would *ask* the patient what the stresses and strains and unhappy thoughts were that wore him down.

Ross disliked the present-day tendency toward accusing patients of developing convenient symptoms. This tends to shatter the person's self-esteem and to make him angry with the physician. For instance, Ross had a patient who hated to live in London. The man developed an indigestion which gave him an excuse to move to the suburbs. Some psychiatrists might have said that the dyspepsia was the result of the patient's unconscious desire to effect an escape, but Ross doubted this, and anyway, he had no desire to blurt out this accusation. Even if it were true, it could only upset and disturb the fellow and make him angry or ashamed.

Many neurotic persons, in order to live with any comfort, have to blind themselves to the defects of their nature: They have to find excuses for their worthlessness and their failures in life. As Ross said, if a physician were suddenly to take away these excuses he would leave the man feeling as if his clothes had been stripped from him. The man's only response would probably be one of anger.

All this does not mean that at times the physician must not show a patient why he has failed: without such enlightenment a cure may be impossible. But all should be done with kindliness, tact, and sympathy. Often, a good technic is gradually to get the person himself to confess. For instance, if a woman has been telling me how trying her husband is, after a while, I may ask, "And you, being human, do you not at times annoy or hurt him? The best of us lose our temper at times." Addressed in this way, the woman usually says, "Yes, at times I am a hellion, and then I don't see how he puts up with me." After this confession, the physician can plead for better behavior without angering the woman.

The need for listening. All wise psychiatrists emphasize the need for the physician's doing a lot of listening while he lets the patient do a lot of talking. I am sorry to say that many people have told me of physicians and some few psychiatrists who did all the talking. Obviously, a man who does not listen cannot help his patients, and he cannot go on learning medicine from them. About all he can become in time is a pompous ass, whose medical education has largely come to an end.

It is hard to see how anyone can tell a stranger why he did this or that. The man who would attempt it must be very sure of his theories of human behavior. He must believe strongly in his dogmas of symbolism. Because I do not always understand all of my own motives, I cannot see how anyone else could ever tell me what they are or were. I know that the psychiatrist uses certain technics to find out what the subconscious motives and thoughts of a person were, and I grant that in this way he can sometimes learn much, but still I think that much that has been written on the subject is unscientific and fantastic, and I am sure it will not stand the test of time.

One of the best stories I know to illustrate the folly of *telling* patients instead of *listening* to them is that of the internist who scolded a nicely dressed woman of forty, saying, "I know your type: childless, pampered, bridge playing, always in the house. You need more often to get out in the open air, and you need more excitement." She did not bother to tell him that, she, the wife of a rum runner, spent her evenings in the car with a machine-gun across her knees!

The psychotherapist should not scold. During psychotherapy the physician must often point out the unwisdom of certain phases of the patient's behavior. He may note that a certain course of action has led to disaster, or he may express fear that, if a course is followed, it will bring further trouble. He may occasionally have to scold a bit but he can always do this in a bantering, friendly way which will not give offense. Many a time, when chiding a woman for doing something she had promised not to do, I have said, "You know you ought to be spanked, but still I like you."

No matter what a patient confesses, the physician must never act like an outraged parent or a goody-goody young parson. Many a woman has said to me, "I confessed that to my doctor but he is so religious and straight-laced that all he did was to give me hell." I do not feel that as a physician I need be concerned with my patients' morals; to me in the office saint and sinner are alike—what I am concerned with is their health. An occasional patient is very grateful when he or she finds a physician who will listen to a story of misbehavior and its consequences without turning a hair or showing any sign of disgust or dislike or disapproval. Sometimes the person goes away "cured" largely because the doctor was not horrified or disgusted.

Some patients have said to me years after I saw them, "You know, that day in the office, I think you saved me from suicide; you made me well again by doing just one thing, and I'll bet you do not know what it was. What you did was to make me feel that after all I had told you you still liked me. You treated me in the same friendly manner as you did when I came in. You did not once recoil in disgust, and you never looked down your nose at me. The fact that you still seemed to look on me as a friend was all I needed to regain my self-respect and my willingness to go on living. I felt clean again, and I went back to my old place in life." Some patients will explain this years later by saying "You accepted me."

Many a nice person with a bad inferiority complex is greatly helped by receiving a physician's friendship. A young woman will keep saying to herself, "Well, if that man in his position likes me and treats me as a friend, I cannot be as awful as I thought I was. Perhaps I *am* nice as he says I am." As the old proverb has it, "And while doing good we never know how much good we do." Often we never know that we helped a soul out of purgatory.

The wrongness of saying "go get a man." A wrong thing some of us do is to tell a single woman or a widow to go get herself a man and have sexual intercourse. The physician who says this must know very little about the needs of women. Their need is not so much for physical sex as for a constant love, tenderness, and companionship. They want someone to go out with and enjoy things with, and someone to give security and a home. The physician who advises an "affair" fails also to think of all the distresses that might come to the fine and sensitive woman if the man in the case were to tire of the liaison and drop her cruelly.

The wrongness of saying "go get married." Bad can be the advice to go and get married. It may be particularly bad advice for a schizoid man or woman who, on attempting to adjust to a sexual life, can go over the edge into a bad psychosis. As I point out in Chapter 14, it is bad to advise the homosexual man or woman to marry. Usually this results only in the cruel victimization of some innocent and unsuspecting person. Occasionally a man or woman is rescued from a life of neurosis or alcoholism by marriage to a devoted person, but that person, if he or she assumes the burden, runs a terrible risk, and that risk should be taken without urging from any physician.

The non-psychiatric physician must sometimes take care of a mildly psychotic patient. Obviously, the non-psychiatric physician will not want to be treating psychotic patients of the type who need special care, and he should not be treating them. But, often, as a country physician, or even as a specialist or consultant, he will run into one of these cases. Then it may be hard to pass the person on to a psychiatrist, if only because the family clings to the hope that if someone will cure a constipation, a headache, a pain, or a tired feeling, the loved one will straighten out mentally. Usually, today, in such cases, the physician makes the mistake of trying to do what the patient wants. Only occasionally does he recognize the seriousness of the situation and try to do something adequate about it.

A schizoid person can sometimes be helped by a kindly physician who will talk over his difficulties with him. The person with a mild manic-depressive tendency can be much helped by learning what his nature is and why sometimes he does too much and at other times he feels so tired and dull and ill.

If one is interested and friendly, a psychotic person will sometimes discuss the reasons for his or her behavior. For instance, a psychotic young woman of wealth, who spent much of her life in asylums told me why she had often tried to commit suicide. She said it all started when on a steamer she fell in love with a nice-looking steward. By the time she reached Southampton she had become obsessed with the idea that she had let her distinguished family down and had disgraced them; she felt that only her death could wipe out the stain.

How should a physician talk to a man who is psychically disturbed? Many a physician, not trained in psychiatry, when faced by a person who is mentally disturbed, wonders how he should talk to him. Usually the best way is to talk logically and in a friendly way just as one would do if the man were sane. Actually, as Clifford Beers maintained, much of a psychotic person's reasoning is logical; his trouble is that some of his premises are wrong. If a psychotic person likes the doctor and trusts him, he may talk to him, at least at times, as sensibly as anyone would.

To get help for handling the mentally troubled, physicians should read Beers' *The Mind That Found Itself.* There they will be impressed with the need for carrying out scrupulously every promise made to an insane person. To deceive him is to upset him still further and to do great harm. Mildly psychotic persons are particularly watchful for signs of untruthfulness or inconsistency in what their doctor says, and when they feel that they have been deceived they are done with that physician.

ne should never get into an argument with a mentally disturbed pa-
t. If the man feels that he has heard Christ talking to him he is not
going to give up the idea simply because a physician tells him it is silly.

Muncie has given a helpful description of how a physician might go
about talking to a paranoiac. The first step is to establish some rapport,
and this can be done by listening to the story with patience and friendliness. The doctor should behave like any courteous person listening to
someone telling of some religious or political belief; he will appear to be
open minded and neutral, but at no time will he give the man the impression that he has been converted to his views. Rather, he will keep
asking for more facts of observation, saying, "We will try to interpret
them later." Some physicians have tried the technic of first agreeing
with the man's views to lead him on, and later telling him that he was all
wrong. Naturally, this only angers the man.

After the doctor has satisfied the patient that he is friendly and
anxious to help, he may start suggesting that there may be some other
· explanation for the facts observed. This must not be done in an argumentative way. If the patient should concede a point or two he may be
complimented on his intelligence and fairness in dealing with the problem. But with all this, Muncie said that one can seldom overthrow a
patient's delusional system, and this is especially true for the paranoiac.
The only thing that may be accomplished is to leave the man less disturbed for a while.

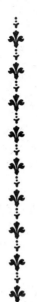

CHAPTER 29

Treatment of
the Psychotic Patient

SOME OF THE TECHNICS USED in the treatment of patients with psychoses are mentioned briefly in this chapter. The non-psychiatric physician should know something about the technics that psychiatrists are now using, if only because every so often a friend or an old patient will ask for advice as to what to do with a relative who has become queer or difficult to handle. Where can the family go for help, or how can they get the patient into a sanatorium? Where can they find a good psychiatrist? What will he probably do in the way of treatment? What are shock treatments? What is prefrontal lobotomy, and in what types of cases is it used?

Once the patient is in good hands the relatives may come again to ask such questions as, "What are the chances of ultimate recovery, or should we give permission for this or that treatment." Although the wise physician will then say, "You are now in the hands of a good man, a specialist in this field, and you had better take his advice," he will be able to help much if he can give the family some idea of what is planned.

The need for consulting a psychiatrist. A fine thing the family physician or specialist can do is to get a psychotic or pre-psychotic person *quickly* into the hands of a psychiatrist before much trauma has been done by poor handling. As I have been pointing out in this book, the doctor is not likely to do this unless he has been taught to recognize quickly the patient who has something worse than an anxiety neurosis or a chronic nervous exhaustion.

I am distressed sometimes, on looking over the record of a patient who evidently for some time was going insane, to note that even neuropsychiatrists were too reluctant to diagnose a psychosis and to write the word into the record. I realize that it is unpleasant, unpopular, and perhaps even legally dangerous to call a patient psychotic; the man's family may be much offended and the other physicians on the case are likely to hoot at the diagnosis, but commonly, because no one has the courage or knowledge to make it, the patient, for long, is wrongly treated. Often he gets operated on again and again. If the first internist or psychiatrist to see him had only had the courage to write down "schizoid personality with abdominal hallucinations" the surgeons might have stayed their hands.

Unfortunately today, many a psychotic, psychopathic, or hysterical patient never gets into the hands of a good psychiatrist; he has to be taken care of by general practitioners, many of them out in the country where they cannot get expert help. Since this must be, every practitioner ought to have some ideas about recognizing the psychotic person, and some ideas of handling him and talking to him. Often the physician needs some information about these problems, if only so that he can give advice to the distracted family. Some ideas about talking to the mentally disturbed patient are to be found in the previous chapter. What is needed today is a good booklet on emergency psychiatry.

Most physicians should have some knowledge of what the early symptoms of a psychosis are. They need to know when to say, "This is worrisome." Some idea of how to recognize the common psychoses is to be found in Chapters 14 and 15. Often it is the family who can see most clearly that the patient has overstepped the bounds of sanity *or of what was sanity for him.* Sometimes the family has difficulty in perceiving that there has been a significant worsening of the situation, because the person has always been queer, eccentric, difficult, choleric, or unpredictable in his behavior. No one, then, can say just when he went over the line. Many years ago, in California, when my brilliant but always eccentric Chief began to go insane, the first difference I noted in him was that after a tantrum he was not sorry or apologetic as he formerly had been.

Once the presence of a psychosis is recognized, the questions arise: Where can help be obtained, and can the patient be cared for at home? If not, should he go to a private or a state institution? Will the cost of private care be prohibitive? Will the person have to be committed, and if so, how is this done and by whom? Can he commit himself for a while?

On finding a psychiatrist. If only because most physicians do not know about these things, they will have to get help from a psychiatrist. The next question is, where can they find a good one? In big cities, they can find several kinds of psychiatrists, with different trainings, interests, abilities, and human qualities. In the country or a small city they may not be able to find any qualified person. The names of diplomates in psychiatry can be found in the directory of specialists published by A. N. Marquis and Company of Chicago. I fear this book is not available to many physicians or laymen.

Obviously it may be difficult to find a good psychiatrist. There are only some 5,000 in the United States, and many of them are not available for private practice. Some are employed by the states, the armed forces and the Veterans' Administration; some are working in private institutions, in university clinics, or in big stores, and some are psychoanalysts who are interested only in a special type of patient. Furthermore, as is the case with all physicians, some are much abler than others; some were born for their job and know how to handle people well; some are more sensible, friendly, kindly, and easy to meet, and some are more reasonable in their charges. Several of my patients have had to consult four or five psychiatrists before they found one who helped at all. It is unfortunate that often the physician who refers a patient does not know the psychiatrist personally; he does not know what sort of a human being he is.

Most of the psychiatrists I know are splendid men, admirable in every way, but my patients have told me of others who were very disappointing to them, and of no assistance. Some, with their accusations and curious interpretations of symptoms, upset the patient badly and did only harm. Evidently, there is still need for a better choice of men for this specialty, and there is much need for their better training. As several able teachers of psychiatry have pointed out, no one should go into this field who is not well balanced himself. A tendency to psychosis in the doctor, or much psychosis in his family may give him a more sympathetic understanding of psychotics, but too often it is likely to fill him with curious theories and ideas. It may also make him so shy and ill at ease that he has to hold his patients off at arms' length. As William Menninger admitted in his splendid book on military psychiatry, the Army had its troubles with such psychiatrists. They had human failings, just like the rest of us, and some were so odd that they had to be shifted about until some place could be found for them in which they could do the least amount of harm.

The type of psychiatrist whom most mildly troubled patients need is a man who preferably was well trained first in internal medicine and perhaps neurology and who does not belong to any "school." He will look into the everyday life problems of his patients much as a general practitioner might do, only he will do it with more skill, developed through years of special study.

On trying to find a suitable asylum. Difficulties are encountered when a physician tries to find a sanatorium for a patient, and especially a sanatorium that will not quickly clean out the family bank account. Usually the names of the biggest and best known of the nearby private sanatoriums can be obtained by looking at the advertisements in the State Medical Journal. Help can be obtained by writing to the National Committee for Mental Hygiene or the secretaries of the state Mental Hygiene Societies, or the State Mental Health Authorities. See the lists of names in Appendix 1. Other useful lists of this type are to be found in the book by Phillip Polatin and E. C. Philtine (1949).

The simpler forms of special therapy. Psychiatrists use several types of therapy. In the office some men practice a sort of psychotherapy much like that used by non-psychiatrists. First, an effort is made to unearth the principal mental difficulties of the patient, in his home and in his office, and then an effort is made to get him to do something helpful about his troubles. Some analysis may be made to find out what sort of man he is: what his up-bringing was, and what his resentments and fears and worries are. If the problem is at all difficult the patient will be asked to return at intervals for talks, during which he will receive guidance, supervision, and encouragement. Perhaps a social service worker will be sent to his home to study his environment and to learn about the problems of the family.

If, for a time, the patient needs to be removed from his environment and placed under close supervision he can be put into a sanatorium. There he can be protected from himself and others; he can be kept away from alcohol and drugs; he can get rest and sleep; he can perhaps calm down and become sensible again; he can get psychotherapy; he can be taught regular habits of living, and he may be kept busy in a shop.

Persons a psychiatrist cannot help. It must be remembered that even the ablest of psychiatrists cannot be expected to help several types of patients. He cannot do much to help a man who is of low mentality, maniacal, depressed, markedly schizophrenic, paranoiac, or suffering from a psychopathic personality. As Yaskin (1936) pointed out, there is little a psychiatrist can do with a patient when he cannot find any mental cause for the symptoms. Often I have heard an intelligent and cooperative patient say, "I wish there was something hurtful on my mind that I could tell you about, but search as I will, I cannot think of any. I guess I was just born jittery, like my mother before me."

Group psychotherapy. In some clinics group psychotherapy is now being tried out, and with considerable success. It saves much time, and the patients are taught in a general way what the neurotic person's common sins and errors are, and what can be done about them. It helps some persons to see that others have succumbed to the weaknesses he has, and that they are reforming and getting better.

Contact with other neurotics also takes away some of the feeling of isolation of the mentally sick, and the feeling that the individual's problem is unique and insoluble. It may help the patient to see someone else confessing to a bad habit or to some way of thinking which he, by himself, might never have had the courage to talk about.

Narco-analysis. Sometimes when it is impossible to get a highly nervous person to talk, a psychiatrist will give him just enough of some barbiturate to take away his wariness and his reluctance to give his history. Some psychiatrists use sodium pentothal in a solution of 2.5 or 5 per cent concentration. This is run into a vein until the desired stage of sedation is secured. Usually something less than 0.5 gm. of the drug is needed. Other men use about 2 grains (0.13 gm.) of sodium amytal injected intravenously. Some men are enthusiastic about this treatment while others doubt if it is of much value.

Hypnosis. Erickson has written a good description of treatment by hypnosis. He doubted if the patient need fear any injurious or detrimental effects, even from repeated hypnotizations. No one can be hypnotized against his will or without his cooperation. No one can be made to do a criminal act under hypnosis, and no one can be kept indefinitely in a trance. · Most normal persons can be hypnotized. The schizophrenic is resistant.

It is well first to explain to the person what he or she may expect. A woman to be hypnotized may be made to lie on a couch. She will be told to gaze on an object held in such a position as to tire her extrinsic eye muscles. Somnolence and relaxation are suggested in a monotone. After the patient has fallen "asleep," questions may be asked and suggestions implanted. There are various depths to the trances, and usually a shallow one is sufficient. It is easy to wake the person; usually all one needs to do is to tell her to wake. (See Psychosomatic Medicine, January, 1943.) When in a deep trance the subject may be able to recall forgotten events. According to Charcot and Janet, hypnosis is an artificial hysteria, or a mental dissociation, during which suggestibility is likely to be increased.

Most psychiatrists are not enthusiastic about the use of hypnosis. Its effects are likely to be transitory, and all it is is a way of treating by suggestion. Some men fear that it may do harm.

The continuous warm bath. Patients who come into a hospital in a state of hypomanic excitement can sometimes be calmed down with the help of a continuous warm bath. They lie on a canvas sling which is stretched across the tub.

Long-continued sedation. Another method of handling the hypomanic patient, when he or she comes in, is to give enough of some barbiturate several times in every twenty-four hours to maintain sleep for several days. From time to time the patient wakes a bit to take food and to empty the bladder and the bowels. In the Army some utterly fatigued and nervously shocked men were given rest in this way for several days until they had calmed down.

Sedative drugs. The mildly manic or somewhat psychotic patient who cannot rest or sleep usually does not react well to barbiturates. Instead of sleeping he may become more upset and may get bad nightmares. Usually he must be quieted with either chloral or paraldehyde. The former can be given in the form of somnos of which an ounce or more will probably have to be given.

Paraldehyde may be given iced with syrup of wild cherry floated over it. It can be given rectally in from 8 to 10 ounces of milk or syrup of acacia. For extreme restlessness in the cases of psychotic patients, doses larger than 4 gm. may have to be used. The physician will have to feel his way. The amount of soporific needed will depend on the degree of the patient's excitement. When a patient is nauseated or vomiting it is useless to give any medicine by mouth, and then sodium amytal may have to be given intravenously in doses of 0.5 or 1 gm. The drug comes in ampules. This may quiet the vomiting center. In mild cases nembutal can be given in rectal suppositories, each containing 3 grains.

On committing a patient. Few physicians know much about committing a patient and few want to get mixed up with this unpleasant business, but every so often a family physician or even a specialist will have to help an old patient with the problem of taking care of a relative who has become too troublesome to keep at home, or who has become violent, or is molesting the neighbors, or writing threatening letters, or is refusing to eat or sleep or bathe or void his excreta in the proper place. Such a person must be taken to either a private or a public institution, and arrangements will have to be made for keeping him there until he can safely be let out.

The laws about the commitment of patients vary in different states. Fortunately, in some the patient who has suddenly become violent can be admitted to an asylum without the help of a judge and an insanity commission. After he has been studied for a while some more permanent arrangement can be made for him. An abstract of the regulations for commitment will be found in Appendix 2 at the end of this volume.

Many families, dreading to put a loved one into a state institution, place him in a private one. They keep him there until their money is all gone, at which time if he is still unable to go out into the world, they are forced to send him to a state institution. Then they wish that, since they were going to have to take this step anyway, they had taken it at the beginning, before they used up all their money.

I have had several people tell me that a relative got better care and more attention and treatment in a fine state institution than in the poorly run or inadequately staffed private institution which they happened to choose.

Types of persons who need hospitalization. Obviously, the persons who need hospitalization are the ones who cannot safely be taken care of at home or cannot be left at large. Manic persons may attack someone, or they may stray away from home and get into all sorts of adventures. Some alcoholics who go from one spree to another eventually have to be locked up. The woman with an agitated depression often has to be put into an institution because at home she soon demoralizes the family by keeping them up all night. Some depressed persons have to be cared for in an institution if only to keep them from committing suicide. Senile oldsters may set fires and may get into all sorts of malicious mischief. Some bad paranoiacs have to be locked up because they are likely to shoot some innocent person on the street. Many harmless psychotics can be cared for at home. Today many psychotic persons are being cared for at home after having been quieted by shock treatments or a prefrontal lobotomy or topectomy.

Getting a disturbed patient to an institution. When the problem comes up of getting a patient to an institution, the family may want to try deception and a shanghai-ing technic. But this is most unwise as was shown so well by Beers. As he said, when, under false pretenses, his brother enticed him into an asylum and locked the door on him, he could not believe that one who loved him could have done such a thing. Accordingly, he came to the, for him, logical conclusion that the man who had done this was not his brother but an imposter who looked like him. For several years he tried to figure out some way of proving that the apparent imposter was his brother, and during this time his recovery was delayed by the fact that he had no affectionate and trusting contact with his family.

Many a time when I have talked quietly and honestly to a mentally disturbed person and perhaps have found someone whom he liked and trusted to take him to an asylum, he has gone there without making any trouble. What I did was to get him to admit that he was ill and in need of help and perhaps in need of such care as would keep him from wasting the family savings or perhaps hurting someone. It is wonderful how reasonable some psychotics can be for a time when appealed to by someone whom they trust and like. The family must then respect scrupulously every promise they or the doctor have made to the patient. For instance, a man may promise to go to the asylum if his sister-in-law, whom he has always liked and trusted, will take him; but he may stipulate that if certain other members of the family whom he does not like or trust are to mix into the affair, the deal is off. Mildly psychotic persons are even more insistent than are the sane that those about them deal with them honestly and in a friendly way. They sense and keenly resent the dislike many people have for them, and they resent any subterfuges designed to get them to do what people want them to do. A sane man might see that the doctor and relatives lied because they thought they were acting for the best, but the psychotic may not be able to see this or to forgive it.

The problems of finding a haven for some patients. A hundred times in my years of practice I have been distressed by the fact that as yet in America there is a dearth of intermediate places for the patient who, while too unreasonable or "difficult," or in occasional short spells too uncontrollable or psychopathic to be handled at home or in an ordinary hospital or rest home, is apparently so sane, or so sane for most of the time, that one cannot bear to think of locking him up, or especially locking him up with the demented, the noisy, and the disoriented. It would be too cruel. Some of the alcoholics and the patients with psychopathic personalities belong in this group of persons for whom today there are no suitable protective refuges.

When sober and sensible, a psychopathic or alcoholic woman may be interesting, pleasant, and even a delightful companion, but next day she may get drunk and wreck the family automobile, or at a party she may start cursing like a fishwife; she may throw things and wreck valuable furniture, or she may forge a check, beat up her little sister, or go on a disgraceful binge with a truck driver.

Thousands of families are cursed by such problem children, and I have never learned of any good way of handling the situation. One of my friends, in the course of a few years, spent over $150,000 trying to save and rehabilitate a son with this sort of instability. The last I heard of the son he was in the state prison where he should have been allowed to go when he was sixteen. Eventually society could no longer tolerate his misdeeds, even when the father was always there, willing to pay well for the losses and hurts of the people who had been robbed and victimized.

It would seem as if some day society must establish a sort of non-punitive colony on some island where these people can live together: A place where there will be no alcohol, no morphine, no money to steal or to gamble away, no checks to forge, and no guns to shoot with. The sad feature today is that these bad little children in adult bodies have to live among pitfalls which they do not know how to steer clear of.

The prevention of suicide. Those who take care of psychotics and particularly depressed persons must always be awake to the danger of suicide. A patient will often seem to be doing so well, and he will seem so perfectly sane, that vigilance will be relaxed, and then out of the window he will go.

Many hysterical persons or women who have been fighting with a husband will attempt suicide but perhaps in a half-hearted way. Their main purpose probably is to upset or disgrace the recalcitrant lover or husband, or they may be trying to get sympathy or to retrieve love. Some will say what is true, that suicide would be a good way out, and would free some relative from a terrible burden; but, at the last minute, the person loses his nerve and does not do a resolute and thorough job.

It is often said that the person who talks of suicide, or threatens it, or much fears it will never take his life, but one cannot count on this.

Electric shock treatment. Today, in many cases, good results are being obtained with electric shock treatments. This technic is safer and much less frightening and distressing than was the old one in which insulin or metrazol was given and violent convulsions were produced. Today the patient lies on his bed or on a table. He will probably be given an injection of curare to cut down on the amount of the spasm in his muscles which comes when the current is sent through his brain. Electrodes are applied to his temples and the special current is turned on for a moment. Persons standing beside the bed hold the man down as he stiffens. After the treatment the patient rests for a while. The shock does not appear to be very disturbing to the patients because most of them keep coming back again and again for more. Those who are very fearful can be given a preliminary injection of pentothal sodium.

For a while after the treatments there is likely to be some impairment of memory. The best results apparently are obtained in cases of depression, either mild or severe. Good results are obtained, also, in cases of "involutional melancholia," of anhedonia, and of some manic states, and in a few cases of early schizophrenia. According to most of the users of this technic, it is not of much use in cases of advanced schizophrenia or of psychoneurosis. It is said that 80 per cent of the depressed patients are better for the treatment. It does not appear to have any permanent deleterious effects on the brain.

Psycho-analysis. As most physicians know, there are several schools of psychiatry, some of which are far apart in their teachings and beliefs. Men in the psycho-analytic school base their activities on the teachings of Freud, who was full of ideas about early sex traumas. As Ross used to say, "Freudian analysis has become crystallized into a somewhat hard body of doctrine in which its practitioners believe with a sincerity which is found elsewhere only among the most dogmatic religions. It is difficult for the analyzed to escape submitting to the doctrines held by the analyzer." In *Oxford Medicine* one reads, "The most casual study of the writings of the majority of psychoanalysts will convince an unprejudiced observer that the analyst finds what he suggests." Often he will not suspect that he has made the suggestion.

To the untutored and skeptical, many of the ideas of the analysts seem bizarre, improbable, unbelievable, and certainly unprovable. What the patient does or says is interpreted with the help of an astounding symbolism. Probably most men will never be convinced that this symbolism is correct. Most of them will believe that it arises in the imagination or training of the analyst. Lowrey (1946) has said that the patient is not aware of the symbolic nature of what he dreams or thinks or does. This is what one would suspect.

One objection many a psychiatrist has to the thinking of the analysts is that they often pass up the simple and logical explanation for a thought or behavior and, instead, drag in some remarkable and unprovable theory. For instance, a man who loves the luxury of a hot bath may be told that he is trying to get back to the old comfort of his fetal life in the amniotic fluid!

Many psychiatrists have little faith in what can be done for a patient with a long analysis, and some see little to be gained from this lengthy and expensive technic. They would restrict its use to only a few cases. As Ross used to say, he seldom felt the need for a long analysis because usually, in one or two interviews, he could learn all he thought he needed to know about a patient's troubles. As he said, "Why use a steam hammer to crack nuts?" or "Why x-ray the whole man to find a little foreign body, when you know about where it is located?" Ross admitted that he doubtless could learn much more about a patient's psychology with the help of a long analysis, but he was not sure that the added information would enable him to do a better job of helping the man. In many cases psycho-analysis is hardly needed because the patient's troubles are not buried in his subconscious mind. He knows perfectly well what they are and always have been; and if he can't tell the doctor about them, his family can. Strecker said that a psychoanalyst tries to dredge up from the depths of the patient's mind a vast quantity of material representing abortive attempts to break his old parental bonds. This idea would seem improbable in the case of the many persons who never had any trouble with parental bonds.

Sadler has said, "I fear there is something of a tendency, especially in the practice of younger psychiatrists, unconsciously to manipulate the history so as to make the case conform to the text-book pictures of some one of our diagnostic entities." Spitz and many others have doubted many of the interpretations published by psycho-analysts.

Neilsen and Thompsen told in their book of a woman who, because of a phobia that there was broken glass in her food, went to a psychiatrist who promptly assured her that this could have only one significance and that was fear of labor pains. By way of treatment, she was advised to break off relations with her fiancé so that there could never be any danger of pregnancy! Many such interpretations are to be found in every number of most journals on psycho-analysis. Some psychiatrists look on this sort of thing with wonderment. What I puzzle over is that never in all my forty-five years of talking to mentally troubled women have I heard of such ideas as penis envy or a desire to get back into the womb or to bite off the father's penis. Yet these ideas are everywhere in the psychiatric literature.

Psycho-analysis is usually conducted with the patient lying on a couch and the physician seated behind him. In this way it is easier for the person to talk freely. He is told to say anything that comes into his mind regardless of how irrelevant it may seem to be. As this is done, certain trends of thought become manifest. There may be signs of hostility, fear, feelings of dependency, sexual fantasies, suspicions, or jealousies. Efforts are made to correlate these feelings with the earliest experiences of childhood. The reliving of these emotional experiences and the insight gained thereby are supposed to enable the patient to purge his mind of the pathologic material. One idea is that psychic energy which was expended in repressing the pathologic material can be freed and turned into more constructive channels. According to Wertham, in psycho-analysis the patient has first to be made to see that he suffers not so much from life, as from the conflict that rages within him.

It is hoped by the analyst that the patient will discover many things that he never knew about himself. It is hoped, also, that he will accept the interpretations made and will use them for the rearrangement of his life. Some persons feel so much resentment at the unpleasant accusations leveled against them and so much distrust of the analysis that they will not try to change their attitudes. In many publications today one reads of the patient's hostility to the analyst, and when one hears what he was accused of, one can easily see why he was angry.

To illustrate how things sometimes go, a patient of mine, a constitutionally frail girl who for years had suffered from terrible menstrual storms, bravely managed to keep earning her living in spite of the pain. Her kindly home surgeon, knowing the girl's great desire for marriage and children, although forced several times to operate, had always saved her ovaries and uterus. Finally, because of frequent flooding and much disabling pain, hysterectomy had to be performed. This so depressed the girl that her doctor sent her to a psychiatrist. He immediately outraged her by telling her that her dysmenorrhea, her flooding, and her hysterectomy had all been the result of her secret desire to lead a riotous sexual life without any danger of getting pregnant! Knowing the girl well, I much doubt if this was true, but even if it had been true, how could one expect her to react favorably to such an insulting accusation? Actually, the girl became so much worse under the "treatment" that she soon stopped it. Later she got well with the help of a kindly general practitioner who gave her sympathy, reassurance, and estrogens.

As some psychiatrists have pointed out, one difficulty with a long course of psycho-analysis is that at the end of it, although the patient may know all about his early sex traumas, he may still be just as odd and psychopathic as he was at the beginning. Thus, William Ellery Leonard told in his book, *The Locomotive God,* that, after much psycho-analysis, he was satisfied that the seed of his troubles was sown when, at the age of four, he was frightened by a locomotive. But still, after getting this information, he was unable to go more than 50 yards from his house. Similarly, a wealthy homosexual man I know was analyzed for years by nationally known experts, but in the end he was just as homosexual and just as unhappy about it as he was at the beginning. Another patient, after being analyzed for two years, was told that she was a Peter Pan who had never grown up. As she said, "I told the doctor that the first day I went to him. I am still that, and so what? What now do I do about it?"

Obviously, only well-to-do persons are likely to be able to afford the luxury of a two-year analysis. According to Jelliffe, it is not likely to help persons of low intelligence, or those who are hypomanic, depressed, schizophrenic, or suffering from hysteria, or compulsion neuroses. Lowrey (1946) found that neurasthenics do not respond well. Maurice Levine wrote that psycho-analysis is contraindicated in illnesses mainly physical in origin, in the cases of persons of defective intelligence or of those past middle age whose emotional patterns are pretty well set or of those suffering from paranoia, schizophrenia, and manic-depressive psychosis. It can be helpful in some of the neuroses, hysteria, anxieties, organ neuroses, phobias, and some cases of drug addiction, alcoholism, and marital derangement.

General semantics. There is a group of psychiatrists who talk of using the technic of Korzybski in helping the neurotic or psychotic person. The idea is that most of his troubles are due to fuzzy thinking, and this is based largely on a poor use of words. It is thought that if a muddle-headed neurotic woman could only be made to see that most of her questions which she keeps constantly asking herself are unanswerable because they are so badly stated, and if she could be made to put her questions logically and clearly so that they could be answered, she might no longer be concerned about them; she might see that she was fussing over something of no consequence.

There is no question that Korzybski's book, *Science and Sanity,* contains much that is valuable and worth studying by every educated man. Unfortunately, the English is abstruse and hard to read or to understand. Certainly, no neurotic or psychotic person is likely ever to wade through the volume or to use it to clarify his thinking.

Prefrontal lobotomy or leukotomy. In recent years, largely through the influence of Freeman, thousands of persons suffering from schizophrenia or severe anxiety have submitted to the operation of leukotomy. After making a couple of trephine holes in the front of the skull the surgeon inserts an instrument and severs many of the tracts running to the front of the brain. In many cases the results are good, and the patient quiets down and is able to go home.

A good report on what has been accomplished is to be found in the New England Journal of Medicine for August 11, 1949, pp. 248-249. The report was from the Yale University News Bureau. There were 294 patients studied after the operation. Most of them had been suffering from severe forms of schizophrenia, and most had been in an asylum for periods averaging five years. Some 61 per cent showed improvement in mental health; 36 per cent could be sent home, and 25 per cent were able to go back to full time work. An additional 38 per cent were working part time. Some 85 per cent had lost their most disturbing traits.

The only sad result of the operation is that these persons have been deprived of some vital spark or of the "integrity of their personality." They are better because they have lost something, not because they have gained something. Several writers have warned against doing the operation on anyone who is not in great need of it, because there can be no question that it injures the personality and takes away something that is important.

The operation is performed sometimes on persons who are complaining bitterly of pain or discomfort, but here, the last state may be worse than the first. The person may become untidy, dirty, and very unpleasant.

Topectomy. Recently a new operation called topectomy has been proposed which appears to have advantages. In this operation small areas of cortex are removed, usually from a frontal lobe or from both of them. It often helps the patient, apparently without markedly injuring his personality. Unfortunately some of the patients after the operation suffer from convulsive seizures.

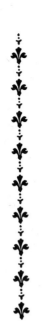

APPENDIX 1

State Mental
Hygiene Societies

ALABAMA SOCIETY FOR MENTAL HYGIENE
Mrs. William S. Pritchard, Sec'y.
309 N. 23rd St.
Birmingham, Alabama

ARKANSAS MENTAL HYGIENE SOCIETY
Mrs. R. M. Cheatham, Sec'y.
1210 Summit Ave.
Little Rock, Ark.

MENTAL HEALTH SOCIETY OF NORTHERN
CALIFORNIA
Mr. S. G. Bloomfield, Exec. Sec'y.
1095 Market St.
San Francisco 3, Calif.

SOUTHERN CALIFORNIA SOCIETY FOR
MENTAL HYGIENE
Mrs. Helene M. Lipscomb, Exec. Dir.
3780 West 6th St.
Los Angeles 5, Calif.

CONNECTICUT SOCIETY FOR MENTAL HY-
GIENE
Miss Frances Hartshorne, Exec. Sec'y.
152 Temple St.
New Haven 10, Conn.

DELAWARE SOCIETY FOR MENTAL HYGIENE
Mr. H. Edmund Bullis, Exec. Dir.
1404 Franklin St.
Wilmington 19, Del.

HAWAII SOCIETY FOR MENTAL HYGIENE
Mrs. Margaret D. Hackfield, Exec. Sec'y.
810 N. Vineyard St.
Honolulu, T. H.

ILLINOIS SOCIETY FOR MENTAL HYGIENE
Dr. Rudolph G. Novick, Medical Director
123 W. Madison St.
Chicago 2, Ill.

INDIANA MENTAL HYGIENE SOCIETY
Mr. Walter W. Argow, Exec. Sec'y.
800 Underwriters Bldg.
Indianapolis 4, Ind.

IOWA SOCIETY FOR MENTAL HYGIENE
Dr. Norman D. Render
c/o State Hospital
Clarinda, Iowa

KANSAS MENTAL HYGIENE SOCIETY
Mr. W. W. Wilmore, Sec'y.
1134 Topeka Ave.
Topeka, Kansas

LOUISIANA SOCIETY FOR MENTAL HEALTH
Mr. Lloyd Rowland, Exec. Sec'y.
816 Hibernia Bank Bldg.
New Orleans 12, La.

619

MARYLAND MENTAL HYGIENE SOCIETY
Mrs. Gertrude Nilsson, Exec. Dir.
8 West 25th St.
Baltimore 18, Md.

MASSACHUSETTS SOCIETY FOR MENTAL
    HYGIENE
Mr. William H. Savin, Exec. Sec'y.
41 Mt. Vernon St.
Boston 8, Mass.

MICHIGAN SOCIETY FOR MENTAL HYGIENE
Mr. Harold G. Webster, Exec. Sec'y.
153 E. Elizabeth St.—Rm. 645
Detroit 1, Michigan

MINNESOTA MENTAL HYGIENE SOCIETY
Mr. Edward I. Morse, Exec. Sec'y.
309 E. Franklin Ave.
Minneapolis 4, Minn.

MISSOURI ASSOCIATION FOR MENTAL HY-
    GIENE
Mrs. Elizabeth Lingenfelter, Sec'y.
1020 McGee St.
Kansas City 6, Mo.

NEBRASKA MENTAL HEALTH ASSOCIATION
Dr. Juul C. Nielsen, Supt.
Hastings State Hospital
Ingleside, Neb.

NEVADA MENTAL HYGIENE SOCIETY
Miss Theodora Fogg, Sec'y.
140 North Virginia St.
Reno, Nevada

MENTAL HYGIENE SOCIETY OF NEW
    JERSEY
Rev. Robert D. Smith, Temp. Chairman
808 West State St.
Trenton 8, N. J.

NEW YORK COMMITTEE ON MENTAL HY-
    GIENE
Mr. Lowell Iberg
105 East 22nd St.
New York 10, N. Y.

NORTH CAROLINA MENTAL HYGIENE SO-
    CIETY
Miss Elsie L. Parker, Exec. Sec'y.
P. O. Box 2599
Raleigh, N. C.

OHIO MENTAL HYGIENE ASSOCIATION
Mrs. Marion S. Wells, Exec. Sec'y.
1014-15 Huntington Bank Bldg.
Columbus 15, Ohio

OKLAHOMA COMMITTEE FOR MENTAL
    HYGIENE
Mr. W. James Logan, Exec. Sec'y.
P. O. Box 1672
Oklahoma City 3, Oklahoma

MENTAL HEALTH ASSOCIATION OF OREGON
Mr. Melvin L. Murphy, Exec. Dir.
229 Park Bldg.
Portland 5, Oregon

DIVISION ON MENTAL HEALTH, PENNSYL-
    VANIA CITIZENS ASSOCIATION FOR
    HEALTH AND WELFARE
Mr. Ross W. Sanderson, Jr., Consultant
    on Mental Health
311 S. Juniper St.
Philadelphia 7, Pa.

RHODE ISLAND SOCIETY FOR MENTAL HY-
    GIENE
Mrs. Elizabeth Bosquet, Exec. Sec'y.
100 North Main St.
Providence, R. I.

SOUTH CAROLINA MENTAL AND SOCIAL
    HYGIENE SOCIETY
Mrs. Richard Ellis, Sec'y.
Richland County Health Dept.
Columbia, S. C.

SOUTH DAKOTA MENTAL HEALTH ASSOCIA-
    TION
Mrs. Faith M. Watson, Sec'y.
712 Sixth St.
Brookings, South Dakota

TENNESSEE MENTAL HYGIENE SOCIETY
Mrs. Richard McNabb
4175 Lyons View Pike
Knoxville, Tenn.

TEXAS SOCIETY FOR MENTAL HYGIENE
Mrs. Elizabeth F. Gardner, Exec. Sec'y.
1617 Watchill Road
Austin 21, Texas

UTAH SOCIETY FOR MENTAL HYGIENE
Mr. Veon G. Smith, Exec. Sec'y.
156 Westminster Ave.
Salt Lake City 15, Utah

VERMONT SOCIETY FOR MENTAL HYGIENE
Miss Harriet Parker, Sec'y.
311 North Ave.
Burlington, Vt.

MENTAL HYGIENE SOCIETY OF VIRGINIA
Mr. F. W. Gwaltney, Exec. Sec'y.
P. O. Box 1991, 9 No. 12th St.
Richmond 19, Va.

WASHINGTON SOCIETY FOR MENTAL HY-
    GIENE
Mr. George F. Ault, Exec. Dir.
408 Seaboard Bldg.
Seattle 1, Wash.

WISCONSIN SOCIETY FOR MENTAL HEALTH
Dr. Esther H. de Weerdt, Exec. Dir.
405 E. Grand Ave.
Beloit, Wisc.

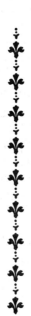

APPENDIX 2

Commitment
Procedures [1]

The following report was prepared by the Group for the Advancement of Psychiatry and is a valuable summary of the status of commitment in the United States.

Every psychiatrist has concern for the procedure of committing psychiatric patients to hospitals and often is involved in this. All of us in psychiatry are aware that many undesirable features of the commitment procedure exist in many of our states. Because each state has its own commitment law, these vary widely and few practicing psychiatrists have opportunity to evaluate or compare the many different laws.

In this Report the Committee on Forensic Psychiatry of the Group for the Advancement of Psychiatry has collected the data about the laws of each state and pointed out the undesirable features. Recommendations are made regarding the features of an ideal "certification" law. The work of this Committee has been reviewed by the entire membership of 150 psychiatrists of the Group for the Advancement of Psychiatry who have given this report their full endorsement. It is hoped that this Report may receive the attention of lawmakers, interested groups of citizens concerned with the improvement of their own state law, as well as of psychiatrists, in order that the improvement of our certification laws may be speeded up.

FACTUAL DATA AND CONCLUSIONS [2]

1. THE ESSENTIAL VARIETIES OF COMMITMENT LAWS.
   a. By jury (21 states)
      1. Mandatory—Texas—Mississippi.

---

[1] Reprinted in part by permission of the Group for the Advancement of Psychiatry. From Report No. 4, April 1948.

[2] Flaschner, F. N., Analysis of Legal and Medical Considerations in Commitment of the Mentally Ill, Yale Law Journal, 56:1178-1209, August, 1947.

2. Optional (19 states)—Alabama, Colorado, Delaware, Georgia, Illinois, Iowa, Kansas, Kentucky, Maryland, Massachusetts, Michigan, Minnesota, Montana, Oklahoma, Tennessee, Vermont, Washington, Wisconsin, Wyoming.

b. By certification of two physicians (6 states)—Louisiana, Vermont, Rhode Island, Pennsylvania, Maryland, New Hampshire.
(NOTE) in Pennsylvania and New Hampshire the physicians' certificate requires certification by law judge or magistrate.

c. By standing Commissions (appointees for term designated by Court)—(6 states), Iowa, Nebraska, North Dakota, South Dakota, Virginia, West Virginia.

d. Non-judicial authority with 2 physicians (3 states), Connecticut, Maine, North Carolina.

e. Judge and Commission (3 men usually including a physician and lawyer) (6 states), Colorado, Florida, Georgia, Pennsylvania, Rhode Island, Wyoming.

f. By Judge and 1 physician (8 states), Alabama, Arkansas, Idaho, Kansas, Missouri, New Mexico, Ohio, Oregon.

g. By Judge and 2 physicians (23 states), Arizona, California, Connecticut, Illinois, Indiana, Kentucky, Louisiana, Massachusetts, Michigan, Minnesota, Montana, Nevada, New Jersey, New York, Oklahoma, Pennsylvania, Rhode Island, South Carolina, Tennessee, Utah, Washington, Wisconsin, Wyoming.

2. THE ESSENTIALS OF A SATISFACTORY COMMITMENT LAW.

a. Minimum legal formalism.

b. Devices which aim to get maximum patient participation in treatment which includes intramural detention.

c. Minimal psychic traumatization in admission procedures.

d. Removal of stigmata, resulting from archaic legal phraseology.

3. THE MOST COMMON ASPECTS OF BAD COMMITMENT LAWS.

Historically the commitment in early statutes was limited to the dangerously insane. This has tended to perpetuate the stigma of criminality upon mental illness. "The mentally ill person may be arrested by a sheriff with a warrant, charged with insanity by a judge, detained in a jail pending a hearing, tried in open court before a jury, remanded to jail pending a vacancy in a mental hospital and finally transported to a hospital by a sheriff. While this procedure in each detail may not be followed by any jurisdiction, it represents a pattern of existing practices which are especially objectionable."[3]

The use of the jury in commitment procedures developed during the latter half of the 19th Century. This was in part due to a notorious case which occurred in Illinois in 1860. Mrs. E. P. W. Packard, the wife of a Calvinist minister who differed violently with her husband on religious matters had been committed involuntarily. On her release, she maintained that she had been railroaded into the institution. In Illinois she obtained the right to a jury trial for every patient already committed. This gave impetus to the use of the jury in commitment procedures.

The worst features of contemporary commitment laws are:

a. Legal service and notice to the patient.

b. Insistence of personal appearance in court.

c. Exposure of patient as public spectacle and the public record of such.

d. Emphasis of lay judgment as in trial by jury. Identification of mental illness and criminality by similarity of procedure.

e. The common acceptance of certification of mental illness as tantamount to legal incompetence rather than a clear separation of these as different issues affecting the rights of the person.

---

[3] Flaschner. Loc. Cit.

f. Use of anachronistic terminology.

g. Inquiry into patient's financial status at time of commitment.

4. The states that seem to have the most satisfactory commitment laws are those states empowering commitment by certificate of 2 physicians: Louisiana, Vermont, Rhode Island, Pennsylvania, Maryland, New Hampshire.

5. The states which have the most unsatisfactory laws are Texas and Mississippi which require trial by jury and to an extent less obnoxious are those states which utilize the permissive trial by jury on petition of patients.

6. STATES WHICH PROVIDE FOR VOLUNTARY ADMISSIONS.

At present all states except Alabama, Florida, Mississippi, Missouri, North Dakota, Georgia. Since 1939 the following ten states have adopted voluntary admissions:—Arizona, Arkansas, Idaho, Louisiana, Montana, Nebraska, Nevada, New Mexico, Tennessee, Wyoming.

The merits of voluntary admission are self evident. The Committee is not sufficiently informed regarding legislative development to assert categorically the reason why such admissions are still not used in some states. It is, however, our impression that the factor is largely economic. This is suggested by the fact that three states now provide for the voluntary admission of only the patients who pay.

7. JAILS USED FOR THE RETENTION OF MENTALLY ILL PATIENTS.

The extent to which this practice is used is unknown statistically. The Committee made inquiries from the National Jail Association and the Federal Bureau of Prisons and from these collateral sources it would seem that the practice of retaining mentally ill persons in jail is widespread.

8. THE TREND TOWARD REFORM OF TERMINOLOGY.

Pennsylvania was the first state (1923) to substitute "Mental illness" for the term insanity. Nine other states followed:—Connecticut, Illinois, Iowa, Nebraska, Nevada, New York, North Carolina, Ohio, Oregon.

The term "parole" is still in wide use throughout the country.

RECOMMENDATIONS BY THE FORENSIC COMMITTEE ON COMMITMENT PROCEDURES IN GENERAL

1. TRANSPORTATION OF MENTALLY ILL PATIENTS.

The Committee believes that the use of regular peace officers should be eliminated as much as possible and suggests the possibility of delegating or deputizing state hospital or clinic personnel especially trained for this purpose.

2. COMMITMENT AND RELEASE PROCEDURES.

The Committee recommends the complete repeal of all types of commitment and release procedures which retain the pattern of criminal procedures.

3. FINANCIAL STATUS OF HOSPITAL PATIENTS.

In keeping with the principle that the treatment of mental illness is a state obligation, the Committee believes that the status of indigence and the ability to pay should not be determined initially by court procedure but only after commitment and by fiscal agents employed by the state hospital system.

4. CONTROL OF PROPERTY.

Commitment procedures should be completely divorced from incompetency procedures.

5. INVOLUNTARY FORMAL COMMITMENTS.

The Committee believes that the certification by 2 physicians now employed in 6 states is the ideal method of procedure. The Committee is unable to see any particular purpose in requiring the physicians to have certificates certified by a law judge or magistrate as required in Pennsylvania and New Hampshire. The Committee believes that they should not advocate that all certificates be made by psychiatrists, except in such areas where psychiatric talent is practicably available.

The Committee believes that there is no need for the protection of the patient by the use of legal devices beyond the scope of habeas corpus and the provisions exemplified in the Maryland Law of 1944. The Committee is opposed to the practice of a jury adjudicating any phase of commitment or discharge and is also opposed to any procedure whereby the patient is served personal notice or required to appear in open hearings. The Committee does realize the need and usefulness of legal notice to kin and the practice of representation of the patient by proxy.

6. EMERGENCY COMMITMENTS.

Twenty-two states have emergency commitment laws. The period of detention ranges from 2 to 30 days. In the period from 1936 to 1946 eight states revised their commitment laws. At present 25 states have temporary observational commitments with detention ranging from 10 to 90 days. Four of these states permit renewals and in 5 all patients are on temporary detention by certification and not formal commitment. The Committee believes that there is no realistic therapeutic or legal value in temporary commitments. More legal formality in commitments (temporary commitments) may create even greater impediments to curing the patient. Any legal artifice setting conditions of time and of treatment tends to prevent the doctor from orienting the patient to his internal psychic problem. Temporary commitments or similar legal devices in practice tend to be reduced in time to routine circumventions and token compromises. Given enough time they deteriorate to the level of meaningless rituals. Our Committee subscribes to the belief that indeterminate commitment serves the best interest of the patient.

No acutely disturbed patient should be delivered to or retained in a jail but should be admitted on an emergency basis to the nearest psychopathic or state hospital. When certifying physicians are not available the admission to the psychopathic or state hospital should be left to the decision of the admitting psychiatrist of such hospital. The usual machinery for certification should be implemented within 72 hours after the admission thereto. In the absence of a welfare worker, a relative or health officer, it should be the duty of the local peace officer to initiate this emergency admission.

7. VOLUNTARY ADMISSIONS.

The Committee would encourage all measures permitting the more extensive use of voluntary admissions and recommends that the period to which the applicant pledges should be not less than 15 days.

At present, provisions for voluntary admission do not exist in the following states: Alabama, Florida, Mississippi, North Dakota, Georgia, Missouri. It is noted that the tendency in the direction of voluntary admissions has been progressively developed. Ten states have enacted laws for the same since 1939. Voluntary admissions should not be limited to patients who pay.

The application of a voluntary patient implies a contract between the patient and the superintendent and on occasions in which the applicant is regarded as incompetent, the legal guardian or close relative should be permitted to arrange for the admission. Such procedure is provided for in four states: Illinois, Arkansas, Ohio and Utah.

It is clear that voluntary admission should not be denied a patient even when insight is dubious. "A person who is a fit subject for mental treatment should not be denied the easy method for admission merely because he may be too indecisive, weak-minded or incompetent to sign his own papers." (Flaschner) Loc. Cit.

8. UNIFORM COMMITMENT LAW.

The Committee recommends a uniform law embodying the following general features:

   a. Certification by 2 qualified physicians.
   b. Safeguard of patients' rights to petition for release by court hearing as exemplified by the present Maryland law.

    c. Emergency admissions.
    d. Voluntary admissions.

9. PRIVATE SANITARIA.

The Forensic Committee has learned that only 17 states require licensing regulation and inspection of private hospitals. Such measures should be a universal practice and the enactment of laws pertaining to the licensing of private institutions should be sponsored by G. A. P.

10. TERMINOLOGY.

The Committee believes that all statutes should delete the term "commitment" in place of which should be substituted the term "certification"; "insanity" and "lunacy" should be replaced by the term "mental illness," and the terms "feeble-minded" or "weak-minded" should be abandoned.

The Committee believes that the term "parole" should be abandoned and in its place the term "convalescent status" or "convalescent leave" should be substituted.

11. PATIENT'S RIGHTS.

The Committee believes that all mental patients detained in either public or private institutions should be granted the following fundamental rights:

    a. Communication with persons outside.
    b. Periodic physical and psychiatric examination.
    c. Discharge as soon as possible.
    d. Civil rights guaranteed by law unless revoked by the same.
    e. Use of the very best existing medical techniques of therapy.

12. STATE DEPARTMENTS OF MENTAL HYGIENE

The Committee believes that for the successful implementation of the reforms necessary in mental health and in the laws relating to mental illness it is essential to promote improvements in the administration in the various states. We would advocate that because of the scope of the problem and the social importance of mental disease there be created in every state a separate department of Mental Hygiene and that there be created an administrative head of such a department who is a recognized leader in psychiatry. His appointment and tenure of office must be stabilized by statute and maintained free of political influence.

APPENDIX 3

State Mental
Health Authorities

ALABAMA
Dr. D. G. Gill
State Health Officer
State Department of Health
Montgomery, Alabama

ALASKA
Dr. E. Earl Albrecht
Commissioner of Health
Territorial Department of Health
Juneau, Alaska

ARIZONA
Dr. J. P. Ward
Director
State Department of Public Health
Phoenix, Arizona

ARKANSAS
Dr. T. T. Ross
State Health Officer
State Board of Health
Little Rock, Arkansas

CALIFORNIA
Dr. Wilton L. Halverson
Director of Public Health
State Department of Public Health
San Francisco, California

COLORADO
Dr. R. L. Cleere
Executive Director
State Department of Public Health
Denver, Colorado

CONNECTICUT
Dr. Stanley H. Osborn
Commissioner of Health
State Department of Health
Hartford, Connecticut

DELAWARE
Dr. M. A. Tarumianz
Superintendent
State Board of Trustees
Delaware State Hospital
Farnhurst, Delaware

DISTRICT OF COLUMBIA
Dr. Daniel L. Seckinger
Health Officer
District of Columbia Health Department
Washington, D. C.

FLORIDA
Dr. Wilson T. Sowder
State Health Officer
State Board of Health
Jacksonville, Florida

GEORGIA
Dr. T. F. Sellers
Director
Department of Public Health
State Office Building
Atlanta, Georgia

HAWAIIAN ISLANDS
Dr. C. L. Wilbar, Jr.
President
Territory of Hawaii Board of Health
Honolulu, Hawaii

IDAHO
Mr. L. J. Peterson
Administrative Director of Public
    Health
Department of Public Health
Boise, Idaho

ILLINOIS
Dr. Roland R. Cross
State Director of Public Health
State Department of Public Health
Springfield, Illinois

INDIANA
Mr. Arthur T. Loftin
Deputy Director
Indiana Council for Mental Health
Radio Center Building
State Fair Grounds
Indianapolis 5, Indiana

IOWA
Dr. Wilbur Miller, Director
The Psychopathic Hospital
The State University of Iowa
Iowa City, Iowa

KANSAS
Dr. F. C. Beelman
Secretary and Executive Officer
State Board of Health
Topeka, Kansas

KENTUCKY
Dr. Bruce Underwood
State Health Commissioner
State Department of Health
620 South Third Street
Louisville, Kentucky

LOUISIANA
Mr. Jesse H. Bankston
State Hospital Board
Baton Rouge, Louisiana

MAINE
Mr. David H. Stevens
Commissioner
State Department of Health and Welfare
Augusta, Maine

MARYLAND
Dr. Robert H. Riley
Director
State Department of Health
2411 North Charles Street
Baltimore 18, Maryland

MASSACHUSETTS
Dr. Clifton T. Perkins
Commissioner
Department of Mental Health
100 Nashua Street
Boston, Massachusetts

MICHIGAN
Mr. Charles F. Wagg
Director
Department of Mental Health
Lansing, Michigan

MINNESOTA
Dr. A. J. Chesley
Secretary and Executive Officer
Minnesota Department of Health
University Campus
Minneapolis 1, Minnesota
(Legally designated agency:
Director of Public Institutions)

MISSISSIPPI
Dr. Felix J. Underwood
Secretary and Executive Officer
State Board of Health
Jackson, Mississippi

MISSOURI
Dr. Buford Hamilton
Director
Division of Health
Jefferson City, Missouri
(Legally designated agency: Depart-
    ment of Public Health and Welfare)

MONTANA
Dr. George H. Freeman
Superintendent
State Department of Mental Hygiene
Montana State Hospital
Warm Springs, Montana

NEBRASKA
Dr. Frank D. Ryder
Director of Health
Department of Health
Lincoln, Nebraska

NEVADA
Acting State Health Officer
State Department of Health
Carson City, Nevada

NEW HAMPSHIRE
Dr. Anna L. Philbrook
Director of Child Guidance Clinics
Board of Trustees
New Hampshire State Hospital
Concord, New Hampshire

NEW JERSEY
Dr. Sanford Bates
Commissioner
State Department of Institutions and
  Agencies
Trenton 7, New Jersey

NEW MEXICO
Dr. James R. Scott
Director
Department of Public Health
Santa Fe, New Mexico

NEW YORK
Dr. Frederick MacCurdy
Commissioner
State Department of Mental Hygiene
Albany, New York

NORTH CAROLINA
Dr. J. W. R. Norton
Secretary
State Board of Health
Raleigh, North Carolina

NORTH DAKOTA
Dr. Russel O. Saxvik
State Health Officer
State Department of Health
Bismarck, North Dakota

OHIO
Judge John Lamneck
Director
State Department of Public Welfare
Columbus, Ohio

OKLAHOMA
Dr. Grady F. Mathews
Commissioner of Health
State Health Department
Oklahoma City, Oklahoma

OREGON
Dr. Harold M. Erickson
State Health Officer
State Board of Health
Portland, Oregon

PENNSYLVANIA
Dr. William C. Brown, Secretary
State Department of Welfare of the
  Commonwealth of Pennsylvania
Harrisburg, Pa.

PUERTO RICO
Dr. Juan A. Pons
Commissioner of Health
Insular Department of Health
San Juan, Puerto Rico

RHODE ISLAND
Mr. Edward P. Reidy
Director
State Department of Social Welfare
40 Fountain Street
Providence, Rhode Island

SOUTH CAROLINA
Dr. C. C. Odom
Superintendent
State Hospital
Columbia, South Carolina

SOUTH DAKOTA
Dr. G. J. Van Heuvelen
Superintendent
State Board of Health
Pierre, South Dakota

TENNESSEE
Dr. R. H. Hutcheson
Commissioner of Public Health
Department of Public Health
Nashville, Tennessee

TEXAS
Dr. George W. Cox
State Health Officer
State Department of Health
Austin, Texas

UTAH
Dr. John W. Spies
State Health Commissioner
State Department of Health
Salt Lake City 1, Utah

VERMONT
Mr. T. C. Dale
Commissioner
State Health Department
Burlington, Vermont

VIRGINIA
Dr. Joseph E. Barrett
Commissioner
State Department of Mental Hygiene
  and Hospitals
Clinic Building
12th and Marshall Streets
Richmond, Virginia

VIRGIN ISLANDS.
Dr. John S. Moorhead
Commissioner of Health
Department of Health
Charlotte Amalie, Virgin Islands

WASHINGTON

Dr. J. A. Kahl
Acting State Director of Health
State Department of Health
Seattle, Washington

WEST VIRGINIA

Dr. N. H. Dyer
State Health Commissioner
State Department of Health
Charleston, West Virginia

WISCONSIN

Mr. John Tramburg
Director
State Department of Public Welfare
State Capitol Building
Madison 2, Wisconsin

WYOMING

Dr. Franklin D. Yoder
State Health Officer
State Department of Health
Cheyenne, Wyoming

Bibliography

Adler, H. F.; Atkinson, A. J., and Ivy, A. C.: A Study of the Motility of the Human Colon: An Explanation of Dysynergia of the Colon, or of the "Unstable Colon." Am. J. Digest. Dis. 8:191, 1941.

Alcohol, Science and Society; 29 lectures at Yale Summer School of Alcohol Studies. Quart. J. Stud. on Alcohol, 1945.

Aldrich, C. A., and Aldrich, M. M.: Babies are Human Beings. An Interpretation of Growth. New York, The Macmillan Co., 1938. (Very good.)

Allen, F. H.: Psychotherapy with Children. New York, W. W. Norton and Co., 1942.

Alpers, B. J.: Personality and Emotional Disorders Associated with Hypothalamic Lesions. Psychosom. Med. 2:287, 1940.

Altmann, M.; Knowles, E., and Bull, H. E.: A Psychosomatic Study of the Sex Cycle in Women. Psychosom. Med. 3:199, 1941.

Alvarez, W. C.: Hysterical Type of Nongaseous Abdominal Bloating. Arch. Int. Med. 84:217, 1949.

Alvarez, W. C.: An Introduction to Gastroenterology. New York, Paul B. Hoeber, Inc., 1948.

Alvarez, W. C.: Cerebral Arteriosclerosis with Little Strokes That Cause a Slow Death. Am. J. Nursing 47:169, 1947.

Alvarez, W. C.: The Migrainous Personality and Constitution: The Essential Features of the Disease. A Study of 500 Cases. Am. J. M. Sc. 213:1, 1947.

Alvarez, W. C.: What Is the Matter with the Person Who Is Always Tired? Northwest Med. 46:437, 1947.

Alvarez, W. C.: What to Do in a Rebellious Case of Migraine: A List of the Drugs Being Used Today. Gastroenterology 9:754, 1947.

Alvarez, W. C.: Cerebral Arteriosclerosis with Small, Commonly Unrecognized Apoplexies. Geriatrics 1:189, 1946.

Alvarez, W. C.: A Rare Syndrome of Crisis-like Abdominal Pain. Gastroenterology 4:296, 1945.

Alvarez, W. C.: Heartburn. Gastroenterology 3:1, 1944.

Alvarez, W. C.: Nervousness, Indigestion and Pain. New York, Paul B. Hoeber, Inc., 1943.

Alvarez, W. C.: The Irritable Digestive Tract. Gastroenterology 1:95, 1943.

Alvarez, W. C.: Constitutional Inadequacy. J.A.M.A. 129:780, 1942.

Alvarez, W. C.: New Light on the Mechanisms by Which Nervousness Causes Discomfort. J.A.M.A. 115:1010, 1940.

Alvarez, W. C.: When Should One Operate for "Chronic Appendicitis?" J.A.M.A. 114:1301, 1940.

Alvarez, W. C.: Lessons to Be Learned from the Results of Tonsillectomies in Adult Life. J.A.M.A. 80:1513, 1923.

Alvarez, W. C.: Migraine. Chapter in Oxford Medicine, Vol. 6.

Alvarez, W. C.: Headache. Chapter in Oxford Medicine, Vol. 6.

Anderson, O. D.; Parmenter, Richard, and Liddell, H. S.: Some Cardiovascular Manifestations of Experimental Neurosis in Sheep. Psychosom. Med. 1:93, 1939.

Anomaly, The Invert and His Social Adjustment. Baltimore, Williams and Wilkins Co., 1927.

Appel, Kenneth E., and Strecker, Edward A.: Practical Examination of Personality and Behavior Disorders, Adults and Children. New York, The Macmillan Co., 1936.

Arthur, J. K.: Jobs for Women over 35. New York, Prentice-Hall, Inc.

Bahn, C. A.: The Psychoneurotic Factor in Ophthalmic Practice. Am. J. Ophth. 26:369, 1943.

Baker, Louise M.: Out on a Limb. Whittlesey House Publications, New York, McGraw-Hill Co., 1946. (A merry story of a woman who lost a leg in girlhood.)

Bakwin, R. M., and Bakwin, Harry: Psychological Care During Infancy and Childhood. New York, D. Appleton-Century Co., 1943.

Bard, Philip: On Emotional Expression after Decortication. Psychol. Rev. 41:309, 1934.

Bard, Philip: A Diencephalic Mechanism for the Expression of Rage with Special Reference to the Sympathetic Nervous System. Am. J. Physiol. 84:490, 1928.

Barton, Betsy: And Now to Live Again; New York, D. Appleton-Century Co., 1944. (A story of a girl badly crippled in an accident, who decided to get out and live again.)

Beaumont, Henry: The Psychology of Personnel. New York, Longmans, Green and Co., 1945.

Beers, Clifford W.: A Mind That Found Itself. New York, Doubleday, Doran and Co., 1935. (The classic.)

Bennett, A. E.: Faulty Management of Psychiatric Syndromes Simulating Organic Disease. J.A.M.A. 130:1203, 1946.

Bennett, A. E., and Semrad, E. V.: Common Errors in Diagnosis and Treatment of Psychoneurotic Patients—Study of 100 Case Histories. Nebraska M. J. 21:90, 1936.

Bennett, A. E., and Wilbur, C. B.: Convulsive Shock Therapy in Involutional States after Complete Failure with Previous Estrogen Treatment. Am. J. M. Sc.: 208:170, 1944.

Benson, A. C.: The House of Quiet. New York, E. P. Dutton and Co., 1906. (Depression; good.)

Bergler, E.: Unhappy Marriage and Divorce. New York, International Universities Press, 1946.

Bostock, John: How Civilization Manufactures Neuroses: A Survey of 200 Consecutive Cases. M. J. Australia 1:444, 1938.

Bourne, G., and Wittkower, E.: The Psychologic Treatment of Cases with Cardiac Pain. Brit. Heart J. 2:25, 1940.

Bowman, K.: Study of Prepsychotic Personality. Am. J. Orthopsychiat. 4:473, 1934.

Bradley, Charles: Schizophrenia in Childhood. New York, The Macmillan Co., 1941.

Brandt, Robert: A Tentative Classification of Psychological Factors in the Etiology of Skin Diseases. J. Invest. Dermat. 14:81, 1950.

Brookhart, J. M., and Day, F. S.: Reduction of Sexual Behavior in Male Guinea Pigs by Hypothalamic Lesions. Am. J. Physiol. 133:225; 133:551, 1941.

Brooks, Lee M., and Brooks, Evelyn C.: Adventuring in Adoption. Chapel Hill, N. C., University of North Carolina Press, 1939.

Brown, Clifford A.: Forty Years of Silence. Francestown, N. H., Marshall Jones, 1946. (Mr. Brown became deaf at the age of ten.)

Brown, Henry Collins: A Mind Mislaid. New York, E. P. Dutton and Co., 1937. (Well written.)

Brown, J. W.; Kirkland, H. B., and Hein, G. E.: Central Nervous System Involvement during Mumps. Am. J. M. Sc. 215:434, 1948.

Brown, S. F.: Advising Parents of Early Stutterers. Pediatrics 4:170, 1949.

Calkins, E. E.: Louder, Please! The autobiography of a deaf man. Boston, Little, Brown and Co., 1924. (The author has been deaf from childhood.)

Calvin, J. K.: Enuresis in Children. M. Clin. North America 12:131, 1928.

Campbell, C. Macfie: Emotional Factors in Health and Disease. Tr. & Stud., Coll. of Physicians, Philadelphia 6:16-34, 1938, 4th series.

Campbell, C. Macfie: The Role of Instinct, Emotion and Personality in Disorders of the Heart. J.A.M.A. *71:*1621, 1918.

Carlson, Earl R.: Born That Way. New York, The John Day Co., 1941. (A Spastic.)

Carmichael, Leonard (ed.): Manual of Child Psychology. New York, John Wiley and Sons, 1946.

Casals, Mary: The Stone Wall: An Autobiography. Chicago, Eyncourt Press, 1930. (Homosexual.)

Caughey, J. L.: Cardiovascular Neurosis: A Review. Psychosom. Med. *1:*311, 1939. (Bibliography of 143 titles.)

Chavanne, Fleury: Oreille et hystérie. Paris, J. B. Baillière et fils, 1901.

Cheney, Clarence O: Dementia Praecox. Oxford Med. 7:389.

Chevigny, Hector: My Eyes Have a Cold Nose. New Haven, Conn., Yale University Press, 1946. (Blind.)

Chevigny, Hector, and Braverman, Sydell: The Adjustment of the Blind. New Haven, Conn., Yale University Press, 1950.

Cleckley, H.: The Mask of Sanity. St. Louis, Mo., C. V. Mosby Co., 1950. (A wonderful discussion of persons with a psychopathic personality.)

Clerf, L. H., and Braceland, F. J.: Functional Aphonia. Ann. Otol., Rhin. & Laryng. *51:*905, 1942.

Cobb, Stanley: When Is a Psychosis Not a Psychosis? Am. J. Psychiat. *102:*705, 1946.

Cohn, Alfred E.: The Cardiac Phase of War Neuroses. Am. J. M. Sc. *158:*453, 1919.

Coleman, J. V.; Hurst, Allan, and Hornbein, Ruth: Psychiatric Contributions to Care of Tuberculous Patients. J.A.M.A. *135:*699, 1947.

Cone, R. E.: Psychosomatic Problems in Urology. J. Urol. *56:*146, 1946.

Conner, L. A.: The Psychiatric Factors in Cardiac Disorders. J.A.M.A. *94:*447, 1930.

Conner, L. A.: The Rehabilitation of Cardiac Patients Through Organized Effort. J.A.M.A. *89:*496, 1927.

Conrad, A: The Psychiatric Study of Hyperthyroid Patients. J. Nerv. & Ment. Dis. *79:*505, 1934.

Cordes, Fred, and Horner, Warren: Hysteric Amblyopia. Am. J. Ophth. *16:*592, 1933, or Tr. Pacific Coast Oto-Ophth. Soc. *20:*92, 1932.

Curran, E. A.: Personality Factors in Counseling. New York, Grune and Stratton, Inc., 1945.

Davidson, G. M.: Further Observations on Hallucinations of Smell. Psychiatric Quart. *19:*692, 1945.

Davidson, G. M.: Concerning Hallucinations of Smell. Psychiatric Quart. *12:*253, 1938.

Davis, K. B.: Factors in the Sex Life of 2200 Women. New York, Harper and Bros., 1929.

Davison, F. W.: Otolaryngologic Symptoms of Psychoneuroses. Laryngoscope, *55:*52, 1945.

Day, G.: Observations on the Psychology of the Tuberculous. Lancet *2:*703, 1946.

de Lenoir, Cecil: The Hundredth Man. New York, Claude Kendall, 1934. (The story of a morphine addict.)

Dell, Floyd: The Case of Floyd Dell, a Study in the Psychology of Adolescence. (Several revealing "novels.")

Denker, Peter G.: Psychosomatic Medicine: Results of Treatment of Psychoneuroses by the General Practitioner. New York State J. Med. *46:*21, 1946.

Despert, J. Louise: Urinary Control and Enuresis. Psychosom. Med. *6:*294, 1944.

Dey, F. L.: Changes in Ovaries and Uteri in Guinea Pigs with Hypothalamic Lesions. Am. J. Anat. *69:*61, 1941.

Dickinson, R. L., and Beam, L.: A Thousand Marriages. Baltimore, Williams and Wilkins Co., 1931.

Drake, Frank R.: Religion and Psychiatry. Am. J. M. Sc. *217:*111, 1949.

Dry, T. J.: The Irritable Heart and Its Accompaniments. J. Arkansas M. Soc. *34*:259, 1938.

Dumas, Alexander, and Keen, Grace: A Psychiatric Primer for the Veteran's Family and Friends. Minneapolis, Minn., University of Minnesota Press, 1945.

Dunbar, H. F.: Emotions and Bodily Changes: Survey of Literature. 3rd ed. New York, Columbia University Press, 1946.

Dunlap, H. F., and Moersch, F. P.: Psychic Manifestations Associated with Hyperthyroidism. Am. J. Psychiat. *91*:1215, 1935.

Ebaugh, F. S., and Rymer, C. A.: Psychiatry in Medical Education. New York, The Commonwealth Fund, 1942. (How psychiatry is being taught.)

English, O. S., and Pearson, G. H. J.: Emotional Problems of Living. New York, W. W. Norton and Co., 1945.

Felix, R. H.: An Appraisal of the Personality Types of the Addict. Am. J. Psychiat. *100*:462, 1944.

Foss, H. L., and Jackson, J. A.: The Relationship of Goiter to Mental Disorders. Am. J. M. Sc. *167*:724, 1924.

Fox, H. M., and Schnaper, N.: Psychiatric Casualties in General Hospitals Overseas. Am. J. Psychiat. *101*:316, 1944.

Frank, R. T.: Dyspareunia, a Problem for the General Practitioner. J.A.M.A. *136*:361, 1948.

Frederics, Diana: A Strange Autobiography. New York, The Dial Press, 1939. (Homosexual.)

Freeman, W., and Watts, J. W.: Psychosurgery. Springfield, Ill., Charles C Thomas Co., 1942.

Freyhan, F. A.: Psychiatric Realities, an Analysis of Autistic Trends in Psychiatric Thinking. J. Nerv. & Ment. Dis. *106*:482, 1947.

Fry, C. C. (with the collaboration of E. G. Rostow): Mental Health in College. New York, The Commonwealth Fund, 1942.

Gantt, W. H.: Experimental Basis for Neurotic Behavior. New York, Paul B. Hoeber, Inc., 1944.

Garrison, Karl C.: The Psychology of Exceptional Children. New York, Ronald Press, 1940.

Gesell, Arnold: Mental Growth of the Preschool Child. New York, The Macmillan Co., 1925.

Gesell, Arnold: The Retarded Child: How to Help Him. Bloomington, Ill., Public School Publishing Co., 1925.

Gesell, Arnold, and Amatruda, C. S.: Developmental Diagnosis. 2nd ed. New York, Paul B. Hoeber, Inc., 1947.

Gibbs, C. E.: Sex Development and Behavior in Female Patients with Dementia Praecox. Arch. Neurol. & Psychiat. *11*:179, 1924.

Gibbs, C. E.: Sex Development and Behavior in Male Patients with Dementia Praecox. Arch. Neurol. & Psychiat. *9*:73, 1923.

Gilfond, Duff: I Go Horizontal. New York, The Vanguard Press, 1940. (Story of a gifted woman with a terrible headache.)

Gleeson, W., and Gildea, E. F.: A Study of the Personalities of 289 Abnormal Drinkers. Quart. J. Stud. on Alcohol *3*:409, 1942.

Goldman, R. L.: Even the Night. New York, The Macmillan Co., 1947. (Deaf and partly paralyzed, he earns a living by writing.)

Goldstein, Kurt: Language and Language Disturbances: Aphasic Symptom Complexes and Their Significance for Medicine and Theory of Language. New York, Grune and Stratton, 1948. (Very good.)

Goodhart, J. F.: On Common Neuroses, or the Neurotic Element in Disease and Its Rational Treatment. Philadelphia, Blakiston Co., 1892.

Granich, Louis: Aphasia, A Guide to Re-training. New York, Grune and Stratton, Inc., 1947.

Graves, Alonzo: The Eclipse of a Mind. New York, The Medical Journal Press, 1942. (Insanity—a fine study.)

Greene, James S.: Psychophonasthenia Syndrome, Ann. Otol., Rhin. & Laryng. *50:*1177, 1941.

Greene, James S., and Small, S. M.: Psychosomatic Factors in Stuttering. M. Clin. North America *28:*615, 1944.

Grinker, R. R.: Hypothalamic Functions in Psychosomatic Inter-relations. Psychosom. Med. *1:*19, 1939.

Guerbé: Líctere Emotif Manifestation hysterique. Paris, These, 1898.

Hahn, E. F.: Stuttering, Significant Theories and Therapy. Stanford University, Calif., Stanford University Press, 1943.

Hall, Radclyffe: The Well of Loneliness. New York, Covici Friede, 1932. (Homosexual.)

Hamill, R. C.: Disability, Damages, or Disease. M. Clin. North America *20:*1499, (May) 1926.

Harrison, Charles Y.: Thank God for My Heart Attack. New York, Henry Holt and Co., 1949. (A good description of a coronary thrombosis.)

Harrison, F.: The Hypothalamus and Sleep. Baltimore, Williams and Wilkins Co., 1940.

Hathaway, Mrs. Katharine B.: The Little Locksmith. New York, Coward-McCann, 1943. (The beautifully written story of a little hunchback.)

Hathaway, Mrs. Katharine B.: The Journals of the Little Locksmith. New York, Coward-McCann, 1946.

Hawk, Sara S.: Speech Therapy for the Physically Handicapped. Stanford University, Calif., Stanford University Press, 1950.

Hayes, E. W.: Tuberculosis As it Comes and Goes. Springfield, Ill., Charles C Thomas, 1947. (Written by a doctor who had it.)

Hayward, Emeline P., and Woods, A. H.: Mental Derangements in Hypothyroidism. J.A.M.A. *97:*164, 1931.

Head, Henry, and Holmes, Gordon: Sensory Disturbances from Cerebral Lesions. Brain. *34:*102, 1911.

Head, Henry; Rivers, W. H. R., and Sherren, J.: The Afferent Nervous System from a New Aspect. Brain *28:*99, 1905.

Heckman, Helen E.: My Life Transformed. New York, The Macmillan Co., 1928. (Deaf and dumb from infancy, she was taught to speak.)

Heiner, Marie Hays: Hearing Is Believing. Cleveland, Ohio, World Publishing Co., 1949. (A deaf woman's campaign to persuade the deaf to use hearing aids.)

Hench, P. S., and Boland, E. W.: Management of Chronic Arthritis and Other Rheumatic Diseases among Soldiers of the United States Army. Ann. Int. Med. *24:*808, 1946.

Henderson, A. T.: Psychogenic Factors in Bronchial Asthma. Canad. M. A. J. *55:*106, 1946.

Henderson, D. K.: Psychopathic States. New York, W. W. Norton and Co., 1939.

Henry, G. W., and others: Sex Variants: A Study of Homosexual Patterns. New York, Paul B. Hoeber, Inc., 1941.

Hillyer, Jane: Reluctantly Told. New York, The Macmillan Co., 1926. (A woman who was wildly insane.)

Hoch, A.: Study of the Mental Makeup in the Functional Psychoses. J. Nerv. & Ment. Dis. *36:*230, 1909.

Hoch, A.: Constitutional Factors in the Dementia Praecox Group. Rev. of Neurol. and Psychiat. *8:*463, 1910.

Holmes, T. H.; Goodell, Helen; Wolf, Stewart, and Wolff, Harold G.: The Nose: An Experimental Study of Reactions Within the Nose in Human Subjects During Varying Life Experiences. Springfield, Ill., Charles C Thomas, 1950.

Hoopes, G. Gertrude: Out of the Running. Springfield, Ill., Charles C Thomas, 1939. (A cripple in a wheel chair.)

Horsley, J. P.: Narco-Analysis. New York, Oxford University Press, 1943.

Hunt, E.: Skin Affections Underlying Pruritus of the Vulva and Anus. Lancet
    1:592, 1936. (A study of 300 cases.)
Ingram, W. R.: The Hypothalamus, a Review of the Experimental Data. Psycho-
    som. Med. *1*:48, 1939.
"Inmate Ward 8": Behind the Door of Delusion. New York, The Macmillan Co.,
    1932. (A newspaper editor who was a bad alcoholic.)
Janet, P.: Psychological Healing. London, Allen and Unwin, Ltd., 1925.
Jayson, L. M.: Mania. New York, Funk and Wagnalls Co., 1937.
Johnson, George T.: Evaluations of Psychoanalysis. Am. J. M. Sc. *200*:837, 1940.
Johnson, W. O.: Emotional Disturbances with Pelvic Symptoms. South. Surgeon
    8:373, 1939.
Johnson, Wendell: People in Quandaries; The Semantics of Personal Adjustment.
    New York, Harper and Bros., 1946.
Kahn, Eugene: Psychopathic Personalities. New Haven, Conn., Yale University
    Press, 1931.
Kallmann, F. J.: Genetic Theory of Schizophrenia, an Analysis of 691 Schizo-
    phrenic Twin Index Families. Am. J. Psychiat. *103*:309, 1946.
Kallmann, F. J.: The Genetics of Schizophrenia; A Study of Heredity and Re-
    production in the Families of 1,087 Schizophrenics. New York, J. J. Augustin,
    1938.
Kanner, Leo: Child Psychology. 2nd ed. Springfield, Ill., Charles C Thomas, 1949.
Katz, L. N.; Winton, S. S., and Megibow, R. W.: Psychosomatic Aspects of Car-
    diac Arrhythmias: A Physiological Dynamic Approach. Ann. Int. Med. *27*:261,
    1947.
King, Marian: The Recovery of Myself. New Haven, Conn., Yale University
    Press, 1931. (The story of an insane person.)
Kitching, Howard: Sex Problems of the Returned Veteran. New York, Emerson
    Books, Inc., 1946.
Klapman, J. W.: Group Psychotherapy. New York, Grune and Stratton, 1946.
Klauder, J. V.: Psychogenic Aspects of Skin Diseases. J. Nerv. & Ment. Dis.
    84:249, 1936.
Knight, R. P.: Functional Disturbances in the Sexual Life of Women. Bull.
    Menninger Clin. *7*:25, 1943.
Kolb, Lawrence, and Ossenfort, W. F.: The Treatment of Drug Addicts at the
    Lexington Hospital. South. M. J. *31*:914, 1938.
Kozol, H. L.: Pre-traumatic Personalities and Psychiatric Sequelae of Head Injury.
    Arch. Neurol. & Psychiat. *56*:245, 1946.
Kraines, S. H.: The Therapy of the Neuroses and Psychoses: A Sociopsychobio-
    logic Analysis and Resynthesis. Philadelphia, Lea and Febiger, 1941. (Good
    for the non-psychiatrist.)
Kraines, S. H.: Mechanism and Treatment of Neurotic Symptoms, Especially of
    the Ear, Nose and Throat. Arch. Otolarying. *33*:579, 1941.
Leonard, William Ellery: The Locomotive God. New York, Century Co., 1927.
    (An eccentric who could not go far from his home.)
Leonard, William Ellery: Two Lives. New York, Viking Press, Inc., 1933. (An
    eccentric who married a mentally deranged woman.)
LeVay, A. D.: Psychosomatic Approach to Orthopedic Surgery. Lancet *1*:125, 1947.
Levine, Alexander: Enuresis in the Navy. Am. J. Psychiat. *100*:320, 1943.
Lewis, Abigail: An Interesting Condition. The Diary of a Pregnant Woman. New
    York, Doubleday and Co., 1950.
Lewis, Nolan D. C.: Psychic Phenomena in Association with Cardiac Failure.
    Arch. Neurol. & Psychiat. *37*:782, 1937.
Lewis, Nolan D. C., and Pacella, Bernard L.: Modern Trends in Child Psychiatry.
    New York, International Universities Press, 1945.
Lidz, Theodore, and Whitehorn, J. C.: Psychiatric Problems in a Thyroid Clinic.
    J.A.M.A. *139*:698, 1949.

Lindemann, Erich: Symptomatology and Management of Acute Grief. Am. J. Psychiat. *101*:141, 1944.
Lindemann, Erich: Hysteria As a Problem in a General Hospital. M. Clin. North America *22*:591, 1938.
Linduska, Noreen: My Polio Past. Chicago, Pellegrini and Cudahy, 1947.
Loeser, Louis H.: The Sexual Psychopath in Military Service: A Study of 270 Cases. Am. J. Psychiat. *102*:92, 1945.
Loftus, T. A.; Gold, Harry, and Diethelm, Oskar: Cardiac Changes in the Presence of Intense Emotion. Two Case Reports. Am. J. Psychiat. *101*:697, 1945.
Lowrey, L. G.: Psychiatry for Social Workers. New York, Columbia University Press, 1946.
Luck, V. J.: Psychosomatic Problems in Military Orthopedic Surgery. J. Bone & Joint Surg. *28*:213, 1946.
MacDonald, Betty: The Plague and I. Philadelphia, J. B. Lippincott Co., 1949. (A story of tuberculosis.)
Macy, J. W., and Allen, E. V.: A Justification of the Diagnosis of Chronic Nervous Exhaustion. Ann. Int. Med. *7*:861, 1934.
Maier, N. R. F.: Frustration; The Study of Behavior without a Goal. New York, McGraw-Hill Book Co., 1948.
Maine, Harold: If a Man Be Mad. New York, Doubleday, Doran and Co., 1947. (The remarkable story of the workings of an alcoholic's mind.)
Mainzer, F., and Krause, M.: The Influence of Fear on the Electrocardiogram. Brit. Heart J. *2*:221, 1940.
Maniac, The, by Himself to His Doctor. London, Rebman, Ltd., 1909.
Marañon, M. G. Le facteur émotionel dans la pathogenie des états hyperthyroidiens. Ann. de méd. *9*:81, 1921.
Martin, N. A.: Psychogenic Deafness. Ann. Otol. Rhin. & Laryng. *55*:81, 1946.
McDermott, N. T., and Cobb, Stanley: A Psychiatric Survey of 50 Cases of Bronchial Asthma. Psychosom. Med. *1*:203, 1939.
McFarland, R. A., and Goldstein, H.: Biochemistry of the Psychoneuroses: A Review. Am. J. Psychiat. *93*:1073, 1937.
McGregor, H. G.: The Emotional Factor in Visceral Disease. New York, Oxford University Press, 1938.
McKinney, Fred: The Psychology of Personal Adjustment. 2nd ed. New York, John Wiley & Sons, 1941. (For college students.)
Menninger, K. A.: Observations of a Psychiatrist in a Dermatology Clinic. Bull. Menninger Clin. *11*:141, 1947.
Menninger, W. C.: The Emotional Factors in Pregnancy. Bull. Menninger Clin. *7*:15, 1943.
Mezzrow, Milton Mezz, and Wolfe, Bernard: Really the Blues. New York, Random House, Inc., 1946. (A vivid autobiography of an addict and musician.)
Miller, N. F.: Hysterectomy: Therapeutic Necessity or Surgical Racket? Am. J. Obst. & Gynec. *51*:804, 1946.
Minnesota Personality Inventory. The Psychological Corporation, 522 Fifth Avenue, New York 18.
Mitchell, J. H.; Curran, C. A., and Myers, Ruth N.: Some Psychosomatic Aspects of Allergic Diseases. Psychosom. Med. *9*:184, 1947.
Mittelman, B.: Psychogenic Factors and Psychotherapy in Hyperthyreosis and Rapid Heart Imbalance. J. Nerv. & Ment. Dis. *77*:465, 1933.
Mittelman, B., and Wolff, H. G.: Affective States and Skin Temperature: Experimental Study of Subjects with Cold Hands and Raynaud's Syndrome. Psychosom. Med. *1*:71, 1939.
Moodie, William: The Doctor and the Difficult Child. New York, The Commonwealth Fund, 1940. (Good.)
Moorhead, J. J.: Traumatic Neuroses. M. Clin. North America. *28*:663, 1944.
Moorman, L. J.: Initial Management of Tuberculosis with Special Reference to the Psychology of the Patient. Ann. Int. Med. *13*:849, 1939.

Morgan, L. O.: Alterations in the Hypothalamus in Mental Deficiency: Psychosom. Med. *1:*496, 1939.

Myerson, Abraham: The Constitutional Anhedonic Personality. Am. J. Psychiat. *102:*774, 1946.

Myerson, Abraham: The Attitude of Neurologists, Psychiatrists and Psychologists Towards Psychoanalysis. Am. J. Psychiat. *96:*623, 1939.

Myerson, Abraham: Traumatic Neuroses. M. Clin. North America *22:*637, 1938.

Myerson, Abraham: Neuroses and Neuropsychoses. The Relationship of Symptom Groups. Am. J. Psychiat. *93:*263, 1936.

Myerson, Abraham: The Inheritance of Mental Diseases. Baltimore, Williams and Wilkins Co., 1925.

Myerson, Abraham: The Foundations of Personality. Boston, Little, Brown and Co., 1921.

Myerson, Abraham: The Nervous Housewife. Boston, Little, Brown and Co., 1920.

Neuropsychiatry for the General Medical Officer. U. S. War Dept. Technical Bull. (TB Med. 94). Washington, D. C., Government Printing Office, 1944.

Newman, H. H.; Freeman, F. M., and Holzinger, K. J.: Twins: A Study of Heredity and Environment. Chicago, University of Chicago Press, 1947.

Nijinsky, V.: The Diary of Vaslav Nijinsky, edited by Romola Nijinsky. New York, Simon and Schuster, Inc., 1936. (A man going insane.)

North 3-1: Pick Up the Pieces. New York, Doubleday, Doran and Co., 1929. (The story of a dipsomaniac.)

Oliver, John R.: The Ordinary Difficulties of Everyday People. New York, Alfred A. Knopf, Inc., 1935.

Oppenheimer, B. S., and Rothschild, M. A.: The Psychoneurotic Factor in the Irritable Heart of Soldiers. J.A.M.A. *70:*1919, 1918.

Owen, Emerson D. (North 3-1 pseud.): Pick Up the Pieces. New York, Doubleday, Doran and Co., 1929. (The story of a dipsomaniac.)

Pastorelli, France: Strength Out of Suffering; a translation of Servitude et Grandeur de la Malade. Boston, Houghton Mifflin Co., 1936. (The story of a bedridden woman and her relations to her family. This teaches much.)

Pearson, G. H. J.: Emotional Disorders of Children, a Case Book of Child Psychiatry. New York, W. W. Norton and Co., 1949.

Pearson, G. H. J.: Some Psychological Aspects of Inflammatory Skin Lesions. Psychosom. Med. *2:*22, 1940.

Penrose, L. S.: A Study in the Inheritance of Intelligence. Brit. J. Psychol. Gen. Sect. *24:*1, 1933.

Pepper, O. H. Perry: A Note on the Placebo. Am. J. Pharm. *117:*409, 1945; Tr. & Stud. Coll. Physicians, Philadelphia *13:*81, 1945.

Pickworth, F. A.: New Outlook on Physiology of Mental and Emotional States. Brit. M. J. *1:*265, 1938.

Pierce, S.W., and Pierce, J. T.: The Layman Looks at Doctors. New York, Harcourt, Brace and Co., 1929. (A depressed woman and how she was treated.)

Plagemann, Bentz: My Place to Stand. New York, Farrar, Straus and Co., 1949. (By a polio victim.)

Polatin, Phillip, and Philtine, Ellen C.: How Psychiatry Helps. New York, Harper and Bros., 1949. (Useful lists of helpful agencies.)

Pollock, H. M.: Malzberg, Benjamin, and Fuller, R. G.: Hereditary and Environmental Factors in the Causation of Manic-Depressive Psychoses and Dementia Praecox. Utica, New York, State Hospitals Press, 1939.

Pollock, L. J.: Phobias and Neurology of the Viscera. M. Clin. North America *12:*31, 1928.

Psychosomatic Medicine, Symposium on. M. Clin. North America Vol *28:* May, 1944.

Ranson, S. W.: The Hypothalamus As a Thermostat Regulating Body Temperature. Psychosom. Med. *1:*486, 1939.

Ranson, S. W.: The Hypothalamus: Its Significance for Visceral Innervation and Emotional Expression. Trans. & Stud. Coll. Physicians, Philadelphia 2:222, 1934.

Ranson, S. W., and Magoun, H. W.: The Hypothalamus. (Ergebn. d. Physiol.) 41:56, 1939.

Rapaport, David: Diagnostic Psychological Testing. Vols I and II. Chicago, Year Book Publishers, Inc., 1945-1946.

Rapaport, David; Schafer, Roy, and Gill, Merton: Manual of Diagnostic Psychological Testing. Publication of Josiah Macy Foundation, 1944. Chicago, Year Book Publishers, Inc., 1945.

Read, G. D.: Childbirth without Fear, New York, Harper and Bros., 1944.

Read, G. D.: Observations on a Series of Labours with Special Reference to Physiological Delivery. Lancet 1:721, 1949.

Rennie, T. A. C.: What Can the Practitioner Do in Treating the Neuroses? Bull. New York Acad. Med. 22:23, 1946.

Richardson, H. B.: Patients Have Families. New York, The Commonwealth Fund, 1945.

Richardson, La Vange Hunt: The Personality of Stutterers. (Psychological Monographs 56: No. 7, whole No. 260.) Evanston, Ill., The American Psychological Association, 1944.

Ripley, H. S., and Wolf, Stewart: Intravenous Use of Sodium Amytal in Psychosomatic Disorders. Psychosom. Med. 9:264, 1947.

Rivers, T. M.: Virus Diseases of the Nervous System. J.A.M.A. 132:427, 1946.

Roberts, Katherine E., and Fleming, Virginia V. D.: Persistence and Change in Personality Patterns. Washington, D. C., Society for Research in Child Development, National Research Council, 1943.

Robertson, G. G.: Nausea and Vomiting of Pregnancy: A Study in Psychosomatic and Social Medicine. Lancet 2:336, 1946.

Robinson, G. Canby: The Patient As a Person. A Study of the Social Aspects of Illness. New York, The Commonwealth Fund, 1939.

Rogers, C. R.: The Clinical Treatment of the Problem-Child. Boston, Houghton Mifflin Co., 1939.

Rogerson, C. H.: Psychological Factors in Skin Diseases. Practitioner 142:17, 1939.

Roman, Charles A.: Man Remade, or Out of Delirium's Wonderland. Chicago, Reilly and Britton, 1909. (Dipsomania.)

Root, J.: Horrors of Delirium Tremens. New York, Josiah Adams, 1844. (A good description of "snakes.")

Rosenberger, A. J., and Moore, J. H.: The Treatment of Hysterical Deafness. Am. J. Psychiat. 102:666, 1946.

Rosenzweig, Saul, and Hoskins, R. G.: A Note on the Ineffectualness of Sex Hormone Medication in a Case of Pronounced Homosexuality. Psychosom. Med. 3:87, 1941.

Ross, T. A.: War Neuroses. Baltimore, Williams and Wilkins Co., 1942.

Ross, T. A.: The Mental Factors in Medicine. Brit. M. J. 2:209, 1938.

Ross, T. A.: The Common Neuroses. London, Edward Arnold and Co., 1924.

Rothman, Steven: The Role of the Autonomic Nervous System in Cutaneous Disorders. Psychosom. Med. 7:90, 1945.

Rowntree, L. G.: Psychosomatic Disorders As Revealed by 13,000,000 Examinations of Selective Service Registrants. Psychosom. Med. 7:27, 1945.

Ruesch, Jergen; Harris, R. E., and others: Chronic Disease and Psychological Invalidism: A Psychosomatic Study. New York, Psychosomatic Medicine Monographs, 1946.

Russell, Harold: Victory in My Hands: The True Story of One Man's Triumph. (The handless veteran who acted in The Best Years of Our Lives presents his warm, friendly story.)

Sadler, William S.: Mental Mischief and Emotional Conflicts, Psychiatry and Psychology in Plain English. St. Louis, C. V. Mosby Co., 1947.

Sadler, William S.: Modern Psychiatry. St. Louis, C. V. Mosby Co., 1945.

Saslow, George: The Emotional Problems of the Chronically Ill. Minn. Med. *33*:673, 1950. (The psychology of the tuberculous.)

Saul, Leon J.: Some Observations on the Relations of Emotions and Allergy. Psychosom. Med. *3*:66, 1941.

Schatia, Viva: The Incidence of Neurosis in Cases of Bronchial Asthma. Psychosom. Med. *3*:157, 1941.

Schnur, S.: Cardiac Neurosis Associated with Organic Heart Disease. Am. Heart J. *18*:153, 1939.

Schultz, Gladys Denny: Widows, Wise and Otherwise. A Practical Guide for the Woman Who Has Lost Her Husband. Philadelphia, J. B. Lippincott Co., 1949.

Seabrook, William: No Hiding Place, An Autobiography. Philadelphia, J. B. Lippincott Co., 1942. (Story of an alcoholic.)

Seabrook, William: Asylum. New York, Harcourt, Brace and Co., 1935. (A very well written story of an alcoholic.)

Seguin, C. A.: Erasistratus, Antiochus and Psychosomatic Medicine. Psychosom. Med. *10*:355, 1948.

Selliger, Robert V.: Alcoholics Are Sick People. Baltimore, Alcoholism Publications, 1945.

Semenov, Herman: Deafness of Psychic Origin and Its Response to Narcosynthesis. Trans. Am. Acad. Ophth., p. 326, 1946-47.

Shaffer, L. R.: The Psychology of Adjustment. Boston, Houghton Mifflin Co., 1936.

Shirley, Hale F.: Psychiatry for the Pediatrician. New York, The Commonwealth Fund, 1948.

Shurly, Burt R.: Some Psychologic Problems in Otolaryngology. Trans. Am. Laryng. Rhin. & Otol. Soc. *33*:374, 1927.

Slater, E. T. O.: Psychopathic Personality As a Genetical Concept. J. Ment. Sc. *94*:277, 1948.

Slater, Eliot: The Neurotic Constitution, a Statistical Study of 2,000 Neurotic Soldiers. J. Neurol. & Psychiat. *6*:1, 1943.

Slater, Eliot, and Slater, Patrick: The Heuristic Theory of Neurosis. J. Neurol., Neurosurg. & Psychiat. *7*:49, 1944.

Smythe, L. H.; Hastings, E. W., and Hughes, Joseph: Immediate and Follow-up Results of Electro-Shock Therapy. Am. J. Psychiat. *100*:351, 1943.

Spearman, C.: The Abilities of Man. New York, The Macmillan Co., 1927.

Spock, Benjamin: The Common Sense Book of Baby and Child Care. New York, Duell, Sloan and Pearce, Inc., 1945, 1946.

Spock, Benjamin, and Huschka, Mabel: The Psychological Aspects of Pediatric Practice. (Reproduced from the Practitioners Library of Medicine and Surgery, by the New York State Committee on Mental Hygiene, Courtesy of the Appleton-Century Co.), New York, 1939.

Stanka, Hugo: Occupational Hazards and Psychoses of Psychiatrists. Am. J. Psychiat. *102*:788, 1946.

Stern, Edith M., and Hamilton, S. W.: Mental Illness, A Guide for the Family. New York, The Commonwealth Fund, 1942. (Most useful to families.)

Stokes, J. H.: Functional Neuroses As Complications of Organic Disease: An Office Technic of Approach, with Special Reference to the Neurodermatoses. J.A.M.A. *105*:1007, 1935.

Stokes, John H., and Beerman, Hermann: The Psychosomatic Correlations in Allergic Conditions. Psychosom. Med. *2*:438, 1940.

Stokes, J. H., and Pillsbury, D. M.: The Effect on the Skin of Emotional and Nervous States. Theoretical and Practical Consideration of a Gastro-Intestinal Mechanism. Arch. Dermat. & Syph. *22*:962, 1930.

Strain, Frances B.: The Normal Sex Interests of Children. New York, Appleton-Century-Crofts Co., 1948.

Strange Confession of Monsieur Mountcairn, The: Privately Printed, 1928. (Remarkable homosexual.)

Strauss, Alfred A., and Lehtinen, Laura E.: Psychopathology and Education of the Brain Injured Child. New York, Grune and Stratton, Inc., 1947.

Strecker, E. A.: Their Mothers' Sons: The Psychiatrist Examines an American Problem. Philadelphia, J. B. Lippincott Co., 1946.

Strecker, E. A., and Palmer, H. T.: The Recognition and the Management of the Beginnings of Mental Disease. Oxford Medicine 7:2.

Strindberg, August (Translated by E. Schleussner): The Confession of a Fool. New York, Viking Press, 1925. (A paranoiac.)

Susselman, Samuel; Feldman, Fred, and Barrera, S. E.: Intravenous Injection of Sodium Amytal As a Test for Latent Anxiety. Arch. Neurol. & Psychiat. 56:567, 1946.

Sweet, Clifford: Enuresis, a Psychologic Problem of Childhood. J.A.M.A. 132:279, 1946.

Sweet, Clifford; Jacobus, L. R., and Stafford, H. E.: The Child-Parent Relationship; The Child in the Family. J.A.M.A. 116:38, 1941.

Symons, Arthur: Confessions. New York, Jonathan Cape and Harrison Smith, 1930. (Story of a person going insane.)

Symons, Arthur: Christian Trevalga. (Written when his mind was slipping.)

Symons, Arthur: Spiritual Adventures. London, Archibald Constable and Co., 1905. (A fine writer going insane.)

Taylor, Norman: Flight from Reality. New York, Duell, Sloan and Pierce, Inc., 1949.

Terman, L. M.: The Gifted Child Grows Up. Vol. 4. Stanford University, Calif., Stanford University Press, 1947.

Terman, L. M.: Genetic Studies of Genius. Vol. I. Stanford University, Calif., Stanford University Press, 1926.

Terman, L. M., and Merrill, M. A.: Measuring Intelligence. Boston, Houghton Mifflin Co., 1937.

Thompson, Florence S., and Galvin, George W.: A Thousand Faces. Boston, The Four Seas Co., 1920. (The story of insanity.)

Thompson, G. N.: Physical Manifestations in Mental Disease. J. Nerv. & Ment. Dis. 102:280, 1945.

Thorndike, E. L., and others: The Measurement of Intelligence. New York, Columbia University Press, 1927.

Thornton, Janet, with Knauth, M. S.: The Social Component in Medical Care; a Study of a Hundred Cases from the Presbyterian Hospital in New York. New York, Columbia University Press, 1937.

Thrasher, Frederick: The Gang; A Study of 1313 Gangs in Chicago. 2nd ed. Chicago, University of Chicago Press, 1936.

Tiebout, H. M.: Therapeutic Mechanisms of Alcoholics Anonymous. Am. J. Psychiat. 100:468, 1944.

Towle, Charlotte: Common Human Needs: An Interpretation for Staff in Public Assistance Agencies. Publ. Assistance Report No. 8. Washington, D. C., Government Printing Office, 1945.

Trudeau, Edward L.: An Autobiography. New York, Doubleday Co., 1915. (Trudeau, who suffered terribly from tuberculosis and was given up to die, cured himself and thereby started the cure of millions of others.)

Vidal, Lois: Magpie; The Autobiography of a Nymph Errant. Boston, Little, Brown and Co., 1934. (A hypomanic woman who went wandering.)

Vincent, John: Inside the Asylum. London, Allen and Unwin, Ltd., 1948. (An unusual autobiography. Well done.)

Wall, J. H.: A Study of Alcoholism in Women. Am. J. Psychiat. *93:*943, 1937.

Wall, J. H., and Allen, D. B.: The Results of Hospital Treatment of Alcoholism. Am. J. Psychiat. *100:*474, 1944.

Walsh, M. N., and Kierland, R. R.: Psychotherapy and the Treatment of Neurodermatitis. Proc. Staff Meet., Mayo Clin. *22:*578, 1947.

Warters, Jane: Achieving Maturity. New York, McGraw-Hill Book Co., 1949. (Contains valuable lists of books.)

Weill, Blanche C.: Through Children's Eyes. New York, Island Workshop Press, 1940. (Very good.)

Weirauch, Anna E.: The Scorpion. New York, Greenberg Publisher, Inc., 1934. (Story of a homosexual woman.)

Weiss, Edward, and English, O. Spurgeon: Psychosomatic Medicine, The Clinical Application of Psychopathology to General Medical Problems. 2nd ed. Philadelphia, W. B. Saunders Co., 1949.

Wengraf, Fritz: Psychosomatic Symptoms Following Hysterectomy. Am. J. Obst. & Gynec. *52:*645, 1946.

White, B. V.; Cobb, S., and Jones, C. M.: Mucous Colitis. Psychosomatic Medicine Monograph No. 1. Washington, D. C., National Research Council, 1939.

White, Paul D.: The Treatment of Heart Disease Other Than by Drugs. J.A.M.A. *89:*436, 1927.

White, Paul D.; Cohen, M. E., and Chapman, W. P.: Electrocardiogram in Neurocirculatory Asthenia, Anxiety Neurosis, or Effort Syndrome. Am. Heart J. *34:*390, 1947.

White, Paul D., and Glendy, R. Earle: The Growing Importance of Cardiac Neurosis. Ann. Int. Med. *10:*1624, 1937.

Wilbur, D. L., and Mills, J. H.: How Accurate Is the Diagnosis of Functional Indigestion? Ann. Int. Med. *12:*831, 1938.

Wile, Ira S., and Winn, M. D.: Marriage and the Modern Manner. New York, Century Co. (A good book to help persons who are trying to adjust to marriage.)

Willius, F. A.: Cardiac Clinics, Cardiac Neurosis. Proc. Staff Meet., Mayo Clin. *12:*683, 1937.

Winton, S. S., and Wallace, Leon: An Electrocardiographic Study of Psychoneurotic Patients. Psychosom. Med. *8:*332, 1946.

Witmer, Helen L. (ed.): Pediatrics and the Emotional Needs of the Child. New York, The Commonwealth Fund, 1947.

Witmer, Helen L. (ed.): Teaching Psychotherapeutic Medicine; An Experimental Course for General Physicians. Given by Walter Bauer and others. New York, The Commonwealth Fund, 1947.

Witmer, Helen L.: Psychiatric Interviews with Children. New York, The Commonwealth Fund, 1946.

Wittkower, E., and Davenport, R. C.: The War Blinded; Their Emotional, Social and Occupational Situation. Psychosom. Med. *8:*121, 1946.

Wolf, Anna W. M.: The Parent's Manual. New York, Simon and Schuster, Inc., 1941.

Wolf, Gerald A., Jr., and Wolff, Harold G.: Studies on the Nature of Certain Symptoms Associated with Cardiovascular Disorders. Psychosom. Med. *8:*293, 1946.

Wolff, Harold G.: Headache and Other Head Pain. New York, Oxford University Press, 1948. (A classic.)

Woltman, Henry W.: Neuropsychiatric Geriatrics. Arch. Ophth. *28:*791, 1942.

Wood, Paul: Da Costa's Syndrome (or Effort Syndrome). Brit. M. J. *1:*767, 805, 845, 1941.

Woodhead, Barbara: The Psychological Aspect of Allergic Skin Reactions in Childhood. Arch. Dis. Childhood *21:*98, 1946.

Woodson, Marion Marie (Inmate Ward 8, pseud.): Behind the Door of Delusion. New York, The Macmillan Co., 1932. (A newspaper editor who was a bad alcoholic.)

Yaskin, J. C.: Cardiac Psychoses and Neuroses. Am. Heart J. *12:*536, 1936.

Yost, Edna: Normal Lives for the Disabled. New York, The Macmillan Co., 1944.

Ziegler, L. H.: Psychosis Associated with Myxedema. J. Neurol. & Psychiat. *11:*20, 1930.

Ziegler, L. H.: Clinical Phenomena Associated with Depressions, Anxieties and Other Affective or Mood Disorders. Am. J. Psychiat. *8:*849, 1929.

Index

Folios in *italic type* indicate main discussions.